Principles and Practice
of Psychiatric Rehabilitation

Principles and Practice of
Psychiatric Rehabilitation

An Empirical Approach

Patrick W. Corrigan
Kim T. Mueser
Gary R. Bond
Robert E. Drake
Phyllis Solomon

THE GUILFORD PRESS
New York   London

Paperback edition 2009

Last digit is print number: 9 8 7 6 5 4 3 2

The authors have checked with sources believed to be reliable in their efforts to provide information that is complete and generally in accord with the standards of practice that are accepted at the time of publication. However, in view of the possibility of human error or changes in medical sciences, neither the authors, nor the editor and publisher, nor any other party who has been involved in the preparation or publication of this work warrants that the information contained herein is in every respect accurate or complete, and they are not responsible for any errors or omissions or the results obtained from the use of such information. Readers are encouraged to confirm the information contained in this book with other sources.

Library of Congress Cataloging-in-Publication Data

Principles and practice of psychiatric rehabilitation : an empirical approach / Patrick W. Corrigan ... [et al.].
     p. ; cm.
   Includes bibliographical references and indexes.
   ISBN 978-1-59385-489-8 (hardcover : alk. paper)
   ISBN 978-1-60623-344-3 (paperback : alk. paper)
   1. Mentally ill—Rehabilitation. 2. Mentally ill—Services for. I. Corrigan, Patrick W.
   [DNLM: 1. Mental Disorders—rehabilitation. 2. Mental Health Services. 3. Needs Assessment. WM 30 P9565 2007]
   RC439.5.P74 2007
   616.89—dc22

                                                                        2007025665

To acquaintances, colleagues, and friends with psychiatric disability who have taught us much about the challenges of mental illness and ways to overcome these disabilities so the individual can continue to achieve life goals

About the Authors

Patrick W. Corrigan, PsyD, is Professor of Psychology at the Illinois Institute of Technology. Previously, he directed the Center for Psychiatric Rehabilitation at the University of Chicago for 15 years. He is also chief of the joint research programs in psychiatric rehabilitation. These programs are research and training efforts dedicated to the needs of people with psychiatric disability and their families. Dr. Corrigan has been principal investigator of federally funded studies on rehabilitation, team leadership, consumer-operated services, and supported employment. He also serves as principal investigator of the Chicago Consortium for Stigma Research, the only National Institute of Mental Health–funded research center examining the stigma of mental illness. Dr. Corrigan's research on stigma includes a study on self-stigma, a nationally representative survey on affirmative action, and a cross-cultural examination of the stigma of employers in Hong Kong, Beijing, and Chicago. He is also a prolific researcher, having authored 10 books and more than 200 papers.

Kim T. Mueser, PhD, is a licensed clinical psychologist and Professor in the Departments of Psychiatry and Community and Family Medicine at Dartmouth Medical School. Dr. Mueser's clinical and research interests include psychiatric rehabilitation for persons with severe mental illnesses, intervention for co-occurring psychiatric and substance use disorders, and the treatment of posttraumatic stress disorder. His research has been supported by the National Institute of Mental Health, the National Institute on Drug Abuse, the Substance Abuse and Mental Health Services Administration, and the National Alliance on Schizophrenia and Depression. He has published numerous journal articles and book chapters, and has coauthored 10 books, including *The Complete Family Guide to Schizophrenia* (with Susan Gingerich), which received the National Alliance on Mental Illness

NYC Metro Ken Book Award for outstanding contributions to better understanding of mental illness.

Gary R. Bond, PhD, is Chancellor's Professor of Psychology at Indiana University–Purdue University Indianapolis, where he served as director of the PhD program in clinical rehabilitation psychology for 14 years. His research has aimed at identifying evidence-based practices for individuals with severe mental illness, with a primary focus on supported employment and assertive community treatment. Drawing on his work in developing scales measuring fidelity of program implementation, he has examined factors influencing successful implementation of these practices. Dr. Bond has received over 50 external grants and contracts and five national awards for research and training. His publications include over 170 journal articles and book chapters. He has consulted with local and state mental health planners throughout the United States and with mental health researchers in other countries, including Japan, Hong Kong, Australia, Spain, the Netherlands, Finland, Northern Ireland, England, and Canada. Dr. Bond is codeveloper of the Evidence-Based Practice Supported Employment Implementation Resource Kit.

Robert E. Drake, MD, PhD, is the Andrew Thomson Professor of Psychiatry and Community and Family Medicine and the Vice Chair and Director of Research in the Department of Psychiatry at Dartmouth Medical School. He is also the director of the New Hampshire–Dartmouth Psychiatric Research Center. Dr. Drake works as a community mental health doctor and researcher, and his research focuses on co-occurring disorders, vocational rehabilitation, health services research, and evidence-based practices. He has written 15 books and over 350 papers.

Phyllis Solomon, PhD, is Professor of Social Work in the School of Social Policy and Practice and Professor of Social Work in Psychiatry in the School of Medicine at the University of Pennsylvania. She is past director of the Social Work Mental Health Research Center at the School of Social Policy and Practice, a National Institute of Mental Health (NIMH)-funded social work development center focused on researching clinical service and service system interventions for adults with severe mental illness and their families. Dr. Solomon has conducted research on services and service delivery systems for adults with severe psychiatric disorders, with a primary focus on peer-provided services, family interventions, and the intersection of the criminal justice and mental health systems. Her research has been funded by a number of federal agencies, including NIMH and the Substance Abuse and Mental Health Services Administration, and she has published extensively on these studies and on issues related to psychiatric rehabilitation. She has received numerous awards for her contributions to mental health policy and practice.

Preface

Who are people with psychiatric disabilities? How do these disabilities interrupt the successful achievement of their life goals? Does rehabilitation help them overcome these challenges so that they can accomplish their personal aspirations? What are the fundamental principles that guide rehabilitation as well as the basic practices that embody these principles? What is the evidence that supports these principles and practices? The goal of this text is to answer complex questions like these. We seek to educate the reader on the various frameworks for understanding the disabilities that challenge many with mental illness. The heart of the text is to describe the repertoire of services, interventions, and resources that help people overcome their disabilities. Without limitations caused by these disabilities, people with serious mental illness are able to achieve the kind of life goals inherent in most adult development.

AN EVOLVING PERSPECTIVE

What is exciting about psychiatric rehabilitation is the current speed with which the paradigm is developing. In just the past decade, constructs related to recovery, hope, empowerment, and well-being have joined with intervention strategies that teach skills and provide support to help people achieve personal goals. It is important to note that the kind of goals that drive psychiatric rehabilitation fall into the same set of aspirations as those that are a priority for all adults: employment, residence, relationships, and health (both physical and mental). One mistake that is often made when describing those with psychiatric disabilities and their treatments is to somehow frame their life problems and objectives as *different* from and *less* than the "norm." One lesson that is stressed throughout this text is that the challenges posed by psychiatric disabilities are not qualitatively distinct from, but rather fall on a continuum with, the rest of the population. Hence, the broad set of practices that comprise psychiatric rehabilitation are equally meaningful for the general population in dealing with the day-to-day problems that occur in everyone's lives.

Two principles—empowerment and recovery—are central to modern approaches to rehabilitation. People with disabilities should have personal power over all aspects of their lives and rehabilitation. This kind of self-determination assures the development of life decisions that are consistent with a person's overall sense of self. Misguided programs that take away personal decision making not only undermine the possible benefits of rehabilitation but may actually cause harm.

Related to empowerment is the idea of recovery—the idea that people with psychiatric disabilities can and do recover. Recovery is a complex phenomenon with multiple models used to explain it; two of these models (*recovery as outcome* and *recovery as process*) are discussed here. Recovery as outcome means that the symptoms, dysfunctions, and impairments experienced by people with mental illness will remit and they will experience a personally satisfying life. Long-term follow-up research that tracks people with serious mental illnesses for 30 years or more shows that large numbers of individuals overcome their disabilities and recover. Recovery is also viewed as a process—namely, recovery reintroduces such important values as hope and well-being back into rehabilitation. For too long, mental health services have been dominated by a gloomy prognosis that robbed people of their future. Serious mental illnesses such as schizophrenia were known as the "kiss of death" diagnosis, in which a person's plans for the future were set aside so that he or she could assume the feckless role of patient. This perspective is now replaced with a more hopeful one in which people are able to master their disabilities and pursue their individual priorities. Principles like recovery and empowerment, therefore, have a central position as the field of rehabilitation continues to mature.

Many of the barriers associated with psychiatric disabilities are not solely due to impairments resulting from illness. These barriers also evolve from the societal stigma of having a psychiatric disability. Many people with psychiatric disabilities are unable to find satisfactory jobs or good housing because of the prejudice of employers and landlords. The book regularly highlights the interactions of stigma and disability in society and provides strategies for overcoming both.

AN EVIDENCE BASE

Like many other areas of health care, mental illness and psychiatric rehabilitation have had their share of principles and practices touted as important to the field but with no research data to support them. As a result, people with psychiatric disabilities whose treatment is based on these principles and practices may receive irrelevant services or participate in iatrogenic treatments that cause them harm. For example, approaches such as mesmerism, phrenology, and psychoanalysis have no utility in understanding disabilities and yield no benefits for addressing the needs of people with serious mental illness. Interventions like hydrotherapy, hypnosis, and insulin shock therapy actually harmed people. Examples like these were based on the good intentions of mental health providers who relied solely on their clinical experience to support their perspectives. In retrospect, we find that good intentions and clinical lore are not sufficient for discerning what is and is not helpful in treating serious mental illness.

The practices highlighted in this text rest on a sound evidence base (i.e., these approaches have survived empirical test across multiple studies). Although evidence-based approaches to the development of rehabilitation practices are not a new idea, what is new is the public embrace of evidence and research in identifying practices. Mental health authorities are now looking closely for the evidence base to discover effective interventions. Over the next decade, we expect to find more practices that have met the evidence standard. Equally important in the evidence-based agenda are dissemination strategies. How do real-world providers learn evidence-based approaches and then incorporate them into day-to-day practices? Future research on technology transfer that tests dissemination strategies will be equally important. Specification of how practices vary with macro variables such as ethnicity and the public mental health system will play a prominent role in the further development of dissemination.

THE TEXT'S FORMAT

The book is divided into four parts representing the major thematic concerns of psychiatric rehabilitation. Part I introduces the reader to overall concerns of psychiatric rehabilitation. Prominent here is a comprehensive consideration of the symptoms, impairments, and dysfunctions that lead to disabilities. Also, fundamental to understanding the disabilities of mental illness is a description of the insidious impact of stigma and discrimination on the lives of people with psychiatric disabilities. Part I ends with a description of the fundamental principles and practices of rehabilitation. As an overview, Chapter 3, "Definition of Psychiatric Rehabilitation," seeks to provide a solitary snapshot of the whole field so that the reader understands how the various principles and practices hold together.

Part II provides summaries of 10 services that currently comprise rehabilitation. These are organized around domains important to most adults: work, continuing education, housing, and family. Each chapter begins with a literature-based review of the problems that occur in domains because of psychiatric disabilities. Treatment aspects necessary for positive outcomes are reviewed next. Research that supports these assertions is summarized and specific guidelines for implementing these practices are then reviewed. Each chapter also includes personal examples—case histories that illustrate practices or principles outlined in the chapter.

Implementing evidence-based practices can vary for special populations and problems. For example, people with psychiatric disabilities who also abuse alcohol and other substances are likely to have a more severe disease course and prognosis. Part III highlights the special populations of concern and the additional principles and practices that are needed for this group.

Evidence-based practices are not adopted in a vacuum; they are implemented within communities that diverge greatly in terms of ethnicity and with service systems that vary in terms of infrastructure and other resources. Part IV reviews three areas related to system considerations. One chapter addresses practical strategies for tackling the stigma of mental illness. Without these strategies, stigma can strangle community efforts to develop effective rehabilitation programs. Another chapter reflects the impact of ethnic and other diversity issues on rehabilitation. Program development and evaluation has only just begun to examine the interface between rehabilitation and diversity. As rehabilitation perspectives mature, we expect to adopt more sophisticated models of difference and rehabilitation practices. The last chapter examines political and administrative influences on program development and implementation. This chapter reviews the statutes and administrative regulations that guide rehabilitation.

WHO IS OUR READER?

We had three groups of readers in mind as we wrote this text. First, we wished to educate students of psychiatric rehabilitation. Several academic disciplines are dedicated to understanding psychiatric disabilities; they are embedded within psychology, social work, occupational therapy, and psychiatry programs. Students who will be future practitioners will benefit from the book's cautious review of principles and practices. Some students are also training as social scientists. The text's focus on evidence-based approaches is an excellent model for nascent investigators.

Students here may also include people with psychiatric disabilities. As addressed in several places in the book, consumers who are acting as providers—prosumers—offer a special relevance and elegance to rehabilitation programs. There seems to be an affirmative action to hire more people with psychiatric disabilities as job specialists, education coaches, and case managers. Information in this text would enhance the career goals of these students.

This text is also meant to be a source book for practitioners. The book is a comprehensive review of rehabilitation principles and practices. The practitioner with this book on the shelf has a well-organized resource to review when questions emerge. This book is equally relevant for administrators whose responsibility includes identifying the best interventions. The literature review in this book provides the research foundation that is essential for administrative decisions.

Acknowledgments

Feedback from a number of experts in the field was incorporated into the development of this book. These include Leslie Alexander, Stephen Bartels, Deborah Becker, Silvia Bigatti, Amy Blank, Mary Brunette, Mark Davis, Jeffrey Draine, Jovier Evans, Howard Goldman, Ingrid Goldstrom, Hea-Won Kim, Tania Lecomte, Harriet Lefley, Sally MacKain, Edie Mannion, Joe Marrone, Stanley McCracken, Susan McGurk, David L. Penn, Bernice Pescosolido, Jo Phelan, Carlos Pratt, Stanley D. Rosenberg, William Torrey, and Yin-Ling Irene Wong.

We are also grateful to our families and friends who have been supportive of our work. We thank in particular Georgeen Carson and Abe and Liz Corrigan (P. W. C.); my mother, Sonja Mueser (K. T. M.); Karli Lindig, Risha, and Matt (G. R. B.); my children, Tyler, Keith, and Robyn, and my partner Debbie (R. E. D.); and Barbara Solomon (P. S.).

Contents

Part I

INTRODUCTION

Psychiatric disabilities are complex, with several factors accounting for the life problems experienced by people with these disabilities. We attempt to set the scene for a consideration of disabilities in the introductory chapter by distinguishing the individual sources of disability-related problems from the community sources. Chapter 1 reviews psychiatric research that describes how symptoms, impairments, dysfunctions, and comorbidities influence the phenomenology and prognosis of psychiatric disabilities. For example, the delusions common to many people with schizophrenia can cause significant distress that interferes with the fulfillment of their aspirations. In Chapter 2 the impacts of stigma, prejudice, and discrimination on personal goals are summarized. Together, basic symptoms and research on stigma set the stage for the fundamental and complex definition of psychiatric rehabilitation. Chapter 3 introduces the reader to the basic principles and various practices used in rehabilitation.

Chapter 1

Who Are People with Psychiatric Disabilities?

People with psychiatric disabilities are as complex and diverse a group as the population in general. Hence, the best way to start a discussion on psychiatric rehabilitation is by understanding who is the person with psychiatric disabilities. *People with psychiatric disabilities are not, because of mental illness, able to attain typical, age-appropriate goals for extended periods of time.* This definition contains three parts. First, psychiatric disability is based on a diagnosable mental illness. This chapter reviews important components of psychiatric diagnosis, focusing on those diagnoses that are most relevant to psychiatric rehabilitation. Second, the person is not able to pursue significant life goals because of the mental illness. Examples of important life goals relate to income, work, and vocation; relationships, intimacy, commitment, and family; physical, dental, and mental health; and recreation and spirituality. Third, both the mental illness and its interference with the attainment of goals persist for significant periods of time, in most cases for years.

Four conceptual domains are important for understanding the nature of psychiatric disabilities.

1. *Diagnoses* represent the collections of symptoms and dysfunctions that cohere to form a meaningful psychiatric syndrome. Typically, diagnoses that are the focus of psychiatric rehabilitation include schizophrenia, the mood disorders (such as major depression disorder, MDD; and bipolar disorder, BPD), some anxiety disorders (such as posttraumatic stress disorder, PTSD; and obsessive–compulsive disorder, OCD), and some personality disorders (PD).

2. *Course.* Psychiatric syndromes are not static phenomena. They vary among individuals in terms of the onset and trajectory of the illness. They also vary within the individual over time in terms of the severity of symptoms and dysfunctions.

PERSONAL EXAMPLES

Four Life Stories

Veronica Howard had lived on the streets since she was 18. She had neither a steady job nor a regular income. She preferred the cold pedestrian tunnels under the freeway to the homeless shelters because she was deathly afraid of other people. Veronica wore dirty clothes and had poor hygiene. She also had difficulty managing her diabetes because of her poor diet.

Joel Jenkins was 22 years old when he was brought into the emergency room of the state psychiatric hospital by the police. He was extremely agitated, shouting at imaginary demons and thrashing at the officers. This was his third admission to the hospital in the past 6 months. His parents were frightened of Joel's recurring "craziness" and feared they would soon have to "put him away" in an institution. The police officers in the small town where Joel lived were afraid that the next time they were called to his home, his combativeness during the arrest could escalate into someone's getting hurt. They were also concerned that Joel might be using marijuana, because it was found in his pants pocket during his last arrest.

George Miller rarely comes out of his apartment. It's not that he is afraid of people, but rather that he just seems to have no interest in them. He does not particularly care about working with others, making small talk when he meets neighbors at the park, or joining friends and family over a holiday meal. For that matter, he has no interest in finding a girlfriend or in settling down.

Harriet Osborne wants to get a job, live on her own, find a husband, and settle down to have a family. But she has been hospitalized six times for mental illness and is afraid she will not be able to handle these goals. So instead, she goes to a recreation program each day, where she is bored with the same routine of doing crafts and playing board games.

3. *Co-occurring disorders*. Psychiatric disorders rarely occur in isolation, without associated disorders. Instead, many people with psychiatric disabilities experience multiple disorders, which interact to significantly impede their life goals. Substance use disorders, in particular, frequently occur with serious mental illness and worsen the disease course.

4. *Disabilities* refer to the inability of people to meet life goals that are appropriate for their age and culture. These tend to be macrolevel goals, which include obtaining a satisfactory job, living independently, developing intimate and mature relationships, managing one's physical and mental health needs, and enjoying life through recreational and spiritual pursuits.

Note that it is disability per se that defines a person as being in need of psychiatric rehabilitation. People can have psychiatric disorders—some that are severe and others that are long lasting—that do not interfere with major life goals. What distinguishes rehabilitation from other forms of psychiatric care is the focus on helping people achieve life goals that are blocked by symptoms and dysfunctions. Each of these four conceptual domains is reviewed more fully in the rest of this chapter.

There is one significant problem with all the discussion on diagnoses, symptoms, dysfunctions, and disabilities: The person is reduced to the sum of his or her problems.

Although a pathology perspective is clearly useful for understanding a disorder and its impact on a person, it ignores the individual's strengths, which has several unintended consequences (Rapp, 1998b). Focusing on limitations adds to the person's feeling of incompetence and stigma. Ignoring strengths misses the resources that the person and the rehabilitation team may use to advance the person's goals. Given the importance of a strengths-based perspective, the chapter ends with a fuller discussion of this focus.

PSYCHIATRIC DIAGNOSIS

Many countries use the *International Classification of Diseases and Related Health Problems* (now in its 10th revision and known as ICD-10; World Health Organization, 1992) as a resource for psychiatric diagnosis. Although the ICD-10 is a reference for all disease, the section on mental disorders is specific to psychiatric diagnosis. Psychiatric rehabilitation practitioners in the United States and some other countries rely on the *Diagnostic and Statistical Manual of Mental Disorders* (currently the text revision of the fourth edition [DSM-IV-TR]; American Psychiatric Association, 2000) as the definitive resource on diagnosis. Although there are some minor differences across manuals, researchers have attempted to make sure that the DSM and ICD correspond as the references continue to develop. Diagnosis in the DSM-IV-TR is based on a multiaxial system; the five axes are summarized in Table 1.1.

Axes I, II, and III represent all diagnoses possibly relevant to the person with psychiatric disability, with Axis III reflecting medical conditions other than psychiatric illness

TABLE 1.1. The Five Axes of the DSM-IV-TR Multiaxial Classification System

Axis	Descriptor	Notes
I	Clinical disorders; other conditions that may be a focus of clinical attention	These two axes include all possible psychiatric diagnoses now in the DSM.
II	Personality disorders; mental retardation	
III	General medical conditions	These are physical conditions that are potentially relevant to the onset, trajectory, or impact of an AXIS I or Axis II disorder.
IV	Psychosocial and environmental problems	These represent the external causes and consequences of an Axis I or II disorder. These conditions may affect the understanding, treatment, and prognosis of the psychiatric disorders.
V	Global assessment of functioning	Typically, this is a single index of the person's overall functioning, given his or her psychiatric illness. Axis V frequently represents a score on the 100-point Global Assessment of Functioning Scale (in which 100 is superior functioning in a wide range of activities). It is important to remember that the score represents both distress *and* impaired function due to the psychiatric illness.

Note. Data from the American Psychiatric Association (2000).

that may be relevant to the person's disorder. Axis III (general medical conditions) is especially important for a rehabilitation agenda when people with psychiatric disability are seeking to manage related physical and dental health goals. Axes I and II include psychiatric disorders and represent an ongoing historical distinction in psychiatry between the principal psychiatric disorders (Axis I) and disorders that have otherwise been ignored or reflect some kind of pathology in development and personality (First, Frances, & Pincus, 1997a). Typically, some Axis I diagnoses are the concern of rehabilitation providers, though Axis II disorders can also lead to significant disabilities.

Axes IV and V represent concepts that are clearly relevant to rehabilitation. Axis IV outlines the environmental variables relevant to the cause and impact of the psychiatric disorder. Environmental variables also are important to the treatment and outcome of the psychiatric disorder. Axis V reflects the overall extent of disability by summarizing the effect of mental illness on overall life functioning. Axis V ratings are sometimes confusing because such a rating is a combination of both the distress and the disabilities caused by the mental illness. Impairment of functioning and distress are not always clearly related. Furthermore, it may be difficult to separate distress and impairment caused by the mental illness in an individual with both a mental illness and a medical condition, such as may occur in an individual with epilepsy who is also severely depressed. Axes IV and V provide relatively gross descriptions of these two important areas, which are more thoroughly addressed using other rehabilitation concepts and strategies.

Although the DSM includes diagnoses relevant to all age groups, disorders of interest to psychiatric rehabilitation are generally dominated by adult syndromes. In part, this focus results because the onset of many of the major mental illnesses (e.g., schizophrenia and the mood disorders) occurs in late adolescence or young adulthood. Another reason for the focus on adult disorders is that disabilities (defined as blocked life goals) are most meaningful in adulthood, when various goals like work, relationships, and independent living are ordinarily achieved. Hence, psychiatric disorders related to children (e.g., attention-deficit/hyperactivity disorder or developmental disabilities) and with onset in later life (e.g., Alzheimer's disease) are typically not the focus of psychiatric rehabilitation.

CHARACTERISTIC DIAGNOSES

Diagnoses in the DSM represent syndromes, or collections of symptoms that have meaning in terms of etiology or treatment. In addition, specific disorders tend to be associated with dysfunctions (e.g., poor social skills) that, when combined with symptoms, prevent the person from achieving life goals. Finally, diagnosis is fundamental for answering epidemiological questions—namely, the distribution of mental disorders in the population and associated risk factors. The DSM refers to the various diagnoses as *disorders*. A psychiatric disorder is a *clinically significant* behavioral or psychological syndrome that is associated with *distress* or *dysfunction* or with increased risk of death, disability, pain, or loss of freedom (American Psychiatric Association, 2000). To say that a condition is clinically significant generally means that the condition is severe enough that treatment would be recommended or sought out.

Symptoms and Dysfunctions

Although the DSM is largely silent about the difference between symptoms and dysfunctions, symptoms tend to be the additional negative experiences that occur because of the illness, whereas dysfunctions represent the absence of normal functioning. Both of these are evident in four fundamental spheres of human psychology: affect, perception and cognition, motivation and behavior, and interpersonal functioning. Note that by reviewing symptoms and dysfunctions in terms of these four spheres, we imply that symptoms are not necessarily linked to specific disorders. For example, hallucinations and depression occur in several different disorders. Psychopathology researchers have looked for *pathognomonic* symptoms that indicated a specific diagnosis—that is, the single symptom that unequivocally signaled a specific disorder. For example, Schneider (1959) proposed four first-rank symptoms as unmistakably defining schizophrenia: thoughts experienced as spoken aloud, voices heard commenting on the person, experiencing bodily movements or functions as being under the control of an outside force, and delusional atmosphere (i.e., a general interpretation of life events in terms of false beliefs). However, efforts like this to identify pathognomonic symptoms have largely been unsuccessful. It is the *collection* of symptoms with the corresponding course and disabilities that defines a diagnosis.

Affect

Four types of mood-related symptoms may constitute psychiatric disorder. These are distinguished from the normal range of positive and negative emotions by their severity or length of time experienced. For example, feeling anxious before a test is common and perhaps adaptive, because it motivates a person to be prepared. Feeling anxious about a test all semester is likely to be overwhelming and to interfere with activities outside school. *Anxiety* has both cognitive and physical components. Worry or ruminating over a stressor is the cognitive component. The physiological or autonomic components of anxiety include rapid heartbeat, shortness of breath, profuse sweating, and/or muscle ache, especially in the head and neck. *Depression* is a feeling of sadness or being blue. Commonly associated with depression is anhedonia, the lack of enjoyment in life activities, especially those that were previously enjoyable. On the opposite end of the continuum from depression is *euphoria*, an overwhelming feeling of intense pleasure and well-being that can lead to uncontrollable excitement and problematic behaviors. Finally, some people have significant *anger* problems, marked by sudden and uncontrollable rage, which can escalate into violence.

Alternatively, affective symptoms may appear in terms of disordered modulation. *Inappropriate affect* refers to emotions that are not consistent with a particular situation—for example, uncontrollable laughter when learning of the death of a friend or sobbing while watching a comedy. *Affective lability* means rapid change from one emotion to the next. An emotionally labile person may swing from crying to anger to laughter during the course of a 3-minute conversation. Dysfunctions in affect are also evident in some psychiatric disorders. Most common among these is flat affect, whereby a person responds to normally emotional situations with almost no signs of emotion. For example, a person with flat affect would seem to show no grief at the death of a love one and no joy at winning the lottery.

Perception and Cognition

Distortions in perception are observed in several psychotic disorders that lead to significant disability. These include four types of common hallucinations: auditory (which are the most commonly experienced in schizophrenia and are often reported as voices), olfactory (which are more commonly associated with major depressive disorder and include putrid odors of decay), tactile, and visual. Psychosis is associated with two cognitive symptoms: delusions, which are erroneous beliefs that may include grandiose, religious, persecutory, referential, or somatic content; and disorganized speech, in which syntax and semantics that govern the meaning of discourse are absent and content may approach nonsense. Depression is associated with world- and self-views of helplessness, hopelessness, and worthlessness. Anxiety is often associated with another kind of cognitive symptom: obsessive thought. Obsessions are persistent ideas, impulses, or images that are experienced as intrusive and that cause marked distress.

Two dysfunctions may be observed in the perceptual and cognitive sphere. First, people with some psychiatric disorders may show deficits in attention and other information-processing abilities. These may include problems with maintenance, span, and selectivity of attention. People with manic episodes may have diminished attention because of distractibility, that is, attention easily drawn to irrelevant stimuli. Additional information-processing deficits have been found in such cognitive functions as short- and long-term memory and the executive functions that help people organize individual processes into an efficient decision-making system (Green, 1998). In addition, some people show problems of impoverished thought. They are unable to spontaneously generate many ideas in response to an issue. Alogia, common for a person with impoverished thought, is speech marked by a minimum of words and little initiation of conversation.

Motivation and Behavior

Symptoms and deficits related to motivation manifest themselves in various ways. First, people with mood disorders typically show motivational problems. People with overwhelming euphoria may experience an *expansive* approach to life; that is, there are no limits, including those that seem obvious to others, to what the person might accomplish. Conversely, those who are depressed may be *lethargic* and have difficulty completing everyday activities like those required for basic hygiene and work duties. Some people may experience *inhibitions* because of their disorders. People with significant anxiety disorders may be unable to accomplish daily activities because they avoid situations that make them anxious or because they are overwhelmed with worry. *Disinhibition* is common in some other important disorders in the DSM. These include sexual and eating disorders. Disinhibition-related syndromes of particular concern to psychiatric rehabilitation are the various substance use disorders—for example, inability to inhibit inappropriate impulses because of intoxication.

We also include symptoms involving behavior in relation to motivation. These include disorganized or catatonic behavior found in some persons with psychotic disorders. Catatonic behavior includes opposite ends of the same spectrum: motoric immobility or excessive motoric activity. Grossly disorganized behavior seen in some of the schizophrenias includes childlike silliness or unpredictable agitation. Behavior-related symptoms also include hypomanic activity, which is found in the manic phase of bipolar disorders. This comprises pressure to keep talking, marked increase in goal-directed activity, or excessive involvement in pleasurable activity. Depression is also associated with behavior change: psychomotor agitation, in which the individual paces or cannot sit still, and the opposite, psychomotor retardation, in which the individual moves, thinks, and talks more slowly than usual. Perhaps the major dysfunction most closely related to motivation is avolition, which is characterized by an inability to initiate and persist in goal-directed activities. People manifesting this symptom rarely show little interest in work or social activities.

Interpersonal Functioning

Social relationships are at the heart of psychological functioning and are fundamental to most life goals. Many psychiatric disorders have a significant impact on a person's ability to form or maintain these relationships. Interestingly, most of the symptoms and dysfunctions in interpersonal relationships represent an interaction with the three afore-mentioned spheres of functioning: affect, cognition, and motivation. In terms of affect, social anxiety can cripple a person's abilities to engage in and enjoy interpersonal transactions. Depression can rob a person of any interest in others or make it unrewarding to be around other people. Euphoria can change interactions into overenergetic and unpredictable encounters. A person's anger and rage can fill others with dread or leave them feeling victimized. The hallucinations and delusions of people with such disorders can make it difficult for them to form close and intimate bonds because their perspectives on the world, including a shared reality, fail to correspond with others'.

Symptoms and dysfunctions in cognition also undermine a person's interpersonal experiences (Corrigan & Penn, 2001). They may prevent the person from correctly perceiving the social cues of a situation or from understanding the roles and goals that govern it. Problems with motivation may also impact interpersonal activities. The loss of motivation common to some disorders leaves some individuals with total disinterest in social interactions. People with this deficit, called schizoid symptoms, are not necessarily fearful of others nor have their interpersonal drive been suppressed by depression. Rather, they seem to have no natural desire for any aspect of the multilevel benefits of human interaction.

A significant amount of work has focused on understanding the deficits and dysfunctions related to social functioning (Mueser & Tarrier, 1998) and social skills (Bellack, Mueser, Gingerich, & Agresta, 2004). Social functioning deficits can prevent people from attaining age-appropriate social roles. For young to middle-age American adults, these roles include employee, head of household, spouse, parent, neighbor, and churchgoer. People with some psychiatric disorders lack social skills, which prevents them from achieving social roles. These include interpersonal skills such as basic conversation, assertiveness, conflict management, and dating skills. They also include personal and instrumental skills like hygiene, money management, and basic work skills.

Suicide and Dangerousness

Many people with psychosis or other serious mental illnesses struggle with suicidal thoughts and impulses; hence, this is an important concern of which rehabilitation providers should be aware and ready to intervene. Epidemiological research showed that 13.5% of a 1992 nationally representative sample reported lifetime suicidal ideation, 3.9% a plan for suicide, and 4.6% a previous attempt (Kessler, Borges, & Walters, 1999). Findings from this study also showed that 34% of people with suicidal ideation progressed to plans and that 72% with plans made attempts.

Suicidal ideation or attempts is one of the criteria for the diagnosis of major depression, though not all people who meet this diagnosis are suicidal. The interested reader should review Chapter 4, in which some considerations for suicide assessment are reviewed. Two points are mentioned here:

1. Past suicidal ideation or attempts is important information for determining whether a person is suicidal and for developing an appropriate intervention plan.
2. Risk of suicide does not necessarily mean that a person should be hospitalized or rule out a person's pursuing other rehabilitation goals.

Answers to difficult issues like these need to involve the person with disability, his or her family, and the complete rehabilitation team.

Some people with serious mental illness also pose a danger to others. This danger can vary from the very rare homicide to yelling at loved ones. Epidemiological research suggests that, depending on diagnosis, people with serious mental illness are as much as six times more likely to be violent, as compared with the rest of the population (Corrigan & Watson, 2005; Swanson, Holzer, Ganju, & Jono, 1990). Concomitant use of alcohol and other drugs increases the rate of violence 20- to 30-fold. Moreover, symptoms related to paranoia and threat/control-override also exacerbate violence (Link & Stueve, 1994; Link, Phelan, Bresnahan, Stueve, & Pescosolido, 1999). Interview items that assess threat/control-override include (1) How often have you felt that your mind was dominated by forces beyond your control? (2) How often have you felt that thoughts were put into your head that were not your own? and (3) How often have you felt that there were people who wished to do you harm?

The two cautions about suicide, listed earlier, apply in terms of understanding violence. Past history of violence and threats should be considered in developing an appropriate intervention plan. The presence of anger and threat does not necessarily preclude pursuit of other rehabilitation goals. Rather, the person and his or her rehabilitation team need to make this issue a priority in pursuing life goals. Concerns about violence and danger are discussed more thoroughly in Chapter 18.

Insight into Symptoms

One might think that a person's psychiatric symptoms and related dysfunctions would dominate the person's awareness. It might be assumed that people with mental illness would be concerned about problems with emotion, perception, cognition, motivation, interpersonal relations, or danger and would therefore be highly motivated to participate in treatment to resolve these problems. However, many people with psychiatric diagnoses are unaware that specific experiences are symptomatic of mental illness (Amador & David, 1998). Lack of insight may occur for three reasons. First, it may be the direct result of biological deficits caused by the illness. For example, deficits in the frontal lobes of the cerebral cortex commonly found in some people with schizophrenia are associated with diminished insight. This area of the cortex is associated with metacognitive processes related to the observing self—that is, the cognitive process that helps a person to check on how well he or she is functioning (Amador, Strauss, Yale, & Gorman, 1991; Amador, Flaum, Andreasen, Strauss, Yale, et al., 1994).

Alternatively, not recognizing symptoms as mental illness may offer a secondary gain. Namely, labeling oneself as mentally ill may evoke both public and self-stigma. If a person does not admit that certain experiences are symptoms of mental illness, thereby denying the psychiatric disorder, he or she can escape the stigma (Lally, 1989). Third, what mental health professionals perceive as symptoms may be experienced as copacetic in relation to a person's image of him- or herself. For example, frequent rage and angry interactions with others may be perceived as a normal part of life by some people. This "misperception" of symptoms is especially common in people with personality disorders (Millon, Davis, Millon, Escovar, & Meagher, 2000).

What implications does lack of insight have for treatment? Poor insight into one's disease predicts poor outcome; that is, people who lack insight are less able to use interventions to control their symptoms and meet their life goals (Amador, Strauss, Yale, Flaum, Endicott, et al., 1993). In addition, lack of insight undermines full understanding of and participating in treatment plans (Cuffel, Aford, Fischer, & Owen, 1996; Kemp & David, 1995; Smith, Hughes, & Budd, 1999a). The traditional notion of psychiatric care was that people had to recognize and admit their mental illness if significant benefits from treatment were to occur. Without such recognition, some people might resist participating in effective interventions. That is, people who do not, for example, admit their schizophrenia will not progress until they do so; thus, the provider "should" motivate the person to recognize his or her illness (Corrigan, Liberman, & Engel, 1990). Most rehabilitation providers realize that focusing on disease acceptance can lead to an unnecessary struggle. Rehabilitation providers avoid this battle, instead partnering with the person by helping him or her to identify life goals and develop the rehabilitation plan to achieve them. People can go back to work whether or not they admit they have schizophrenia.

Epidemiology

Psychiatric diagnosis facilitates the goals of epidemiology. Epidemiologists seek to address public health questions about how many people meet the criteria for specific disorders (Robins, 1978; Tsuang, Tohen, & Zahner, 1995). *Incidence rates* represent new cases that emerge in a healthy population within a fixed time frame, often 1 year. *Prevalence rates* represent the proportion of the population that meets the criteria for a disease at a specified point or period of time. Working at the population level allows researchers to also understand the biological, behavioral, psychological, social, and economic variables that predict the risk and course of the disorders. Public health officials use this information to set priorities in treatment policy and to track the impact of specific approaches on a disorder in the population. Prevalence rates for diagnostic groups relevant to psychiatric rehabilitation are presented in Table 1.2 and later in this chapter as specific illnesses are discussed more fully.

Etiology

One purpose of diagnosis in medicine is to classify people with similar disorders into groups that share similar causes. For example, people with respiratory symptoms whose test results suggest a bacterial infection may be diagnosed with pneumonia, which may be effectively treated by antibiotics. Psychiatry has been less successful in developing a diagnostic system that corresponds with etiology. A diagnosis of major depressive disorder, for example, does not automatically suggest a specific set of causes. Despite this limitation, psychiatry has made huge strides in identifying what causes and exacerbates the serious mental illnesses that lead to psychiatric disability. Clearly, research has *not* substantiated the out-of-date notion that mother, father, or some other family member necessarily caused such illness through bad parenting. Instead, research has identified several biological processes that may explain the development of these disorders. A complete discussion of these processes is beyond the scope of this text. In brief, research has suggested two factors that may yield a diagnosis consistent with disorders like schizophrenia:

1. *Genetic.* Population approaches to genetics as well as the newer field of molecular genetics, have clearly implicated genetic inheritance as a primary cause of schizophrenia and the affective disorders. Research at this point seems to support the involvement of a complex multifactorial pattern of inheritance rather than a single gene (Cannon, van Erp, & Glahn, 2002).
2. *Obstetric complications.* Adverse intrauterine events are associated with later

onset of schizophrenia (Crow, 2003). For example, mothers who contract influenza during the second trimester of pregnancy are significantly more likely than comparison groups to give birth to children who later show signs of schizophrenia (Machon, Huttunen, Mednick, Sinivuo, Tanskanen, et al., 2002).

Stress Vulnerability

Biological factors are not sufficient to explain the onset and course of most serious mental illnesses. Researchers have developed a stress vulnerability model that integrates biological vulnerabilities with environmental stressors to explain how serious mental illnesses occur (Green, 1998; Nuechterlein, Dawson, Gitlin, Ventura, Goldstein, et al., 1992). (See Figure 1.1.) According to this model, genetic and other biological factors have many effects, one being that some people are vulnerable to stress. When this vulnerability is overwhelmed, typically in late adolescence or young adulthood, the person experiences prodromal symptoms (the subtle, usually nonpsychotic signs of an illness that precede the first episode). Continued stress yields a full-blown psychotic episode and onset of the disorder. With treatment, the psychosis may remit; however, subsequent stress may cause relapse or residual symptoms.

Research on the model has shown that common events that occur as part of "normal" life development can cause sufficient stress to overwhelm the vulnerable person (Ventura, Nuechterlein, Subotnik, Hardesty, & Mintz, 2000). Such events may include leaving home when launching from one's family of origin, starting a job, or getting married. Moreover, some stressful family interactions can overwhelm the vulnerability (Butzlaff & Hooley, 1998). Protective factors that can diminish a person's vulnerability to stress may prevent subsequent relapses. Broadly speaking, these factors include psychotropic medication, interpersonal and instrumental skills, and social support (Anthony & Liberman, 1992). In some ways, these protective factors provide the basic building blocks for rehabilitation.

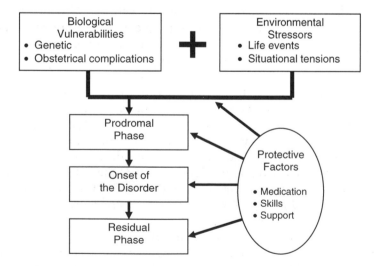

FIGURE 1.1. The stress-vulnerability model. Originally developed to explain the course of schizophrenia, its broad principles are applicable to the other disorders that lead to psychiatric disabilities.

COMMON DIAGNOSES AMONG PSYCHIATRIC DISABILITIES

Four diagnostic syndromes are commonly associated with psychiatric disability: schizophrenia, mood disorders, anxiety disorders, and personality disorders such as borderline personality disorder. We do not mean to imply that these are the only diagnoses relevant to psychiatric rehabilitation. Any of the Axis I diagnoses—other than a solitary diagnosis of substance abuse disorder or developmental disability, childhood disorders, or disorders with onset in elder adulthood such as the dementias—may be considered the cause of psychiatric disabilities and be relevant for psychiatric rehabilitation. Still, these four groups of disorders comprise the vast majority of people with psychiatric disabilities and are therefore most common in rehabilitation practice. The symptoms and dysfunctions that are DSM criteria for the four categories are summarized in Table 1.2. Aspects of each category relevant to psychiatric disability are discussed in the following sections.

Schizophrenia

Schizophrenia is one of the psychotic disorders that lead to psychiatric disabilities. The DSM-IV-TR defines psychosis at various levels. The narrowest definition is restricted to evidence of delusions or prominent hallucinations, with the person not having insight into the pathological nature of the hallucinations. A broader definition includes other positive symptoms such as disorganized speech or grossly disorganized behavior (positive symptoms are the florid signs of psychosis). Most people with schizophrenia are challenged by significant disabilities and unable to achieve life goals in most domains. In fact, inherent to the definition of schizophrenia are *psychotic symptoms that interfere with major life functions*. Schizophrenia is more accurately considered a spectrum disorder—that is, a variety of disorders that may vary in course and outcome but share similar symptoms and dysfunctions. Epidemiological research has shown a 1.5% lifetime prevalence for the various disorders in the spectrum (see Table 1.1).

Schizophrenia itself encompasses several subtypes: *paranoid* type (marked by prominent persecutory or grandiose delusions and/or auditory hallucinations related to the content of the delusions), *disorganized* type (with disorganized speech or behavior, or inappropriate affect), *catatonic* type (a marked psychomotor disturbance that may involve motoric immobility or excessive motor activity), and *undifferentiated* type (referring to people with schizophrenia who do not meet the criteria for one of the three other types). The DSM-IV-TR also lists a fifth subtype, *residual type*, though this type may be better understood as a phase of the disorder. The residual type consists primarily of negative symptoms (discussed below) or positive symptoms of reduced severity. Generally, the distinction between subtypes has not been particularly helpful for rehabilitation plans.

Other diagnoses in the schizophrenia spectrum include *schizoaffective* and *schizophreniform* disorder. Schizoaffective disorder combines a period of schizophrenia with either a major depressive or manic episode. The differential diagnosis between schizoaffective disorder and schizophrenia may have important implications for medication. Individuals with schizoaffective disorders may benefit from mood stabilizers, as well as antipsychotic medication, to address the affective components of their illness. People with schizophreniform disorder meet the diagnostic criteria for schizophrenia, except for length of the disorder. The course of schizophreniform disorder is shorter than that of schizophrenia, lasting between 1 and 6 months. People with schizophreniform disorder typically have a much more benign course than those with schizophrenia. Although not

TABLE 1.2. The Symptoms, Dysfunctions, Course, and Prevalence of Severe Mental Illnesses

Diagnosis	Symptoms and dysfunctions					Lifetime prevalence
	Affect	Perception and cognition	Motivation and behavior	Interpersonal functioning	Other	
Schizophrenia spectrum	• Affective flattening (Neg. syn.) • Inappropriate affect • Emotional lability	• Hallucinations • Delusions • Disorganized speech • Alogia (Neg. syn.) • Poor attention, memory, executive functioning	• Grossly disorganized or catatonic behavior • Avolition (Neg. syn.)	• Unable to attain social roles • Diminished social skills		1.5%[a] (includes schizophrenia and schizophreniform disorder)
Mood disorders MDD	• Depressed mood • Anhedonia	• Ideas of worthlessness • Diminished concentration • Suicidal ideation	• Loss of energy • Psychomotor agitation or retardation	• May diminish interpersonal relationships	• Appetite change • Sleep change	17.1%[b]
BPD	• Elevated mood or irritated	• Ideas of grandiosity • Racing thoughts • Distractibility	• Pressured speech • Increase in goal-directed activity • Excessive pleasurable activity	• May diminish interpersonal relationships	• Decreased need for sleep	1.6%[b]
Anxiety disorders Agoraphobia	• Anxiety about being in multiple "inescapable" situations		• Situations avoided or endured with marked distress	• May diminish interpersonal relationships		5.3%[b]

Disorder	Symptoms				Prevalence
OCD	• Anxiety or distress that results from persistent thoughts or impulses	• Recurrent and persistent thoughts that are difficult to ignore or suppress	• Impulses to perform ego-dystonic actions	• Obsessions and concomitant distress may interfere with reloationships	3.5%[c]
PTSD	• Intense distress around trauma cues • Restricted affect • Irritability	• Intrusive recollections of traumatic event • Recurrent distressing dreams • Inability to recall trauma • Difficulty concentrating • Hypervigilance	• Persistent avoidance of trauma-related thoughts, feelings, places	• Feeling estranged from others	• Difficulty in sleeping	7.8%[b]
Borderline PD	• Affect instability • Marked reactivity of mood • Feelings of emptiness • Intense anger	• Unstable self-ideas • Transient paranoid ideation • Dissociative symptoms	• Avoidance of real or imagined abandonment • Impulsivity in areas like sex, substance abuse, or binge eating	• Unstable interpersonal relationships • Recurrent suicide attempts	2.8%[d]

Note. The list of symptoms and dysfunctions are adapted from DSM-IV-TR (American Psychiatric Association, 2000). The interested reader should consult DSM-IV-TR regarding the number and kind of specific signs that are needed for diagnosis of a specific disorder. Neg. syn., negative syndrome; MDD, major depressive disorder; OCD, obsessive–compulsive disorder; BPD, bipolar disorder; PTSD, posttraumatic stress disorder; PD, personality disorder.
[a] Epidemiologic Catchment Area Study (Regier et al., 1988).
[b] National Comorbidity Survey (Kessler et al., 1994).
[c] Widiger and Weissman (1991).
[d] Angst et al. (2003).

an Axis I disorder, schizotypal personality disorder is frequently included in the schizophrenia spectrum and is also associated with significant impairment.

In addition to spectrum diagnoses and subtypes, schizophrenia has been defined in
terms of *positive* and *negative* symptoms (Andreasen & Olson, 1982; Crow, 1982)
Positive symptoms represent the florid signs of psychosis and the disorder; they include
hallucinations, delusions, grossly disorganized and catatonic behavior, and inappropriate affect. Negative symptoms are sometimes called the deficit syndrome—alogia,
avolition, and affective flattening—and represent the absence of normal functioning
seen in many people with schizophrenia. Typically, positive symptoms are more
episodic and fluctuating over time as compared with negative symptoms. Although
positive and negative symptoms were originally thought to be mutually exclusive syndromes representing different etiological processes (Crow, 1982), research now indicates that people with schizophrenia can manifest both clusters of symptoms (Ho &
Andreasen, 2001). Of more relevance to rehabilitation practitioners, research has suggested that the assessment of positive and negative symptoms has been useful for prognosis and treatment planning. Research suggests that positive, as compared with negative, symptoms respond well to traditional antipsychotics, as well as many of the
atypical antipsychotic medications (Ho & Andreasen, 2001); see Chapter 7 for a more
complete discussion of medication. Noticing this trend, researchers have specifically
sought to improve the impact of some antipsychotics on negative symptoms. Research
also suggests that the prognosis for negative symptoms is worse than for positive symptoms, especially in the psychosocial treatments that often include psychiatric rehabilitation (Crow, 1995). Nevertheless, there is no indication that the presence or severity of
positive and/or negative symptoms precludes an individual from participating in and
benefiting from a rehabilitation program.

Mood Disorders

Symptoms related to mood define major depression. People with this disability either
experience long periods of time with a prominent depressed mood or have significant
anhedonia (i.e., loss of enjoyment of almost all human activities and interactions, including those that were previously reported as pleasurable). In addition, people with major
depression may experience cognitive, motivation, and interpersonal symptoms and
dysfunctions. Many people with major depression also exhibit vegetative signs. These are
changes in major life functions, such as sleep, appetite, and energy. Interestingly, change
can be either an increase or decrease from the person's typical baseline. So, many people
with major depression report sleeping significantly more or not being able to sleep as
much; eating more than usual, which leads to noticeable weight gain, or experiencing a
decrease in appetite; and having little energy or experiencing high levels of agitation.

Mood disorders are among the most common of psychiatric disorders. Approximately 17% of the adult population can, over time, meet the criteria for a major depressive episode (Blazer, Kessler, McGonagle, & Swartz, 1994). Some of these people, however, do not suffer long-term disabilities because of their illness. People with bipolar
disorder are more likely to experience significant disabilities. Typically, people with bipolar disorder experience separate periods of major depression and mania, interspersed
with periods of normal mood. Manic and depressed episodes can last weeks or even
months. Periods longer than several months are atypical, especially in terms of mania,
and may represent a more benign cyclothymic disorder. Conversely, rapid cyclers are people who experience episodes in relatively brief periods. The DSM-IV-TR defines rapid

cycling as four or more mood episodes in a 12-month period. But episodes as short as a few days, followed by an episode of opposite polarity, are not uncommon.

DSM-IV distinguished bipolar disorder of two types: Bipolar I and Bipolar II. Both disorders are marked by interspersed periods of major depression and some version of mania. People with Bipolar I, the more severe of the two types, experience full-blown manic episodes, typically with psychosis. People with Bipolar II disorder experience episodes of major depression plus hypomanic episodes, which include many of the sped-up symptoms and dysfunctions of mania but are less severe; that is, there are no psychotic symptoms, little need for hospitalization, and less impairment of functioning. Although people with both forms of bipolar disorder may experience psychiatric disabilities, those with Bipolar I disorder are more likely to need the assistance of rehabilitation programs.

Anxiety Disorders

Anxiety disorders are frequently viewed by the public as less disabling than the schizophrenias and mood disorders. Epidemiological research tends to support this notion for the general population (Kessler, DuPont, Berglund, & Wittchen, 1999). However, individuals with anxiety disorders may still struggle with significant life disabilities for prolonged periods of time. In addition, anxiety disorders frequently co-occur with one of the schizophrenia disorders or mood disorders, which is likely to yield significant life disabilities (Cosoff & Haffner, 1998). Although any of the anxiety disorders alone can lead to disabilities requiring psychiatric rehabilitation, three in particular may be seen in rehabilitation clients.

The essential features of *obsessive–compulsive disorder* are recurrent obsessions (persistent thoughts that are experienced as intrusive) or compulsions (repetitive behaviors that the person feels driven to perform) that are sufficiently severe to be time-consuming or cause significant impairment. Common examples of obsessions include thoughts about contamination or cleanliness, repeated doubts, a need for order, aggressive impulses, and sexual images. Common compulsions include washing, counting, checking, requesting assurance, or repeating actions. Typically, people with this disorder recognize that their obsessions or compulsions are unreasonable or excessive. The time spent on obsessions or compulsions, as well as the distress they cause, can significantly interfere with persons pursuing their life goals.

Agoraphobia is anxiety about being in places or situations from which escape is difficult or embarrassing. In many instances, this disorder is manifested as an unwillingness to leave one's home so as not to risk situations of this kind. Avoidance of certain situations frequently impairs a person's ability to travel outside the home, thereby undermining work and other independent living goals. *Posttraumatic stress disorder* (PTSD) occurs following exposure to an extreme traumatic stressor that involves actual or threatened death to self or others, which leads to intense fear, helplessness, or horror. The subsequent experience of symptoms may happen immediately after the traumatic event or may be delayed for months or years. The symptoms that correspond with PTSD include some form of reliving the event, accompanied with intense emotional arousal. Research suggests that many persons with a diagnosis of schizophrenia or mood disorder have a history of trauma and PTSD that worsens their disabilities considerably (Mueser, Rosenberg, Jankowski, Hamblen, & Descamps, 2004b). Alternatively, significant trauma and PTSD can interfere with life goals in their own right, leading to a need for rehabilitation. See Chapter 14 for a more complete discussion of trauma and psychiatric rehabilitation.

Personality Disorders

As outlined in the DSM-IV-TR, personality disorders involve the way people relate to and think about their environment and themselves. Symptoms and dysfunctions of the personality disorders are frequently inflexible or otherwise maladaptive manifestations of normal personality traits. Personality disorders are organized into three clusters. Cluster A includes the paranoid, schizoid, and schizotypal personality disorders; individuals meeting criteria for these diagnoses often appear eccentric or odd. Cluster B comprises antisocial, borderline, histrionic, and narcissistic disorders. People with these diagnoses may seem dramatic or emotional. Cluster C includes avoidant, dependent, and obsessive–compulsive personality disorders, in which individuals appear anxious or fearful. Although any of these 10 disorders can lead to significant disabilities and the need for rehabilitation, much has particularly been written about psychosocial services for people with borderline personality disorders (Linehan, 1993).

Borderline personality disorder is marked by a pervasive pattern of instability in social relationships, self-image, and emotions, exacerbated by severe impulsivity. Impulsive behaviors can include self-mutilation or suicide. Because their relationships are so tumultuous, people with borderline personality disorders frequently lack a support network that can help them cope with even the most minor of problems. As a result, minor depression and anxiety can explode into overwhelming stress. People with borderline personality disorder may have significant difficulty in accomplishing employment, relationship, and other independent life goals because of these symptoms and thus may benefit from rehabilitation.

Additional Information for an Accurate Psychiatric Diagnosis

The presence or absence of the criteria listed in Table 1.2, as assessed during a single interview, is usually not sufficient to make a diagnosis. It is almost impossible to decide whether a person presenting with depression and psychotic symptoms at a clinic visit has major depressive disorder, or schizophrenia with depression, schizoaffective disorder, bipolar disorder, substance-induced disorder, or some combination thereof. Complete diagnosis requires two other elements in addition to the assessment of symptoms and dysfunction.

1. *History.* What kind of impact have the symptoms and dysfunctions had on the person over time? The next section of this chapter examines this question in terms of the course of the disorder.
2. *Depth of impact.* How much does the illness interfere with the person's life? Does it lead to an occasional acute crisis, followed by significant periods when symptoms are in remission and life goals are accomplished? Or does the illness significantly disrupt the person and his or her life plan? The chapter ends with a consideration of the various kinds of disabilities that psychiatric disorders may bring.

COURSE OF THE PSYCHIATRIC DISORDER

The symptoms, dysfunctions, and disabilities that constitute psychiatric disorders are dynamic phenomena; that is, they change over a person's lifetime. Key milestones help to explain a disease course, including *onset* of the disorder and the prodromal period leading up to it, ongoing disease *trajectory* once the illness has begun, and *end state*. As outlined in Figure 1.2 for schizophrenia, each milestone may be described as one of two types. The onset may occur over a slow and chronic course, or it may be sudden or acute. The trajectory may be simple and unchanging, or it may represent undulating waves that vacillate between significant symptoms and remission. The end state may be severe and unremitting, or recovery may occur. Each of these is reviewed more fully below.

Disease Onset

The onset of most of the mental illnesses that lead to psychiatric disability and rehabilitation typically occurs in late adolescence or early adulthood. The period preceding the onset of the full-blown disease is known as the prodrome. As outlined in Figure 1.2, the prodromal course may be brief and acute, or it may be chronic and insidious. An acute onset of a disease is a relatively greater shock to individuals and their families. In such a case it is typical that the person was experiencing few psychiatric problems prior to the full-blown set of symptoms characteristic of the illness. The subsequent course of the disease in a person with acute onset is frequently more benign than in a person with chronic onset (Moeller & von Zerssen, 1995).

For those with an insidious and chronic onset, the prodrome can be a brief period of months or can extend over several years. Because it is slow and insidious, the person and his or her family often do not identify the prodrome as signaling psychiatric illness. In this case, the prodrome is marked by attenuated forms of the symptoms that characterize the illness. For example, people who end up with schizophrenia may show such signs as "ideas of reference," the uncertain concern that people might be noticing them, rather than delusions, odd beliefs or magical thinking, and unusual perceptual experiences. The presence of symptoms like these during adolescence or young adulthood does not neces-

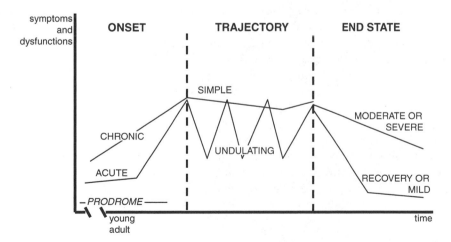

FIGURE 1.2. The different elements of course and their presentations as adapted from Ciompi's (1980) model of schizophrenia. As in most serious mental illnesses relevant to psychiatric rehabilitation, the course here is described as starting in late adolescence or young adulthood. Onset may be an acute change from "normal" functioning or a long prodrome with a chronic increase of symptoms. Trajectory may be simple and relatively flat, *in which* symptoms remain relatively unchanged, or undulating, *in which* symptoms alternate with periods of remission. End state may be total recovery or severe illness, or somewhere in between.

sarily mean that the person's disorder will convert to a full-blown psychotic disorder. Alternatively, these symptoms may signal the onset of the less disabling schizotypal personality disorder.

Early and accurate assessment of the onset of serious disorders like schizophrenia is important in regard to the subsequent impact of interventions. Research has shown that the *duration of untreated psychosis* (the period in which the prodrome is not correctly identified as leading to psychosis) is positively associated with poor outcome in terms of relapse and inversely associated with remission (Crow, 1986; Jablensky, Sartorius, Ernberg, Anker, Korten, et al., 1992; Loebel, Lieberman, Alvir, Mayerhoff, Geisler, et al., 1992). Early intervention programs have been developed and evaluated to treat people soon after psychosis first emerges. A possible goal of programs of this kind is to help people avoid disabilities by learning to manage the illness from the start. Hence, early intervention programs typically do not fall under the rubric of psychiatric rehabilitation. See Edwards and McGorry (2002) for a comprehensive review of the elements of early intervention.

Ongoing Trajectory

Although some serious mental illnesses are short in duration, most relevant to psychiatric rehabilitation is that some can last for years. The trajectory of serious mental illness is described by two patterns. Some people experience a relatively simple or flat trajectory in which symptoms, dysfunctions, and disabilities do not change much from the onset. Alternatively, many people with serious mental illness experience an undulating pattern in which symptoms, dysfunctions, and disabilities wax and wane. Undulating patterns can be regular and episodic, that is, described by regular shifts from disease states to remission (Modestin, Huber, Satirli, Malti, & Hell, 2003). The research is not clear as to what may account for these rhythms, but possible factors include biological patterns (e.g., monthly hormonal changes; Halbreich & Kahn, 2003), social schedules (e.g., regular stresses at work), or anniversaries of earlier traumatic events (Mueser, Rosenberg, Goodman, & Trumbetta, 2002b). Irregular patterns are more common, however, in which recurring waxing and waning are not predictable.

Decreases of symptoms and dysfunctions from the acute and severe level are described by two phases. During the *residual phase*, symptoms and dysfunctions have markedly decreased from the acute level, but the person still experiences problems that result from attenuated versions of the disorder. Hence, the person has fewer psychiatric problems than experienced in the acute phase of the illness but is still likely to be disabled by the disorder. In other instances, a person with serious mental illness experiences a total *remission* of symptoms and dysfunctions during benign periods of the course of the disorder, that is, the person has returned to a preprodromal level. Generally, evidence of remission during the trajectory suggests a better end state than when only residual phases are experienced.

End State

What becomes of people with serious mental illnesses? Early psychiatric models mostly indicated a negative prognosis. Schizophrenia, for example, was thought to result inevitably in a progressive downhill course. Kraepelin (1896) called schizophrenia *dementia praecox*, or a precocious dementia, because he believed that, as in most dementing illnesses, the loss of normal functioning was irreversible. Several long-term follow-up research projects were completed to test this assertion; most of this research was done on schizophrenia. In studies of this type, people with schizophrenia were typically identified while they were in a psychiatric hospital and then followed for 10–30 years to determine the end states of their disorders. Findings from prominent studies of this kind are summarized in Table 1.3. The table lists the criteria used by each study to determine improvement or recovery.

If Kraepelin were correct, we would expect the vast majority of, if not all, people with schizophrenia to still be symptomatic and dysfunctional and to not be working or living independently at follow-up. Instead, each of the studies found that schizophrenia has a heterogeneous range of end states—from severe cases requiring repeated or continuous hospitalization to cases in which a single episode of illness is followed by complete remission of symptoms. The findings reported in these studies as a whole indicate that roughly half of participating subjects recovered or significantly improved over the long term, suggesting that remission or recovery is much more common than originally thought.

Criteria for Recovery

Different dimensions of outcome and end state, such as symptom levels and psychosocial functioning, have generally been found to intercorrelate only to a modest degree (Strauss & Carpenter, 1972, 1974, 1977; Harding, Brooks, Ashikaga, Strauss, & Breir, 1987a, 1987b). For this reason, the choice of which dimensions are used as criteria for recovery is important. Some investigators (e.g., McGlashan, 1984) believe that a study must use multiple dimensions to provide a comprehensive and valid picture. However, one may also argue that the presence of symptoms within an otherwise functional life should not disqualify an individual from being judged "recovered." Psychosocial functioning is arguably a more important criterion of recovery than being symptom-free, and an overreliance on symptom-based criteria, together with the false assumption that symptoms and functioning are strongly correlated, may partially explain why the pessimistic Kraepelinian view of schizophrenia has persisted. Reliance on global ratings of outcome collapses these differences, making the exact nature of outcome unclear.

In many cases, persons with schizophrenia have learned ways to cope with and manage symptoms when they arise. In cautioning against the criterion of presence versus absence of symptoms, Liberman, Kopelowicz, Ventura, and Gutkind (2002) argued that positive symptoms experienced during a given follow-up period may last only days or weeks and may have a minimal impact on social or occupational functioning. In addition, the International Study of Schizophrenia (Harrison, Hopper, Craig, Laska, Siegel, et al., 2001) found that 20% of subjects maintained employment despite persisting symptoms and/or disability. In any case, we certainly should not limit a determination of outcome to positive psychotic symptoms, given that negative symptoms, anxiety, and depression may be much more disabling in a given case than positive symptoms (Liberman, 2002).

COURSE PREDICTORS AND MODIFIERS

Research has identified several factors that either predict or modify the course of serious mental illness, including family history, stress, substance use, some demographic characteristics, and some socioeconomic variables. These are relevant concepts to keep in mind as rehabilitation plans are developed to help people achieve their life goals. However, neither the person with psychiatric disabilities nor the rehabilitation team should feel bound

TABLE I.3. Summary of Long-Term Follow-Up Studies on Schizophrenia

Name of study	% recovered or improved	Average follow-up	Improvement/recovery criteria
Burgholzli Study (Bleuler, 1978)	53%	23 years	5-year "end state" determined through clinical interview by Bleuler.
Iowa 500 Study (Tsuang & Winokur, 1975)	46%	35 years	Marital, residential, occupational, and symptom status rated on 3-point scales and combined into a global measure.
Bonn Hospital (Huber et al., 1980)	56%	22 years	Symptoms and social functioning assessed by exam. Social recovery was defined as full-time employment.
Lausanne Study (Ciompi, 1980)	49%	37 years	M. Bleuler's 5-year "end state" criteria.
Chestnut Lodge (McGlashan, 1984)	36%	15 years	Personal interview in which examiner rated subject on hospitalization, employment, social activity, psychopathology, and a global functioning score that combined these factors.
Japanese Study (Ogawa et al., 1987)	57%	21–27 years	Follow-up interviews emphasizing social relationships and residential status.
Vermont Study (Harding, 1987b, 1987c)	68%	32 years	Interviews using structured instruments for the collection of data on social functioning, hospital records, various symptom-based measures summarized with the Global Assessment Scale.
Cologne Study (Steinmeyer et al., 1989)	36%	25 years	Interviews using the Global Assessment Scale, the Disability Assessment Schedule, the Psychological Impairment Rating Schedule, and the Bonn criteria for categorization of psychopathological outcome.
Maine Sample (DeSisto et al., 1995)	49%	36 years	Criteria replicated the Vermont Study. The Global Assessment Scale provided a global measure of psychological and social status.
International Study of Schizophrenia (Harrison et al., 2001)	56%–60%	15 and 25 years	Bleuler global assessment based on all information on course, symptoms, and functioning.

Note. Data from Corrigan and Calabrese (2005).

by the predictions that correspond with individual factors. The person with serious mental illness who is motivated to achieve work, independent living, and other life goals will be able to achieve these goals, regardless of course modifiers, with appropriate rehabilitation services. Each of these is reviewed more fully below.

Familial History

A person's having biological relatives with serious mental illness is probably the best predictor of disease onset because it is a proxy for probability that the person has inherited the genetic vulnerability (Kendler, McGuire, Gruenberg, Spellman, & Walsh, 1993). For example, having a first-degree parent or sibling with schizophrenia increases a person's likelihood of experiencing schizophrenia 10-fold (Kendler & Diehl, 1993). An individual with an identical twin diagnosed with schizophrenia has a 50% chance that he or she too will contract the disorder (Kendler & Diehl, 1993). Note, however, that only a 50% risk rate in a genetically identical person implicates nongenetic factors such as stress as important in terms of the onset and trajectory of serious mental illness.

Stress

As discussed earlier in this chapter, people with serious mental illnesses are thought to be vulnerable to stress. Psychosocial stressors are frequently implicated in the onset of a disorder, as well as likely to cause relapse when a person is in remission (Bebbington, Wilkins, Jones, Foerster, Murray, et al., 1993; Ventura, Nuechterlein, Lukoff, & Hardesty, 1989). Psychosocial stressors may take the form of everyday life events, that is, the kinds of life demands that correspond with work, independent living, and intimate relationships. Life events are particularly stressful at times of loss (being fired from a job or divorced) or change (moving from one's residence or office). Stressful relationships can also overwhelm a person's vulnerability and cause symptom relapse (Shreiber, Breier, & Pickar, 1995).

Demographic and Socioeconomic Variables

Several demographic variables are associated with the onset and course of a disorder, including gender, age, culture, and ethnicity. Poverty can also be an important variable.

Gender

Men generally have a worse course with schizophrenia than women. The incidence of schizophrenia is higher in men (Castle, Wessely, & Murray, 1993; Iacono & Beiser, 1992). Men with the disorder are less able to live independently, more likely to show social impairment, and more likely to be hospitalized (Angermeyer & Kuehn, 1988; Susser & Wanderling, 1994). This finding may be confounded by the higher frequency of negative symptoms in men, as compared with women (Johnstone, Frith, Lang, & Owens, 1995; Ring, Tantam, Montague, Newby, Black, et al., 1991). Women, however, seem to have a tougher time with major depression. The prevalence rates for women are approximately double the rates for men (Blazer, Kessler, McGonagle, & Swartz, 1994), though the research is unclear as to whether the actual course of major depression varies by gender. Thus far, research has implicated both biological (e.g., endocrinology) and psychosocial (e.g., social roles) factors as relevant to explaining gender differences in depression (Kessler, 2000).

Age

Generally, the younger the person at the onset of the disorder, the worse the trajectory and end state (Johnstone, Owens, Bydder, & Colter, 1989; Winokur, Coryell, Keller, Endicott, Akiskal, et al., 1993). People of a young age at onset are more likely to show negative symptoms when diagnosed with schizophrenia (Andreasen, Flaum, Swayze, Tyrrell, & Arndt, 1990; Hoff, Harris, Faustman, Beal, DeVilliers, et al., 1996). The illness trajectory tends to be marked by significant symptoms or residual dysfunctions for those with early onset (Johnstone et al., 1989). Note, however, that with increasing age, people with schizophrenia show a decrease in positive symptoms (Winokur, Pfohl, & Tsuang, 1987).

There is also a schizophrenia syndrome that is defined in terms of older age, called late onset schizophrenia. The DSM-IV-TR defines late onset as occurring after age 45. Given that the National Institute on Aging (1987) predicted a one-third increase in the number of people over age 45 in the American population, late onset schizophrenia is expected to grow significantly as a problem. Research has suggested that late onset accounts for 23% of cases in a cross section of adults with schizophrenia over 40 (Harris & Jeste, 1988). Unlike the case with earlier onset of schizophrenia, more women than men show late onset patterns (Howard, Almeida, & Levy, 1994; Jeste, Gilbert, McAdams, & Harris, 1995). They are also less likely to ever be married, have a better work history, and show a greater frequency of the paranoid subtype (Jeste et al., 1995). Research at this point is unclear about whether symptoms, dysfunctions, and trajectories vary between groups experiencing early onset and late onset (Jeste et al., 1995).

Culture and Ethnicity

Two interesting trends are noticeable in terms of culture and ethnicity. First, people in developing nations (typically not from European or American countries) show a more benign trajectory and end state in schizophrenia and mood disorders (Jablensky et al., 1992; Susser & Wanderling, 1994). This finding does not seem to be attributable to geographic locale as much as ethnicity and culture. For example, research has shown that immigrants from developing countries with serious mental illness who move to developed countries still have a more benign course of illness than natives of those developed countries (Callan, 1999; McKenzie, van Os, & Fahy, 1995). Research also suggests that these differences are attributable to culture and not to the biological differences that distinguish peoples of developing and developed countries (Jablensky et al., 1992). In particular, agrarian societies are surmised to be less harmful factors in the course of mental illness than industrialized countries.

Within the United States, ethnic differences seem to support the opposite conclusions. That is, people of color, especially African Americans, seem to experience a worse trajectory and end state than the European American majority. African Americans seem to have a worse course, as marked by more involuntary hospitalizations (Sanguineti, Samuel, Schwartz, & Robeson, 1999) and more emergency room admissions (Hu, Snowden, Jerrell, & Nguyen, 1991; Klinkenberg & Calsyn, 1997). Some researchers conclude that these differences are more likely to represent systemic discrimination and prejudice rather than biological or sociocultural limitations of these groups. People of color tend to have worse health insurance in the United States (Scheffler & Miller, 1989). Moreover, ethnic minorities often find the mental health system to be unwelcoming. African Americans and Hispanics are significantly less likely to seek consultation for psychiatric problems as compared with European Americans (Gallo, Marino, Ford, & Anthony, 1995). Differences between U.S. ethnic groups may also be due to poverty.

Poverty

Poorer people with serious mental illness are more likely to experience a worse course. They have worse community outcomes and tend to spend more time in the hospital (Myers & Bean, 1968; van Os, McKenzie, & Jones, 1997). They tend to benefit less from rehabilitation programs and are less likely to meet the criteria for recovery (Cooper, 1961; Gift & Harder, 1985). These differences are not due to cultural or psychological limitations of people who are poor, but rather reflect the important role of economics in the successful rehabilitation of people with mental illness.

Substance Use

People who use and abuse alcohol and other drugs are likely to have a more malignant course and end state. In fact, the impact of co-occurring substance abuse, and the prevalence of this problem among people with psychiatric disabilities, has become a dominant issue among rehabilitation providers. Hence, the problem is described more thoroughly in the next section and corresponding interventions are addressed in Chapter 15.

CO-OCCURRING DISORDERS

Note that schizophrenia, the mood disorders, anxiety disorders, and some personality disorders are the foci of psychiatric rehabilitation. People who *primarily* have substance use disorders or developmental disabilities do not fall under the purview of psychiatric rehabilitation. However, significant numbers of people with the focal disorders experience co-occurring disorders in the substance abuse and developmental disabilities spectra. Concerns about co-occurring substance abuse are especially prominent and are the focus of Chapter 15.

DISABILITIES

Thus far we have defined the symptoms and dysfunctions that constitute disorders that commonly lead to a need for psychiatric rehabilitation, the factors that describe the course of these disorders, and co-occurring disorders that influence course and outcome. *Disabilities* are the definitive focus of psychiatric rehabilitation and are what distinguish it as an approach to services based more essentially on psychopharmacology or psychotherapy. Disabilities may simply be defined as those psychological phenomena that arise from psychiatric illness to block achievement of goals in the key life domains. Perhaps most important about the focus on disability is the way it defines the mission of psychiatric rehabilitation. Other approaches to psychiatric care may focus on diminishing symptoms or dysfunctions. The goal of psychiatric rehabilitation is to help people overcome their disabilities so that they are able to achieve their life goals. People may be able to achieve life goals in this manner while still experiencing significant symptoms and dysfunctions.

Age and Culture Defined

What are appropriate life goals? Consistent with rehabilitation's commitment to personal empowerment, the person with psychiatric disability is best able to answer this question for him- or herself. However, most cultures have age-defined goals that are benchmarks of achievement; these are defined in terms of role attainment in the United States. The prototype young to middle-aged adult in the United States is assumed to pursue and/or accomplish the following goals:

- Launch from family of origin and set up an independent household.
- Complete the necessary education and training to pursue one's vocation.
- Obtain at least an entry-level position commensurate with one's vocational goals.
- Begin to achieve income goals so that one can be self-sustaining.
- Find a mate with whom one can share an intimate and long-term relationship.
- Develop personally meaningful approaches to address recreation and spiritual needs.

Note that we defined these goals as age specific. Hence, we would expect younger adults to be first engaging some of these goals and elder adults to be moving away from them and pursuing other goals. We also defined the goals in terms of culture. Those listed here largely represent a Western European ethos. It is up to rehabilitation providers to understand what the culture-specific goals are within the culture of the people they serve; this issue is discussed more fully in Chapter 20. Suffice it to say here that cultural definition of life goals is likely to change across national borders as well as within ethnically diverse countries. Within the Untied States, for example, launching-from-family goals are likely to differ for African Americans, Hispanics, and Asian Americans. Even with these guidelines, the rehabilitation provider must remember that the ultimate definition of specific goals depends on people's experiences with their culture and their personal desires, given these experiences.

Specific Disability Domains

The absence of symptoms and dysfunctions does not a good life make. Instead, *quality of life* depends on achieving goals in the major life domains (Lehman, 1988; Skantze, Malm, Dencker, May, & Corrigan, 1992). At the minimum, this should include the satisfaction of basic needs such as safe, private, and comfortable housing; stimulating and financially beneficial work; comprehensive physical, dental, and mental health care; sufficient financial resources; transportation and access to facilities throughout one's community; and adequate legal counsel. A quality life also requires some sense of satisfaction with more transcendent desires: support networks including family, friends, and coworkers (or fellow students, depending on the situation); recreation, both alone and with others; intellectual stimulation; and spiritual life (Malm, May, & Dencker, 1981). We summarize a quality life in the rest of this section in terms of six domains: independent living, education and employment, relationships, health, criminal justice, and spiritual life and recreation. Note that these six domains are the heart of the chapters in Part II of this book, "Service Approaches."

Independent Living

Most adults in Western cultures seek to launch from their family of origin to set up a household that reflects their adult tastes and interests. This means renting or buying a residence. Housing goals usually include a safe neighborhood and a residence of reasonable size and amenities and in good condition. Sometimes people with psychiatric disabilities need support from rehabilitation providers to successfully live in their own homes. Rehabilitation providers need to make sure that the institutional demands of their agencies do not interfere with this goal. For example, agency regulations should not limit people's options about the neighborhood where they live or the type of housing they wish to obtain.

An equally important part of independent living is the decision about with whom the person resides. Options include living with family members (either the family of origin or the family created in adulthood—e.g., spouse and children), alone, with friends, or with roommates who help defray costs. In all cases, people need to decide about whom they want to live with. This means rehabilitation providers cannot impose roommates on individuals because of institutional necessity. Adults are changeable creatures; desires about whom we choose to live with change over time. Perhaps a divorce is necessary. Perhaps older parents must move into assisted living and the person with disabilities must learn to live alone. Whatever the reason, rehabilitation providers need to assist people with the evolution of their independent living needs.

Education and Employment

Work serves many goals in American culture. It is the basis on which most adults obtain an income to achieve their independent living goals. It is a source of identity; many people describe themselves in terms of their jobs and develop self-identities that correspond with these descriptions. Work-related issues dominate our conversations with friends and family and take up major portions of our time and energy. Work provides a sense of place within the larger context of society. In no way do we mean *place* to suggest caste, that some jobs denote better status than others. Rather, place is meant in the concrete sense. It defines where a person goes daily and with whom a person associates. Work is frequently the source of vocation: the belief that I, as an individual, am involved in personally meaningful industry. *Industry* does not refer here to an economic sector, but rather to the psychological life function of being industrious or busy. For reasons like these, work is a significant priority for the general adult population and for people with psychiatric disabilities. One study showed that 71% of people with psychiatric disabilities want to work (Rogers, Anthony, Toole, & Brown, 1991a).

Education is the typical path many people take to beginning the accomplishment of work goals. It provides the general credentials, such as a high school or college diploma, that are necessary for most jobs. Education teaches basic skills that are needed to be successful on the job. It may also provide work-specific talents that are necessary for jobs in varying sectors, such as computer skills needed in an information technology position. Education also yields nonspecific products that are important for many young adults. It provides many with a sense of competence and mastery. Intellectual stimulation is also of interest to many adults and may continue in adult education programs after the need for credentials and certification has passed.

Relationships

Most adults have broad and significant interests in interpersonal relationships. They seek to change the form of interaction with their family of origin from one of dependence to launching, becoming independent, and setting up an ongoing, mutually loving relationship with parents and siblings. Adults search for significant others with whom they can be intimate and develop long-standing relationships. In many cases, these intimate relationships yield children, with all the promise and challenges they entail. Adults also seek to extend their network of friends, neighbors, and coworkers.

Health

All adults have physical, dental, and mental health problems that vary in severity. People with psychiatric disabilities seem to have an inordinate amount of significant physical illnesses, which may be related to lifestyle issues (Druss, Marcus, Rosenheck, Olfson, Tanielian, et al., 2000b). Rehabilitation programs seek to help them not only to work closely with the general medical system to address these immediate illnesses, but also to address the lifestyle decisions that may be exacerbating these illnesses. Although, by definition, people with psychiatric disability have significant mental illness, not all mental illness may cause distress. For example, some aspects of mania are experienced as pleasant and some experiences of personality disorder are not viewed as mental illness. Similarly, some hallucinations or delusions may not be disturbing to the individual even though they are signs of psychosis. The rehabilitation provider's task is to assist the person with psychopharmacological and psychotherapeutic interventions for symptoms that are distressing.

Health is not just an issue of avoiding illness. Many adults also seek wellness. This includes issues related to diet and exercise in terms of physical wellness. In addition, it includes those physical, psychological, and spiritual experiences that help a person to achieve what he or she views to be a personally full and meaningful life.

Criminal Justice

An unfortunate result of the symptoms, dysfunctions, and disabilities for some people with serious mental illness may be court involvement. This can occur in both criminal and civil courts and can range from minor misdemeanors to severe violence. Comorbid drug abuse and homelessness often increase a person's involvement in the criminal justice system. The nature of these problems is more fully discussed in Chapter 16; two points are considered here. First, criminal and/or civil court involvement can significantly derail the pursuit of goals in the other five domains. Second, court participation, and the coercion it frequently entails, can be unsettling to most people in its own right. Hence, rehabilitation programs help people navigate the various levels and intricacies of the justice system so they can meet the demands of the judge, cut their ties with the police, and return to their principal goals of independent living, work, relationships, and health.

Spiritual Life and Recreation

Work, relationships, health, and housing are not enough for a meaningful adult life. Recreation provides an opportunity to broaden one's interaction with and enjoyment of the world. Recreation may involve formal planned activities (e.g., hobbies) or spontaneous experiences. Family, friends, and others may be essential for recreation or not necessary. Some recreation requires significant resources, whereas other recreation can be engaged in without such assets. The rehabilitation provider helps a person survey the activities that may be recreational for him or her and then helps that person to access these activities. The rehabilitation provider also engages in problem solving with the person as to how he or she can obtain the necessary resources to enjoy a specific recreation.

Social thinkers have distinguished *religiousness*, participating in a community of people who gather around common ways of worshiping, from *spirituality*, thinking about one's self as part of a larger spiritual force (Hill, Pargament, McCullough, Swyers, Hood, et al., 2000; Zinnbauer, Pargament, & Scott, 1999). A nationwide survey of people with psychiatric disorders showed that 67.5% of respondents viewed themselves as religious and 85.1% as spiritual (Corrigan, McCorkle, Schell, & Kidder, 2003). Findings from this study also showed that both religiousness and spirituality are associated with psychological well-being and diminished psychiatric symptoms. Hence, an important goal of rehabilitation providers is to help individuals with psychiatric disorders to explore their religious and spiritual goals and to access services and people who will assist them in achieving these goals.

STRENGTHS FOCUS

As stated earlier in this chapter, although discussion of diagnosis, symptoms, dysfunctions, course, and disabilities helps the rehabilitation provider better understand the challenges faced by a person, this kind of discussion tends to frame the person as a victim of his or her disabilities without recognizing the individual's positive assets. Each of the areas of symptoms and dysfunctions summarized in Table 1.2 not only suggests problems blocking the achievement of life goals, but also indicates possible strengths on which the person may draw to accomplish his or her goals. Examples of possible strengths are summarized in Table 1.4. Note that this is not meant to be an exhaustive list of strengths. Instead, the rehabilitation provider must actively engage a person to determine what his or her specific profile of strengths might be.

Although affect is frequently distressed by psychiatric illness, people with psychiatric disabilities may have several strengths in this domain. Among others, emotions can impart a certain color to life, which may motivate individuals to act against their symptoms and achieve their goals. People with psychosis often experience diminished perceptual and cognitive abilities. But despite these limitations, they frequently have the ability to understand problems and brainstorm solutions (Corrigan & Toomey, 1995), as well as perceive interpersonal situations correctly (Corrigan, Green, & Toomey, 1994). Among the greatest strengths a person with disabilities may draw upon is motivation. That is, despite the hurdles thrown up by symptoms and dysfunctions, the person wants to achieve work, independent living, relationship, and other goals. Symptoms and dysfunctions often interfere with interpersonal relationships. Nevertheless, most people with serious mental illness have family or friends on whom they can rely. Alternatively, reha-

TABLE 1.4. Possible Strengths That May Correspond to the Domains That Define Symptoms and Dysfunctions

Domains	Possible strengths
Affect	• Experiences the full range of emotions. • Is concerned about emotions that are "out of control" or distressing.
Perception and cognition	• Is able to orient to task at hand. • Is able to problem solve. • Is able to understand the basics of human interaction.
Motivation	• Is motivated to achieve specific goals. • Is motivated to work with rehabilitation programs and other resources to accomplish goals.
Interpersonal functioning	• Has some family members, friends, neighbors, and/or coworkers who provide support and companionship. • Has rehabilitation providers and/or peers who provide support and companionship.

bilitation providers or peers with psychiatric disabilities are also frequently available to step in to offer support and companionship.

SUMMARY AND CONCLUSIONS

Our answer to "Who are people with psychiatric disabilities?" is both simple and multilevel and complex. The simple definition is straightforward: People with psychiatric disabilities are first and foremost persons. They have the same breadth of life goals as others in their culture. Unfortunately, achieving these goals is undermined by the disabilities that arise from serious mental illness.

The complexity of our answer lies in understanding the barriers to achieving life goals. Diagnoses represent mental illness syndromes comprising distressing symptoms and disabling dysfunctions. As a result, people are unable to accomplish social roles and goals in such important life domains as work, independent living, income, relationships, and health. The course of an illness is described by a complex amalgamation of onset, trajectory, and end state. The course of a disorder is exacerbated by several factors, including age of onset, gender, familial history, stress, and substance abuse. Co-occurring substance abuse, in particular, is a frequent phenomenon in psychiatric disability that can have a serious effect on a person's life goals

People with psychiatric disabilities are not well described solely by symptoms, dysfunctions, and disabilities. An equally important part of the picture is strengths. A focus on strengths reminds us that people with disabilities, like everyone else, are complex beings who have many qualities that describe them. A strengths focus also highlights the resources that may be availed as the person engages his or her rehabilitation plan. A combination of the simple picture of the person as person, with the recognition of the individual's strengths and limitations, provides the fullest answer to our opening question: Who are people with psychiatric disabilities?

PERSONAL EXAMPLE

Joel Jenkins Revisited

This chapter began with the complex stories of four people with serious mental illness. What might we make of one of these persons, given the information reviewed in this chapter? How might the concepts reviewed in this chapter expand our understanding of Joel Jenkins and his needs for psychiatric rehabilitation?

Because of his age, Joel is experiencing what is likely to be an early phase of schizophrenia. His symptoms seem to be acute, tumultuous, and problematic for his parents. Frequent hospitalization is likely interfering with the kind of goals that would dominate a 22-year-old's life: completing education, beginning a career, moving out of the home of origin, and building intimate relationships. Instead, his frequent hostile exchanges with parents have yielded significant problems with the police. He is becoming enmeshed in the court system and finding his life options diminished by the demands of the judge. His court troubles are further exacerbated by marijuana use. Smoking pot is both worsening his symptoms and increasing police involvement in his life.

Joel has identified several life goals. He would like to move out of his parents' home and find a place of his own. He recognizes that to do this successfully, he will need to find a job that pays a reasonable salary. He also recognizes that his recurring psychotic symptoms and agitation will likely interfere with these goals in the short term. So in addition to his working with job and housing coaches, the rehabilitation team is helping Joel and his psychiatrist to better manage his antipsychotic medication. Joel is also working on relapse prevention skills to diminish his use of marijuana.

Joel has several strengths. Despite the angry and sometimes violent battles at home with his parents, Joel's mother and father are deeply committed to helping Joel beat his illness. Joel is strongly motivated to get back to work, though admittedly his motivation to decrease marijuana use wanes and waxes. Joel has engaged closely with his rehabilitation job coach to develop a reasonable plan for achieving his vocational goals.

Chapter 2

Stigma and Mental Illness

Serious mental illness and psychiatric disabilities strike with a two-edged sword. On one side are the symptoms, dysfunctions, and disabilities that arise from the disorder to block a person's life opportunities. On the other side are the barriers produced by the stigma of mental illness, which impacts people and life opportunities in two ways. Public stigma influences people in positions of power not to extend various opportunities; for example, landlords decide not to rent to and employers do not hire people with mental illness. Self-stigma occurs when people internalize the stigma of mental illness, which then undermines their self-esteem and self-efficacy.

This chapter reviews the ways in which stigma impacts people with psychiatric disabilities. We review both social-psychological and sociological models, with the former explaining why citizens stigmatize people with mental illness and the latter describing social structures that impede life opportunity. We then elaborate on the impact of public and self-stigma in several life domains, including employment, housing, and health. The chapter begins with a look at the role of media in promoting the stigma of mental illness.

Stigma can be a significant barrier to rehabilitation goals. Hence, rehabilitation providers need to understand the breadth and depth of its impact so that they can develop plans to challenge its effects. Chapter 19 reviews strategies for diminishing stigma. The opposite of lost opportunities that result from public stigma is community integration, actively and affirmatively seeking opportunities for people with mental illness to achieve all life goals. The obverse of self-stigma is personal empowerment, whereby individuals with psychiatric disabilities make the ultimate decisions about the pursuit of life goals. The role of community integration and personal empowerment are briefly reviewed at the end of this chapter and more fully developed in Chapter 19.

PERSONAL EXAMPLE

Celeste Robinson Can't Get Work

Celeste Robinson had been struggling with the challenges of schizophrenia since it disrupted her college education some 12 years earlier. Despite being hospitalized eight times, she was finally able to graduate from State U with a bachelor's in Business Administration. She had completed an internship at an accounting firm with the support of a local job coach. She also had much better control over her psychotic symptoms after starting an atypical antipsychotic medication. She thought that with medication and regular meetings with a counselor, she would be able to handle a full-time job at an entry-level position.

Celeste lined up four interviews with local businesses through the placement office at the university. During the first meeting, the employer noticed that she had several gaps in her resume. When asked about it, Celeste reported that those were periods when she took time off from school to treat her illness.

"You were in the psychiatric hospital?" asked the interviewer.

"Only two of those times. Mostly, I just needed some time away from the pressures of school while I learned to adjust to my medication."

"Well, at least you're through that stage in your life," the interviewer said.

Celeste responded, "Oh, yes, sir. With Dr. Halpin's assistance and careful monitoring of both my warning signs and my meds, I have total control over the illness."

"My goodness, you still have this thing?"

"Well, yes, in some ways. Some of the problems with schizophrenia continue."

The employer was noticeably shocked by this information. "Schizophrenia! I didn't know you had schizophrenia. I didn't think people could live outside the hospital with that kind of illness." The interviewer then looked at his watch and said, "Well, our time is up. You are one of several applicants we are talking to. We will get back to you next week."

Unfortunately, the firm did not. Celeste learned quickly that if she did not produce alternative explanations for blanks in her resume, other employers were similarly likely to bar job opportunities.

THE MEDIA AND STIGMA

Large surveys that employ representative samples of the population have shown that the stigma of mental illness is still prevalent (Angermeyer & Matschinger, 2003; Pescosolido, Monahan, Link, Stueve, & Kikuzawa, 1999). Pescosolido and colleagues (1999) completed a study of an American probability sample using the General Social Survey (GSS) of 1996. Their results showed that, depending on the psychiatric disorder (e.g., depression, substance abuse, or schizophrenia), a third to about three-quarters of survey participants viewed people with mental illness to be violent toward others. Of more concern, a comparison of these GSS data with a sample collected in 1950 (Star, 1955) suggested that the stigma may be worsening (Phelan, Link, Stueve, & Pescosolido, 2000). Almost twice the number of people in the 1996 survey endorsed the violence stigma, as compared with the 1950 sample. In trying to account for this difference, the investigators opined that the greater influence of mass media—especially television and newspapers—may lead to increasing stigma. Wahl (1995) summarized the media effects in terms of three categories: entertainment, news, and advertising.

The entertainment industry frequently uses two stigmatizing images of people with mental illness. First is the violent and out-of-control psycho killer. Media watch studies have shown that more than two-thirds of television shows and films that include a character with mental illness portrayed that person as violent (Gerbner, 1985; Signorelli, 1989; Wahl & Roth, 1982). Psycho-killer films like *Nightmare on Elm Street* and *Friday the 13th* define an entire industry that promotes this stigma. Alternatively, the entertainment industry presents people with mental illness as comical buffoons. This is seen in films like *The Dream Team*, in which Michael Keaton, Christopher Lloyd, and Peter Boyle were alternately described as "nutty psychiatric patients," "a motley crew of lunatics," or "crazoids who hit the streets." Jim Carrey's *Me, Myself, and Irene* is the 2000 Farrelly Brothers film that combines the violent and buffoonish images of mental illness. In the film, Carrey portrays a police officer with a split personality who bounces between comic figure and possessed demon. "From gentle to mental" was the tagline used to market the film.

The news media can also be guilty of perpetuating stigmatizing images. Surveys show that newspaper stories repeatedly present people with mental illness in a violent light. As many as 75% of stories dealing with mental illness focus on violence (Shain & Phillips, 1991). Although more recent research suggests that the prevalence of these kinds of stories is diminishing (Wahl, Wood, & Richards, 2002), at least a third of news stories continue to focus on the dangerousness of people with mental illness. This is an especially troublesome finding, given the credibility that seemingly accompanies news pieces. For example, an article on the front page of the *Reader* in Chicago, asks whether Lee Robin, who killed his wife and daughter in a psychotic frenzy, is still a monster after more than a dozen years of court-ordered hospitalization. The article is all the more sobering given that the *Reader* has a long and honored reputation in Chicago journalism of doing only high-quality and carefully considered pieces. Unfortunately, this kind of ill-considered language continues. In the July 10, 2002, daily of *The Trentonian* (New Jersey), the paper described a recent fire at Trenton Psychiatric Hospital with the headline "Roasted Nuts."

Advertising frequently uses stigmatizing images of mental illness to sell products. There was a time in American history when merchants used disrespectful images of people of color to hawk their wares. Consider the restaurant chains that were called *Little Black Sambo's* or *Aunt Jemima's Pancake House*. Today, most Americans would be horrified at advertisers that used any version of racial prejudice to promote their products. Yet it is still common to hear radio spots talk about "crazy deals that could get you put away" or television commercials presenting "maniac salesmen out of control." One human resource development firm distributed a flyer on spotting the "nuts and flakes" that get in the way of efficient and productive business.

WHY INDIVIDUALS STIGMATIZE PEOPLE WITH MENTAL ILLNESS

What is it about people that allow media to so easily promote stigma about individuals with mental illness? Research on mental health stigma may be organized into a social-cognitive model like the one in Figure 2.1 (Corrigan, 2000). This model seeks to explain the relationship between discriminative stimuli and consequent behavior by identifying the cognitions that mediate these constructs. In a simple version of the model, persons with severe mental illness signal the public about their mental illness: "That person talking to himself on the park bench must be crazy." These signals yield stereotypes and prejudice about persons with mental illness: "Crazy people are dangerous." Stereotypes and prejudice lead to behavioral reactions or discrimination: "I'm not going to allow danger-

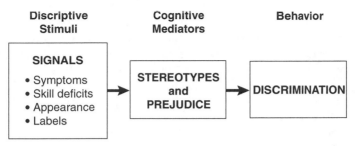

FIGURE 2.1. How signals lead to stereotypes and discrimination. Note that this model parallels a cognitive-behavioral model with discriminative stimuli, cognitive mediators, and behavior.

ous people like that to move into my neighborhood." Below, we take a closer look at each of the elements of this model.

Signals That Lead to Stigma

Erving Goffman (1963) defined stigma as a discrediting mark of one group (typically the minority) that results in another group (the majority) stealing some of the rights and privileges that correspond with their humanity. In this framework, those with mental illness join the many groups that have experienced stigma, prejudice, and discrimination: ethnic groups such as people of color in the United States, women, religious groups, less educated or impoverished people, gays and lesbians, people with physical disabilities, and people who are overweight. As outlined in Figure 2.2, what Goffman calls stigma are the signals that evoke stereotypes, prejudice, and discrimination. This section focuses on stigma as signal; the role of stereotypes, prejudice, and discrimination is discussed more fully later in the chapter.

The general public must infer mental illness from four signals: psychiatric symptoms, social skills deficits, poor physical appearance, and labels (Penn & Martin, 1998). Many of the symptoms of severe mental illness—inappropriate affect, bizarre behavior, lan-

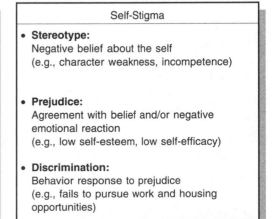

FIGURE 2.2. The distinction between public stigma and self-stigma.

guage irregularities, and talking to self aloud—are manifest indicators of psychiatric illness that frighten the public. Research has shown that symptoms like these tend to produce stigmatizing reactions (Link, Cullen, Frank, & Wozniak, 1987; Penn, Guyan, Daily, Spaudling, Garbin, et al., 1994; Socall & Holtgraves, 1992). Moreover, poor social skills that are a function of psychiatric illness also lead to stigmatizing reactions. Deficits in eye contact, body language, and choice of discussion topics (Bellack, Morrison, Mueser, Wade, & Sayers, 1990a; Mueser, Bellack, Douglas, & Morrison, 1991a) potentially mark a person as "mentally ill" and lead to stigmatizing attitudes. Finally, research suggests that personal appearance may also lead to stigmatizing attitudes (Eagly, Ashmore, Makhijani, & Longo, 1991; Penn, Mueser, & Doonan, 1997b). In particular, diminished physical attractiveness and personal hygiene may be manifest indicators of mental illness, leading to stereotypical responses from a person's community (e.g., "That unkempt person walking down the street must be a mental patient."

Note, however, the potential for misidentifying someone as mentally ill based on the first three types of these signals. What may be eccentric behavior that is not characteristic of a psychiatric disorder (e.g., the musician singing aloud a piece from an upcoming concert) could be misunderstood as mental illness. Social skills vary on a continuum, such that a deficit in skills may represent shyness rather than mental illness. Physical appearance may also lead to false positives about judging someone as mentally ill. Many street people with a slovenly appearance are believed to be mentally ill when, in actuality, they are instead poor and homeless (Koegel, 1992; Mowbray, 1985). Just as these three signs may yield false positives, so the absence of these signs often lead to false negatives. Many people are able to conceal their experiences with mental illness without those around them being aware. Goffman (1963) more fully developed this point when he distinguished between discredited and discreditable stigma. The former occurs when people have a mark that is readily perceivable. Examples of a discredited group include persons from a cultural minority with an apparent physical trait that leads them to believe that their differentness is obvious to the public (e.g., African Americans who have dark skin). Persons with discreditable stigma, however, can hide their condition; they have no readily manifest mark that identifies them as part of a stigmatized group. For example, one's sexual orientation cannot be discerned by a manifest marker. The public frequently cannot determine whether a person is mentally ill by merely looking at him or her. Only in those cases in which a person is acutely ill and floridly psychotic might he or she be accurately identified as "mentally ill."

Juxtaposing concerns about false positives with the idea that the stigma of mental illness may be hidden poses a question: What, then, is the mark that leads to stigmatizing responses? Several carefully constructed studies suggest *labels* as the key signals leading to stereotypes, prejudice, and discrimination (Jones, Farina, Hastorf, Markus, Miller, et al., 1984; Link, 1987; Scheff, 1974). People who are known as "mentally ill" are likely to be victims of mental illness stigma. Labels can be obtained in various ways: Others can tag a person with a label (a psychiatrist can inform someone that Ms X is mentally ill), individuals can label themselves (a person can decide to introduce himself as a psychiatric survivor), or labels can be obtained by association (a person observed coming out of a psychologist's office may be assumed to be mentally ill).

Is It Disease or Label?

During the 1960s questions arose regarding whether the disabilities associated with mental illness originate entirely from medical conditions, or whether the labels attached to mental illness exacerbate the problem. This dilemma divided many mental health providers and researchers into factions supporting the medical model versus labeling theory. Thomas Scheff (1975), a leading proponent of the latter view, described the difference in perspectives: "Labeling theory is a sociologistic theory, in that it deals only with social processes. . . . Labeling theory is the antithesis of the medical model thesis" (pp. 75–76). The key principle in Scheff's labeling theory is that the label "deviant" (i.e., mentally ill) leads society to treat the labeled individual as deviant (Scheff, 1966, 1972). Common responses to the label "mental illness" included fear and disgust, leading people to minimize contact and socially distance themselves from anyone marked in this way. In addition, the person with mental illness is exposed to adverse reactions (such as prejudice and discrimination) from others, which facilitates the process of his or her socialization into the role of the mental patient (Braginsky, Braginsky, & Ring, 1969; Goffman, 1963). This causes the individual with mental illness to exhibit continued deviant behavior, fitting the label and stabilizing the mental illness (Scheff, 1966). Thus, the label of mental illness can become a self-fulfilling prophecy in which the person acts "crazy" in order to meet expectations of the public mark (Scheff, 1972). This kind of self-fulfilling prophecy leads to continued stigma.

Critics have countered labeling theory on several grounds. Some argue that aberrant behavior, and not the label per se, is the source of negative responses from the public (Gove, 1982; Huffine & Clausen, 1979; Lehman, Joy, Kreisman, & Simmens, 1976). Others have argued that the impact of stereotypes on persons with mental illness is temporary, posing only a minor and brief problem for the person with mental illness (Gove, 1980; Gove & Fain, 1973; Karmel, 1969). Gove and Fain (1973) counter labeling theory's concept of secondary deviance, arguing that psychiatric relapse is due solely to the recurrence of the mental disorder; it is not impacted by the label. According to Gove (1975), the label does not elicit negative societal reactions. Rather, negative reactions are due to the bizarre behavior displayed by persons with mental illness. Other researchers concluded that generally there is no negative reaction toward people labeled mentally ill (Crocetti, Spiro, & Siassi, 1971).

In an effort to resolve differences between labeling theory and Gove's medical model, Link and colleagues (1987) conducted a study in which label and aberrant behavior were manipulated in a series of vignettes. Results indicated that members of the general public were likely to stigmatize a person labeled mentally ill even in the absence of any aberrant behavior if they held the belief that people with mental illness are dangerous. Link and colleagues (1987; Link, Cullen, Struening, Shrout, & Dohrenwend, 1989) posed a *modified labeling theory* to make sense of the diverse literature, concluding that psychiatric labels are associated with negative societal reactions that exacerbate the course of a person's disorder. This represents a middle ground between Scheff's original labeling theory and Gove's medical explanation. Aberrant behavior causes negative reactions from society, which lead the public (and the individual him- or herself) to label mental illness negatively; this can exacerbate the existing disorder for the individual. Although the debate over the mechanics of labeling remain unresolved, it seems clear that stigma worsens the lives of people suffering from mental illness. (Link & Cullen, 1983; Mechanic, McAlpine, Rosenfield, & Davis, 1994).

Public and Self-Stigma

As stated earlier, public stigma is distinguished from self-stigma as a reaction of the general population to people with mental illness. Three components from the social-psychological paradigm in Figure 2.1 make up this model, as outlined in Figure 2.2: stereotypes, prejudice, and discrimination. Social psychologists view *stereotypes* as knowledge structures that are learned by most members of a social group (Augoustinos, Ahrens, & Innes, 1994; Esses, Haddock, & Zanna, 1994; Hilton & von Hippel, 1996; Judd & Park, 1993; Krueger, 1996; Mullen, Rozell, & Johnson, 1996). Stereotypes are especially efficient means of categorizing information about social groups. Stereotypes are considered "social" because they represent collectively agreed-upon notions of groups of persons. They are "efficient" because people can quickly generate impressions and expectations of individuals who belong to a stereotyped group (Hamilton & Sherman, 1994). Stereotypes about mental illness include dangerousness, incompetence, and character weakness.

Just because most people have knowledge of a set of stereotypes does not imply that they agree with them (Jussim, Nelson, Manis, & Soffin, 1995). For example, many persons can recall stereotypes about different racial groups but do not agree that the stereotypes are valid. People who are *prejudiced*, on the other hand, endorse these negative stereotypes ("That's right; all persons with mental illness are violent.") and generate negative emotional reactions as a result ("They all scare me!") (Devine, 1988, 1989, 1995; Hilton & von Hippel, 1996; Krueger, 1996). Prejudice is also viewed as a general attitude toward a group. In contrast to stereotypes, which are beliefs, prejudicial attitudes involve an evaluative (generally negative) component (Allport, 1954; Eagly & Chaiken, 1993).

Prejudice, which is fundamentally a cognitive and affective response, leads to *discrimination*, the behavioral reaction (Crocker, Major, & Steele, 1998). Prejudice that produces anger can lead to hostile behavior (e.g., physically harming members of a minority group) (Weiner, 1995). In the case of those with mental illness, angry prejudice may lead to withholding help or replacing health care with services provided by the criminal justice system (Corrigan, 2000). Fear leads to avoidance; for example, employers do not want persons with mental illness nearby so they do not hire them (Corrigan, Larson, Watson, Barr, & Boyle, 2006). As outlined in Figure 2.2, stereotype, prejudice, and discrimination are manifested differently, depending on whether the public is considering stigma or the person. The specific impacts of public and self-stigma are reviewed in the following sections.

THE IMPACT OF PUBLIC STIGMA

The public endorsement of stigma impacts many people, with four groups being of special importance: people with mental illness, their families, service providers, and the general public. Perhaps of greatest concern is the harm that public stigma causes *people who are labeled mentally ill*. Rather than broadly considering the effect of stigma manifested by the general public, our review focuses on specific power groups, people in functional roles that have significant implications for the life goals of people with mental illness. These may include landlords, employers, members of the criminal and civil justice systems, health care providers, legislators, and policy makers. *Family members and friends* are also impacted by public stigma (Corrigan, Watson, & Miller, 2004b; Phelan, Bromet, & Link, 1998; Wahl & Harman, 1989). They may experience shame, blame, or contamination because of their relationship with relatives identified with mental illness. Moreover, representatives of many of the various *provider groups* involved in mental health services have reported harm from public stigma. People working in these professions are frequently disrespected by colleagues (Dickstein & Hinz, 1992; Gabbard & Gabbard,

1992; Persaud, 2000). Finally, public stigma negatively impacts the *general public*. Citizens are not able to benefit from a large segment of society when they discredit its members with stigma.

Most researchers and advocates agree: People with mental illness suffer the greatest impact from stigma. Moreover, stigma will greatly hinder a person's rehabilitation goals. In this section, we focus on three such examples of negative impact. First, stigma robs people of rightful life opportunities. Two that are especially relevant to the lives of people with mental illness are employment and housing. Second, stigma interacts with the perception of violence to cause people with mental illness to have a distorted experience with the criminal justice system. Third, the general health care system seems to withhold appropriate medical treatments because of mental illness stigma. We consider each of these areas in turn.

The Loss of Rightful Life Opportunity

Stereotype, prejudice, and discrimination can rob people labeled mentally ill of important life opportunities that are essential for achieving life goals. Two goals, in particular, are central to the concerns of people with serious mental illness (Corrigan, et al., 2006): (1) obtaining competitive employment and (2) living independently in a safe and comfortable home. Stigma's role as a barrier to obtaining good jobs and housing may be understood in terms of Link's modified labeling theory. That is, these problems may occur partially because of the disabilities that result from serious mental illness (Corrigan, 2001). Many people with serious mental illness lack the social and coping skills to meet the demands of a competitive work force and independent housing. Yet the problems of many people with psychiatric disability are further exacerbated by labels and stigma. People with mental illness are frequently unable to obtain good jobs or find suitable housing because of the prejudice of key members in their communities: employers and landlords. Several studies have documented the public's widespread endorsement of stigmatizing attitudes (Bhugra, 1989; Brockington, Hall, Levings, & Murphy, 1993; Greenley, 1984; Hamre, Dahl, & Malt, 1994; Link, 1987; Madianos, Madianou, Vlachonikolis, & Stefanis, 1987; Rabkin, 1974; Roman & Floyd, 1981). These attitudes have a deleterious impact on obtaining and keeping good jobs (Bordieri & Drehmer, 1986; Farina & Felner, 1973; Farina, Fellner, & Boudreau, 1973; Link, 1982, 1987; Olshansky, Grob, & Ekdahl, 1960; Wahl, 1999a; Webber & Orcutt, 1984) and leasing safe housing (Aviram & Segal, 1973; Farina, Thaw, Lovern, & Mangone, 1974; Hogan, 1985a, 1985b; Page, 1977, 1983, 1995; Segal, Baumohl, & Moyles, 1980; Wahl, 1999). Classic research by Farina (Farina & Felner, 1973) poignantly illustrates the nature of the problem. A male confederate, posing as an unemployed worker, sought a job at 32 businesses. The same work history was reported at each of the job interviews, except that 50% also included information about a past psychiatric hospitalization. Subsequent analyses found that interviewers were less friendly and less supportive of hiring the confederate when he added his psychiatric hospitalization.

Two considerations could conceivably provide an alternative perspective on the conclusions drawn from this body of research. First, although some landlords and employers endorse stigma, this prejudice has no *meaningful* effect on the housing and work problems of people with mental illness. Instead, these problems solely arise from the cognitive and behavioral dysfunctions that result from the disorders. Although research has not tested this assumption directly, studies have shown a parallel connection between attitudes and behavior—that is, that stigmatizing attitudes about mental illness impact access to care. Stigma has been shown to decrease participation in rehabilitation and other ser-vices that assist people in obtaining their life goals (Leaf, Bruce, & Tischler, 1986; Leaf, Bruce, Tischler, & Holzer, 1987; Sirey, Bruce, Alexopoulos, Perlick, Friedman, et al., 2001). Second, some may believe that prejudice was a problem 10–30 years ago when many of these studies were completed, but that stigma has greatly diminished because of more public knowledge about mental illness. Actually, analyses of 1996 General Social Survey data, reviewed earlier in this chapter, showed the opposite. A U.S. probability sample in 1996 was more likely to endorse stigmatizing attitudes than a similar group in 1956 (Phelan et al., 2000). Hence, the potential for landlords and employers to discrimi-nate against people with mental illness is exceedingly present.

The Reaction of the Criminal Justice System

With the stigma attached to mental illness intensifying over the last four decades (U.S. Surgeon General, 1999; Martin, Pescosolido, & Tuch, 2000), the number of people with mental illness entangled in the criminal justice system also rose significantly. The preva-lence rate of serious mental illness among people in jails, currently between 6 and 15% (Teplin, Abram, & McClelland, 1996; Ditton, 1999; Lamb & Weinberger, 1998; Teplin, 1984, 1990), has risen 154% over the past 20 years (Travis, 1997). Recent studies have shown that as many as 6% of individuals considered suspects by police have a serious mental illness (Engel & Silver, 2001; Teplin & Pruett, 1992). LaGrange (2000) surveyed officers of a large metropolitan area police department and found that 89% had had con-tact with citizens with mental illness in the previous year. For a person with mental ill-ness, police officers are often the first point of contact with the criminal justice system. An officer's determination has an influence on whether persons with mental illness receive adequate psychiatric care or are further processed into the criminal justice system.

   Unnecessarily criminalizing mental illness is one way in which the criminal justice system reacts to people with mental illness, contributing to the increasing proportion of people with serious mental illness in jail (Watson, Ottati, Corrigan, & Heyrman, in press). As Teplin (1984) points out, persons exhibiting symptoms and signs of serious mental illness are more likely than others to be arrested by the police. This selective pro-cess continues if the person is taken to jail. Those suffering from mental illness tend to spend more time incarcerated than persons without mental illness (Steadman, McCarty, & Morrisey, 1989). Treating a person with mental illness like a criminal, instead of like someone who is sick and in need of treatment, not only has implications for the life, lib-erty, and well-being of individuals with mental illness, but also affects the larger commu-nity. As noted before, public fear of individuals with mental illness has increased over the past 40 years (Martin et al., 2000; Phelan, Link, Moore, & Stueve, 1997; Phelan et al., 2000), resulting in a higher degree of preferred social distance from persons with mental illness. The growing intolerance of offenders in general has led to harsher laws and ham-pered effective treatment planning for mentally ill offenders (Lamb & Weinberger, 1998; Jemelka, Trupin, & Chiles, 1989).

   Persons with mental illness are not always encountered as the perceived wrongdoers by members of the criminal justice system, but sometimes as witnesses or victims of crime. Research on helping behavior suggests that officers who believe that individuals are responsible for their own illness may be less willing to provide appropriate assistance (Weiner, 1995). This may occur in situations in which an individual needs help in access-ing mental health or other social services. If an offense has occurred, officers who blame individuals for their illness may be more inclined to arrest the person, even if a referral to mental health services would be more appropriate. Officers may also be less willing to assist individuals with mental illness who are victims of crime (Mastrofski, Snipes, Parks, & Maxwell, 2000). Similarly, officers who view individuals with mental illness as incompetent may be less willing to accept the information they provide as credible. This may cause police to disregard useful information from witnesses and potential suspects. It may also cause them to fail to believe and assist victims of crime. As this review shows, the attitudes and beliefs held about mental illness by police officers, the gatekeepers of the criminal justice system, may have significant consequences in terms of safety and quality of life for both the general public and the individual with mental illness.

The Reaction of the General Health Care System

A research program by Benjamin Druss and colleagues seems to indicate that people with psychiatric disabilities are less likely to benefit from the depth and breadth of the American health care system than people without these illnesses. Druss and colleagues completed two studies on archival data suggesting that people with mental illness receive fewer medical services than those not so labeled (Desai, Rosenheck, Druss, & Perlin, 2002; Druss & Rosenheck, 1997). Moreover, studies by Druss and colleagues suggest that individuals with mental illness are less likely to receive the same range of insurance benefits as people without mental illness (Druss, Allen & Bruce, 1998; Druss & Rosenheck, 1998). Clearly, the data reported by his group and others (Berk, Schur, & Cantor, 1995; Mark & Mueller, 1996) identify a disparity in services across groups that are identified as mentally ill or not mentally ill. However, the findings from this research are unclear as to whether this disparity is due to stigma on the part of health care providers and insurers or reflects economic and sociocultural variables that interact with the experience of mental illness. One study by Druss and colleagues (Druss, Bradford, Rosenheck, Radford, & Krumholz, 2000a) seems to implicate stigma more directly.

Previous research has used rates of procedures for cardiovascular disorders as an index of differential service rate by race (Ayanian, Udvarhelyi, Gatsonis, Pashos, & Epstein, 1993; Wenneker & Epstein, 1989) and gender (Ayanian & Epstein, 1991; Krumholz, Douglas, Lauer, & Pasternak, 1992) bias. For this reason, Druss and colleagues (2000) examined the likelihood of a range of medical procedures after myocardial infarction in a sample of 113,653. As compared with the rest of the sample, these investigators found that people with comorbid psychiatric disorder were significantly less likely to undergo percutaneous transluminal coronary angioplasty. Once again, mental illness is indicated as a barrier to receiving appropriate care.

Nevertheless, the body of research by Druss and colleagues illustrates the difficulty of research that seeks to examine the impact of stigma. Although it is not unreasonable to conclude that people with mental health diagnoses receive less quality health care and coverage because of stigma, we cannot exclude a number of other variables that may also account for this disparity. People with mental illness, for example, often find themselves in impoverished socioeconomic classes that traditionally receive less adequate care. Note, however, that these socioeconomic variables do not rule out stigma as a relevant variable. Link and Phelan (2001) argued that some sociocultural differences between people with mental illness and the rest of the population may represent *structural stigma*. That is, because of a history of stigmatizing mental illness, certain social structures develop that reflect prejudice against this group. Inability to pass meaningful insurance parity bills is an example of structural stigma. Structural stigma is discussed more fully later in this chapter. Research to examine the impact of social structures needs to include more macro

PERSONAL EXAMPLE

Lillian Johnson Thinks, "I'm Mentally Ill, So I Must Be Bad"

Lillian Johnson had heard her fair share of jokes and stories about "the mentally ill." TV shows had taught her that "they" were either people to be feared or silly folks to be laughed at. She even recalls, with some shame, a period in high school when she had tormented a classmate because he had been sent away to the psycho ward for a month.

When Lillian was 22, she experienced severe, unexplained depression. She was unable to sleep much, had almost no appetite, wondered whether being dead was better, and had little energy. Her family physician referred her to a psychiatrist who, concerned about her increasing suicidal statements, talked Lillian into admitting herself into a hospital. Her first reaction to the other patients on the ward was denial. "Not me. I'm not like them. I'm not crazy. This is all a mistake. Just a temporary thing."

Unfortunately, Lillian was not able to control her symptoms easily. She experienced some reprieves from the loss of energy and inability to sleep. But every year or so thereafter, the symptoms seemed to come back and the need for another hospitalization or some kind of break from regular life became apparent. With the waxing and waning course, stigma began to set in.

"Maybe everything they say about mentally ill people is true. They can't really take care of themselves. They are unpredictable. They are suited for nothing but living in transient hotels on welfare. And now I am one of them."

Slowly, she internalized the stigma and made more self-defeating statements: "I must be weak because I am mentally ill!" Her self-esteem suffered, as well as her public face. "People can surely tell I am one of those 'mentals.' No wonder nobody wants to hang out with me." In addition, her self-efficacy diminished. "Someone who is mentally ill and weak like me is not capable of getting a career. I just need to accept my lot in life, that I should go to day programs where I play bingo all day."

---

social science theories and methods to illustrate these effects; this kind of perspective is reviewed later in this chapter.

THE IMPACT OF SELF-STIGMA

Living in a culture steeped in stigmatizing images, persons with mental illness may accept these notions and suffer diminished self-esteem, self-efficacy, and confidence in their future as a result (Corrigan, 1998; Holmes & River, 1998). Persons with mental illness like Kathleen Gallo have written eloquently about this kind of self-stigma.

> I perceived myself, quite accurately unfortunately, as having a serious mental illness and therefore as having been relegated to what I called "the social garbage heap." . . . I tortured myself with the persistent and repetitive thought that people I would encounter, even total strangers, did not like me and wished that mentally ill people like me did not exist. Thus, I would do things such as standing away from others at bus stops and hiding and cringing in the far corners of subway cars. Thinking of myself as garbage, I would even leave the sidewalk in what I thought of as exhibiting the proper deference to those above me in social class. The latter group, of course, included all other human beings. (1994, pp. 407–408)

First-person narratives such as this, as well as other subjective data, provide a compelling illustration of the impact of stigma on a person's self-esteem (Davidson, 1992; Estroff, 1989; Strauss, 1989). Qualitative data of this sort have been augmented by quantitative surveys of persons with mental illness. For example, studies of persons with mental illness and their families demonstrated that diminished self-esteem is a significant problem (Wahl, 1999a; Wahl & Harman, 1989).

First impressions about the stigma of mental illness suggest that people with psychiatric disability, living in a society that widely endorses stigmatizing ideas, will internalize these ideas and believe that they are less valued because of their psychiatric disorder (Link & Phelan, 2001). Like public stigma, self-stigma includes prejudice and its components. First, persons who agree with the prejudice concur with the stereotype: "That's right—I am weak and unable to care for myself." In addition, self-prejudice leads to negative emotional reactions. Prominent among these are low self-esteem and poor self-efficacy. Self-esteem is typically operationalized in this kind of research as the rating of agreement of personal worth on Likert scale items (Corrigan, Faber, Rashid, & Leary, 1999a; Rosenberg, 1965). Self-efficacy is defined here as the expectation that one can successfully perform a certain behavior in a specific situation (Bandura, 1977, 1989) and is often assessed with self-report measures (Sherer & Adams, 1983).

Self-prejudice may also lead to related behavioral responses. Low self-efficacy and demoralization have been shown to be correlated with individuals' failing to pursue work or independent living opportunities at which they might other wise succeed (Link, 1982, 1987). Obviously, this kind of self-stereotype, self-prejudice, and self-discrimination will significantly interfere with a person's life goals and quality of life; this impact is discussed more fully below. However, it is also important to remember that self-stigma is not universal.

Diminished Self-Esteem Is Not Inevitable

Many persons with mental illness are aware of the stereotypes about people with mental illness in general. However, awareness of stigma is not synonymous with internalizing it (Crocker & Major, 1989). Although persons with mental illness report being aware of the negative stereotypes about them (Bowden, Schoenfield, & Adams, 1980; Kahn, Obstfeld, & Heiman, 1979; Shurka, 1983; Wright, Grofein, & Owens, 2000), they do not necessarily agree with these stereotypes (Hayward & Bright, 1997). Hence, not every person with a mental disorder reacts to the stigma of mental illness with loss of self-esteem. On the contrary, some individuals are energized by prejudice and express righteous anger. Others neither experience lowered self-esteem nor become righteously angry; instead these individuals seem to ignore the effects of public prejudice altogether.

Long-standing theories have represented self-stigma as the automatic result of being a member of a stigmatized group (Allport, 1954/1979; Erikson, 1956; Jones et al., 1984). Accordingly, African Americans, women, and persons with physical disabilities would all be expected to have lower self-esteem as compared with the majority. Several studies have shown, however, that people of color and other ethnic minorities do not have lower self-esteem than the white majority (Hoelter, 1983; Jensen, White, & Gelleher, 1982; Porter & Washington, 1979; Verkyuten, 1994, 1995; Wylie, 1979). Nor are women shown to have lower self-esteem than men (Maccoby & Jacklin, 1974; Wylie, 1979). Similar results have been found in persons with mental illness, even though they are aware of the stigmatizing views about them. Despite such awareness, several studies have been unable to find a sharp decline in self-esteem in this group (see Hayward & Bright, 1997, for a review).

Crocker and colleagues (Crocker & Lawrence, 1999; Crocker & Major, 1989) highlight an even more amazing trend in stigma and self-esteem. Several stigmatized groups showed higher self-esteem than the majority; participants in these studies included persons of color (Hoelter, 1983; Jensen et al., 1982; Porter & Washington, 1979) and people with disabilities (Fine & Caldwell, 1967; Willy & McCandless, 1973). It seems that being stigmatized somehow stimulates psychological reactance (Brehm, 1966), suggesting that rather than complying with the perceived threat of stigma and viewing oneself poorly, an individual opposes the negative evaluation and positive self-perceptions emerge. Research on empowerment supports this concept, revealing persons with psychiatric disability who, despite this disability, have positive self-esteem and are not significantly encumbered by a stigmatizing community. Instead, they seem to be energized by the stigma to righteous anger (Corrigan et al., 1999a; Rogers, Chamberlin, Ellison, & Crean, 1997a). Righteous anger is evident in many of the narratives of persons with serious mental illness: "I was angry that I'd been crazy, but I was even more angry at the inhumane, hurtful, degrading, and judgmental 'treatment' I'd been subjected to" (Unzicker, 1989, p. 71; see also Davidson, Stayner, & Haglund, 1998; Estroff, 1995).

In addition to those who view mental illness stereotypes as unjust, persons who believe them to be irrelevant also experience no reduction in self-esteem due to stigma. Persons with intact self-esteem respond to stigma with indifference or indignation, depending on their identification with the generic group of people with mental illness. Those with high group identification show righteous anger. Those who do not identify with the group are indifferent to stigma.

The Impact on Accessing Services

Self-stigma may have another unfortunate effect: People may chose not to seek out treatment so that they are not identified with the stigmatized group (Corrigan, 2004). Research has shown that the psychiatric symptoms, psychological distress, and life disabilities caused by many mental illnesses are significantly remedied by a variety of psychopharmacological and psychosocial treatments. Unfortunately, research also suggests that many people who meet the criteria for treatment, and who are likely to improve after participation, either choose not to seek services or fail to fully adhere to treatments once they are prescribed. Results from the Epidemiologic Catchment Area (ECA) study show that only 60% of people with schizophrenia participated in treatment (Regier, Narrow, Rae, Manderscheid, Locke, et al., 1993). The National Comorbidity Survey (NCS) showed similar results (Kessler, Berglund, Bruce, Koch, Laska, et al., 2001). Less than 40% of the 6.2% of respondents with serious mental illness in the previous year received stable treatment, with young adults and individuals living in more urban/suburban areas being more likely to have unmet needs.

Many people choose not to pursue mental health services because they do not want to be labeled "mental patients" or suffer the prejudice and discrimination that the label entails. Results gleaned from the Yale arm of the Epidemiological Catchment Area data (Leaf et al., 1986) indicated that respondents with psychiatric diagnoses were more likely to avoid services if they were unreceptive to treatment (e.g., agreeing that people should not seek care if they have a mental or emotional problem) or believed family members would have a negative reaction to these services. A second study by the same group showed similar results; namely, that negative attitudes inhibit service utilization in those at risk for psychiatric disorder (Leaf et al., 1987). Results from the NCS suggest several beliefs that might sway people's decisions against accepting treatment (Kessler et al.,

2001). These include concerns about what others might think and the desire to solve their own problems. Hence, perceptions of and identification with existing stereotypes about mental illness can hinder persons in getting much needed help, which may make their lives unnecessarily more difficult.

UNDERSTANDING STIGMA AT THE SOCIETAL LEVEL

Thus far, this chapter has provided an overview of psychological models of stigma, descriptions of cognitive-behavioral processes engaged in by individuals that harm people with mental illness (public stigma) or themselves (self-stigma). The individual level of analysis provides only half the picture of the egregious impact of stigma. Sociologists have also discussed how political, economic, and historical forces create societal-level phenomena that diminish the life opportunities of people with mental illness and hence become stigma (Link & Phelan, 2001; Pincus, 1999; Rubinstein, 1994; Wilson, 1987). As outlined in Figure 2.3, two levels of stigma in society have been identified: institutional policies and social structures. The key distinction between this form of stigma, and stigma at an individual level of analysis, is the emergence of societal forms and structures that restrict the life opportunities of people with mental illness. Although concepts related to institutional and structural stigma have a prominent role in explaining racism and sexism, related models have not been well developed in explaining mental illness stigma other than in an important article by Link and Phelan (2001).

Institutional Policies and Stigma

Pincus (1999) argues that stereotypes and prejudice can have a major impact on people of color when they are enacted into rules that impede their opportunities. These rules can be embodied in formal legislation at various levels of government, like the Jim Crow laws of the late 19th and the first half of the 20th centuries that robbed African Americans of their right to vote. They can be company policy, such as in the practices of banks that do not provide mortgages to minorities in order to redline neighborhoods. They can be less formal polices, such as those followed by restaurant chains like Denny's, which instructed its employees to provide a lesser grade of service to people of color. In each case, there is one person (e.g., a CEO of a company) or a group of people (e.g., a legislative bloc) in positions of power with a prejudicial agenda who promote this agenda by enacting policies that discriminate against a particular group.

INSTITUTIONAL POLICIES	SOCIAL STRUCTURES
Prejudice of people in leadership positions ↓ Translated into laws and regulations that discriminate against people with mental illness	The effects of prejudice and discrimination: • historically • politically • economically Structures • Lack of parity in health benefits appropriations

FIGURE 2.3. Societal levels of stigma: Institutional policies and structural stigma.

PERSONAL EXAMPLE

Elmer Rodriguez: "The System Is Against Me"

Elmer Rodriguez was excited about the new voucher system that had been introduced by the state mental health authority. To give control to consumers of rehabilitation services, they would be given vouchers, which they could turn in to service providers to fund the rehabilitation program that would best meet their life goals. Elmer went down to the Metro Building on the first day the vouchers became official. Unfortunately, he was unable to find the staff responsible for the office when he got there. It seemed that no one in the governor's office had yet assigned staff from the nearby Medicaid program to administer the voucher system. In addition, legislators from the Black Caucus were concerned that the new voucher priorities might undermine the Medicaid priorities of some of their constituents. Hence, the legislators were holding up movement on the mental health vouchers until this question was resolved.

Nine months later, Elmer got his first appointment with an accounts representative. He had done his homework, reviewing the service options in the area, and met the agent with a list of options. Top on the list was the Little Village Rehab Program, which provided an excellent supported employment program; Elmer thought this kind of program would be essential for him to meet his vocational goals. Unfortunately, the agent reported that Little Village was not certified for vouchers. All that was available for Elmer in his part of town was a sheltered workshop where clients were paid for piece work in assembling card stock. The nearest supported employment program was in Westside, which was a 2-hour, one-way bus ride for Elmer. Despite the state's seemingly progressive agenda, Elmer's rehabilitation plans were blocked by unforeseen structures.

Similar examples are evident in regard to people with mental illness, especially in government institutions. Research has shown state laws that restrict the rights of people with mental illness in terms of such fundamental opportunities and privileges as jury service, voting, holding public office, marriage, and parenting (Hemmens, Miller, Burton, & Milner, 2002). In fact, findings from this survey suggest that the restriction of familial rights may be worsening for people with mental illness (e.g., a person's mental illness may be used in divorce court and child custody hearings to rule against that person), despite an increasing concern about prejudice in this arena. Another study shows that mental illness continues to be used as a rationale for restricting medical licensure (Hansen, Goetz, Bloom, & Fenn, 1998). The results suggested that it was the label of mental illness, rather than evidence of current psychiatric disability, that led to the restriction of medical practice.

Social Structures and Stigma

Typically, institutional stigma arises from the prejudices of individuals in power who enact legislation and administrative rules that discriminate against people with mental illness (Pincus, 1996, 1999; Wilson, 1987). Sociologists have also identified structural stigma that develops historically as the result of the economic and political injustices wrought by prejudice and discrimination. Once again, this concept has mostly been used to explain racism and sexism. Pincus (1999), for example, describes the disparity of insurance rates across white and black communities. Although agents may explain this as the result of higher rates of street crime in lower-income black communities, it nevertheless results in higher premiums for people of color. The key element of structural stigma is not the *intent* but rather the *effect* of keeping certain groups in a subordinate position. Hence, there is not clearly a prejudicial group in power maintaining structural stigma; rather, it is the product of historical trends in discrimination.

Inability to achieve parity in mental health insurance with general medical coverage may be an example of structural stigma related to mental illness (Feldman, Bachman, & Bayer, 2002). Although the failure of legislatures to endorse parity may be affected by the individual prejudices of some representatives and senators (Corrigan & Watson, 2003), it also reflects the insidious effects of structural stigma. For example, several decades of history in which insurance benefits for physical illness have surpassed those for mental illness leads to the assumption that greater benefits for mental illness will produce diminished benefits for physical illness, an assumption, by the way, that may not be borne out by actuarial evidence. The significantly lower rate of federal monies for mental health research, as compared with other areas of health research, is another example of structural stigma (Link & Phelan, 2001). The latter example also shows the circular nature of structural stigma. Knowledge about mental illness that will diminish stigma, and hence lead to more enlightened policies about funding research, cannot be increased, because funding agencies are not supporting studies in the psychiatric arena at the same rate as for other, general medical conditions.

THE OPPOSITE OF STIGMA: COMMUNITY INTEGRATION AND PERSONAL EMPOWERMENT

The problem with focusing on stigma is that it renews the description of what is wrong with the life of people with psychiatric disabilities. Just as a strengths focus is essential for a full picture of the person with disabilities, so too is the obverse of stigma necessary to fully appreciate the goals of psychiatric rehabilitation. Public stigma, prejudice, and discrimination rob people of life opportunities in their community. Community integration is the affirmative vision specifying that the public is responsible for helping people achieve their life goals. Self-stigma fills individuals with doubt, harms their self-esteem, and undermines their confidence. Personal empowerment asserts that ultimate control over the life of the person with psychiatric disabilities belongs solely to that person. We end this chapter with a more complete discussion of the elements of community integration and personal empowerment.

Community Integration

Correcting the community biases and structures that prevent full integration will require affirmative actions. Affirmative action was originally thrust on the American political scene as an executive order signed by Lyndon Johnson directing federal contractors to develop a hiring plan that would increase the number of women and minorities in all job categories. This plan was seeking to resolve the historical disparities in hiring practices that kept women and people of color out of the better categories of work. Affirmative action may be more broadly construed as any official effort that seeks to decrease structural and other forms of stigma by purposively and strategically increasing the opportunities of a stigmatized group. Two examples come to mind in terms of mental illness. Reasonable accommodations for people with psychiatric disabilities promote community integration. An important clause of the Americans with Disabilities Act (ADA), reasonable accommodations are those provisions that employers must supply to employees with disabilities so that those employees can competently do their jobs. (See Chapter 21 for a more thorough discussion of the ADA.) The provision of these accommodations may not put an undue burden on employers and their businesses. Common examples of such accommodations include wheelchair accessibility so that people with ambulatory disabilities can easily navigate their work environments. More difficult to define have been accommodations for people with psychiatric disabilities (MacDonald-Wilson, Rogers, Massaro, Lyass, & Crean, 2002; Mechanic, 2003). These have included the provision of flexible schedules and job coaching so that people with mental illness can cope with the stress of job demands.

The U.S. Supreme Court's ruling in *Olmstead v. L.C.* is an example of court decisions that have led to affirmative actions for people with mental illness that promote community integration. In this case, the State of Georgia was found to be in violation of the ADA because it did not provide community services to psychiatric inpatients (Cohen, 2001; Herbert & Young, 1999). In particular, the Court found that states could not avoid their duties under the ADA because they did not appropriate sufficient funds to support community programs for all people with psychiatric disabilities in need of these services. To comply with the ruling, states must develop comprehensive plans to end unnecessary institutionalization (Bazelon Center, 1999). Hence, the Supreme Court is requiring affirmative actions that challenge these kinds of structural stigmas that have evolved over time. Chapter 19 more fully explores specific strategies that can undermine stigma and promote community integration.

Personal Empowerment

Empowerment has been defined as personal control over all domains of one's life, not only in decisions related to mental health care, but also in decisions related to such important areas as vocation, residence, and relationships (McLean, 1995; Rappaport, 1987; Segal, Silverman, & Temkin, 1995). Research on the construct of empowerment has led to a better understanding of effective services and their impact on quality of life (Corrigan & Garman, 1997). Rosenfield (1992), for example, found that consumer empowerment correlated with quality of life. Rogers and colleagues (1997a) completed a more comprehensive series of studies on mental health consumer empowerment with their Empowerment Scale. An unpublished analysis of the scale yielded seven factors that describe the construct: self-efficacy, powerlessness, self-esteem, effecting change, optimism/control over the future, righteous anger, and group/community action (Rogers et al., 1997a). These factors are intercorrelated and seem to correspond to two superordinate factors that describe the impact of empowerment on persons with schizophrenia and on their communities (Corrigan et al., 1999a): (1) The impact of empowerment on the self is such that, despite societal stigma, empowered consumers endorse positive attitudes about themselves. They have good self-esteem, believe themselves to be self-efficacious, and are optimistic about their future. (2) The impact of empowerment on the community is manifested by the consumer's desire to affect his or her stigmatizing community. Consumers believe they have some power within society, are interested in effecting change, and wish to promote community action.

Note that the terms *empowerment* and *disempowerment* indicate a continuum (Corrigan et al., 1999a; Rogers et al., 1997a). At the positive end of the continuum are people with psychiatric disability who, despite their disability, have positive self-esteem and are not significantly encumbered by a stigmatizing community. At the negative end are people who report being unable to overcome all the pessimistic expectations about mental illness. One might think that a book in which empowerment plays such a central role would summarize the research in an affirmative voice, describing what people with mental illness, service providers, and the community at large may do to promote personal power. Unfortunately, much of the research and literature on empowerment looks at the negative impact of its absence—what happens when a person with mental illness is disempowered (Corrigan & Garman, 1997; Rapp, Shera, & Kisthardt, 1993). Hence, we have chosen to intertwine what is *known about disempowerment* with what we see as the *vision of empowerment*, where appropriate.

SUMMARY AND CONCLUSIONS

The loss of life opportunities experienced by people with psychiatric disabilities does not stem solely from the symptoms and dysfunctions of their illness. Public reaction in the form of stigma may also produce significant hurdles for a person. Moreover, internalizing this stigma may fill the person with doubt, further undermining his or her efforts to successfully achieve life goals. Public stigma can undermine rehabilitation goals related to work, education, health, and housing. It can exacerbate the problems in interactions between people with psychiatric disabilities and the police. Self-stigma can block people from seeking psychiatric and rehabilitative services that might assist them with their goals. It can harm a person's sense of self-esteem and self-efficacy. Stigma is also a sociological phenomenon. Institutional and social structures, including the public mental health system, may intentionally and unintentionally prevent people with mental illness from fully enjoying their rights as citizens, including their right to access the public mental health system.

Service providers need to be aware of rehabilitation goals that decrease stigma. These include community integration that seeks to replace public stigma with a commitment to helping people achieve *their* goals in *their* communities. They also include personal empowerment, which is an essential process of rehabilitation (i.e., the person has entire control of his or her life). Community integration and personal empowerment underpin all rehabilitation practices. As a result, the reader will see frequent mention of these principles throughout this book. In addition, rehabilitation providers need to join with advocates and people with psychiatric disabilities to directly challenge the stigma of mental illness. Chapter 19 discusses strategies for accomplishing these goals.

Chapter 3

Definition of Psychiatric Rehabilitation

WHAT IS PSYCHIATRIC REHABILITATION?

Psychiatric rehabilitation has been broadly defined as "the systematic utilization of a combination of specific modalities to assist in the community rehabilitation of persons with psychiatric disabilities" (Rutman, 1997, p. 4.). Bachrach (1992) defines psychosocial rehabilitation as "a therapeutic approach that encourages a mentally ill person to develop his or her fullest capacities through learning and environmental supports" (p. 1456). These are but two of many definitions in the literature, which differ according to whether they focus on goals, methods, philosophy, or linkages to the broader field of rehabilitation. In an early conceptualization, Anthony (1982) drew an analogy between rehabilitation for psychiatric and physical disabilities, suggesting that the goals were similar, although the methods differed because of differences in functional limitations. A widely cited definition is, "To help persons with psychiatric disabilities to increase their ability to function successfully and to be satisfied in the environments of their choice with the least amount of ongoing professional intervention" (Anthony, Cohen, Farkas, & Gagne, 2002, p. 101). In common usage, *psychiatric rehabilitation* is limited to programs for adults with severe mental illness (SMI) (i.e., specifically excluding children). In this context, *adults* include the entire spectrum from adolescence to older adulthood, in recognition of the need to tailor service to developmental stage.

Historically, psychiatric rehabilitation had its major impetus in the formation of maverick psychosocial rehabilitation centers outside the mainstream mental health system, starting in the 1950s (Dincin, 1975). Growing out of this tradition is a definition of psychiatric rehabilitation in pragmatic, concrete terms as "giving people with psychiatric disabilities the opportunity to work, live in the community, and enjoy a social life, at their

50

> ## ORGANIZATIONAL EXAMPLE
> ### *Thresholds*
>
> Located alongside high-rises and other residences in an affluent neighborhood of Chicago, the home base for the Thresholds does not look like a psychiatric rehabilitation center. It appears to be a large residence, which it once was. Once inside, you may be struck by the apparent chaos of simultaneous diverse activities on every floor of the building. In the lobby, you step aside as a group of members (i.e., consumers) assemble as a mobile work crew for cleaning government buildings. In the basement, a coffee shop is open for business. On the first floor, a peer-led medication education group is meeting. Nurses from the local university are conducting routine physicals in another room. Adding to the swirl of activity on the first floor, the Mothers' Group offers training and support to mothers with schizophrenia in childcare for their preschoolers. On the second floor, some members are preparing the noon-day meal, while the members' council is planning the summer camping program. On the upper floors, workers hold individual counseling sessions. "Education" meets on the fourth floor, providing tutorial help for members preparing for their GEDs. Elsewhere, Community Scholars help members enroll in local community colleges. That evening, Thresholds is trans-formed into a drop-in center, with board games, food, and music. As you learn more about Thresholds, you discover that these impressions are only a small part of its scope—they do not include the Thresholds Bridge assertive community treatment teams, the large network of housing programs and many other services.
>
> Thresholds embodies the core principles of psychiatric rehabilitation (discussed below). For example, all of its programs have *a focus on real-world issues* (work, housing, income support) with attention to *members' personal goals and preferences*. Interventions aim at both *skills training* (sometimes through formal classes, but more often through experiential learning) and *environmental modification*. Threshold staff members work together in *teams* that provide the entire spectrum of psychiatric rehabilitation services, including mental health case management, vocational services, and residential services. All of Thresholds' pro-grams aim at *community integration* and, especially for the Bridge programs, the intention is to provide time-unlimited services, in recognition of the importance of *continuity of services*.

own pace, through planned experiences in a respectful, supportive, and realistic atmo-sphere" (Rutman, 1993, p. 1). This simple definition captures the focus of psychiatric rehabilitation as grounded in *normalizing roles and relationships, practical, realistic ele-ments* of everyday living, and *experiential activities* (Rutman, 1997).

For many contributors to the psychiatric rehabilitation field who stress the formal structured elements of psychiatric rehabilitation interventions as described in later chap-ters, the origins of psychiatric rehabilitation owe a huge debt to the work of Paul and Lentz (1977) in the implementation of a social learning program for long-term residents of a psychiatric hospital.

In years past, a distinction was drawn between *psychiatric* rehabilitation, which was originally associated with the medical model, and *psychosocial* rehabilitation, based on a social rehabilitation model (Flexer & Solomon, 1993). Psychosocial rehabilitation was originally construed as a set of services apart from mental health treatment, both physi-cally and philosophically. The reference to "psychosocial" reinforces a core value of focusing on the person–environment interaction, but the term is also misleading and sometimes misunderstood because it is so encompassing. For this reason, *psychiatric rehabilitation* has gained favor as a more descriptively useful label. A second reason for abandoning the psychosocial/psychiatric distinction is the evidence that separating rehabilitation from mental health treatment is counterproductive (Drake, Becker, Bond, & Mueser, 2003a). In practice, treatment and rehabilitation often are intertwined, although "treatment" refers specifically to medications and psychotherapy, whereas "rehabilitation" is associated with programs aimed at employment, housing, and other aspects of community functioning.

In common parlance, the term *psychiatric rehabilitation* has been used in ways that are misleading or unduly restrictive. Thus, it may be useful to note what we do *not* mean by *psychiatric rehabilitation*. It is not a program or a place, even though the term is used colloquially in that fashion. Neither is the broader concept of psychiatric rehabilitation adequately defined by a set of specific services funded by a particular source, such as Medicaid (through the Medicaid Rehabilitation Option) or a targeted program initiative designated by a state mental health agency (Barton, Steiner, & Giffort, 2001).

To restate our definition in terms of the concepts introduced in Chapter 1, psychiatric rehabilitation can be understood as systematic efforts to help adults with psychiatric disabilities move forward in their recovery process. The rest of this book articulates specific psychiatric rehabilitation *practices* that have been proven effective or, when the evidence is lacking, practices that represent our best understanding of how to help in that process. Common to these practices are a set of fundamental concepts, which are summarized in the following section.

PERSONAL EXAMPLE

Alan and the Benefits of Psychiatric Rehabilitation

Like many consumers, Alan is shy and withdrawn and does not offer many opinions when asked about his preferences. In their first meeting, his case manager, Beth, resists her first inclination to tell Alan what he needs to do, but, rather, patiently tries to draw Alan out. Currently living with his parents, Alan finally admits that, although scared of the prospect, he desperately would like to live in his own apartment. Over the next few meetings, Alan also discloses that he hates his medications and doesn't understand why he needs to take them. A high school dropout, Alan does not know what he wants to do, but he would like to have a car and a stereo. He is also terribly lonely and isolated. However, Beth identifies many strengths that Alan has, including a well-groomed appearance, consistency in keeping appointments, and cooperativeness. Together, Beth and Alan begin devising a rehabilitation plan. Beth takes her lead from Alan, identifying his priorities while clarifying and providing information. She asks Alan if he would like to include his parents in the planning process. With Alan's permission, Beth consults with the nurse on the treatment team to arrange a meeting with Alan and his parents to explain the purpose of his medications as well as their side effects. Because Alan has identified independent living as his primary goal, Beth and Alan list this as the first goal, and they identify the substeps required to achieve that goal. In subsequent weeks, they begin searching the local community for an affordable apartment. The ramifications of moving out of his parents' home are also discussed. Beth offers to help Alan develop independent living skills (cooking, shopping, using public transportation) once he moves out. In the other areas he has identified, Beth and Alan also begin developing realistic plans, recognizing that it may be best not to make too many changes all at once.

FUNDAMENTAL CONCEPTS IN PSYCHIATRIC REHABILITATION

Many different classifications of the core principles of psychiatric rehabilitation have been proposed over the years (Anthony et al., 2002; Bond & Resnick, 2000; Cnaan, Blankertz, Messinger, & Gardner, 1988; Cook & Hoffschmidt, 1993; Dincin, 1995a; Hughes & Weinstein, 1997b; Pratt, Gill, Barrett, & Roberts, 1999). A comparison of these lists leads to several conclusions: First, some authors have included items reflecting practitioner attitudes and behaviors fundamental to *any* effective helping relationship, such as *conveying hope* (Dincin, 1975), *treating clients with respect* (Hughes & Weinstein, 1997b), *individualizing services* (Pratt et al., 1999), and delivering them in a *culturally competent* manner (Hughes & Weinstein, 1997b). Although these elements are sometimes classified as critical components of psychiatric rehabilitation practice, we conceptualize them as part of a set of core psychiatric rehabilitation practitioner *competencies* (Hoge, Paris, Adger, Collins, Finn, et al., 2005), as discussed below. Second, although most lists generally converge toward a set of common principles, some reflect a specific theoretical point of view (Anthony et al., 2002). Third, some commonly identified principles are more specific to a historical model of psychosocial rehabilitation as a separate entity from mental health treatment (e.g., "social rather than medical supremacy"; Cnaan et al., 1988). Fourth, a strong theme that comes through in reading the psychiatric rehabilitation literature is that many of these approaches have evolved in the absence of a strong theoretical framework (Hogarty, 1995). It is not an exaggeration to say that psychiatric rehabilitation has been the antithesis of theory-based practice (Cnaan, Blankertz, Messinger, & Gardner, 1989). Hence, Anthony et al. (2002) list *eclecticism* as one of the core principles and Dincin (1995a) refers to the *pragmatism* of psychiatric rehabilitation, reflecting the fact that many of its most widely practiced approaches have been developed through a trial-and-error process. In our view, the source of initial inspiration for a program practice is not as important as whether research shows it to be effective. Finally, another important distinction in defining program principles is whether these principles refer to *philosophy and values* or if the principles are meant to inform the *operational elements of practice*. Our view is that a set of principles should accomplish both: They should be consistent as a broader set of values, as well as having concrete implications for how programs are organized and delivered. Nevertheless, some principles are stated in terms of values (e.g., self-determination), and others are more representative of the practice level (e.g., skills training).

During the 1980s, leaders of the psychiatric rehabilitation field were surveyed regarding perceptions of core principles (Cnaan, Blankertz, Messinger, & Gardner, 1990). Using factor analysis, the investigators identified 13 principles, each defined by a minimum of three behavioral items, labeled as follows: equipping clients with skills, self determination, utilizing environmental resource, social change, differential assessment and care, commitment from staff, emphasis on employment, emphasis on the here and now, early intervention, social rather than medical emphasis, normalization, emphasis on strengths, intimate environment of service. Later surveys of practitioners and consumers on these principles yielded differences in ratings of importance, particularly between experts and consumers, but identified no additional principles (Cnaan, Blankertz, & Aunders, 1992).

Since this survey was completed, many changes have occurred within the psychiatric rehabilitation field. Given the proliferation of new approaches to psychiatric rehabilitation, we may not find strong consensus among psychiatric leaders today. Nonetheless, guided by the diverse sources discussed in this chapter, in addition to the Cnaan surveys, we suggest the following principles, summarized in Table 3.1.

TABLE 3.1. Psychiatric Rehabilitation Principles

• Self-determination	• Environmental modification and supports
• Attention to consumers' personal goals and preferences	• Integration of rehabilitation and treatment
	• Multidisciplinary team
• Real-world focus	• Continuity of services
• Focus on strengths	• Community integration
• Skills training	• Recovery orientation

Self-Determination

The first principle recognizes the primary role for the consumer in his or her own illness management and recovery process (Mueser et al., 2002a). Some psychiatric rehabilitation programs refer to consumers as "members," stressing their role as active participants in the rehabilitation program (Dincin, 1975). Consumer self-help activities are one expression of this self-determination principle (Solomon, 2004).

Attention to Consumers' Personal Goals and Preferences

Psychiatric rehabilitation is organized around consumer goals, choices, and preferences. There are three aspects of this principle: First, in terms of rehabilitation goals, the goal-setting process begins with a dialogue between the psychiatric rehabilitation professional and the consumer, incorporating the consumer's aspirations into the overall rehabilitation goal (Anthony et al., 2002). Collaboration is particularly important in rehabilitation planning, because practitioners often misjudge consumer goals and preferences (Crane-Ross, Roth, & Lauber, 2000; Noble, Honberg, Hall, & Flynn, 1997; Tanzman, 1993). The personal goals that consumers identify (e.g., to have friends, a decent place to live, and meaningful work) differ from treatment goals typically recorded in medical charts for reimbursement purposes, such as "attending day treatment," or "taking medications as prescribed" (Adams & Grieder, 2004).

Second, the attention to consumer preferences extends to the decisions about which psychiatric rehabilitation services consumers are to receive. Instead of "placing" consumers in programs, practitioners provide information to allow consumers to make informed choices about the array of possible rehabilitation options, including, for example, whether services are provided individually, in a group setting, or in some other modality. The role of consumer preferences is congruent with the findings from the literature on evidence-based medicine, which suggest that when patients are provided good information about treatment options, they make better decisions and are more involved in the treatment process (Drake, Rosenberg, Teague, Bartels, & Torrey, 2003c; Wennberg, 1991). Moreover, decisions about rehabilitation options are not one-time decisions, but instead a continuous process guided by changing goals and realities.

Third, psychiatric rehabilitation practitioners attend to consumer preferences in helping them achieve their stated goals—for example, in helping consumers to find jobs in the occupations they desire (Becker, Drake, Farabaugh, & Bond, 1996) and to obtain their preferred types of housing (Carling, 1995).

Real-World Focus

Consumers aspire to the same things as do individuals without disabilities—to have friends, to work, to live on their own, to have a car and other possessions, and so forth

(Rapp & Goscha, 2006). Following from the principle of consumer choice, the content and design of psychiatric rehabilitation programs reflect such aspirations. Hence, most approaches to psychiatric rehabilitation have a focus on practical problems in everyday living (Dincin, 1995b).

Focus on Strengths

In many service settings, consumers are bombarded by "spirit-breaking" messages reinforcing the negative expectations of patienthood and the stigma of mental illness (Deegan, 1990). In contrast, the strengths-based philosophy recognizes the unique capabilities and potentialities of each individual that provide a foundation for pursing personal goals (Rapp & Goscha, 2006).

Skills Training

Psychiatric rehabilitation approaches help consumers to acquire and apply skills needed to achieve community adjustment (Anthony & Liberman, 1986). The methods for skills training vary widely, ranging from informal, experiential methods (Vorspan, 1988) to structured, curriculum-driven behavioral approaches (Wallace, Liberman, MacKain, Blackwell, & Eckman, 1992). Increasingly, psychiatric rehabilitation skills training has incorporated cognitive interventions (Penn & Mueser, 1996), including strategies to compensate for cognitive impairments (Velligan, Prihoda, Ritch, Maples, Bow-Thomas, et al., 2002). The *locus* of training also varies, with evidence favoring the view that training *in vivo*, that is, in the specific setting in which the skills are used, is more effective than training in a clinic setting (Glynn, Marder, Liberman, Blair, Wirshing, et al., 2002; Tauber, Wallace, & Lecomte, 2000). Along with providing skills training in environments where the skills are actually used, many psychiatric rehabilitation approaches emphasize situational assessment approaches over conventional assessment methodologies. *Situational assessment* refers to evaluating an individual's actual performance in the environment where it is pertinent rather than inferring it from a test. For example, situational assessment of vocational behaviors examines behavior in actual work settings (Bond & Dietzen, 1993).

Environmental Modification and Supports

Although skills training aims at helping consumers cope by improving their inner resources, in many cases the key to success involves resources outside the consumer. Thus, interventions often involve selecting and modifying environments to maximize the likelihood that consumers will succeed. For example, the best strategy for helping a consumer with poor hygiene to obtain employment may be to find a job in a recycling center, where hygiene is unimportant, rather than attempting to modify the person's personal habits (Becker & Drake, 2003). Another common example of environmental modification is helping consumers to move out of emotionally charged living situations (Dincin, 1995a). The most common expression of this principle, however, is direct provision of individualized support in the environments where these skills are used (e.g., where consumers work and live). Support may be offered through a variety of mechanisms, including professional, peer, and "natural" supports, the latter referring to family members, friends, coworkers, and others who are not affiliated with the mental health system (McHugo, Drake, & Becker, 1998; Rapp & Goscha, 2004).

Integration of Rehabilitation and Treatment

First articulated in the assertive community treatment model, this principle states that consumers benefit most when a multidisciplinary team provides help in a holistic fashion, comprehensively addressing all of their psychosocial and mental health needs. Traditional practice has separated rehabilitation services from mental health treatment, resulting in fragmented services and poor employment outcomes (Noble et al., 1997). Similarly, mental health and substance abuse treatment are typically provided in an uncoordinated fashion by entirely separate programs (Drake, Essock, Shaner, Carey, Minkoff, et al., 2001a). However, rehabilitation services are most effective when closely integrated with mental health treatment interventions (Drake et al., 2003a). Historically, there has been an "uneasy alliance" between psychiatry and psychiatric rehabilitation (Bachrach, 1992). Yet this collaboration is essential. Because the large majority of consumers with SMI require psychotropic medications, a critical element in this principle of integration is the provision of medications with psychosocial interventions (Hogarty, 2002), following evidence-based principles of medication management (Miller, Crismon, Rush, Chiles, Kashner, et al., 2004).

Multidisciplinary Team Approach

An integration of treatment and rehabilitation implies that psychiatric rehabilitation is provided by a multidisciplinary team that meets frequently enough to ensure a high level of communication (Stein & Test, 1980a). Some descriptions of psychiatric rehabilitation emphasize the skills and competencies of individual practitioners, conveying the impression that one-on-one contact with consumers lies at the heart of the work of psychiatric rehabilitation. Certainly, the formation of strong relationships in rehabilitation is critical (Dincin, 1975), but this does not mitigate the role of collaboration among the various disciplines necessary to provide comprehensive and integrated rehabilitation and treatment (e.g., psychiatry, nursing, social work, vocational rehabilitation, and substance abuse counseling).

Continuity of Services

The importance of providing continuity of services over time is another fundamental principle (Test, 1979; Ware, Dickey, Tugenberg, & McHorney, 2003). Because psychiatric disabilities involve chronic conditions, time-limited interventions are generally ineffective. Maintaining continuity in relationships by providing timely and predictable support is a key element in successful psychiatric rehabilitation programs.

The principle of continuity of services sounds discordant in the context of self-determination, especially for psychiatric rehabilitation programs, such as drop-in centers and clubhouse programs, which stress the voluntary nature of membership. In such programs, one way this principle is expressed is through systematically reaching out to those who have stopped participating (Beard, Malamud, & Rossman, 1978).

Community Integration

Psychiatric rehabilitation embraces the principle of normalization, promoting illness self-management and normal adult roles in the participants' communities (Bond, Salyers, Rollins, Rapp, & Zipple, 2004). Programs embracing this principle avoid the use of stepwise approaches, in which individuals first adjust to protected settings, such as sheltered workshops, segregated housing arrangements, and day treatment programs, as preparation for eventual full integration (Carling, 1995).

Recovery Orientation

As discussed in Chapter 1, the overarching goal of psychiatric rehabilitation is to promote the recovery process for each consumer. By extension, psychiatric rehabilitation programs strive to provide recovery-oriented services. A recovery orientation promotes a sense of hope, personal directedness, goal orientation, and optimism.

Other Principles

Many other elements ideally would be included in the list of core concepts of psychiatric rehabilitation. For example, psychiatric rehabilitation practices are most effective when they include family members and other significant others (Mueser et al., 2002a). In addition, some authors have suggested that an outcome orientation is integral to psychiatric rehabilitation, referring to the continuous quality improvement processes that are found in most, if not all, successful organizations (Rapp & Poertner, 1992).

To summarize, we have not yet reached the point of an empirically validated and exhaustive list of psychiatric rehabilitation principles. However, the 11 principles listed in Table 3.1 are supported by the literature and endorsed by many psychiatric rehabilitation practitioners. These principles represent a synthesis of viewpoints emerging from a diverse history, to which we now turn.

HISTORY OF THE FIELD OF PSYCHIATRIC REHABILITATION

The history of psychiatric rehabilitation includes both the spread of programs and practices and the development of the conceptualization of psychiatric rehabilitation as a coherent field. Regarding the spread of psychiatric rehabilitation practices, they have evolved in many diverse forms. Although some of the better-known models have well-articulated program philosophies, in everyday practice most programs include many eclectic, pragmatic elements. The diversity of goals, consumers served, community characteristics, funding mandates, staffing patterns, local norms, and many other factors also influence the character of programs as they evolve in particular settings (Bachrach, 1988).

Regarding the original conceptualization of psychiatric rehabilitation, no one was more influential than Bill Anthony. His work helped to legitimize psychiatric rehabilitation as a field, which, he argued, should have equal status with rehabilitation for physical disability within vocational rehabilitation. Anthony and Liberman (1986) provided a vulnerability–stress conceptual framework for psychiatric rehabilitation, asserting that skills training was a foundation for psychiatric rehabilitation interventions.

Psychiatric rehabilitation developed from many sources. To understand the context for its development, we have embedded this chronology within the cycle of "reform movements" in mental health (Goldman & Morrissey, 1985; Morrissey & Goldman, 1984; U.S. Department of Health and Human Services, 1999), as shown in Table 3.2.

This historical review is intended as a partial antidote to the tendency for each era's leaders to "have us believe that all psychiatric care was morally and scientifically benighted until they developed a more compassionate approach to rehabilitation, hous-

TABLE 3.2. Historical Reform Movements in Mental Health Treatment in the United States

Reform movement	Era	Setting	Focus of reform
Moral treatment	1800–1850	Asylums	Humane, restorative treatment
Mental hygiene	1890–1920	Mental hospitals or clinics	Prevention, scientific orientation
Community mental health	1955–1970	Community mental health centers	Deinstitutionalization
Community support	1975– present	Community support programs	Mental illness as a social welfare problem (e.g., housing, employment)
Psychosocial rehabilitation	1960–1990	Psychosocial rehabilitation centers	Limitations of medical model and recognition of central role of rehabilitation
Consumer movement	1990– present	Consumer organizations	Recovery as a guiding concept in the design of programs
Evidence-based practice	1998– present	Community	Use of evidence in all stages of service provision

Note. Adapted from U.S. Surgeon General's Report on Mental Health (1999).

ing, family intervention, recovery, or whatever" (Becker & Drake, 2003, p. 6). Of course, it should be understood that this account is by necessity an oversimplification. For one thing, national trends do not give the nuanced stories for each state (Torrey, Erdman, Wolfe, & Flynn, 1990). Because state mental health agencies have always had primary responsibility for establishing and promoting mental health policy, a more historically accurate account would consist of different chronologies for each state, to say nothing of community variations.

Historical Origins of Psychiatric Rehabilitation

The roots of psychiatric rehabilitation can be traced back to the moral treatment movement starting in the late 18th century. Appalled by the widespread inhumane treatment of mental patients, Philippe Pinel in France and William Tuke in England relocated patients to retreats in the countryside, treated them with kindness and respect, and organized daily routines around social contact, exercise, and productive activity. In the United States, Dorothea Dix was a leader in founding mental hospitals with these principles in mind, so that individuals with mental illness would not be consigned to jails, poorhouses, or life on the streets, as was common in the 1800s (Sharfstein, 2000).

A precursor to later ideas about using normalized settings as alternatives to institutionalization evolved in the village of Gheel, Belgium. In the 13th century, Gheel became the destination for religious pilgrimages for cures for mental illness. In the 1800s, because of the large number of pilgrims, the church began appealing to townspeople to house them. Thus, a boarding system developed in which host families took in pilgrims.

This custom evolved into the establishment of permanent residences for individuals with mental illness, who lived in the homes of ordinary townspeople (Bloom, 1984). Geel's approach foreshadowed some 20th-century ideas about crisis housing as an alternative to institutionalization (Stroul, 1988).

Originating in the late 19th century in the United States, the mental hygiene movement was a reaction to deterioration of the quality of care in public institutions, where overcrowding and underfunding ran rampant (U.S. Department of Health and Human Services, 1999). The ideals of this movement combined the concepts of public health, scientific medicine, and social progressivism. Despite the innovative ideas born of this era, the lack of effective treatments for mental illness resulted in great pessimism and continued neglect for patients in large state inpatient facilities.

Pharmaceutical Breakthroughs and Deinstitutionalization

Deinstitutionalization

During the 1950s there were a number of pharmaceutical breakthroughs profoundly affecting the treatment of severe mental illness, especially the discovery of chlorpromazine and other antipsychotics as a treatment for schizophrenia, but also the development of antidepressants and mood stabilizers. These new medications led to a new view of mental illness and the inevitability of long-term hospitalization. Beginning in the 1950s, a combination of economic, legal, and humanitarian factors, in addition to the widespread use of these new medications, led to deinstitutionalization, that is, the transferring of patients out of state psychiatric hospitals in the United States. The resident population of state and county mental hospitals in the United States, which peaked at 559,000 in 1955, declined to fewer than 60,000 by 1998 (Lamb & Bachrach, 2001). Geller (2000) and many others have noted that those discharged from psychiatric hospitals who did not return to live with their families often relocated in institution-like facilities in the community.

Role of Antipsychotic Medications

Within the psychiatric field, many believed (and still believe) that antipsychotics were the only effective treatment for schizophrenia and that psychotherapy did not contribute to improved client outcomes, except to the extent that they improved adherence to medications. Supporting the view of psychotherapy (as it was conceptualized at the time) as having a negligible impact was one early hospital study comparing antipsychotic medications to "milieu therapy" (group activities promoting support on hospital wards) and psychodynamically oriented psychotherapy (May, 1968). This study found that antipsychotics were helpful in controlling symptoms, whereas the two psychotherapy approaches were not. In fact, many studies have documented that antipsychotics are far more effective than placebo treatment in reducing relapse and hospitalization rates and controlling positive symptoms of schizophrenia (Davis, 1980). However, the actual consequences of deinstitutionalization made it abundantly clear that medications alone were not sufficient to address the needs of individuals with schizophrenia or other severe mental illnesses.

A landmark experiment by Hogarty and Goldberg (1973) helped to clarify the potential synergistic roles of psychosocial interventions and antipsychotic medications. This two-factor design examined four conditions: placebo alone, placebo and sociotherapy, drug alone (chlorpromazine), and drug and sociotherapy. Sociotherapy involved a combination of psychosocial interventions, including supportive therapy, social case-work, and rehabilitation counseling. With its focus on the practical problems of community functioning, sociotherapy, resembled what later would be called clinical case management (Hogarty, 2002). As expected, the group receiving drugs did significantly better in avoiding relapse than those receiving the placebo. The most important finding, however, was that the group receiving both antipsychotic medications and sociotherapy had the best long-term outcomes, including better instrumental role functioning (that is, working in competitive jobs and in homemaker roles). Those receiving sociotherapy and the placebo actually fared worse than those receiving the placebo alone (Hogarty, Goldberg, & Schooler, 1974). The negative results for this latter group were unexpected. On the basis of this and other studies, Hogarty (2002) concluded that consumers who were "withdrawn, disorganized, anxious, and less insightful" (p. 30) are vulnerable to relapse if they receive high-expectation psychosocial services in the absence of adequate medications. A later study by Hogarty, Schooler, Ulrich, Mussare, Herron, et al. (1979) using depot medications (injections) suggested that the positive impact of sociotherapy was not merely the result of its influence on medication adherence. The current view in psychiatry is that psychotropic medications are a critical component of treatment, but that provision of medications in the absence of psychosocial interventions is insufficient (Lehman, Kreyenbuhl, Buchanan, Dickerson, Dixon, et al., 2004).

Transitional Housing Strategies

In the early stages of deinstitutionalization, the majority of discharged patients were relatively high functioning and most returned to live on their own with their families, but by the mid-1960s, individuals with more serious impairments (compounded by the consequences of long-term institutionalization) were increasingly being released without any consideration of their housing needs, often with disastrous results (Torrey, 1983).

Starting in the 1950s, psychiatric hospitals began developing a variety of transitional housing models for consumers making the transition from comprehensive care provided by the hospital back to the community (Geller, 2000). (In later years, community agencies assumed the role of operating residential programs.) The underlying philosophy for helping psychiatric patients return to the community involved training them in a gradual, stepwise fashion to gain the skills necessary to function in normal society. Discharged patients were first transferred to supervised group homes ("halfway houses"), later to a less supervised setting, and eventually to unsupervised independent housing (Ridgway & Zipple, 1990). Two experimental programs evaluating strategies for bridging the transition to community living deserve note (Fairweather, Sanders, Cressler, & Maynard, 1969; Paul & Lentz, 1977).

An early transitional housing approach with documented effectiveness was the *lodge* model (Fairweather et al., 1969). This approach involved developing a cohesive group of patients on an inpatient ward and subsequently relocating them to a "lodge" in the community. The lodge served as a self-contained society in which discharged patients lived, worked, and socialized together. The lodge model is still active today in a few states (Krepp, 2000), but the model never achieved the national expansion Fairweather envisioned (Fairweather, 1980), partly because short inpatient stays today make some elements of the model obsolete.

Many varieties of halfway houses were developed, some as highly structured as the Fairweather models, but ranging widely in philosophy and rule making. Despite an early positive review of the halfway house literature (Rog & Raush, 1975), this approach has not been studied rigorously (Cometa, Morrison, & Ziskoven, 1979). Transitional housing approaches have proved to be problematic for a number of reasons, as discussed in Chapter 8.

Behavioral Strategies and Skills Training

As described by B. F. Skinner, all behavior is determined by its consequences of reward and punishment (Skinner, 1938). On the basis of this seemingly simplistic notion, Skinner and other proponents of behaviorism exerted enormous influence on psychology, education, and treatment services in the United States, especially in the first few decades after World War II. A direct application of behaviorist principles was the *token economy*, first applied to "back ward" psychiatric inpatients in a state hospital (Ayllon & Azrin, 1968). This demonstration study showed that individuals with schizophrenia who were believed to be so "unmotivated" that they were incapable of self-care would respond dramatically to contingencies systematically applied within a controlled environment. Using very similar techniques, the "social learning" program developed by Paul and Lentz (1977) for long-term inpatients with multiple behavioral problems was experimentally compared with usual inpatient care. This study showed that behaviorist principles could greatly facilitate the discharge and community tenure of psychiatric inpatients.

The use of the token economy is recognized as an effective modality (Lehman et al., 2004). However, because the token economy requires control over rewards and punishments, it is difficult to implement outside institutional settings and therefore has never achieved the wide scale adoption its developers believed it warranted (Paul & Menditto, 1992). A related approach that continues to be used in community settings for substance abuse treatment is *contingency management*, which involves giving monetary awards to participants with substance use disorders for such behaviors as remaining abstinent for a period of time or looking for employment (Budney, Sigmons, & Higgins, 2001; Drebing, Van Ormer, Krebs, Rosenheck, Rounsaville, et al., 2005).

Starting in the late 1970s, the field of psychiatric rehabilitation was also influenced by the development of systematic skills training programs for individuals with schizophrenia and other disorders by groups such as the UCLA (University of California, Los Angeles) group headed by Bob Liberman, the Center for Psychiatric Rehabilitation headed by Bill Anthony, and a group headed by Alan Bellack (now at the University of Maryland). Whereas token economies often focus on the elimination of undesired behavior (e.g., aggressive behavior, inactivity), skills training programs aim more at acquisition and application of skills needed to successfully function in society (e.g., carrying on a conversation). Many of the practices described in this book (e.g., illness management, integrated dual disorders treatment, family psychoeducation) incorporate skills training as an essential component.

Community Mental Health Movement

In 1963, the Community Mental Health Centers Act authorized the creation of a network of community mental health centers (CMHCs) (U.S. Congress, 1963). This bill was revolutionary, reversing a century of federal policy of noninvolvement in state services for the mentally ill marked by a presidential veto of the Indigent Insane Bill in 1854, which was Dorothea Dix's attempt to fund asylums to promote moral treatment (Sharfstein, 2000). The initial legislation established five essential CMHC services: inpatient care, outpatient care, emergency services, partial hospitalization, and consultation and education (Bloom, 1984). These centers were intended to address the comprehensive mental health needs for the community, not only for individuals with SMI, but for those with ill-nesses across the spectrum of psychiatric disorders. In addition to treating psychiatric conditions directly, CMHCs were intended to prevent or ameliorate their development through consultation and educational efforts. Another key element of the legislation was the objective of treating individuals near their homes, rather than in remote state hospi-tals. This legislation and later amendments eventually led to the funding of 789 CMHCs throughout the United States (Torrey, 2001).

Despite initial optimism, most CMHCs were unprepared to serve people with SMI for several reasons. First, most mental health professionals were not trained to work with people with SMI. Second, many professionals incorrectly assumed that antipsychotic medications by themselves would be sufficient to enable people with SMI to cope with community living. Second, CMHCs were typically limited to facility-based services, with the assumption that discharged patients would seek their services as necessary. This assumption also proved wrong: A 1986 national survey found that 937,000 (78%) of 1.2 million persons with schizophrenia living outside institutions were not receiving any CMHC-based outpatient treatment (Torrey, 2001), either because they never made it to an initial appointment or because they dropped out soon thereafter (Axelrod & Wetzler, 1989). A main factor was that most CMHC practitioners preferred working with less dis-abled consumers, having been trained in the insight-oriented psychotherapeutic ap-proaches popular at that time. Even in early studies, it was apparent that insight-oriented psychotherapeutic approaches were not helpful in addressing problems of everyday liv-ing, whereas more practical approaches were (Gunderson, Frank, Katz, Vannicelli, Frosch, et al., 1984; Vitale & Steinbach, 1965). Intensive insight-oriented approaches often have adverse effects for individuals with schizophrenia (Drake & Sederer, 1986a).

One of the most enduring legacies of the CMHC Act was the mandated establish-ment of partial hospitalization programs, modeled partly after the day hospital concept first described in the 1950s (Geller, 2000). Since the establishment of CMHCs, partial hospitalization has been a central feature of mental health programming in the United States (Krizay, 1989). A national survey estimated there were 1,000 such programs in 1980 (Parker & Knoll, 1990). Often referred to as "day treatment," partial hospitaliza-tion arose as an alternative to inpatient hospitalization, providing comprehensive, multi-disciplinary services to consumers with SMI (Casarino, Wilner, & Maxey, 1982) for lower costs than inpatient care (Endicott, Hertz, & Gibbon, 1978). Although day treat-ment has demonstrated effectiveness for its original purpose as an alternative to hospital-ization (Marshall, Crowther, Almarez-Serrano, Creed, Sledge, et al., 2001), it is now often used to provide rehabilitative services rather than hospital diversion (Fishbein, 1988; Rosie, 1987). It continues to be widely used as a long-term treatment option, in large part because it is handsomely reimbursed (Riggs, 1996). For decades, authors have expressed serious reservations about the use of day treatment as a rehabilitation approach (Anthony & Liberman, 1992; Creed, Black, & Anthony, 1989; Pryce, 1982). There is no evidence of any rehabilitation benefits of long-term day treatment for con-sumers with SMI (Marshall et al., 2001). Despite the espousal of rehabilitative goals, day treatment does not help people move out of treatment settings and into normal adult roles in the community.

In addition to the aforementioned inadequacies, CMHCs failed to address a wide range of pressing needs relating to housing, employment, socialization, and other areas of functioning. The phenomenon of "revolving-door" clients—those who return frequently to psychiatric hospitals—was one consequence of their limited treatment focus. More than half of all psychiatric patients released from state hospitals returned within 2 years

(Weiden & Olfson, 1993). These trends suggested the need for new, comprehensive psychosocial approaches to augment traditional CMHC services and to complement pharmacological treatments (Talbott, 1978).

Community Support Program

By the early 1970s it was very clear that the community mental health movement, with its focus on symptom control and stabilization, had failed miserably to address the psychosocial needs of individuals with SMI (Drake, Green, Mueser, & Goldman, 2003b). By 1975 federal legislation increased the number of "essential" CMHC services from 5 to 12, expanding both the populations served (to include children and individuals with substance use disorders) and the range of programs offered (e.g., transitional living facilities for persons with mental illness) (Torrey, 1988).

The National Institute of Mental Health (NIMH), the federal agency formed in 1946 to formulate and lead mental health policy for the nation and to promote research, training, and quality services, held a series of conferences to promote the development of *systems of care*. Participants at these meetings helped to formulate a new set of program principles, which became the foundation for the *community support program* (CSP) approach (Turner & TenHoor, 1978). The contributions of psychiatric rehabilitation leaders attending these meetings, as well as the growing knowledge base from the field of psychiatric rehabilitation, influenced the formulation of CSP principles.

The CSP approach identified fundamental modifications to the CMHC model necessary for ensuring effective services for individuals with SMI. Whereas CMHCs typically provided *episodic* services, with consumers receiving assistance primarily when in crisis, the CSP approach advocated a *continuous* system of care. CSP features included the identification of a core service agency responsible for the comprehensive needs of consumers and performing 10 basic functions (Stroul, 1986; Turner & TenHoor, 1978):

- Outreach (locating consumers, informing them of available services, and ensuring access)
- Assistance in meeting basic needs (food, clothing, shelter, safety, medical and dental care, income assistance)
- Mental health care (diagnostic evaluations, medication management, counseling)
- 24-hour crisis assistance (including temporary housing)
- Psychosocial and vocational services
- Rehabilitative and supportive housing
- Consultation and education (to families, friends, landlords, etc.)
- Natural support systems (recognizing and involving self-help groups, churches, community organizations)
- Protection of consumer rights (including grievance procedures)
- Case management

Thus, CSP popularized a new type of mental health worker—the case manager. As discussed in Chapter 6, the case manager's role is to ensure that consumers receive services needed for community reintegration, primarily through linking consumers to appropriate services (Mueser, Bond, Drake, & Resnick, 1998a). Exemplifying the CSP approach was the assertive community treatment (ACT) model (Stein & Test, 1980a). ACT is a comprehensive individualized approach to treatment and rehabilitation employing assertive outreach, small client–staff ratios, attention to details of everyday living, frequent contact with consumers, and provision of service without a time limit. ACT uses a multidisciplinary treatment team that makes most contacts in the consumer's home and community, rather than in agency offices.

Formed in 1977, the CSP Branch at NIMH provided significant leadership in the shift in CMHCs toward the aforementioned principles. In 1992, NIMH was reorganized and the Substance Abuse and Mental Health Services Administration (SAMHSA) was created. The CSP branch moved to SAMHSA, where it was renamed the Center for Mental Health Services.

The CSP approach coincided with the expansion of community residential programs. Unlike the earlier transitional housing model, the CSP approach defined a new paradigm consisting of an array of housing alternatives with flexible time limits and no fixed linear progression (Ridgway & Zipple, 1990). By the mid-1980s, a national survey identified 4,500 community residential programs for people with SMI (Carling, 1988). Most of these programs were first funded during the 1980s, as prompted by additional CMHC requirements for residential services.

Supported Approaches

One of the most influential offshoots of the CSP movement was the growing emphasis on helping individuals in normal community settings outside the protected mental health settings. In the 1980s, as a logical extension to the CSP movement, "supported" approaches to achieving rehabilitation goals were first defined in the literature as more realistic alternatives to protected approaches (e.g., day treatment) and transitional approaches (e.g., transitional group homes). Supported approaches address the key areas of housing, employment, and education. In each of these areas, the strategy is to help consumers achieve normal adult roles in integrated settings of their own choosing by providing the professional and informal support needed to succeed in those settings. For example, *supported housing* involves identifying affordable housing and providing ongoing support for consumers to live independently in their own apartments. Proponents of supported housing have criticized transitional housing approaches for requiring individuals to complete a series of residential moves that are stressful, artificial, often contrary to personal preferences, and not always culminating in independent living (Carling, 1993).

Whereas the concept of supported housing originated within the mental health field, supported employment was first developed in the field of special education in the early 1980s as a more effective, humane, and cost-effective alternative to sheltered workshops for individuals with developmental disabilities (Wehman & Moon, 1988). Subsequently, supported employment was adapted for individuals with psychiatric disabilities (Becker & Drake, 2003; Danley & Anthony, 1987). *Supported employment* is intended for people with the most severe disabilities; it is defined as paid work that takes place in normal work settings with provision for ongoing support services (Final Regulations, State Supported Employment Services Program, 1987). As an extension of the supported employment concept, *supported education* was developed as a set of strategies to help consumers obtain education and training (in colleges, technical schools, community centers, and other educational settings not located within mental health or rehabilitation settings) in order to have the skills and credentials needed to obtain jobs with career potential (Carlson, Eichler, Huff, & Rapp, 2003; Mowbray, 2000).

Consistent with the psychiatric rehabilitation principle of environmental support as a means to promoting recovery, supported approaches have been developed for others areas of role functioning. Thus, Davidson and colleagues (Davidson, Shahar, Stayner,

Chinman, Rakfeldt, et al., 2004), have coined the term *supported socialization* to describe strategies to help consumers achieve social integration, consonant with their aspirations (Angell, 2003).

Legacy of CSP

The NIMH CSP Branch had a catalytic effect on mental health services throughout the United States. Its extramural research funding fostered evaluations of innovative programs (Anthony & Blanch, 1989). These studies showed the challenges of implementing programs according to well-defined program models (Brekke, 1988). The CSP Branch also helped nourish the consumer movement, as discussed below.

Although the CSP principles have had an enormously positive influence on community services for persons with psychiatric disabilities, one criticism was, and continues to be, that too often CMHCs have interpreted CSP principles to mean that CSP programs should assist consumers by creating protected settings within CMHCs, rather than supporting consumers to live and work and interact within the larger community (Bond, Saylers, Rollins, Rapp, & Zipple, 2004). In many CMHCs, prevocational programs have been surrogates for competitive jobs; group homes and mental health center-owned apartments have replaced normal tenancy; and recreation has been dominated by day treatment-sponsored affairs.

Psychosocial Rehabilitation Center Movement

Most authors acknowledge the role of the psychiatric rehabilitation center movement in the spread of psychiatric rehabilitation (Anthony et al., 2002; Becker & Drake, 2003; Dincin, 1975; Flexer & Solomon, 1993; Grob, 1983; Pratt et al., 1999; Rutman, 1987). While the U.S. mental health system was changing radically from an institution-based system of care to CMHC-based, and later CSP-based, system of care, the field of psychiatric rehabilitation developed, originally in parallel to and relatively independently of the mental health establishment. By the 1990s, however, these two fields merged.

Clubhouse Model

The origin of the field of psychiatric rehabilitation can be traced to the founding of Fountain House in New York City. In the 1940s, the precursor to Fountain House was a self-help group for patients discharged from Rockland State Hospital. With help from a charitable organization, the group acquired a mansion to serve as its meeting place. A charismatic social worker, John Beard, was appointed its first director, and his ideas were galvanizing (Beard, Propst, & Malamud, 1982). Operating outside the mental health system, the center became known as a *clubhouse*, because its identity evolved from a central meeting place for members to socialize. Many of the core values associated with psychiatric rehabilitation can be attributed to the clubhouse movement, including assumptions such as that individuals with SMI have an important role and responsibility for their own rehabilitation, that consumers do have the ability and the right to live normal lives, and that psychiatric rehabilitation should be a voluntary "membership" and not a series of appointments. In the clubhouse model, staff and member roles are blurred; if you visit a clubhouse, you may not be able to tell consumers from staff members. Beard et al. (1982) believed the clubhouse should make every member feel wanted and needed, in recognition of the basic human need for belongingness (Maslow, 1970).

Another basic human need is to be productive. Fountain House pioneered two key vocational concepts: the *work-ordered day* and *transitional employment* (Beard et al., 1982). With the work-ordered day, members participate in work units, performing chores around the clubhouse (e.g., preparing noonday meals, cleaning the building). Beard et al. (1982) theorized that a major benefit of the utilization of work crews is that members feel *needed* for the successful functioning of the clubhouse, in contrast to their usual feelings of worthlessness in most areas of their lives. Transitional employment placements consist of temporary, part-time community jobs commensurate with members' stamina and stress tolerance and designed to acclimate members to work and increase their self-confidence. These placements are arrangements with community employers and negotiated by clubhouse staff.

In 1977, Fountain House established a national training program on the clubhouse model. With the assistance of this training program, the number of clubhouses grew to 230 worldwide over the next decade. By the 1980s it became apparent that model diffusion was occurring, with many different types of programs describing themselves as clubhouses departing widely from the Fountain House model. In 1989, attendees at an international seminar on the clubhouse model endorsed 35 standards contained in the International Standards for Clubhouse Programs (Propst, 1992). To help ensure adherence to these standards, the Faculty for Clubhouse Development was established to conduct site visits and determine which programs would be accredited as "official" clubhouses. In 1994, the International Center for Clubhouse Development (ICCD) was established at Fountain House to serve as the umbrella organization for accredited clubhouses. ICCD's 2002 directory listed 250 clubhouses worldwide, similar to the number reported in a 1996 survey (Macias, Jackson, Schroeder, & Wang, 1999), of which about two-thirds were deemed "in substantial compliance" with the 35 clubhouse standards. This number does not include an unknown number of other programs described as clubhouses but not included in the ICCD directory. Among the 173 U.S. clubhouse programs responding to the 1996 survey, 72% were affiliated with a CMHC, 90% had work units, and 82% had a transitional employment program, with a mean of 12 transitional employment placements per clubhouse (Macias et al., 1999).

Other Psychosocial Rehabilitation Centers

Starting in the 1960s, the success of Fountain House spawned a national network of independent psychosocial rehabilitation centers, all originally located in urban areas. By 1975 this group included Thresholds (Chicago), Hill House (Cleveland), Horizon House (Philadelphia), Independence Center (St. Louis), Portals House (Los Angeles), Friendship House (Hackensack, New Jersey), Center Club (Boston), and Council House (Pittsburgh) (Dincin, 1975). Although sharing some of the Fountain House ideology, the centers began innovating and adopting diverse approaches relating to social rehabilitation (including recreational activities), vocational rehabilitation, housing, academic education, psychoeducation regarding illness and medications, physical health, intensive case management, supportive counseling, and family support (Weinstein & Hughes, 1997). For example, whereas the bedrock of the Fountain House approach is experiential learning, some agencies began implementing rehabilitation guided by a structured skills training model. Another difference was that some did not adopt the strident ideology of separation of rehabilitation and medical treatment found in the early years of Fountain House's development. These comprehensive centers introduced many programmatic innovations—in housing, outreach to new populations (e.g., mothers with SMI and their children, those who were hearing impaired and mentally ill, young adults), and new program services (e.g., academic tutoring, camping) (Dincin, 1995b).

In 1971, there were only 13 comprehensive psychiatric rehabilitation agencies in the United States (Weinstein & Hughes, 1997). Starting in the 1980s, psychiatric rehabilitation moved into the mainstream of community mental health, with psychiatric rehabilitation programs often part of the core offerings of CMHCs (Barton et al., 2001). The evolution of psychiatric rehabilitation programs has been shaped by funding sources, notably Medicaid, as discussed in Chapter 21. The number of psychiatric rehabilitation programs in the United States is unknown. On the basis of a national directory compiled in 1980 (International Association of Psychosocial Rehabilitation Services, 1990), Weinstein and Hughes (1997) concluded that there were 1,334 psychiatric rehabilitation programs serving an estimated 121,000 individuals daily in 1980. These authors estimated that the number had grown to 2,000 organizations by 1997.

Even when a psychiatric rehabilitation program is affiliated with a mental health center, there may be a physical, if not ideological, separation between the psychiatric rehabilitation program and the center's outpatient services (Bond, Dietzen, Vogler, Katuin, & McGrew, 1995; Lucca & Allen, 2001). And it is certainly true that there is great diversity among programs described as providing psychiatric rehabilitation services, regardless of what definition of psychiatric rehabilitation is used (Anthony, Cohen, & Farkas, 1982; Bond et al., 1995b; Burt, Duke, & Hargreaves, 1998; Lucca & Allen, 2001). In fact, some leaders within the psychiatric rehabilitation field have encouraged pluralism and eclecticism in the interests of innovation (Hughes & Clement, 1999; O'Brien & Anthony, 2002).

A converging finding across several state surveys is the relative dearth of vocational services in psychiatric rehabilitation, despite its roots in the primacy of work found in Fountain House (Bond et al., 1995b; Connors, Graham, & Pulso, 1987; Lucca & Allen, 2001). Social and recreational activities appear to be the common denominator of programs. Other surprising deficits found in one survey included substantial discrepancies between average membership enrollment and daily attendance, low percentages of peer-managed activities, and the predominance of services in traditional clinical settings (Lucca & Allen, 2001).

United States Psychiatric Rehabilitation Association

The practice of psychiatric rehabilitation today reflects the heterogeneity of its diverse roots. A unifying force is the International Association of Psychosocial Rehabilitation Services (IAPSRS), founded in 1976 as an organization of psychiatric rehabilitation agencies, practitioners, consumers, family members, and others dedicated to promoting, supporting, and strengthening community-oriented rehabilitation services through its annual conference, newsletter, publications, and lobbying efforts. Its membership numbers more than 400 organizations in addition to approximately 1,500 individual members. In 2003, IAPSRS split into two organizations, the United States Psychiatric Rehabilitation Association (USPRA), and Psychosocial Rehabilitation Canada/Réadaptation Psychosociale Canada (PSR/RPS Canada).

Consumer Movement

Because of the strong ethic of consumer empowerment in the clubhouse model, it is not surprising that the consumer self-help movement has historically had ties to psychiatric rehabilitation programs. Fountain House, in fact, evolved out of a self-help group. The term *self-help group* encompasses many different types of groups and organizations. Some self-help groups have been short-lived, and others have had an enduring impact. Some are single groups; others have evolved into organizations with extended networks. We can distinguish three different functions of self-help groups: mutual aid/peer support, consumer-operated services, and advocacy.

Mutual Aid/Peer Support

The best known of all self-help groups is Alcoholics Anonymous (AA) and its offshoots. Examples of peer support self-help organizations specifically for individuals with psychiatric disabilities are Recovery, Inc., founded in the 1930s and perhaps the oldest existing self-help organization for mental health consumers in the United States (Low, 1967) and an Australian-based self-help organization known as GROW (Roberts, Salem, Rappaport, Toro, Luke, et al., 1999). Reliable estimates of the number of peer support groups and their memberships are difficult, given their sometimes transitory existence, fluid memberships, and other definitional ambiguities, as well as lack of empirical data. A 1980 survey found that 3% of respondents with schizophrenia reported participating in self-help groups (Lieberman & Snowden, 1993).

Consumer-Operated Programs

Some groups have developed drop-in centers, offering friendship, social and recreational activities, and practical assistance (Trainor, Shepherd, Boydell, Leff, & Crawford, 1997). Other consumer-operated programs include consumer-run businesses (Krupa, 1998).

Consumer Advocates

During the 1980s mental health self-help activities started to coalesce into a national movement, sometimes referred to as the *ex-patient movement*, with the formation of an estimated 500 groups (Chamberlin, Rogers, & Sneed, 1989). These groups have advocated for patient rights, speaking out on failings of the mental health system, including issues related to involuntary treatment, the use of seclusion and restraint in hospitals, and lack of access to resources. The National Mental Health Consumers' Self-Help Clearinghouse in Philadelphia and the National Empowerment Center in Lawrence, Massachusetts, are two organizations representing this movement.

Family members have also been involved in developing self-help groups. Since its inception in 1979, the National Alliance on Mental Illness (NAMI), an organization for families, has grown to 1,200 state and local affiliates in the United States and a membership of 210,000 (*www.nami.org*). NAMI has become active on many fronts, including sponsoring anti-stigma campaigns, providing psychoeducational through its Family-to-Family program, and promoting the Program for Assertive Community Treatment.

Prosumers

Another trend influenced by the consumer movement has been the development of the role of *prosumers*, or consumers who are employed as direct service providers (Manos, 1993), for example, in case management (Felton, Stastny, Shern, Blanch, Donahue, et al.,

1995) and in supported employment (Mowbray, Bybee, & Collins, 2000) and supported housing (Besio & Mahler, 1993) programs. Prosumers have also been referred to as *consumers as colleagues*, to stress equality and respect for them as coworkers in psychiatric rehabilitation efforts (Solomon, Jonikas, Cook, & Kerouac, 1998). The role of prosumers appears to be far more accepted today in the professional community than even a decade ago. For example, Georgia's state mental health plan includes the hiring of 200 peer support specialists statewide.

Studies suggest that prosumers approach the role of case management differently than nonconsumer professionals, drawing more on their self-management techniques and role modeling in their interventions with service recipients (Lyons, Cook, Ruth, Karver, & Slagg, 1996; Paulson, Herinckx, Demmler, Clarke, Cutler, et al., 1999), and their presence in team meetings influences the way issues are discussed (Solomon & Draine, 1998). Gaining acceptance as a full-fledged member of a case management team is sometimes difficult (Basto, Pratt, Gill, & Barrett, 2000). The relative dearth of randomized controlled trials in this area suggests caution in overstating the positive impact of prosumers (Solomon & Draine, 2001).

Evidence-Based Practice

As we have been emphasizing in this chapter, the psychiatric rehabilitation field includes a panoply of approaches, many of them adapted from existing program models or invented *de novo* by program leaders. It is regrettable that probably more often than not, programs have been shaped by the funding streams that dictate how long services are offered, with whom, and when (Riggs, 1996; Clark, 1998), as discussed in more detail in Chapter 21. A great many of the influences on psychiatric rehabilitation practice have nothing to do with knowledge about what works.

Fortunately, over the past three decades, we have witnessed amazing strides in the development of effective service models for people with SMI. Yet even with the accumulation of positive research evidence, the psychiatric rehabilitation field, until recently, continued to espouse a pluralistic philosophy with a multiplicity of approaches considered "best practices" (Hughes & Weinstein, 1997a). In the 1990s a consensus started to emerge that some practices had achieved a sufficient critical mass of evidence warranting the designation "evidence-based practices" (EBPs), defined as "interventions for which there is consistent scientific evidence that they improve client outcome" (Drake, Goldman, Leff, Lehman, Dixon, et al., 2001b, p. 180). For example, Mueser, Drake, and Bond (1997c) identified five practices with the most compelling evidence at that time. In 1998, based on systematic literature reviews and expert surveys, the Schizophrenia Patient Outcomes Research Team (PORT) issued an influential report with 35 recommendations for psychopharmacological and psychosocial interventions for individuals with schizophrenia (Lehman, Steinwachs, & PORT Co-Investigators, 1998a). Paired with this report was a study of usual practice showing abysmally low rates of congruence with these recommendations (Lehman, Steinwachs, & PORT Co-Investigators, 1998b). An update of the PORT recommendations was issued in 2004 (Lehman et al., 2004). Other surveys have also repeatedly shown poor conformance between PORT recommendations and the services consumers actually receive (West, Wilk, Olfson, Rae, Marcus, et al., 2005).

Also in 1998, the Robert Wood Johnson Foundation sponsored a national consensus panel of mental health services researchers, consumers, family advocates, clinicians, and administrators, who identified six evidence-based practices for individuals with SMI (Drake et al., 2001). These six practices were (1) supported employment, (2) assertive community treatment, (3) illness management and recovery, (4) family psychoeducation, (5) integrated dual disorders treatment, and (6) medication management according to protocol. Supported employment and assertive community treatment are briefly described above; all six are described in detail in later chapters.

An important defining characteristic of an EBP is that it is well defined according to a set of operationally defined principles and therefore can be and has been replicated faithfully in diverse settings. Accordingly, *fidelity scales*, which are measures that assess the degree to which a particular program meets the standards of a program model (Bond, Evans, Salyers, Williams, & Kim, 2000a), have been developed for each of the EBPs. Two of these scales have been well validated (Bond, Becker, Drake, & Vogler, 1997; Teague, Bond, & Drake, 1998). A working hypothesis, that programs with high fidelity are more likely to achieve desired consumer outcomes, has been supported in some studies (Becker, Smith, Tanzman, Drake, & Tremblay, 2001b; McHugo, Drake, Teague, & Xie, 1999).

From the start, the list of practices identified in the Robert Wood Johnson Foundation meeting proved to be highly influential in shaping subsequent mental health policy in the United States at the federal, state, and local levels (Ganju, 2003). Evidence-based practice was promoted through two high-visibility federal reports that reinforced the need to increase access to effective services (New Freedom Commission on Mental Health, 2003; U.S. Department of Health and Human Services, 1999). However, the Robert Wood Johnson panel further concluded that simply identifying EBPs is not sufficient to ensure their adoption. A more systematic approach to dissemination was needed.

In 1999, the National EBP Project was launched to address the fact that dissemination of EBPs was hampered by the lack of comprehensive, easily accessible information on their implementation (Drake, Mueser, Torrey, Miller, Lehman, et al., 2000a; Mueser, Torrey, Lynde, Singer, & Drake, 2003d). In the first phase of this project, teams of researchers, practitioners, and consumers created "implementation resource kits" for each of the six EBPs (Torrey, Drake, Dixon, Burns, Rush, et al., 2001). The contents of these resource kits included materials to facilitate practice implementation, such as workbooks, key research articles, fidelity scales, and introductory and instructional videotapes. Accompanying these resource kits was a training-consultation model that included the following elements: (1) an implementation steering committee composed of key stakeholders (e.g., agency administrators, program leaders, family members, and consumers) who would guide the process, (2) introductory presentations intended to build enthusiasm, (3) skills training for practitioners, (4) systematic assessment of model fidelity, (5) ongoing consultation, and (6) measurement of key consumer outcomes (Torrey, Finnerty, Evans, & Wyzik, 2003). A recent study found encouraging outcomes for this complementation model (McHugo, Drake, Whitley, Bond, Campbell, et al., in press).

Evidence-based practice in mental health is part of a larger evidence-based medicine movement, which has quickly become a dominating influence in medical care. It has been described as the integration of best research evidence with clinical expertise and patient values (Institute of Medicine, 2001). Thus, evidence-based practice is not simply a list of approved practices but also incorporates the values of self determination, shared decision making, and individualization of services (Drake et al., 2003c; Essock, Goldman, Van Tosh, Anthony, Appell, et al., 2003). Further work is much needed to identify additional evidence-based practices as well as to continue refining the practices identified at the Robert Wood Johnson meeting.

CONTRIBUTIONS FROM ACADEMIA

Many individuals representing numerous agencies have contributed to the development of the concepts and practices described in this book, including administrators and practitioners in community settings, individuals within state mental health agencies, leaders within the consumer movement, and family members. Also influencing the field have been the contributions of researchers and educators in university settings. We mention five university-based groups among many that have made significant contributions.

The Center for Psychiatric Rehabilitation at Boston University was an early leader in the development of psychiatric rehabilitation theory and continues to influence the field. The center's director, William Anthony, played an important initial role in legitimizing the psychiatric rehabilitation field through his seminal papers (Anthony, 1977, 1982; Anthony, Buell, Sharratt, & Althoff, 1972). The first center funded by NIMH to focus specifically on psychiatric rehabilitation, the Center has been funded continuously since 1979. From the start, Anthony's conceptualization of psychiatric rehabilitation was heavily influenced by client-centered therapy and the work of Carkhuff (1972). Anthony and his colleagues developed a systematic client-centered approach to the psychiatric rehabilitation process for the individual practitioner, which includes identifying the overall rehabilitation goal, conducting a functional assessment, developing a rehabilitation plan, and providing skills training (Anthony et al., 2002). Anthony (1994) does not consider his approach to be a model, but rather a "technology" that can be superimposed on virtually any practice in almost any setting—including psychiatric hospitals, day treatment, clubhouses, and case management programs. Over the years this technology has been elaborated and refined in a series of training modules that have been disseminated worldwide (Farkas & Anthony, 1989). Another contribution of this group has been the "Choose-Get-Keep" model of psychiatric rehabilitation, which stresses the importance of consumer choice in the rehabilitation process (Danley & Anthony, 1987). Although originally developed for application to vocational rehabilitation, it has also been applied to other areas, such as housing programs for homeless persons with mental illness (Shern, Tsemberis, Anthony, Lovell, Richmond, et al., 2000) and case management (Goering, Wasylenki, Farkas, Lancee, & Ballantyne, 1988). Anthony has also popularized the concept of recovery as an organizing principle for conceptualizing psychiatric rehabilitation (Anthony, 1993).

The Dartmouth Psychiatric Rehabilitation Center, established in 1987 as a public academic liaison between the state mental health agency and Dartmouth Medical School, has had a major influence on the development of science-based approaches to psychiatric rehabilitation. Headed by Robert Drake, not only has the Center been the leader in defining and evaluating several of the most important psychiatric rehabilitation practices, such as supported employment (Becker & Drake, 2003) and integrated dual disorders treatment (Mueser, Noordsy, Drake, & Fox, 2003b), but Drake and his colleagues have also been the leaders of the evidence-based practice movement (Drake et al., 2000a), as discussed above.

Under the leadership of Robert Liberman, the UCLA Center for Research on Treatment and Rehabilitation of Psychosis has been developing and refining skills training modules since 1977. This research group has placed strong emphasis on theory-driven research, based on the stress-vulnerability model of SMI and social learning approaches to rehabilitation, and on rigorous empirical validation of the effects of their treatment methods on outcomes. They have developed modules for a wide range of skill areas, including vocational, dating, independent living, and medication management skills. In addition to wide scale dissemination of these modules this group has been noteworthy for its attention to the problem of generalization of skills learned in the clinic setting.

The University of Kansas School of Social Welfare, under the direction of Charles Rapp, has exerted a major influence on the psychiatric rehabilitation field through the strengths-based model of case management (Rapp & Goscha, 2006). Its staff has excelled in transforming the Kansas mental health system into a recovery-oriented, community-based system of care with a focus on outcomes. This group is known for its excellence in supported employment, supported education, and case management services. Another contribution of this group has been the identification of the central role of supervisors in determining the quality of services.

Chaired by Kenneth Gill, the Department of Psychiatric Rehabilitation and Behavioral Health Care at the University of Medicine and Dentistry of New Jersey (UMDNJ) is the only academic department in the United States devoted to psychiatric rehabilitation and the only one that provides every level of postsecondary education from the postsecondary certificate program through the doctoral level (Pratt & Gill, 2001). It enrolls more than 150 students each semester in its various degree programs.

Gill and his colleagues at UMDNJ have been leaders in developing the Psychiatric Rehabilitation Educators Group. In 2001, UMDNJ sponsored the first of what has become an annual meeting of educators in the fields of psychology, psychiatry, social work, rehabilitation counseling, and other mental health fields. Gill and other psychiatric rehabilitation educators also participated in the 2004 Annapolis Coalition on Behavioral Health Workforce Education, which aimed at the identification and assessment of work force competencies in mental health and substance abuse treatment (Hoge, Morris, Daniels, Huey, Stuart, et al., 2005).

COMPETENCIES OF PSYCHIATRIC REHABILITATION PRACTITIONERS

There have been many attempts to define the competencies needed to be an effective psychiatric rehabilitation practitioner (Coursey, Curtis, Marsh, Campbell, Harding, et al., 2000b; Friday & McPheeters, 1985; Gill, Pratt, & Barrett, 1997; Hoge, Jacobs, Belitsky, & Migdole, 2002; Hoge et al., 2005; Hughes & Weinstein, 1997b; Jonikas, 1994; Spaulding, Harig, & Schwab, 1987; Trochim & Cook, 1993; Young, Forquer, Tran, Starzynski, & Shatkin, 2000). Only recently have there been attempts to measure systematically the practitioner competencies (Casper & Oursler, 2003; Marrelli, Tondora, & Hoge, 2005; Chinman, Young, Rowe, Forquer, Knight, et al., 2003). Although some evidence has been found for factor validity and discrimination between novice and more experienced practitioners, using self-report inventories developed by these researchers, to date no rigorous research has shown that the knowledge, attitudes, and skills of practitioners relate to successful rehabilitation outcomes. Moreover, the conclusion of one expert panel is telling: It was unable to identify the unique competencies needed to be an effective psychiatric rehabilitation practitioner, as distinct from those needed to be effective in working with populations other than persons with psychiatric disorders (Sechrest & Pion, 1990). Indeed, the vocabulary for selecting new staff with native talents to work with this population has often been intuitive and imprecise. Thus, the description in this section is based primarily on clinical opinion. We discuss knowledge, attitudes, and skills in turn.

Knowledge

The knowledge base important for psychiatric rehabilitation practitioners includes both theoretical and practical knowledge. Content domains include abnormal psychology, psychopharmacology, counseling approaches, assessment, and information about psychiatric rehabilitation models and the history of deinstitutionalization. Practical knowledge includes the workings of the service systems (vocational rehabilitation, Social Security Administration, Medicaid, public housing, etc.) and information about local community resources.

Attitudes

Many observers have emphasized the importance of a core set of values and attitudes as a precondition to effectiveness. It is frequently noted that staff who are afraid of mental illness or who do not like people with SMI are poorly suited for this work. Dincin (1975) noted the importance of maintaining an attitude of hopefulness and optimism. Other desirable traits often mentioned include high energy, flexibility, persistence, creativity, problem-solving ability, orientation toward growth, and "street smarts" (Engstrom, Brooks, Jonikas, Cook, & Witheridge, 1992). On the basis of a qualitative study of managers of successful case management programs, Rapp (1993b) concluded that a particular constellation of values and attitudes were facilitative of positive consumer outcomes. Rapp's "principles of client-centered performance management" are (1) venerate the people called "clients," (2) create and maintain the focus, (3) possess a healthy disrespect for the impossible, and (4) learn for a living.

Skills

The range of skills needed to be an effective psychiatric rehabilitation practitioner is extensive, for example, as outlined by Coursey et al. (2000b). One fundamental set of skills involves empathic listening and motivational interviewing (Miller & Rollnick, 2002). Skills that facilitate positive, trusting relationships with consumers are fundamental, because of the role of a therapeutic alliance in effective psychiatric rehabilitation (Gehrs & Goering, 1994).

Characteristics of Psychiatric Rehabilitation Practitioners

A national survey in the early 1990s documented the characteristics of individuals working in the field (Blankertz & Robinson, 1996). The survey found that 34% provided day rehabilitation services (including clubhouses and social rehabilitation), 24% were case managers, 16% provided residential services, and only 6% provided vocational services. (The remaining 20% were supervisors or had less easily classified job titles.) The average age was 38, 65% were female, and 74% were European American. Of the individuals surveyed, 38% had a bachelor's degree, another 26% had a master's or doctorate, and 36% had not completed a bachelor's degree. Among college graduates, the predominant majors were as follows: psychology (27%), social work (16%), social sciences (6%), education (6%), and nursing (5%). Case manager surveys have found higher educational attainment, but a similar trend toward feminization of the work force (Boyer & Bond, 1999; Ellison, Rogers, Sciarappa, Cohen, & Forbess, 1995).

Given the ambiguities about the specific competencies needed, it is not surprising that there is little research on the effectiveness of training approaches to impact the skills needed to be an effective psychiatric rehabilitation professional, through either preservice or inservice training. In a survey of 81 mental health employers, 34% rated their bachelor's-level employees as unprepared (Gill et al., 1997). Gill concluded that academic curricula generally do not prepare students to work as psychiatric rehabilitation specialists.

Certification

Until recently, there have been no shared standards for what skills and competencies workers in the psychiatric rehabilitation field should have. Intended to "foster the growth of a qualified, ethical, and culturally diverse psychiatric rehabilitation workforce through a test based certification program and enforcement of a practitioner code of ethics," the Psychiatric Rehabilitation Certification Program of the United States Psychiatric Rehabilitation Association (USPRA) is directed by the Certification Commission, which was chartered in 2001. The CPRP examination is a 3-hour test with 150 multiple-choice items covering seven practice domains: Interpersonal Competencies; Professional Role Competencies; Community Resources; Assessment, Planning, and Outcomes; Systems Competencies; Interventions; and Diversity. Over 2000 professionals hold a CPRP and the CPRP credential is recognized by regulations defining and/or qualifying mental health practitioners in 12 states (*www.uspra.org*).

SUMMARY AND CONCLUSIONS

We have defined psychiatric rehabilitation as *systematic efforts to help adults with psychiatric disabilities move forward in their recovery process*. Over the last three decades, many different models have been developed, some based on specific ideologies, others developed in response to funding initiatives, and still others developed on a trial-and-error basis. In its evolution, the field has moved away from some early assumptions related to the concepts of *asylum* (consumers are best served in enclaves apart from mainstream community life), *separation of rehabilitation and medical models* (psychiatric rehabilitation programs should distance themselves from mental health treatment), and *transitionalism* (consumers are best helped through gradualistic, stepwise programs of preparation for community living). Many of these ideas have died hard, just as in an earlier era many practitioners stubbornly maintained their faith in psychodynamic interventions as a way to help consumers with SMI in the face of overwhelming evidence to the contrary. In fact, many practices continue to be offered despite the lack of evidence for their effectiveness, or worse, evidence that they interfere with the recovery process. As much as it is possible, this book aims at identifying and elaborating evidence-based psychiatric rehabilitation practices. However, our focus is not limited to these practices, for several reasons.

First, in addition to EBPs, we also describe *current psychiatric rehabilitation practices*, recognizing that these often fall far short of the ideal (Lehman et al., 1998b). We intend to make clear when there are deficiencies in current practice, which include (1) lack of access to practices that should be available (Hall, Graf, Fitzpatrick, Lane, & Birkel, 2003), (2) promotion of practices, such as day treatment, that are demonstrably less effective than evidence-based alternatives, and (3) inadequate implementation of evidence-based practices (Bond, 1991; Moser, DeLuca, Bond, & Rollins, 2004; Rosenheck, Neale, Leaf, Milstein, & Frisman, 1995).

Second, we include descriptions of *promising approaches*, which are interventions that have not been researched enough to warrant the label of evidence-based. So, for example, future studies may change the current tentative and cautious assessment of the effectiveness of some of the cognitive strategies described in Chapter 12.

Third, *consumer-run alternatives* represent a special category that warrants attention, despite an inadequate empirical base. Because of their voluntary nature, consumer-run approaches are difficult to evaluate using randomized controlled trials. Nonetheless, these "value-based services" should be encouraged as a complement to the formal mental health system (Frese, Stanley, Kress, & Vogel-Scibilia, 2001; Tracy, 2003). The history of mental health reform also suggests that consumer advocacy has had a tremendously positive effect on keeping priorities straight.

Fourth, we include *practices that address critical domains of functioning and/or critical issues*, even though at this point the literature is insufficient to designate any specific model or models as the best. In this category we include psychiatric rehabilitation approaches addressing housing, social networks, education, physical health, involvement with the criminal justice system, and trauma as examples. In each of these areas, program models have been developed and in some cases have been studied in rigorous research designs. Yet their status as evidence-based practice is in doubt. In the meantime, psychiatric rehabilitation programs must address these issues as best they can; the history of community mental health amply documents the disastrous consequences of ignoring such problems.

Part II

SERVICE APPROACHES

Human beings are complex, with individual aspirations varying across many domains. Hence, psychiatric rehabilitation is a vast and complex enterprise that includes individual practices across the breadth of life domains. Part II begins with a discussion on assessment, strategies for collecting information on strengths and disabilities that influence a person's life course. Our review presents assessment as an ongoing task that continues with the person throughout his or her involvement in rehabilitation. Nine separate chapters then review the discrete practices of rehabilitation. They address such basic needs as housing and employment. They include strategies to facilitate illness management and cognitive rehabilitation. They note the importance of other people in generally assisting in social relationships, as well as more specifically addressing the needs of the family and peers. These chapters specify the tools available to both the individual with disabilities and the rehabilitation team in helping a person master his or her disabilities and achieve personal hopes and goals.

Chapter 4

Rehabilitation Assessment

Assessment is the cornerstone of all intervention for persons with psychiatric disabilities. Understanding an individual's needs is the first step toward identifying the areas that are most important to address, and in evaluating the success of rehabilitation efforts. Therefore, assessment is involved in all aspects of rehabilitation, and skill in assessing individuals' needs is a prerequisite to effective work with people with psychiatric disabilities.

We begin this chapter with a discussion of the functions of assessment in psychiatric rehabilitation. Next, we discuss basic values and assumptions underlying the assessment process, such as the collaborative nature of assessment. We then discuss different methods for assessing rehabilitation needs, such as self-report and interview-based approaches, and consider the advantages and disadvantages of each. Next, we discuss the various domains of assessment for psychiatric rehabilitation, such as symptoms and adaptive functioning. Finally, we discuss treatment planning, monitoring treatment outcomes, and tailoring intervention to meet continuing or emerging needs.

FUNCTIONS OF ASSESSMENT

Assessment serves four broad, overlapping functions in psychiatric rehabilitation: (1) identification of treatment and rehabilitation needs; (2) assessment of the strengths and weaknesses of the individual, his or her family (or broader social network), and the environment; (3) developing a rehabilitation plan; and (4) monitoring progress and altering the rehabilitation plan as needed.

Identification of Rehabilitation Needs

Identifying psychosocial needs involves posing the question, What needs to be changed in order to reduce the impact of the psychiatric disability on the individual's life and his or her adjustment in the community? The different dimensions of personal life experience that can be influenced by psychiatric disability span a broad range, including mood (e.g., depression, anxiety, happiness), enjoyment of life, involvement in work or school, satisfaction with close relationships, self-care skills, substance abuse, health, and aggression. Adequate functioning across these different life areas is considered important to an individual's quality of life (Huxley, 1998).

In addition to an assessment of these broad areas of functioning, more specialized assessment may be conducted to evaluate the effect of specific symptoms or abilities on functioning. For example, examining the frequency and nature of specific psychotic symptoms may provide valuable information about an individual's anxiety or depression, because psychotic symptoms are often associated with these negative moods (Mueser, Douglas, Bellack, & Morrison, 1991c). Similarly, social skills assessment may be conducted to pinpoint specific skills that need to be taught in order to improve aspects of a person's social functioning (Bellack, Mueser, Gingerich, & Agresta, 2004). Specialized assessment may also be conducted to determine whether cognitive impairments contribute to functional, social, or vocational problems (Spaulding, Sullivan, & Poland, 2003).

Assessment of Strengths

Historically, psychiatric and psychosocial assessment has focused primarily on psychopathology and deficits and has neglected the role of strengths and capabilities. Although such a focus may address many of the problems experienced by people with a psychiatric disability, lack of attention to people's strengths can make them feel discouraged and inadequate. In addition, by not taking stock of personal strengths, the rehabilitation provider is not able to take full advantage of the individual's assets in working toward rehabilitation goals. To address these problems, the rehabilitation field has shifted toward capturing a more comprehensive picture of an individual's functioning, including his or her personal assets and strengths (Rapp, 1998b).

Strengths are broadly conceived as attributes that can be used to help an individual achieve personally valued goals. These attributes may be personal, social (i.e., residing in others with whom the individual has contact), or in the nonsocial environment. Examples of *personal strengths* include intelligence, determination, punctuality, affability, and a good sense of humor. Examples of *social strengths* include the support of a family member and interest in and enjoyment of the person by a friend, a loving partner, or concerned member of the clergy. Examples of *environmental strengths* include a local health club with a discount for people of low incomes, a pharmacy that provides daily pillboxes for medications, a local library, or a local inexpensive Internet café.

Helping people to become aware of their strengths can make them feel better about themselves and more hopeful about their future, while increasing their options for achieving rehabilitation goals. In the process of establishing rehabilitation goals, an inventory is taken of the person's strengths, while noting weaknesses, and a rehabilitation plan is formulated for achieving those goals by capitalizing on those strengths.

Development of a Rehabilitation Plan

For almost every conceivable rehabilitation goal, a variety of options are available for achieving that goal. Research evidence is often useful in identifying effective rehabilitation interventions. For example, research has shown that supported employment is more effective than other vocational rehabilitation models for helping people with psychiatric disabilities to find and keep competitive jobs (see Chapter 9). Similarly, research evidence indicates that social skills training is effective in helping people improve their social relationships (see Chapter 10). However, not everyone who participates in supported employment is successful in getting to work, and not everyone who receives social skills training improves his or her social relationships. Therefore, treatment planning requires an understanding about which interventions have been found to be effective for improving specific areas of functioning, as well as flexible, creative thinking to identify other ways of helping people achieve their goals when evidence-based practice is not helpful or to address areas of functioning for which evidence-based practices do not yet exist.

Monitoring Progress toward Goals

The final function of assessment is to monitor progress in achieving rehabilitation goals and to modify the plan as needed to address stubborn problems or emergent needs. Without ongoing monitoring of progress, it is impossible to know whether an individual is benefiting from rehabilitation. For practitioners, this lack of information can either be demoralizing (e.g., they may believe they are not helping the individual) or misleading (e.g., they believe they are helping the person when, in fact, they are not). For people with a psychiatric disability, the failure to monitor progress toward goals implies that the treatment team does not view these goals as important. This can lead individuals to devalue the importance of their own goals or can make them pessimistic about their ability to achieve their goals. Regular monitoring of goals, and modifying rehabilitation plans as needed, reinforces the importance of those goals as the basis for the therapeutic relationship (Bordin, 1976; Solomon, Draine, & Delaney, 1995b).

CORE VALUES IN PSYCHIATRIC REHABILITATION ASSESSMENT

A number of core values underlie the practice of psychiatric rehabilitation and are critical to the success of the assessment process. These values include collaboration, shared decision making, and consumer-centered goals identification.

Collaboration

The assessment of a consumer's needs and strengths and establishing rehabilitation goals is a collaborative process. Collaboration is important for many reasons. First, the goal of psychiatric rehabilitation is to help consumers overcome the effects of mental illness on their life, and therefore they must naturally be involved in deciding what changes are desired and how they should be accomplished. Second, active collaboration between the practitioner and the consumer, and with significant others such as family members, improves the likelihood of achieving rehabilitation goals by garnering support for working toward those goals and avoiding the problem of people working at cross-purposes with one another. And third, working together to establish goals facilitates development of a therapeutic alliance with the consumer and, along with it, trust, validation, and hope for the future (Goering & Stylianos, 1988).

Shared Decision Making

Shared decision making is a natural corollary of the principle of collaboration. Psychiatric treatment, like all medical care, has traditionally been delivered in a hierarchical fashion in which the provider simply instructs the "patient" on what to do. Over time, as options have increased and medical decision making has become more complex, there has been a movement toward sharing the decision-making process between the treatment provider and the recipient (Wennberg, 1988). Similarly, in psychiatric treatment and rehabilitation there has been a shift toward shared decision making between mental health practitioners and consumers (Fenton, 2003).

Shared decision making means that consumers are involved in making decisions about their treatment and rehabilitation, with the expectation that such collaboration leads to greater satisfaction with services and better outcomes (Hamann, Leucht, & Kissling, 2003). However, in order to make informed decisions, consumers need information about the nature of their problems and different options for addressing them (Mueser et al., 2002a). Shared decision making is always a goal of rehabilitation assessment. Often, as consumers become better informed about their psychiatric disability and the options for achieving goals, they become increasingly able to make their own decisions and to become directors of their own care. Rehabilitation providers must strive to nurture the decision-making capacity of the consumers with whom they work, and resist the temptation to make all the decisions for them, including those decisions for consumers who seem uninterested or incapable of being involved in their own treatment.

Consumer-Centered Goals

It should be evident from the preceding value that consumers' preferences about rehabilitation goals are of paramount importance. Consumers, like everyone else, differ in what they think is important. One consumer may place a high priority on returning to school or getting a job, and another may emphasize improving social relationships. Focusing on the goals that are most important to the consumer is the best way to enlist his or her involvement in goal setting and rehabilitation planning (Rapp, 1993a).

Although establishing consumer-centered goals is important, this does not mean that the practitioner should not also address other concerns that may have a bearing on the consumer's welfare. For example, a consumer may not believe that his use of drugs and alcohol is a problem, but the clinician may suspect that it interferes with functioning, such as in areas that the consumer wants to improve. Similarly, a consumer may believe that medication is not helpful, but the provider may be aware that the consumer is more cognitively disorganized and prone to symptom relapses when she does not take medication. During the assessment process the clinician can work toward instilling motivation to work on problems such as substance abuse or medication adherence by exploring with consumers whether those (or other) behaviors interfere with attaining their goals. When people perceive that certain behaviors interfere with their goals, they often become motivated to change those behaviors (Corrigan, McCracken, & Holmes, 2001c). Instilling motivation in this fashion is referred to as *motivational interviewing* (Miller & Rollnick, 2002) (see Chapter 15 for more discussion of motivational interviewing).

ASSESSMENT METHODS

A number of different methods can be used to conduct a rehabilitation assessment, including interviews with the consumer, the use of self-report questionnaires, obtaining information from informants (such as family members, inpatient staff, residential workers), and role-play or situational assessments. Each of these assessment approaches has advantages and disadvantages, which are discussed below.

Consumer Interviews

Interviewing involves obtaining information about an individual's needs and strengths by asking questions and engaging in conversations in specific topic areas. Interview-based approaches vary in their degree of structure, ranging from an unstructured format to fully outlined approach. An unstructured format is one in which the interview is organized around particular themes, but specific questions and follow-up probes are not used to elicit information. Semistructured and structured interviews differ mainly in the extent to which specific probes and follow-up questions are included as part of the interview. Structured interviews usually include specific questions to elicit information about particular areas of functioning and often specify follow-up questions as well. Semistructured interviews often provide specific guidance about initial and follow-up questions, without scripting the precise wording or constraining the interviewer in asking those questions.

Unstructured interviews also differ from more structured interviews in the coding of the consumer's responses. Information concerning an individual's functioning is often summarized descriptively in unstructured interviews, whereas semistructured and structured interviews usually provide a quantitative method for summarizing information. For example, with the use of the Structured Clinical Interview for the *Diagnostic and Statistical Manual of Mental Disorders*, 4th edition (DSM-IV) (First, Spitzer, Gibbon, & Williams, 1997b), an instrument for establishing psychiatric diagnoses, specific symptoms are rated on a 3-point scale: 1 = not present, 2 = not clear, 3 = definitely present. A psychiatric diagnosis is then established by ascertaining which specific symptoms of the disorder the individual has and whether other factors such as substance use can account for the symptoms. For another example, the quality of specific aspects of social functioning or the severity of psychiatric symptoms is often rated on a fixed scale, with low numbers representing better functioning or less severe symptoms.

There are a number of advantages to structured interviews over unstructured interviews. First, when the questions to be asked are specified, differences between interviewers due to style or specific wording can be minimized. Eliminating interviewer differences improves the precision of the assessment. Second, structured interviews tend to be more comprehensive than unstructured interviews because they are designed to tap different areas of functioning related to rehabilitation. This specificity is difficult to achieve without providing clear guidelines to the interviewer. Third, summarizing assessment data quantitatively, as provided in semistructured and structured interviews but not unstructured interviews, facilitates the comparison of different consumers with one another, as well as the evaluation of changes in a consumer's functioning over time. It may be useful to be able to compare the functioning of different consumers for treatment planning purposes, such as forming a group of consumers who want to learn how to cope better with their symptoms of depression. It is important to be able to evaluate changes in functioning over time in consumers to determine whether they are making progress toward achieving their desired goals.

Although there are important advantages of structured interviews over unstructured ones, there are also some disadvantages. More training is usually required to learn how to use structured or semistructured interviews. Structured interviews necessarily constrain the interview because of the focus on particular areas of functioning. These interview formats may not provide much leeway to delve into other areas of functioning, some of which may be important to consumers. In addition, structured interviews are not available for assessing every area of functioning, and unstructured formats may be required to understand consumers' functioning in some areas. Considering their advantages and disadvantages, effective rehabilitation assessment usually involves a combination of unstructured and structured interviewing.

Self-Report Questionnaires

Self-report questionnaires are usually paper-and-pencil or computer-based questionnaires in which consumers respond to a series of specific questions about symptoms, functioning, or satisfaction in particular domains. Responses to these questions are provided in either a yes/no format or on a continuum, such as on a 4-point scale ranging from 1 (not a problem), to 4 (severe problem). Like the data obtained in structured interviews, the quantitative data gathered in self-report questionnaires can be summarized to provide an index of functioning in a particular area.

Self-report questionnaires are used to evaluate functioning in a wide range of areas. For example, distress related to depression, anxiety, or health concerns can easily be rated with self-report questionnaires. Substance use problems are often rated with self-report questionnaires, as well as engagement in high-risk behaviors, such as sexual behaviors that may increase the risk of contracting infectious diseases.

Self-report questionnaires have a number of distinct advantages. They tend to be efficient because they require the practitioner only to give the consumer instructions and to score the questionnaire (although additional time may be needed to explain questions). A related advantage is that self-report questionnaires can be used in group settings of consumers because everyone can complete a questionnaire at the same time. Self-report questionnaires can be especially useful as an alternative to directly asking people about certain behaviors that are considered socially undesirable. For example, research has shown that individuals are more likely to acknowledge the use of drugs and certain sexual behaviors (e.g., homosexual behavior) when completing a computer-based self-report assessment than when responding to a live interviewer (Turner, 1998).

Despite these advantages, there are some disadvantages of self-report questionnaires. Written self-report questionnaires require good reading skills, which not all consumers have. Some computer-administered questionnaires provide a solution to this difficulty by asking the questions aloud, although these devices are not routinely available at this time. Another disadvantage of self-administered questionnaires is that there is no opportunity to correct misunderstandings that may occur when completing the questionnaire because there is little interaction with the practitioner. In addition, some areas of functioning may be more difficult for individuals to rate than others. For example, psychotic symptoms, especially delusions, are difficult to assess with self-report questionnaires, as is cognitive impairment. Finally, some consumers may be reluctant to report socially undesirable behaviors even in self-report questionnaires. For example, consumers often underreport their use of drugs and alcohol (Barbee, Clark, Craqanzano, Heintz, & Kehoe, 1989), high-risk sexual behavior (Cournos & McKinnon, 1997), and lack of medication adherence (Weiden, Mott, & Curcio, 1995).

Informant-Based Assessments

Informant-based assessments involve obtaining information about a consumer's functioning from someone who knows him or her well, such as a family member, friend, or another treatment provider. People are often not very accurate observers of their own behavior. The accuracy of self-observation may be further compromised when an individual has significant cognitive impairments or when he or she has altered perceptions of reality (such as psychotic symptoms), both of which are common challenges for individuals with psychiatric disabilities. Obtaining information from others who know the consumer well is a useful strategy for overcoming the many limitations of assessments based on consumers' self-reported functioning.

Informant-based assessments are generally conducted with interviews, and, like consumer-based interviews, they may vary in their degree of structure. Also like consumer-based interviews, structured interviews with informants have several advantages over unstructured assessments; for example, they standardize the way in which information is elicited and they yield quantitative data that can be used for treatment planning and outcome evaluation. Because significant others and clinicians tend not to be privy to the internal experiences of consumers, informant-based assessments are limited to areas of functioning that can be directly observed. Thus, informant-based assessments can be used to judge an individual's social appropriateness, degree of connection and association with others, work performance, independent living skills, substance use and consequences, and leisure time.

The major advantage of informant-based assessments is that they provide an independent perspective on the consumer's functioning, which can be useful in understanding how an individual fits into his or her social context. At the same time, an independent perspective on the consumer's functioning is not necessarily more objective; informants can have their own personal biases that may distort information in particular ways. For example, informant ratings may be biased by the person's desire to portray the consumer in a positive or negative light, depending on the nature and quality of relationship with the consumer.

Another advantage of informant-based assessments is the potentially greater awareness informants may have of the social norms within the community in which the consumer lives. Some individuals with psychiatric disabilities have significant difficulties in social cognition (Penn, Corrigan, Bentall, Racenstein, & Newman, 1997a), which includes the ability to perceive and understand common social conventions. Not understanding social norms can make it difficult for an individual to rate his or her own social functioning with respect to community norms. Informant-based ratings can bypass this problem.

Despite the advantages of informant-based assessments, several disadvantages should be noted. Many consumers are unable to identify an informant who can provide information about their functioning. Even when informants are identified, they may be difficult to contact or require multiple efforts to successfully contact. In addition, some consumers can, but are unwilling to, identify an informant who can be contacted.

Informant ratings based on clinicians' observations may be somewhat easier to obtain, because their jobs involve working with consumers and they are therefore easier to identify. However, because of the many demands on mental health practitioners' time, it can be difficult to enlist their cooperation in providing information about consumers' functioning. In addition, rehabilitation providers vary greatly as to their knowledge of consumers' functioning in the community, and they may therefore be able to provide very limited amounts of information about some consumers.

Role-Play or Situational Assessments

Role-play or situational assessments are evaluations conducted in simulated or real-life situations. For example, role-play tests are often used to evaluate social skills by seeing how an individual performs in a pretend social interaction (Bellack et al., 2004;

Liberman, DeRisi, & Mueser, 1989b; Patterson, Moscona, McKibbin, Hughs, & Jeste, 2001). Several standardized and well-validated measures of social skills and problem solving have been developed and validated for persons with psychiatric disabilities (Bellack, 2006; Donahoe, Carter, Bloem, Hirsch, Laasi, et al., 1990). Situation-based assessments of work performance involve evaluating an individual in either a simulated work situation or an actual work-related interaction (Bond & Friedmeyer, 1987). The person's performance can then be evaluated, providing detailed information about specific skills and problems related to functioning in particular areas. Rehabilitation efforts can then focus on those areas identified in the assessment.

Role-play and situational assessments have the advantage of providing the most detailed information about specific strengths and areas of impairment, as compared with other assessment methods. This information can be helpful in rehabilitation planning inasmuch as greater specificity helps to narrow the focus of rehabilitation efforts. It can also be useful in determining whether certain rehabilitation approaches are successful at improving the most immediate focus of intervention, specific functional abilities (McKibbin, Brekke, Sires, Jeste, & Patterson, 2004). The primary disadvantage of these types of assessments is that they are time-consuming, and many mental health practitioners lack the time, resources, and skills to perform such assessments. Thus, in many settings, direct assessments of functional abilities are not conducted in routine rehabilitation practice, but may be included in research on rehabilitation programs.

SPECIFIC DOMAINS OF ASSESSMENT

In this section we discuss the wide range of domains important to rehabilitation assessment and treatment planning. For each domain, we first discuss its relevance to psychiatric rehabilitation. Then we describe the nature of the domain, followed by specific assessment strategies and instruments.

Diagnosis

Psychiatric diagnosis often has important treatment indications for individuals with psychiatric disabilities (see Chapter 1). The most important implication is that diagnosis is strongly related to a determination of which medications are most likely to reduce symptoms and prevent relapses. Specifically, abundant evidence shows that antipsychotic medications are most effective in the treatment of schizophrenia and schizoaffective disorder (Davis, Barter, & Kane, 1989; Davis, Chen, & Glick, 2003), mood stabilizing medications (such as lithium and valproic acid) are most effective for the treatment of bipolar disorder (Goodwin & Jamison, 2007), and antidepressant medications are most effective for the treatment of depression and anxiety disorders (such as panic disorder and obsessive–compulsive disorder) (Schatzberg, Cole, & DeBattista, 2007). Thus, knowing an individual's diagnosis can help clinicians select the most promising pharmacological interventions.

In addition to providing guidance for pharmacological treatment, diagnostic information can be helpful in identifying specific psychotherapeutic approaches. Some types of psychotherapy have been developed to specifically address symptoms and functioning in a particular diagnostic group. For example, specific cognitive-behavioral treatment approaches have been developed to address a range of different disorders, such as schizophrenia and schizoaffective disorder (Kingdon & Turkington, 2004), bipolar disorder (Newman, Leahy, Beck, Reilly-Harrington, & Gyulai, 2002), major depression (Beck, Rush, Shaw, & Emery, 1979), social anxiety disorder (Heimberg & Becker, 2002), panic disorder (Barlow, 2002), posttraumatic stress disorder (Foa & Rothbaum, 1998), obsessive–compulsive disorder (Clark, 2004), and borderline personality disorder (Linehan, 1993b). Aside from pharmacological and psychotherapeutic treatment recommendations, psychiatric diagnosis is of less importance for rehabilitation planning.

Assessment Instruments

Both self-report questionnaires and standardized interviews can be used to diagnose psychiatric disorders. With respect to major clinical disorders, self-report questionnaires are most useful for screening disorders, which are followed up with interviews to confirm a suspected disorder. For example, the Psychiatric Diagnostic Screening Questionnaire (Zimmerman & Mattia, 2001a) was developed to screen for the broad range of psychiatric disorders across a variety of clinical populations, such as persons presenting for treatment at medical settings, substance abuse treatment settings, and mental health centers, and has been shown to be strongly predictive of diagnoses based on structured interviews (Zimmerman & Mattia, 2001b; Zimmerman, Sheeran, Chelminski, & Young, 2004). The strong consensus in the field is that interviewing an individual is necessary in order to firmly establish a psychiatric disorder, which often needs to be supplemented with additional information provided by significant others such as family members or other treatment providers. The importance of obtaining additional information from people who know the individual well is especially high when diagnosing schizophrenia, schizoaffective disorder, and bipolar disorder inasmuch as these disorders often involve a lack of insight, as characterized by symptoms such as paranoia and grandiose delusions. Great skill is involved in diagnostic and other clinical interviewing, and there are many helpful books on this topic (Hersen & Turner, 2004; Rogers, 2001; Shea, 1988).

In the United States, the clear "gold standard" for assessing diagnosis is the Structured Clinical Interview for DSM-IV (SCID; First et al., 1997b). The SCID is the most widely used diagnostic assessment instrument in research studies of persons with psychiatric disabilities in the United States. Briefer versions of the SCID have been developed to aid in the diagnosis of psychiatric disorders in specific clinical settings, such as the Primary Care Evaluation of Mental Disorders (PRIME-MD). Extensive work has been conducted to develop and validate efficient interview instruments that can be used by nonclinicians to establish psychiatric disorders, mainly for large-scale epidemiological studies requiring numerous interviews. For example, the Diagnostic Interview Schedule (Helzer & Robins, 1988) has been used extensively in epidemiological studies, although it has less sensitivity and specificity for detecting psychiatric disabilities than clinical interviews such as the SCID (Malgady, Lloyd, & Tryon, 1992). Various interview instruments for diagnosing major psychiatric disorders are described in Table 4.1.

As with clinical disorders, a variety of semistructured interviews have been developed in order to diagnose personality disorders according to DSM-IV or *International Classification of Diseases*, 10th edition (ICD-10) criteria. Some of the most commonly employed interview instruments for assessing personality disorders are summarized in Table 4.2. In addition to these interview instruments, numerous self-administered personality tests have been designed to measure different dimensions of personality, in both the general and clinical populations, such as the Revised NEO Personality Inventory (Costa

TABLE 4.1. Instruments for Diagnosing Major Psychiatric Disorders

Instrument	Primary application	Focus	Administration time	Advantages	Disadvantages
Structured Clinical Interview for DSM-IV (First et al., 1997b)	Clinical/research	All Axis I disorders	1–2 hours	• Documented reliability and validity • Covers all major disorders • Considered "gold standard" for diagnosis of psychiatric disorders	• Extensive training required • Limited depth of symptom assessment
Comprehensive Assessment of Symptoms and History (Andreasen, Flaum, & Arndt, 1992)	Research	Psychotic, mood, and substance use disorders	2 hours	• In-depth assessment of psychotic and negative symptoms • Good reliability and validity of data	• Extensive training required • Covers limited range of disorders
Present State Examination—10th Edition (World Health Organization, 1992)	Clinical/research	All Axis I disorders	2–3 hours	• Provides comprehensive assessment of symptoms • Translated into numerous languages and widely used outside the United States • Strong reliability and validity	• Requires extensive training • Does not map directly onto DSM-IV disorders
Composite International Diagnostic Interview (CIDI) (World Health Organization, 1997)	Epidemiological research	All Axis I disorders	1–2 hours	• Can be administered by paraprofessionals • Reliable for current episodes • Moderate training required	• Reliability and validity of data favor DIS over CIDI • Most research conducted outside North America

Instrument	Purpose	Disorders	Time	Strengths	Limitations
Diagnostic Interview Schedule–IV (DIS–IV) (Robins et al., 1995)	Epidemiological research	All Axis I disorders	1–2 hours	• Can be administered by paraprofessionals • Extensive reliability and validity of data • Self-administered version available	• Limited assessment of symptom severity • Complex judgments required about etiology of symptoms
Schedule for Affective Disorders and Schizophrenia (Endicott & Spitzer, 1978)	Research	Schizophrenia and mood disorders	1–2 hours	• Provides extensive information about duration and intensity of symptoms • Strong psychometric properties	• Requires extensive training • Long time to administer
Royal Park Multidiagnostic Instrument for Psychosis (McGorry, Kaplan, Dossetor, Copolov, & Singh, 1988)	Research/clinical	Psychotic disorders	1–2 hours	• Specific focus on psychosis	• Limited psychometric studies conducted
Mini-International Neuropsychiatric Interview (Sheehan, Lecrubier, Sheehan, Amorim, Janavis, et al., 1998)	Clinical	Most major Axis I disorders	15 minutes	• Designed to be administered by paraprofessionals • Brief but accurate identification of major disorders	• More extensive assessment required to confirm diagnoses

& McCrae, 1992), the Millon Clinical Multiaxial Inventory-II (Millon, 1982), and the Minnesota Multiphasic Personality Inventory-2 (Butcher, Dahlstrom, Graham, Tellegen, & Kaemmer, 1989). These self-administered tests are not considered further here because their relevance for rehabilitation of persons with psychiatric disabilities remains to be determined.

Symptomatology

Evaluating symptom severity is important because it is often related to distress, which can interfere with functioning as well as enjoyment of life. In addition, the assessment of symptoms provides an important outcome by which to measure the success of psychiatric treatment and rehabilitation efforts. By definition, individuals with psychiatric disabilities usually experience such disabilities over long periods of time. Although treatment and rehabilitation efforts usually do not eliminate psychiatric disabilities altogether, they may be successful at reducing the severity of symptoms and the suffering associated with them. Therefore, it is important to be able to assess symptom severity in order to determine whether a consumer needs help in managing a particular symptom and whether interventions are successful in reducing its severity.

Assessment Instruments

A wide range of instruments have been developed to evaluate the severity of psychiatric symptoms. In general, these instruments can be divided into self-report and interview-based instruments. Self-report instruments provide a good, valid measure of the severity of mood problems in persons with psychiatric disabilities. For example, the Beck Depression Inventory is the standard self-report instrument in the field and has been shown to be very accurate for the measurement of depression (Beck, Steer, & Garbin, 1988) and as a screening instrument for the detection of major depressive disorder. However, self-report instruments are less useful for measuring psychotic symptoms, negative symptoms, or cognitive impairments. Self-report instruments that query consumers as to the frequency and distress associated with psychotic symptoms, such as the Symptom Checklist-90 (SCL-90; Derogatis, 1977), tend to produce general measures of distress, but not independent measures of the severity of psychotic symptoms.

Psychiatric rating scales based on semistructured interviews have been developed to provide an objective measure of common symptoms. These scales typically contain between 20 and 50 specifically defined items, each rated on a severity scale with 5–7 points. Some scales have been developed to measure the full range of psychiatric symptoms, such as the Brief Psychiatric Rating Scale (BPRS; Lukoff, Nuechterlein, & Ventura, 1986) and the Positive and Negative Syndrome Scale (Kay, Opler, & Fiszbein, 1987), and others have been designed to tap specific dimensions, such as the Scale for the Assessment of Negative Symptoms (Andreasen, 1984) and the Hamilton Depression Rating Scale (Hamilton, 1960).

Interview-based psychiatric rating scales typically include a combination of symptoms elicited through direct questioning and symptoms observed in the course of the interview. For example, on the BPRS, depression is rated by asking questions such as "What has your mood been lately?" and "Have you been feeling down?" Mannerisms and posturing, however, are rated on the basis of the interviewer's observations of the individual's behavior. Psychiatric symptoms scores can either be added for an overall index of symptom severity based on a rating scale, or summarized in subscale scores cor-

TABLE 4.2. Instruments for Assessing Personality Disorders

Instrument	Primary application	Focus	Administration time	Advantages	Disadvantages
Structured Interview for DSM-IV Personality Disorders (Pfohl & Zimmerman, 1995)	Research/clinical	DSM-IV personality disorders	60–90 minutes	• Extensive research supporting reliability and validity • Well-developed probe questions	• Lack of cross-cultural studies • Requires extensive training
International Personality Disorder Examination (Loranger, 1999)	Research/clinical	ICD-10 and DSM-IV personality disorders	3 hours	• Good psychometric data • Attention to cultural issues • In-depth assessment of symptoms	• Length of administration • Unclear validity of DSM-IV Cluster A personality disorders
Structured Interview for DSM-IV Personality Disorders (First et al, 1997b)	Research/clinical	DSM-IV personality disorders	30–45 minutes	• Good diagnostic reliability and validity • Easy to administer and interpret • Little training required	• Does not provide information on symptom severity
Personality Disorder Interview–IV (Widiger, Mangine, Corbitt, Ellis, & Thomas, 1995)	Research	DSM-IV personality disorders	2 hours	• Can be administered by paraprofessionals	• Limited data on validity • Complex questions limit use in psychiatric disabilities
Revised Diagnostic Interview for Borderlines (Gunderson & Zanarini, 1992)	Clinical/research	Gunderson's model of borderline personality disorder	50–90 minutes	• Extensive psychometric data support	• Limited psychometric data • Not a measure of DSM-IV borderline personality disorder
Psychopathy Checklist Revised (Hare, 1991)	Forensic/research	Cleckley's concept of psychopathic personality (Cleckley, 1976)	1.5–2 hours	• Extensive research supports reliability and validity • Provides dimensional ratings	• Requires extensive training to administer • Validity not established in persons with psychiatric disabilities

responding to symptom dimensions such as negative, positive, and affective symptoms. Scales for assessing symptoms in persons with psychiatric disabilities are summarized in Table 4.3.

Social Functioning

Problems of social functioning are a core feature of mental illnesses and are included as part of the diagnostic criteria for some disorders, such as schizophrenia (American Psychiatric Association, 1994). Problems in the quality and extent of social relationships often predate the onset of psychiatric illnesses and continue to hamper the enjoyment of life for many consumers. Because the enjoyment of close personal relationships is an important part of living for most people, improving social relationships is a common goal of psychiatric rehabilitation.

In addition to improving quality of life, better social functioning can also serve as a protective factor for improving the course of the psychiatric illness (Liberman, Mueser, Wallace, Jacobs, Eckman, et al., 1986). Good social functioning and associated social support may be beneficial for several reasons. First, good relationships with others may help give consumers meaning in life, reasons to live, and motivation to take care of themselves. Second, social support can buffer the negative effects of stress, making individuals less vulnerable to stress-induced relapses. Third, having close relationships with other people can provide opportunities for reality testing, which may be especially beneficial for individuals with psychotic symptoms. Abundant evidence documents that people with better social functioning and greater levels of social support experience a more benign course of their mental illness (Buchanan, 1995; Erickson, Beiser, Iacono, Fleming, & Lin, 1989; Wells, Miranda, Bruce, Alegria, & Wallerstein, 2004). Thus, improving social support is an important goal for rehabilitation, and the assessment of social functioning is critical to evaluating the success of the efforts to achieve such improvement.

Assessment Instruments

Interview-based methods are often useful for assessing individuals' social functioning, especially when interviews with consumers can be supplemented with information from significant others. Such information can be especially valuable for consumers who are less aware of how they are perceived by others. When multiple perspectives on an individual's social functioning are obtained, comparing the different reports can permit the "triangulation" of information, yielding the best possible picture of an individual's social functioning.

A wide range of instruments have been developed and validated for assessing the social functioning of persons with psychiatric disabilities. The most rigorous of these instruments are based on interviews with the consumer (and sometimes a significant other as well) and can be relatively time-consuming to administer, requiring on average between 30 and 60 minutes. Many measures of social functioning provide specific subscale scores. For example, the Social Adjustment Scale II (Schooler, Hogarty, & Weissman, 1979) provides subscale scores for the following dimensions of social functioning: family, extended family, friends, romance, leisure/recreation.

Aside from interview-based instruments that delve specifically into different dimensions of social functioning, other instruments provide a more general assessment of the adequacy of an individual's functioning in the community or some other context (e.g., residence). General functioning scales, such as the Multnomah Community Ability Scale

TABLE 4.3. Commonly Used Measures of Psychiatric Symptoms

Scale	Format	No. of items	Symptom focus	Administration time	Advantages	Disadvantages
Interview-based instruments						
Brief Psychiatric Rating Scale, Expanded Version (Lukoff et al., 1986)	Interview	24	General symptoms	20 minutes	• Widely used • Captures broad range of symptoms • Relatively brief	• Requires interviewer training • Limited assessment of negative and cognitive symptoms
Positive and Negative Syndrome Scale (Kay et al., 1987)	Interview	30	General symptoms	30 minutes	• Widely used • Captures broad range of symptoms • Good assessment of negative and cognitive symptoms	• Requires interviewer training
Scale for the Assessment of Negative Symptoms (Andreasen, 1984)	Interview	23	Negative symptoms	20 minutes	• Most in-depth assessment of negative symptoms available	• Requires interviewer training
Comprehensive Psychopathological Rating Scale (Åsberg, Montgomery, Perris, Schalling, & Sedvall, 1978)	Interview	67	General symptoms	35 minutes	• Comprehensive assessment instrument	• Requires interviewer training • Used mainly in Europe
Hamilton Rating Scale for Depression (Hamilton, 1960)	Interview	21	Depression	15 minutes	• Specific focus on depression	• Primary focus on vegetative symptoms of depression
Nurses Observation of Inpatient Evaluation (Honigfeld & Kleff, 1976)	Staff observation	30	General symptoms	10 minutes	• Focus on inpatient symptomatic behavior	• No subjective assessment of symptoms

(continued)

TABLE 4.3. (continued)

Scale	Format	No. of items	Symptom focus	Administration time	Advantages	Disadvantages
Self-report-based instruments						
Symptom Checklist-90-R (SCL-90) (Derogatis, 1977)	Self-report	90	General symptoms	30 minutes	• Covers broad range of symptoms	• Chiefly measures distress
Brief Symptom Inventory (Derogatis, 1993)	Self-report	53	General symptoms	15 minutes	• Covers broad range of symptoms • Briefer than SCL-90	• Like SCL-90, chiefly measures distress
Beck Depression Inventory-II (Beck et al., 1988; Beck, Steer, & Brown, 1996)	Self-report	24	Depression	10 minutes	• Widely used • Sensitive to depression	
Behavior and Symptom Identification Scale (Eisen, Dill, & Grob, 1994)	Self-report	32	General symptoms	10 minutes	• Covers broad range of symptoms	• Chiefly measures distress

(Barker, Barron, & McFarlane, 1994), are most often completed by practitioners who are privy to information about the individual's functioning and are less time-consuming to complete because they do not require direct interviews. The advantage of more general measures of functioning is that they are easy to administer and can provide a useful summary of an individual's functioning in the community. The disadvantage is that because of their global nature they are often unsuitable for pinpointing specific areas in need of rehabilitation. Although more detailed assessment instruments may be more time-consuming, they are also useful in yielding more specific information that can serve as a basis for identifying and planning rehabilitation needs.

Common instruments used for the assessment of social functioning (and the related domains of role functioning and independent living skills) in persons with psychiatric disabilities are summarized in Table 4.4.

Role Functioning

Role functioning refers to the extent to which an individual is able to meet the expectations of socially defined roles, such as worker, student, parent, or spouse. Role functioning is often included as a dimension of social functioning, and it is strongly related to the quality of social relationships and use of leisure time. However, pragmatically it is useful to distinguish role functioning from the quality of social relationships, as impairment in this area of functioning is critical to the definition of disability.

Assessment Instruments

Some aspects of vocational functioning are relatively easily assessed, whereas others are more challenging. The assessment of work is probably most direct. Work can be measured by obtaining information such as the type of job an individual has, the wages and benefits paid, the number of hours worked, and the person's satisfaction with his or her job. Work history information may be similarly obtained, such as prior jobs the individual has worked at, longest duration of competitive employment, wages and hours worked at the last competitive job, and reasons for termination of employment. These measures are readily obtained through direct interview with the consumer.

Some structured interviews of social functioning also contain questions concerning work performance, such as the Social Adjustment Scale-II (Schooler et al., 1979). Observational measures of the quality of vocational functioning have also been developed, such as the Work Behavior Inventory (Lysaker, Bell, Bryson, & Zito, 1993). Observational measures such as these rely on another individual, such as the employer, to complete them. Therefore, these measures are limited to vocational settings in which the consumer has disclosed his or her disability to the employer.

Despite the prominent difficulties many consumers experience in the areas of school, parenting, and spouse or partner relationships, there is a dearth of well-established instruments for evaluating functioning in these domains. For parenting skills, measures developed in the general population can be used, but there have been limited efforts to develop specialized assessments for persons with psychiatric disabilities.

Independent Living and Self-Care Skills

Like difficulties in social relationships and role functioning, difficulty in caring for oneself and living independently is a major problem for many individuals with psychiatric dis-

TABLE 4.4. Commonly Used Measures of Social and Adaptive Functioning

Scale	Respondent	Format	No. of items	Domains	Administration time	Advantages	Disadvantages
Specific Assessment Scales							
Social Adaptive Functions Scale (Harvey et al., 1997)	Staff	Staff report	17	Community living, self-care, social skills, recreation, cooperation	15 minutes	• Brief, broad assessment, easy to complete	• Requires knowledge of consumer daily functioning
Social Behavior Schedule (Wykes & Sturt, 1986)	Staff	Interview/ Staff report	30	Social mixing, symptomatic behavior, leisure, work, activity level	20 minutes	• Broad assessment of social behavior	• Requires knowledge of consumer functioning
Social Adjustment Scale–II (Schooler et al., 1979)	Consumer, relative	Interview	75 (consumer) 68 (relative)	Consumer and relative: instrumental role, finances, household, extended family, social/leisure. Relative only: personal well-being, burden/ satisfaction	45 minutes (each)	• Very comprehensive assessment of social functioning	• Time-consuming to administer • Requires interviewer training
Social Functioning Scale (Birchwood, Smith, Cochrane, Wetton, & Copestake, 1990)	Consumer, relative	Interview	85 (consumer) 86 (relative)	Social, recreation, independence	45 minutes (each)	• Detailed assessment of social functioning	• Time-consuming to administer
Specific Level of Functioning Scale (Schneider & Struening, 1983)	Staff	Staff report	43	Physical functioning, personal care skills, social functioning, community living, work	30 minutes	• Comprehensive assessment	• Requires knowledge of consumer functioning

Instrument	Rater	Format	No. of items	Content areas	Time	Strengths	Limitations
Social and Occupational Functioning Scale (Goldman, Skodol, & Lave, 1992)	Staff	Staff report	1	Social and occupational functioning	5 minutes	• Very brief	• Requires interviewer training • Lacks specificity
Life Skills Profile (Rosen, Hadzi-Pavlovic, & Parker, 1989)	Consumer	Interview	39	Self-care, nonturbulence, social contact, communication, responsibility	20 minutes	• Specifically designed for schizophrenia	
Social Dysfunction Index (Munroe-Blum, Collins, McCleary, & Nuttall, 1996)	Consumer, relative, or staff	Interview	27	Public, self, independent living, occupational, family relationships, other relationships, leisure, health, communication, insight	40 minutes	• Comprehensive assessment	• Requires interviewer training
Cardinal Needs Schedule (Marshall, Hogg, Gath, & Lockwood, 1995)	Consumer, relative, or staff	Interview	Varies	Symptoms, underactivity, side effects, dangerous or destructive behavior, organic symptoms, health, socially embarrassing behavior, independent living, self-care, education, occupation	60 minutes	• Focuses on establishing specific areas in need of rehabilitation	• Limited focus on social relationships
Camberwell Assessment of Needs (Phelan, Slade, Thornicroft, Dunn, & Holloway, 1995)	Consumer	Interview		Housing, independent living, self-care, social, occupation, knowledge of illness, symptoms, childcare, welfare benefits, health	25 minutes	• Separate clinician and researcher versions • Widely used in Europe	
Independent Living Skills Survey (Wallace et al., 2000)	Consumer, staff	Interview	112	Eating habits, grooming, domestic activities, health, cooking, economic skills, transportation, leisure, job-seeking skills	30 minutes	• Specific focus on independent living skills	

(continued)

TABLE 4.4. *(continued)*

Scale	Respondent	Format	No. of items	Domains	Administration time	Advantages	Disadvantages
Specific Assessment Scales (cont.)							
Needs and Resources Assessment Interview (Corrigan, Buican, & McCracken, 1995a)	Consumer	Self-report or interview	52	Housing, health, mental health, social, family, leisure, spiritual, substance use, legal, work	25 minutes	• Broad-based functional assessment	
Client Assessment of Strengths, Interests, and Goals (CASIG; Wallace, Lecomte, Wilde, & Liberman, 2001)	Consumer (CASIG-SR) and informant (CASIG-I)	Interview	Multiple	Health, food preparation, vocational, transportation, friends, leisure, hygiene, personal possessions, medication, quality of life	60 minutes for CASIG-SR and 45 minutes for CASIG-I.	• Interviewer training not required • Useful for treatment planning	• Time-consuming to administer
Global functioning assessment scales							
Multnomah Community Ability Scale (Barker et al., 1994)	Staff	Staff report	17	Social competence, independent functioning, behavioral problems, mood and anxiety	15 minutes	• Very broad assessment	• Requires knowledge of consumer functioning • Limited specificity
Global Assessment of Functioning (American Psychiatric Association, 1994)	Staff	Staff report	1	Global assessment of psychosocial functioning	5 minutes	• Very brief	• Lacks specificity
Role Functioning Scale (Goodman, Sewell, Cooley, & Leavitt, 1993)	Consumer	Interview	4	Work, independent living, social relationships	15–30 minutes	• Good reliability and validity • Behaviorally anchored ratings	• Lacks interview probes • Low specificity

abilities, and often requires extensive supports from treatment providers and family members. As with these other areas, impaired self-care skills are incorporated into the diagnostic criteria of some disorders such as schizophrenia. For these reasons, improving self-care and independent living skills is an important priority of many rehabilitation programs.

Assessment Instruments

The best-validated instrument for assessing these skills is the Independent Living Skills Survey (Wallace, Liberman, Tauber, & Wallace, 2000). This measure includes both a consumer and a staff (or significant other) version and assesses a wide range of specific behaviors related to self-care and independent living. Many other instruments for measuring community functioning also tap some independent living skills, such as the Social and Adaptive Functions Evaluation (Harvey, Davidson, Mueser, Parrella, White, et al., 1997) and the Multnomah Community Ability Scale (Barker et al., 1994) (see Table 4.4).

Substance Abuse

Drug and alcohol abuse is one of the most common comorbid disorders among people with psychiatric disabilities, with about 50% of individuals with a psychiatric disability experiencing problems related to their substance use at some point in their lives (Mueser, Bennett, & Kushner, 1995a; Regier, Farmer, Rae, Locke, Keith, et al., 1990). Substance abuse has a wide range of effects, including relapses and rehospitalizations, legal, economic, and family problems, and increased vulnerability to infectious diseases (Drake & Brunette, 1998). Thus, substance abuse is an important focus of psychiatric rehabilitation. This topic is discussed more thoroughly in Chapter 15.

Assessment Instruments

Because people with psychiatric disabilities are more likely to experience adverse consequences of using small amounts of alcohol and drugs, instruments developed for detecting substance abuse in the general population tend to be of limited value (Carey & Correia, 1998; Corse, Hirschinger, & Zanis, 1995). In recent years a number of instruments have been developed specifically to assess substance abuse in persons with psychiatric disabilities. These instruments include screening instruments, diagnostic instruments, descriptive instruments, and measures of engagement and progress in substance abuse treatment. Some of the most widely used of these instruments are summarized in Table 4.5.

Medication Adherence and Side Effects

Medication is probably the most powerful treatment tool for psychiatric disabilities, having a significant impact on reducing symptoms and preventing relapses in 70–90% of consumers (Schatzberg & Nemeroff, 1998). However, medication adherence is a common problem, with more than half of all consumers being nonadherent to medication at some point in their illness (Corrigan, Liberman, & Engle, 1990). Medication nonadherence is an important contributor to relapse and rehospitalization, as evidenced by numerous studies (Zygmunt, Olfson, Boyer, & Mechanic, 2002). Therefore, improving medication adherence is a common goal for psychiatric rehabilitation.

TABLE 4.5. Instruments for Screening and Assessing Substance Use Problems

Screening instruments

Instrument	Format	Focus	No. of items	Administration time	Sensitivity and specificity in psychiatric disabilities
Dartmouth Assessment of Lifestyle Instrument (Rosenberg, Drake, Wolford, Mueser, Oxman, et al., 1998)	Self-report	Alcohol, marijuana, cocaine	18	10 minutes	High
Alcohol Use Disorder Identification Test (Babor, De La Fuente, Saunders, & Grant, 1989)	Self-report	Alcohol	10	5 minutes	High
Michigan Alcoholism Screening Test (Selzer, 1971)	Self-report	Alcohol	24	10 minutes	Moderate
Drug Abuse Screening Test (Skinner, 1982)	Self-report	Drugs	28	15 minutes	Moderate
CAGE Questionnaire (Mayfield, McLeod, & Hall, 1974)	Self-report	Alcohol	4	5 minutes	Moderate

Descriptive and assessment instruments

Instruments	Format	Focus	Time frame	Administration time	Comments
Alcohol Use Scale, Revised (Drake, Osher, Noordsy, Hurlbut, Teague, 1990; Mueser et al., 2003b)	Clinician rated	Alcohol use problems	Past 6 months	20 minutes (including Drug Use Scale)	• Easy to use for classification and tracking alcohol abuse outcomes

Instrument	Type	Content	Time frame	Duration	Notes
Drug Use Scale, Revised (Mueser et al., 2003b)	Clinician rated	Drug use problems	Past 6 months	20 minutes (including Alcohol Use Scale)	• Easy to use for classification and tracking alcohol abuse outcomes
Time-Line Followback Calendar (Sobell & Sobell, 1992; Mueser et al., 2003b)	Interview	Pattern of substance use over time	Past 6 months	15 minutes	• Useful for treatment planning
Substance Abuse Treatment Scale, Revised (McHugo et al., 1999; Mueser et al., 2003b)	Clinician rated	Stage of treatment: engagement, persuasion, active treatment, relapse prevention	Past 6 months	5 minutes	• Useful for treatment planning
Addiction Severity Index (McLellan, Kushner, Metzger, Peters, Smith, et al., 1992)	Interview	Alcohol use, drug use, medical status, employment, legal status, family/social, psychiatric	Lifetime and past 30 days	70 minutes	• Comprehensive assessment • Persons with psychiatric disabilities score low on many subscales

As in all branches of medicine, powerful medications often have undesirable effects that go along with their beneficial effects, and psychiatric medications are no exception. The side effects of medication can be uncomfortable, and in some cases dangerous. In addition, medication side effects may contribute to nonadherence.

Although medication side effects are common, there are many options available for their management, and effective pharmacological management can often eliminate them. However, in order to effectively address this problem, side effects must first be detected. Therefore, medication side effects are often routinely assessed in individuals receiving pharmacological treatment for their psychiatric disabilities. These assessments are usually conducted by the physician or nurse practitioner who is prescribing the medication. The role of medications in treatment is reviewed in Chapter 7.

Assessment Instruments

Although medication nonadherence is a common problem, accurately measuring adherence is a significant challenge. Almost all approaches to measuring adherence have their limitations, and more accurate approaches are more time-consuming. The most accurate methods for assessing medication adherence involve either pill counts or electronic medication cap devices.

In order to conduct a pill count, consumers are requested to bring their medications to a visit and the provider simply counts the number of pills in each bottle of prescribed medication. The extent to which more pills exist than would be expected, based on the prescribed dosage and frequency, is an indicator of nonadherence. Although this technique can easily be subverted by the consumer's taking pills out and throwing them away, it is nevertheless considered quite accurate, and apparently such attempts to conceal medication nonadherence are comparatively rare. However, obtaining an accurate measure of medication adherence from pill counts can nevertheless be difficult for many reasons, including the availability of free samples, the use of noncountable medications such as inhalers, eye drops, or insulin vials, and medications given with a regular dose and a limited number of PRNs (taken as needed).

Electronic cap devices record the number of times a cap is taken off a medication container, which is also quite a reliable measure of medication adherence. The primary limitation of this approach is the expense of the devices, especially for the majority of consumers who are prescribed multiple types of medication. In addition, many consumers use weekly pillboxes to organize their medications, for which electronic devices cannot be used.

Direct interviews with consumers about their use of medications can be useful, but their accuracy is often questionable. If a consumer indicates that he or she does not routinely take his or her medication, it can be assumed that this report is relatively accurate. Reports of consistent medication adherence, however, are not necessarily accurate. An alternative to direct questioning about medication adherence is to indirectly inquire about the consumer's attitude about medication. Some research indicates that a negative attitude toward medication (such as the belief that it is not beneficial) may be more strongly related to adherence than direct self-reports of adherence (Pratt, Mueser, Driscoll, Wolfe, & Bartels, 2006).

Reports of significant others can also provide useful information about a consumer's use of medication, although, again, veracity depends on their contact with the consumer and their biases. For example, treatment providers may overestimate adherence because they believe that consumers are doing as they are told and following instructions to take medication. Blood levels of some medications can be determined. For example, an important part of monitoring the prescription of lithium for bipolar disorder is to regularly check lithium blood levels in order to prevent high toxic levels from developing. A very low level of lithium can indicate nonadherence. However, blood levels cannot be used to monitor most medications, either because guidelines for therapeutic levels do not exist or because of the expense of the tests. A final indication of medication nonadherence may be unexplained symptom exacerbations.

In practice, as in the assessment of social functioning and substance abuse, using a combination of consumer reports, significant other reports, and behavioral observations can provide the most accurate measure of whether a consumer is taking his or her prescribed medications. Table 4.6 summarizes various instruments and methods for assessing medication nonadherence and their advantages and disadvantages.

Although different classes of psychiatric medications tend to have common side effects, each specific medication has its own unique profile. Two widely used scales for measuring antipsychotic side effects are the Extrapyramidal Side Effects Questionnaire (Simpson & Angus, 1970) and the Abnormal Involuntary Movements Scale (Health, 1975). Other medication side effects are typically monitored by the prescriber, without standardized rating scales.

Quality of Life

The growth of treatment alternatives over the past several decades has led medical and psychiatric care to expand its focus beyond improving the course of disease to addressing quality-of-life issues. This shift is based on the recognition that the benefits of any specific intervention for improving an illness must be weighed against its costs to the individual, which is a personal choice depending on the values and preferences of that person. Thus, the concept of quality of life deals mainly with the enjoyment and appreciation of various aspects of living and is less concerned with the specific psychopathology and impairments that characterize psychiatric disorders (Huxley, 1998).

Assessment Instruments

A wide range of instruments have been developed for the measurement of quality of life, with most including objective and subjective perspectives. As previously mentioned, objective measures of quality of life overlap considerably with measures of community functioning, such as quality of social relationships. In some cases, quality-of-life measures overlap with symptom measures. For example, the Quality of Life Scale (Heinrichs, Hanlon, & Carpenter, 1984) is strongly related to negative symptoms (Bellack, Morrison, Wixted, & Mueser, 1990b), and the overall scale may be better conceptualized as a measure of the deficit syndrome of enduring negative symptoms (Carpenter, Heinrichs, & Wagman, 1988; Mueser, Bellack, Douglas, & Wade, 1991b) than a conventional quality-of-life measure. A number of scales commonly used for the assessment of quality of life are summarized in Table 4.7.

Trauma and Its Consequences

Accumulating evidence demonstrates that people with psychiatric disabilities are more likely to experience traumatic events throughout their lives, both before and after the

TABLE 4.6. Instruments and Methods for Assessing Medication Adherence

Instruments

Scale	Respondent	Format	No. of items	Administration time	Advantages	Disadvantages
Rating of Medication Influences Scale (Weiden, Rapkin, Mott, Zygmunt, Goldman, et al., 1994)	Consumer	Interview	20	20–30 minutes	• Very comprehensive	• Time-consuming • Requires interviewer training
Medication Adherence Rating Scale (Thompson, Kulkarni, & Sergejew, 2000)	Consumer	Questionnaire	10	5 minutes	• Easy to administer • Good reliability and validity	• Still misses many nonadherent consumers
Drug Attitude Inventory (Hogan, Awad, & Eastwood, 1983)	Consumer	Questionnaire	30/10 item versions	10 minutes	• Easy to administer	• Measures attitudes about adherence, not behavior • Unclear validity
Brief Evaluation of Medication Influences and Beliefs (Dolder, Lacro, Warren, Golshan, Perkins, 2004)	Consumer	Questionnaire	8	2–3 minutes	• Very brief • Some validity	• Only moderate internal consistency • Used for older people so far

Other methods for assessing medication adherence

Method	Administration time	Advantages	Disadvantages
Consumer self-reports		• Easy to conduct • Accurate when nonadherence reported	• Often inaccurate
Pill counts	5 minutes	• Often accurate • Simple	• Easy to fake
Electronic cap recorders	5 minutes	• Very accurate • Simple	• Relatively easy to fake • Expensive • Cannot be done with pill organizers
Blood or urine assays		• Objective	• Only moderately accurate • Invasive • Not available for many medications
Prescription refill records			• Probably accurate for missed refills, but timely refills do not necessarily imply adherence

TABLE 4.7. Instruments for Assessing Quality of Life

Instrument	Format	Objective/ subjective	Domains	No. of items	Administration time	Comments
Subjective Quality of Life Profile (Dazord, Astolfl, Guisti, Rebetez, Mino, et al., 1998)	Self-report	Subjective	Functional life, social life, material life, spiritual life	36	15 minutes	• Simplified 17-item version available
Quality of Life Interview (Lehman, Kernan, & Postrado, 1995)	Interview	Both	Housing, daily activities, family, friends, finances, work and school, legal and safety, health	153	45 minutes	• 15-minutes version available • Very widely used instrument
Lancashire Quality of Life Profile (Oliver, 1991)	Interview	Subjective	Work/education, leisure, religion, finances, living situation, legal and safety, family, friends, well-being	100	35 minutes	• Based on the Quality of Life Interview
Quality of Life Scale (Heinrichs et al., 1984)	Interview	Objective	Interpersonal relations, role functioning, intrapsychic foundations, common objects and activities	21	20 minutes	• Requires interviewer training • Strongly related to negative symptoms
Quality of Life, Enjoyment and Satisfaction Questionnaire (Endicott, Nee, Harrison, & Blumenthal, 1993)	Self-report management	Subjective	Health, feelings, leisure, social, work, school, relationships, general activities, household	93	30 minutes	• Mainly studied in depression
Schizophrenia Quality of Life Scale (Wilkinson, Hedson, Wild, Cookson, Farina, et al., 2000)	Self-report	Subjective	Psychosocial, motivation and energy, symptoms, side effects	30	10 minutes	• Brief assessment • Specifically developed for schizophrenia

onset of their psychiatric disorders (Goodman, Rosenberg, Mueser, & Drake, 1997). Traumatic events, such as physical and sexual assault, can have devastating effects on people's lives, such as triggering relapses and rehospitalizations in people with major mental illness (Goodman, Salyers, Mueser, Rosenberg, Swartz, et al., 2001). In addition, exposure to traumatic events can lead to specific psychiatric syndromes that are themselves associated with high levels of suffering and distress, such as posttraumatic stress disorder (PTSD). Because of the effects of trauma on both the quality of life and course of psychiatric disorders, reducing these effects and the potential for future victimization has become an important treatment priority in psychiatric rehabilitation efforts in recent years. Chapter 14 reviews this issue more fully.

Assessment Instruments

A variety of instruments have been employed for assessing trauma exposure and PTSD in people with psychiatric disabilities. Most of these instruments have been drawn from work conducted in the general population, with some adaptations. Table 4.8 summarizes instruments for assessing trauma and PTSD that have been employed with people with psychiatric disabilities. Several studies indicate that reliable and valid trauma and PTSD assessments can be obtained with this population, including people who have psychotic symptoms (Goodman, Thompson, Weinfurt, Corl, Acker, et al., 1999; Meyer, Muenzenmaier, Cancienne, & Struening, 1996; Mueser, Salyers, Rosenberg, Ford, Fox, et al., 2001b).

Both self-report- and interview-based assessments are useful for evaluating trauma history and PTSD in persons with psychiatric disabilities. In many settings, a brief trauma screen and a self-report checklist of PTSD symptoms is sufficient to identify people likely to have a diagnosis of PTSD. Screening assessments should be followed up with a direct interview to confirm the presence of symptoms and to correct any misunderstandings that may have occurred in completing the self-report measure. Although self-report questionnaires alone cannot be used to establish a diagnosis of PTSD, they can be very useful to monitor the effects of treatment.

Cognitive Functioning

Impairment in cognitive functioning is common in persons with psychiatric disabilities. For example, cognitive impairment is pervasive in schizophrenia, with many individuals experiencing at least some decrement in their cognitive functioning following the onset of their disorder (Heaton, Paulsen, McAdams, Kuck, Zisook, et al., 1994). Furthermore, in the absence of intervention, impairment in cognitive functioning tends to be quite stable over the course of psychiatric illness (Gold, 2004) and is strongly related to various domains of functioning, such as independent living (Brekke, Raine, Ansel, Lencz, & Bird, 1997), social relationships (Addington & Addington, 1999), and work (McGurk & Mueser, 2004). Cognitive impairment also occurs in individuals with other disorders. For example, difficulty concentrating is a symptom of major depression in DSM-IV (American Psychiatric Association, 1994). Unlike the case with schizophrenia, cognitive difficulties in people with mood disorders tend to be correlated with depression. Because of the prominence of cognitive impairment in some individuals with psychiatric disabilities, and its association with functional outcomes, evaluating cognitive functioning is of interest to psychiatric rehabilitation. See Chapter 12 for a thorough discussion of cognitive matters.

TABLE 4.8. Instruments for Assessing Trauma Exposure and Related Problems

Instrument	Format	Focus	Administration time	Comments
Trauma history				
Trauma History Questionnaire (Green, 1996a)	Interview	Lifetime trauma history	15 minutes	• Covers broad range of traumatic events
Brief Trauma Questionnaire (Schnurr, Vielhauer, Weathers, & Findler, 1999)	Questionnaire	Trauma history	5 minutes	• Easy to use • Captures most major traumatic events
History of Physical and Sexual Abuse Questionnaire (Meyer et al., 1996)	Interview	Physical and sexual abuse	10 minutes	• Specifically designed for persons with psychiatric disabilities
Conflict Tactics Scales–2 (Straus et al., 1996)	Interview	Aggression and victimization in family and partner relationships	45 minutes	• Examines perceptions of contextual factors related to aggression and victimization
PTSD and related problems				
Posttraumatic Stress Disorder Checklist (Blanchard, Jones-Alexander, Buckley, & Forneris, 1996)	Questionnaire	Screening instrument for PTSD	10 minutes	• Easy to use • Strongly related to diagnoses of PTSD

Measure	Type	Purpose	Time	Characteristics
Posttraumatic Diagnostic Scale (Foa, Cashman, Jaycox, & Perry, 1997)	Interview	Diagnosis of PTSD	30–40 minutes	• Easy to use, validated in general population
Clinician-Administered PTSD Scale (Blake, Weathers, Nagy, Kaloupek, Charney, et al., 1995)	Structured interview	Diagnosis of PTSD	1 hour	• "Gold standard" for assessing PTSD • Requires interviewer training • Validated for psychiatric disabilities
Revised Impact of Event Scale (Horowitz, Wilner, & Alvarez, 1979)	Questionnaire	Assessment of common PTSD symptoms	10 minutes	• Easily completed measure of PTSD symptoms
Trauma-related cognitions				
Posttraumatic Cognitions Inventory (Foa, Ehlers, Clark, Tolin, & Orsillo, 1999)	Questionnaire	Assesses trauma-related thoughts about self and the world	20 minutes	• Useful for cognitive-behavioral treatment of PTSD
World Assumptions Scale (Janoff-Bulman, 1989)	Questionnaire	Measures common assumptions about the world commonly affected by trauma	20 minutes	• Useful for cognitive-behavioral treatment of PTSD

Assessment Instruments

A great variety of measures have been developed to assess specific areas of cognitive functioning in general and clinical populations (Lezak, 2004). The most sophisticated instruments are neuropsychological tests, which are designed to assess particular cognitive functions. These tests are often combined in a comprehensive package of assessments designed to tap a range of cognitive functions in a systematic fashion, such as the Halstead–Reitan Neuropsychological Test Battery (Reitan & Wolfson, 1993). These batteries can be quite time-consuming to administer, requiring upwards of 3–6 hours, and require special education and training to administer and interpret. We do not review these tests here because they have limited relevance to the practice of psychiatric rehabilitation at this time.

Of more practical relevance, briefer instruments have also been developed for detecting cognitive impairment, either in the general population or in persons with psychiatric disabilities. These assessments are usually easier to administer and score and do not require the amount of training required for standard neuropscholoical tests. Some of the more commonly used brief cognitive assessments are summarized in Table 4.9.

Aggression and Violence

The relationship between major mental illnesses such as schizophrenia and aggression and violence has been a topic of great debate over the past several decades. Strong feelings are often aroused in this debate, and for good reasons. Extensive research on the stigma of mental illness demonstrates that inflated public perceptions of violence in people with psychiatric disabilities is the single most important predictor of stigmatizing attitudes about mental illness and of behavioral avoidance of people with psychiatric disabilities (Angermeyer & Matschinger, 2003; Corrigan, Green, Lundin, Kubiak, & Penn, 2001b). Furthermore, the popular media frequently portray persons with psychiatric disabilities as violent, contributing to public perceptions that these portrayals have more than a grain of truth to them (Wahl, 1995).

Although the public often believes that people with disabilities are prone to violence, how well do these beliefs accord with the actual data? The answer is a complex one that continues to be debated among the experts. Research on violence and mental illness can be summarized in the following points: First, most people with a psychiatric disability are not violent, although problems with aggression are not uncommon during the acute periods of a symptom exacerbation (Foley, Kelly, Clarke, McTigue, Gervin, et al., 2005; Swanson, Borum, Swartz, & Hiday, 1999). In fact, people with psychiatric disabilities are more likely to hurt themselves than to hurt other people. Second, people with psychiatric disabilities, particularly schizophrenia, are more likely to engage in aggressive and violent behavior than people who do not have such a disability (Arseneault, Moffitt, Caspi, Taylor, & Silva, 2000; Brennan, Mednick, & Hodgins, 2000). Third, the presence of substance use disorders and antisocial personality disorder in persons with psychiatric disabilities complicates the picture, as these disorders tend to be related to a greater incidence of aggression in both the general population and among persons with psychiatric disabilities (Crocker, Mueser, Clark, McHugo, Ackerson, et al., 2005; Mueser, Crocker, Frisman, Drake, Covell, et al., 2006a; Steadman, Mulvey, Monahan, Robbins, Applebaum, et al., 1998). Thus, the assessment of aggression and violence is a domain of concern in rehabilitation assessment. Chapter 18 directly addresses the management of violent behaviors. The possible involvement of the criminal justice system in this problem is addressed in Chapter 13.

TABLE 4.9. Brief Cognitive Assessments

Instrument	Focus of assessment	Administration time	Comments
Brief Cognitive Assessment (Velligan, DiCocco, Bow-Thomas, Cadle, Glahn, et al., 2004)	Brief assessment of cognitive functioning	15 minutes	• Good psychometric properties • Scores related to performance on neuropsychological battery and community functioning
Brief Assessment of Cognition in Schizophrenia (Keefe, Goldberg, Harvey, Gold, Poe, et al., 2004)	Brief assessment of broad range of cognitive functions	35 minutes	• Strongly related to performance on comprehensive neuropsychological battery • Requires some background in neuropsychology to administer
Repeatable Battery for the Assessment of Neuropsychological Status (Gold, Queern, Iannone, & Buchanan, 1999)	Brief assessment of broad range of cognitive functions	45 minutes	• Strongly related to performance on comprehensive neuropsychological battery • Requires some background in neuropsychology to administer
Mini-Mental State Exam (Folstein, Folstein, & McHugh, 1975)	Screening instrument for severe cognitive impairment	5–10 minutes	• Easy to administer and score • Used mainly to identify gross cognitive impairment
Neurobehavioral Cognitive Status Examination (Kiernan, Mueller, Langston, & Van Dyke, 1987)	Screening instrument for dementia and severe cognitive impairment	45 minutes	• More sensitive to cognitive impairment than Mini-Mental State Exam • Good validity of data

Assessment Instruments

Relatively few instruments have been developed for measuring violence or aggression in persons with psychiatric disabilities. One measure is the Modified Overt Aggression Scale (MOAS) (Kay, Wolkenfeld, & Murrill, 1988), which provides an assessment of verbal, physical, and property aggression. The MOAS has support for its validity in assessing persons with psychiatric disabilities (Mueser, Drake, Ackerson, Alterman, Miles, et al., 1997b; Watts, Leese, Thomas, Atakan, & Wykes, 2003). Some instruments have been developed that have been shown to predict violence in persons with psychiatric disabilities (Monahan, Steadman, Applebaum, Robbins, Mulvey, et al., 2000; Watts, Bindman, Slade, Halloway, Rosen, et al., 2004), but the role of these instruments in psychiatric rehabilitation practice is not yet established. Similarly, the Conflict Tactics Scales-2 (Straus, Hamby, Boney-McCoy, & Sugarman, 1996) provides a rich assessment of aggressive and violent behavior in the context of close relationships, but it is primarily a research tool and requires significant training to administer.

Rehabilitation providers should record a history of aggressive and violent behavior, based on both the consumer's report and those of others. A positive history should be followed up with a more detailed assessment aimed at understanding the circumstances in which the aggressive incidents occurred and evaluating their seriousness. Particular attention should be paid to the possible roles of medication nonadherence, antisocial personality disorder, substance abuse, and interpersonal conflict as factors contributing to aggression and violence, and rehabilitation that may reduce the chances of such incidents recurring.

INTEGRATING ASSESSMENT INTO REHABILITATION

Assessment plays a critical role in the identification of treatment and other needs, and in rehabilitation planning. In addition, ongoing assessment is needed to determine whether rehabilitation efforts are achieving their intended aims. Pragmatically, it is helpful to divide the role of assessment into treatment and rehabilitation planning, and monitoring the effects of rehabilitation interventions.

Treatment and Rehabilitation Planning

The assessment of treatment and rehabilitation needs can be hierarchically organized in terms of the immediacy with which needs must be attended to: urgent matters, clinical needs, and rehabilitation needs.

Urgent Matters

Urgent matters are issues so pressing that they must be attended to immediately in order to protect the person or others. Urgent needs typically involve health, psychiatric, or housing issues. For example, if an individual has a chronic medical condition for which he or she is not receiving treatment, attending to these treatment needs is of utmost importance. Similarly, if a person is seriously injured, such as in an accident or from an attack, attending to the treatment of these injuries is critical.

Urgent matters of a psychiatric nature typically involve threats to the self or others. Threats to the self may be deliberate, as in an actively suicidal person who has either attempted suicide or is formulating concrete plans to do so, or unintentional, as in an individual's refusing to eat or care for him- or herself because of paranoid delusions or gross disorganization. Psychiatric needs that are threats to others often involve either paranoid delusions or hallucinations instructing the person to hurt another.

Urgent matters involving housing typically deal with the loss of housing for a person who was previously stably housed. Housing issues may be less pressing, but are nevertheless important, for individuals who have experienced long bouts of homelessness and for whom it is less likely to have a destabilizing influence in their lives. Another type of urgent matter involving housing arises when a person's housing is threatened by strife with other people, such as family members, roommates, or a landlord.

Clinical Needs

Clinical needs involve the direct manifestation of clinical syndromes that are responsible for a person's psychiatric disability. The severity of specific psychiatric symptoms, relapses, and medication side effects are all clinical needs for which pharmacological management is most important. Although some degree of persistence in clinical symptoms is common in people with psychiatric disabilities, insufficiently treated symptoms or persistent side effects can interfere with the effectiveness of rehabilitation and the goal of improving functional outcomes. For example, if an individual is experiencing the early signs of a relapse, or has actually experienced a symptom exacerbation, getting immediate treatment for these signs and symptoms is important in order to minimize the effects of a relapse on other areas of functioning. For individuals who have unstable and persistent symptoms, it is often unclear as to whether optimal pharmacological treatment is being provided. However, people are most likely to benefit from rehabilitation if their symptoms and side effects are routinely monitored and pharmacological treatment is provided in accordance with standard practice guidelines for their disabilities (Rush, Rago, Crismon, Toprac, Shon, et al., 1999).

Rehabilitation Needs

The distinction between clinical and rehabilitation needs is not a clear one, because rehabilitation services are often directed at helping people cope with or overcome the clinical effects of a psychiatric disorder on their functioning. For example, people may be troubled by persistent cognitive impairments or psychotic symptoms, which can interfere with day-to-day functioning, and rehabilitation efforts may be undertaken to minimize this interference and promote better coping. For practical purposes, addressing the second level of the hierarchy of needs (clinical needs) can include addressing symptoms or side effects due to suboptimal pharmacological treatment, and the third level (rehabilitation needs) involves addressing other clinical needs (such as coping with persistent symptoms) and working toward rehabilitation goals.

There are few established guidelines for prioritizing rehabilitation goals. A wide range of such goals are possible, such as improved family relationships and illness management through family psychoeducation, improving skills for self-management of an illness, pursuing work or educational goals through supported employment or supported education, overcoming substance abuse, improved parenting skills, or greater self-care and independent living skills. Many of these goals can be pursued simultaneously, and the best strategy is to focus first on those goals that the consumer is most motivated to work toward and that are closest to his or her personal recovery goals.

Integrating Assessment into Monitoring Outcomes

Just as assessment is the key to effective treatment and rehabilitation planning, it is also crucial for evaluating the success of those efforts. This is most effectively accomplished by incorporating formal, ongoing, collaborative assessment into the monitoring of rehabilitation efforts. Ongoing assessment involves identifying key indicators of the assessment area and monitoring them on a routine basis. Informal monitoring can occur almost continuously with some rehabilitation goals, but more formal monitoring should also be conducted every 1–3 months.

The ease with which outcomes can be monitored varies significantly from one domain to another. Some domains are quite easy to monitor, such as employment and involvement in school. Other may require specific assessment probes. These probes can be conducted by selecting key outcomes related to the domain of interest. For example, the effectiveness of treatment for substance abuse in a person with a psychiatric disability can be monitored by periodically assessing the person's use of substances. The effectiveness of teaching coping skills can be evaluated by periodically checking the person's perception of his or her coping efficacy. The effectiveness of interventions for PTSD or depression can be monitored by periodically asking the individual to complete a self-rating assessment scale.

Sustained lack of progress toward targeted rehabilitation goals should signal the provider to reconsider the rehabilitation plan, again in collaboration with the consumer. Lack of progress can be addressed a variety of ways: breaking down the goal into smaller and more manageable steps, altering the goal to make it more attainable, establishing a different goal that the consumer is more motivated to work toward, or trying a different rehabilitation approach. The rate of change to be expected depends on the consumer's specific strengths, the nature of the desired goal, and the rehabilitation approach used. Treatment manuals, experience with an approach, and research on the intervention provide the best guidance as to whether the consumer is making progress at a suitable rate or whether the approach needs to be modified or reconsidered.

SUMMARY AND CONCLUSIONS

Assessment in rehabilitation planning is a complex process that involves delving into a wide range of areas of functioning. Effective assessment is crucial to identifying the most important rehabilitation goals and prioritizing those goals. Familiarity with each domain is crucial, because major problems in any one can impede progress toward rehabilitation goals. Yet it is difficult for one provider to have the expertise needed to assess every domain, and thus teamwork is often necessary for performing a comprehensive assessment. Teamwork involves not only the contributions of a multidisciplinary group of providers, but active collaboration with consumers and their significant others. Sharing the responsibilities of assessment and planning, and incorporating ongoing assessment into monitoring progress, ensures that goals and rehabilitation methods are jointly agreed upon and modified as needed over time.

Chapter 5

Illness Self-Management

Helping consumers learn how to manage their psychiatric disabilities in collaboration with others, including understanding the nature and treatment of their mental illness, and developing strategies for minimizing its impact on their lives, is an important goal of psychiatric rehabilitation. Illness self-management is a crucial step for consumers toward achieving a sense of personal wellness and control over their destiny. As illustrated in the personal example below, poor control over a psychiatric disorder can wreak havoc on lives of consumers, and their family members and others as well.

This chapter addresses the role of illness self-management for persons with psychiatric disabilities. Self-management of one's psychiatric disability can be narrowly defined as including the ability to make informed treatment decisions, reducing the impact of distressing or otherwise problematic symptoms, and reducing relapses and rehospitalizations. More broadly, illness self-management approaches also help people to identify and pursue personal goals and to develop a physically and psychologically healthy lifestyle imbued with hope, optimism, and a sense of purpose (or "recovery").

We begin with a review of historical factors that have contributed to the broadly accepted importance of illness self-management, including progress in disease management, shared decision making, and the rise of the consumer self-help movement. We then review the components of illness self-management, and the research evidence supporting those components. Finally, we describe several widely used illness self-management programs, and research evaluating their effectiveness.

PERSONAL EXAMPLE

Jerome Develops a Psychiatric Disorder

Jerome was in his first year of college when he began to have difficulty in concentrating and started to withdraw from others. According to members of his family, Jerome just "wasn't his usual self," and their concerns increased when he performed poorly during his first semester. When his parents tried to talk to Jerome about his problems, he seemed cagey or suspicious. These concerns were only amplified when Jerome stopped going to classes the following semester and confided to friends that his dormitory room had been bugged and his roommate could read his thoughts. School officials contacted Jerome's parents and explained that he needed to see a doctor because he was experiencing psychological problems at school. Jerome refused to see a doctor and insisted that there was a conspiracy against him. Eventually, Jerome stopped eating because he thought his food was poisoned, and he was involuntarily hospitalized.

In the hospital, Jerome was diagnosed with schizophreniform disorder–provisional and informed that medication was an important part of his treatment. It took several weeks for his psychotic symptoms to improve, and he was discharged from the hospital and given an appointment at his local community mental health center. Jerome decided he would not return to school at this time because it was too late to get his second semester back on track, so he returned home to live with his parents.

Jerome missed his appointment at the community mental health center, and when his behavior began to become more disorganized and psychotic again, his family took him to the center to meet with his doctor. Jerome was given a new prescription for antipsychotic medication and again told that taking it was an important part of his treatment. He was also assigned a case manager, who met with him to determine his needs and goals. Jerome told his case manager that he was interested in returning to school at some point, but felt he needed to get his "affairs in order" before that time. The case manager suggested he participate in a social rehabilitation group at the center before returning to school, which Jerome noncommittally agreed to do.

In subsequent months, Jerome continued to be inconsistent in taking medications, disorganized in his speech, and paranoid about his family's intentions toward him. After numerous family arguments and significant tension in the family, it was agreed that Jerome should move out and into a local apartment where supported living services would be available. This was accomplished without incident, but as soon as he was on his own, Jerome stopped taking his medication, which made him more prone to relapses. His behavior was often disorganized and psychotic, which eventually led the mental health center to assign him to an assertive community treatment (ACT) program to ensure that his daily living needs would be met, including taking medication. Jerome had fewer relapses over the next few years. However, he continued to function marginally in terms of involvement in meaningful activities and social relationships and still had one or two relapses per year requiring brief hospitalization.

Although Jerome's cycle of relapses and rehospitalizations was slowed by the outreach and home-based services provided by the ACT team, he had received little help focused on helping him learn how to manage his illness in collaboration with others. Although Jerome had been informed by his psychiatrist that he had schizophrenia, and had repeatedly been told about the importance of taking medication, little effort had been aimed at developing a shared understanding of the nature of Jerome's psychiatric disorder, the principles of its treatment, or how to manage persistent symptoms. Of even greater importance, Jerome had not received assistance in exploring and developing his personal life goals and learning how to manage his disorder in order to achieve those goals.

HISTORICAL PERSPECTIVES ON ILLNESS SELF-MANAGEMENT

Efforts to foster the self-management of psychiatric illnesses in persons with psychiatric disabilities have their historical roots in similar efforts to help people manage chronic medical diseases, the shared-decision-making movement in medicine, and the rise of the mental health recovery movement in rebellion against traditional hierarchical (and coercive) psychiatric treatment.

Disease Self-Management

Lifelong diseases such as diabetes, heart disease, and asthma require ongoing care and management to minimize their disruptive effects on daily living and prevent premature mortality. Modern medicine has learned much about the principles of long-term management of chronic diseases. For example, understanding which foods can dramatically increase blood sugar levels can enable people with diabetes to maintain a steady glucose blood level through dietary monitoring. In addition, advances in medical technology have also improved the outcomes of chronic diseases. For example, through regular monitoring of blood glucose levels and daily administration of insulin, individuals with Type I diabetes can enjoy a normal and long life.

Although increased understanding of the causes of disease and determinants of outcomes have improved long-term prognoses, the gains from these advances can be realized only though teaching patients the principles of managing their illness, and helping them incorporate critical changes into their lifestyle. Thus, in routine medical practice, part of treating individuals with chronic diseases involves teaching them about the nature of those diseases, informing them about lifestyle changes that may promote better disease management, teaching them how to monitor their illness and, when possible, self-administer treatments, and knowing when they need to contact treatment providers in order to address emergent concerns before they become more serious (Hanson, 1986; Masur, 1981; Swezey & Swezey, 1976).

Just as the treatment of chronic diseases has evolved to incorporate teaching self-management as a core part of treatment, so has the management of psychiatric disabilities. Mental health professionals strive to help persons with a psychiatric disability to learn about their mental illness and how to deal with it more effectively. Thus, promoting illness self-management is a natural part of any helping profession that strives to minimize the impact of a chronic disease on functioning and quality of life.

Shared Decision Making

Shared decision making is the process by which important medical decisions are made in active collaboration with the patient/consumer, the treatment provider, and anyone else who may be closely involved with the person, such as family members. Shared decision making is a movement that began in modern medicine (Campbell, Donaldson, Roberts, & Smith, 1996; Wennberg, 1991) and has been rapidly endorsed in psychiatry (Fenton, 2003; Hamann, Leucht, & Kissling, 2003). The rationale for shared decision making is twofold.

First, as the medical technology for treating various diseases has grown, so too has the awareness that deciding which interventions are best for a particular disease is often not straightforward, but rather depends on the personal values and preferences of the individual with the disease. For example, surgery for prostrate cancer may prolong life, but at the cost of compromised sexual function. In such cases, the decision to have surgery or not is better understood as a personal one that depends on what is important to the individual, and is not simply an objective decision that can be made by the treatment provider. All treatments, as well as the decision not to obtain treatment, have their advantages and disadvantages. Therefore, informed decision making requires an individual to learn basic information about the nature of the disorder, the treatment options, and their likely effects, both positive and negative.

Second, low adherence to recommended treatments is a problem throughout all of modern medicine (Blackwell, 1973), including psychiatry (Coldham, Addington, & Addington, 2002). *Psychological reactance* is a concept that refers to an individual's sensitivity to others' efforts to control his behavior (Brehm, 1966). Authoritarian-based, treatment recommendations may precipitate nonadherence in persons who are high in psychological reactance (Fogarty, 1997; Moore, Sellwood, & Stirling, 2000). However, people may be more likely to adhere to treatment recommendations if they are developed in a collaborative way that respects their right to choose the treatments they want. Shared decision making involves providing people with the information they need in order to make informed decisions about treatment, which may ultimately improve adherence to recommended and effective treatments.

The Consumer Movement

According to Frese and Davis (1997), the historical roots of the mental health consumer movement can be traced back to the establishment of the Alleged Lunatic's Friend Society in England in 1845 and the later publication of Clifford Beers's (1923) book, *A Mind That Found Itself*, which chronicled abuses committed in the name of treatment for psychiatric disabilities. More recent influences contributed to the rise in consumerism beginning in the 1970s, including deinstitutionalization, widespread dissatisfaction with traditional psychiatric care, and the growth of self-help approaches for personal problems. Chapter 17 addresses the role of consumer empowerment and peer services.

COMPONENTS OF ILLNESS SELF-MANAGEMENT PROGRAMS

Teaching individuals how to better manage their psychiatric disabilities is a complex enterprise for which a wide range of strategies has been developed. The most commonly employed approaches include educating individuals about mental illness and its treatment, the use of strategies for enhancing medication adherence, relapse prevention training, cognitive-behavioral therapy for persistent symptoms, family collaboration and psychoeducation, self-help and peer support. This section describes the rationale and nature of each of these approaches to self-management and the research evidence supporting them. The use of strategies for improving social relationships and social supports is another, indirect, way of improving illness management. Approaches for accomplishing this are covered in Chapter 10 on social relationships.

Education

People need information about their psychiatric disabilities and the available treatments for them in order to make informed decisions. Education (also called psychoeducation) is the most widely used approach for accomplishing this goal. Educational teaching is distinguished from other teaching approaches, such as cognitive-behavioral approaches, by its reliance on didactic, rather than experiential (e.g., role playing, practicing) teaching methods.

Examples of didactic teaching methods include providing basic information, asking questions to elicit the consumer's experience, asking review questions to evaluate understanding of taught material, using written handouts that summarize pertinent material, and using films and videos to illustrate important points. Practically all consumers are provided with information at some point during their treatment about their psychiatric diagnosis, treatment strategies, and ways in which they can improve the outcome of their illness. This information may be provided by a combination of doctors, nurses, case managers, and other mental health practitioners. Teaching is often done in an unstandardized way, although core curricula and standardized teaching methods have been developed (Ascher-Svanum & Krause, 1991; Weiden, 1999). Therefore, although it is common for some information about psychiatric illness to be provided, it is less certain how much consumers learn and retain it. Similarly, it is often unclear whether providers use a variety of teaching strategies for imparting information about mental illness and its treatment, or whether they rely primarily on didactic lectures.

Education about mental illness is also a common characteristic of most family intervention programs (Anderson, Reiss, & Hogarty, 1986; Falloon, Boyd, & McGill, 1984; Kuipers, Leff, & Lam, 2002; Mueser & Glynn, 1999). Family psychoeducation is aimed at helping family members, including the consumer, learn how to manage the psychiatric disability in collaboration with the treatment team. Therefore, the goals of family psychoeducational overlap with the individual programs for the self-management of illness.

Research

Education is frequently incorporated into comprehensive treatment programs aimed at improving illness self-management for psychiatric disabilities (Atkinson, Coia, Gilmour, & Harper, 1996; Gonzalez-Pinto, Gonzalez, Enjuto, Fernandez de Corres, Lopez, et al., 2004; Hogarty, Greenwald, Ulrich, Kornblith, DiBarry, et al., 1997a; Hogarty, Kornblith, Greenwald, DiBarry, Cooley, et al., 1997b; Hornung, Feldman, Klingberg, Buchkremer, & Reker, 1999). However, research on these programs is not informative as to the specific benefits of education, because any improvements favoring a comprehensive treatment program could be due to other, noneducational components of that program. Understanding the effects of educational interventions may be further clouded by the fact that some programs that are described as "educational" in fact include other treatment components as well, such as systematic training in problem solving (Atkinson et al., 1996).

In a review of research on illness self-management, Mueser and colleagues (2002a) identified 12 randomized controlled trials of specific educational interventions. The results of these studies indicated that education was effective in teaching people with psychiatric disabilities information about their disorders and treatment, but did not improve other outcomes, such as reducing symptom severity or relapses. These findings suggest that educational approaches alone are insufficient for improving the ability of consumers to manage their psychiatric disabilities. Similar conclusions have been reached by other reviews of educational interventions for schizophrenia (Merinder, 2000) and medication adherence (Zygmunt et al., 2002).

However, one interesting study appears to contradict these conclusions. Colom, Vieta, Martinez-Aran, Reinares, Goikolea, et al. (2003) evaluated the effectiveness of a

21-session group psychoeducational program for bipolar disorder as compared with unstructured group meetings. Although the material was taught primarily using psycho-educational methods, the curriculum covered a wide range of topics, including detection and prevention of hypomanic, manic, depressive, and mixed-state episodes, stress management, and problem-solving techniques. Written exercises were completed in the sessions, such as identifying possible triggers for relapses. During the 2-year follow-up, consumers who participated in this program had significantly fewer relapses. The findings, if replicated, suggest that broad-based psychoeducation that includes written exercises may confer a benefit to persons with bipolar disorder.

Enhancing Medication Adherence

Problems with adherence to treatment recommendations are among the greatest challenges faced by mental health practitioners (Fenton, Blyler, & Heinssen, 1997). These problems are especially troublesome with psychotropic medications, which are among the most effective treatments available for psychiatric disabilities (Schatzberg & Nemeroff, 2001). Although estimates vary, there is abundant evidence that the majority of people with a psychiatric disability are not adherent to their prescribed medication at some point in their disorder (Breen & Thornhill, 1998). Therefore, improving medication adherence is a common goal of illness self-management programs.

Strategies for enhancing medication adherence broadly stem from health behavior theories adapted to persons with cognitive and social disabilities. Corrigan (2002) notes that two models have been especially important in guiding treatment approaches. The Health Belief Model emphasizes *value expectancies* (Rosenstock, 1975), which posit that people are more likely to engage in specific health behaviors when they perceive themselves to be unhealthy in some way and that a specific behavior is likely to improve their health or well-being. Lack of insight into having a psychiatric disability could therefore contribute to medication nonadherence (Amador, Strauss, Yale, & Gorman, 1991). Efforts to educate consumers about the benefits of medication, as well as use of motivational interview, are strategies for improving medication adherence based on this model.

The Theory of Reasoned Action points out the importance of *attitudes and supports of significant others* in contributing to health behaviors (Fishbein & Ajzen, 1975). Given the interpersonal nature of health behaviors, efforts to improve medication adherence stemming from this theory emphasize improving consumer skills for engaging with providers, and family psychoeducation for helping family members acting as social supports to understand the benefits of medication. An additional consideration leading to medication adherence strategies has been the cognitive impairments related to psychiatric disabilities. While people in the general population often forget to take their medications, for those with severe cognitive difficulties, the problem of medicication nonadherence is exacerbated. Several strategies have been developed to address this problem, including incorporating the lack of medication into one's daily routine, behavioral tailoring, simplifying the medication regimen, using medication devices to keep track of when and what pills to take, and delivering medication directly to consumers and observing them take it. These strategies are described briefly below.

Psychoeducation involves providing information about the benefits and side effects of medication, as well as correcting common misconceptions, such as the belief that medications are addictive. *Motivational interviewing* is based on Miller and Rollnick's (2002) work with addictive disorders. The essence of motivational interviewing is that people are most likely to change their health behaviors when they see that doing so will help them achieve their personal goals and avoid unpleasant consequences of not changing. Motivational interviewing for medication adherence involves a combination of activities, including making a list of the advantages and disadvantages of taking medication, exploring with individuals the consequences of not taking medication in the past (such as relapses and rehospitalizations; becoming disorganized, psychotic, manic, or depressed), and evaluating whether taking medication can help people achieve personally meaningful goals (Kemp, Hayward, Applewhaite, Everitt, & David, 1996).

The *skills training* approach to improving medication adherence is aimed at helping consumers develop better skills for interacting with their mental health providers, especially whoever prescribes their medication. The assumption underlying this approach is that medication nonadherence is often due to poor skills for interacting effectively with treatment providers (Eckman, Liberman, Phipps, & Blair, 1990), such as the ability to get critical information from their treatment providers or to discuss medication side effects.

Family psychoeducation is aimed at helping families become aware of the benefits of medication and the nature of side effects. Primary goals of family psychoeducation are to enlist the support of family members in helping consumers adhere to their treatment recommendations, including prescribed medication, and to monitor adherence to medication.

Behavioral tailoring involves helping people develop strategies so that they are reminded to take their medication during the course of their daily activities. For example, people who have to take their medication in the morning and the evening could put a rubber band around their medication bottle or pillbox and put their toothbrush through the rubber band in order to remind them to take their medication when they brush their teeth in the morning and evening. Behavioral tailoring is typically combined with psychoeducation about the side effects of medication and is often implemented in one to three sessions (Cramer & Rosenheck, 1999). Home visits may be provided to determine the optimal way of integrating medication into the person's routine.

Simplifying the medication regimen involves reducing the number of medications that need to be taken throughout the day. Over the past decade there has been a trend toward prescribing numerous types of medications, some of which must be taken several times throughout the day (Covell, Jackson, Evans, & Essock, 2002). The natural difficulties of remembering to take medication can be compounded when additional medications are prescribed for medical conditions that occur more frequently in people with psychiatric disabilities than in the general population, such as diabetes (Sokal, Messias, Dickerson, Kreyenbuhl, Brown, et al., 2004). Developing a plan with the consumer to simplify the medication regimen (e.g., taking all one's medication in the evening instead of taking it twice a day) reduces the cognitive demands of having to remember to take medications more frequently.

Two different *medication devices* are commonly used to facilitate medication adherence. The most common device is pill boxes, which contain separate compartments for storing pills to be taken at different times on different days. By preparing pill boxes in advance and putting all the medications that need to be taken together in a place that is clearly labeled, the complexities of having to open multiple pill bottles throughout the day are avoided. Pill boxes are typically set up on a weekly or biweekly basis, often by a pharmacist, nurse, or case manager (although some consumers prepare their own pill boxes). Another medication device is the use of timers (which may be combined with pill boxes) to remind people when it is time to take their medication.

Finally, direct delivery of medication to consumers on a daily basis and monitoring the ingestion of medication are strategies that have been employed on Assertive Community Treatment teams (Stein & Santos, 1998) and by other direct service delivery staff to address medication adherence problems. Since such delivery of medications runs counter to the very goals of illness self-management, we do not consider them further here.

Research

Several studies have been conducted that have focused on strategies for improving medication adherence (Mueser et al., 2002a; Sajatovic, Davies, & Hrouda, 2004; Zygmunt et al., 2002). Behavioral tailoring has been most extensively studied, with four randomized controlled trials showing that it improves medication adherence (Azrin & Teichner, 1998; Boczkowski, Zeichner, & DeSanto, 1985; Cramer & Rosenheck, 1999; Kelly & Scott, 1990). A few studies have examined a standardized motivational interviewing intervention called *compliance therapy*. The first randomized controlled trial of this intervention showed that it improved medication adherence and led to lower symptoms and fewer hospitalizations (Kemp et al., 1996; Kemp, Kirov, Everitt, Hayward, & David, 1998). The lower inpatient treatment costs for consumers who received compliance therapy resulted in an overall net savings for this treatment compared to usual care (Healey, Knapp, Astin, Beecham, Kemp, et al., 1998). However, a second randomized controlled trial founded no benefit for compliance therapy (O'Donnell, Donohue, Sharkey, Owens, Migone et al., 2003). It is not clear why this second study failed to replicate the findings from the first study, although it was not documented in the second study that clinicians showed consistent fidelity to the treatment program.

Only one small-scale study has been examined to evaluate the effects of skills training on improving medication adherence (Dekle & Christensen, 1990). The results of this study were inconclusive. Finally, one controlled trial has demonstrated that simplifying the medication regimen is effective at improving medication adherence (Razali & Yahya, 1995).

In summary, the simplest and most efficient approach to improving medication adherence, behavioral tailoring, has also been found to be the most effective one. The results suggest that cognitive limitations associated with mental illness may contribute to adherence problems that can be overcome by making environmental modifications that incorporate cues to take medication into one's daily routine. This method is similar to other approaches to improving adaptive functioning in persons with psychiatric disabilities by environmental modifications, such as cognitive adaptive therapy (Velligan, Bow-Thomas, Hutchings, Ritch, Ledbetter, et al., 2000; Velligan et al., 2002).

Finally, although the effects of education and motivational enhancement on medication adherence remain unclear, they may nevertheless be important ways of fostering adherence. Consumers have a need and right to know about the side effects of medications so that they can make informed decisions about taking them. Ultimately the goal of psychiatric rehabilitation is for people to regain control over their lives and pursue and achieve personal and meaningful goals. As motivational interviewing helps people explore how changes in personal lifestyle behaviors (e.g., taking medication, using substances) can help them achieve their personal goals, it should be regarded as a potentially useful approach for dealing with the problem of medication nonadherence.

Relapse Prevention Training

Symptom relapses typically occur gradually over a period of several days and weeks. For many individuals, these relapses affect functioning only when they are severe and untreated, and therefore helping consumers prevent relapses is a goal of illness self-management. Symptom relapses are often preceded by subtle changes in cognition, mood, and social behavior, such as difficulties with concentration, feeling more anxious or depressed, and withdrawing from other people. The gradual onset of symptom relapses provides opportunities to teach individuals how to recognize their early signs of relapse and to take action to avert a full-blown relapse.

Relapse prevention training is a systematic approach to educating people about the nature of relapses, the early warning signs of relapses, how to identify possible triggers of relapses (such as holidays), identifying and monitoring personal early warning signs, and establishing a relapse prevention plan for responding to early warning signs of relapse. Because relapses often involve the loss of insight into the illness, involving significant others in developing a relapse prevention plan is common practice (and is a common component of family psychoeducational programs; see Chapter 11). Plans for responding to the early signs of a relapse can vary, but they often include contacting a member of the treatment team in order to obtain a temporary increase in medication, which is often a useful way of staving off a relapse (Herz, Glazer, Mirza, Mostert, & Hafez, 1989). The steps in developing a relapse prevention plan are summarized in Table 5.1.

TABLE 5.1. Steps of Relapse Prevention Training

1. Whenever possible, strive to develop a relapse prevention plan in collaboration with both the consumer and a significant other, such as a family member or another person who spends time with the consumer.

2. Discuss what a relapse is (a return or significant worsening of symptoms that interferes with functioning) and how having relapses and hospitalizations has affected the consumer's life and attainment of desired goals. Explain that relapses usually occur gradually over time and that developing a relapse prevention plan can minimize the chances or severity of future relapses.

3. Describe how stressful experiences can sometimes trigger relapses. Drawing from a discussion of one or two previous relapses, help the consumer identify some triggers of past relapses, such as increased school or work expectations or conflict with others. Stopping taking medication or using alcohol or drugs can also be identified as triggers.

4. Explain that relapses are usually preceded by small changes called "early warning signs of relapse." These signs include changes in feelings (such as anxiety or depression), thinking (such as concentration problems or disorganization), social connections (such as avoiding people), beliefs (such as paranoia or believing others are talking about the person), and sensory experiences (such as hearing voices). Based on past relapses, help the consumer identify two or three personal early warning signs of relapse.

5. Talk over and agree on a plan for responding to the early warning signs of a relapse. The plan should include who should monitor early warning signs, what steps need to be taken if early warning signs are detected (e.g., talk over the concern, problem solve about possible stresses, call the case manager, arrange for a special appointment to see the medication prescriber).

6. Write down the plan, rehearse the plan (in a role play) with people who are important to implementing it, give copies of the plan to people who need to know it (such as family members, the case manager), and identify a place where the consumer can post the plan.

7. If another relapse occurs, meet to review how the relapse prevention plan worked, reinforce the steps and strategies of the plan that worked well, and explore whether any changes are needed to make the plan even more effective.

Relapse prevention training has a long history in treating both substance abuse and mental health disorders (Herz, 1984; Marlatt & Gordon, 1985). Early detection of a relapse can either avert a relapse altogether or reduce the severity of a relapse and its impact on functioning. Relapse prevention training gives consumers greater mastery over their psychiatric disabilities by providing them with skills for minimizing problems related to relapses and rehospitalizations.

Research

The results of multiple randomized controlled trials of teaching relapse prevention strategies support its effectiveness (Mueser et al., 2002a). The relapse prevention programs studied have varied in their length and comprehensiveness. For example, Perry and colleagues (Perry, Tarrier, Morriss, McCarthy, & Limb, 1999) developed a 6-week relapse prevention program aimed at teaching people with bipolar disorder how to prevent recurrent episodes and showed that their program was effective over 1- and 2-year follow-ups. In contrast, Herz and colleagues (Herz, Lamberti, Mintz, Scott, O'Dell, et al., 2000) developed a relapse prevention program for people with schizophrenia, which involves weekly meetings over a 1-year period and support groups, aimed at helping people to track, recognize, and respond to the early warning signs of a relapse, and at improving their ability to manage common triggers of relapse, such as increased stress. This program was shown to reduce both relapses and rehospitalizations.

In addition to the research focusing on relapse prevention in persons with psychiatric disabilities, there is extensive research showing that family psychoeducation is also effective at preventing relapses and rehospitalizations (Dixon, McFarlane, Lefley, Lucksted, Cohen, et al., 2001; Pitschel-Walz, Leucht, Bäuml, Kissling, & Engel, 2001). One of the common ingredients of family psychoeducation programs is teaching family members how to recognize and respond to the early warning signs of a relapse. Thus, relapse prevention training can be conducted in the context of individual or group work with the consumer or through psychoeducation.

Coping Skills Training and Cognitive Restructuring

Consumers with psychiatric disabilities often experience persistent, troubling symptoms, such as psychotic symptoms (e.g., hallucinations, delusions), mood problems (e.g., depression, anxiety), negative symptoms (e.g., apathy, anhedonia), and cognitive difficulties (e.g., problems with concentration and memory). These symptoms can be both psychologically distressing and contributors to functional impairment. Helping people to cope with or overcome persistent symptoms is an important goal of most rehabilitation programs. Coping skills training and cognitive restructuring are two commonly used approaches to helping consumers manage or overcome persistent symptoms. Each is briefly introduced here and discussed more fully in Chapter 12, including the research evidence that supports them.

Coping skills training is a broad approach to enhancing the ability of people to manage persistent symptoms through the identification and practice of specific coping strategies. The approach evolved from research on how people with persistent symptoms successfully manage their symptoms. These accounts, and research on the use of various coping strategies among people with psychiatric disabilities, show that the more coping strategies a person reports using, the greater their coping efficacy (Falloon & Talbot, 1981; Mueser, Valentiner, & Agresta, 1997e). Therefore, an important aim of enhancing coping skills is to increase the number and variety of coping strategies people are able to use for managing persistent symptoms (see Table 5.2).

Cognitive restructuring is a set of cognitive-behavioral techniques that help people to examine thoughts and beliefs that contribute to negative feelings or dysfunctional behavior and to challenge and change those thoughts when they are inaccurate (Beck, 1995). The primary assumption underlying the use of cognitive restructuring is that people's emotional reactions to situations are determined by both their thoughts and their beliefs about those situations, as well as more general beliefs about themselves and the world. Thus, two people may react to the same situation in very different ways, depending on their individual thoughts and beliefs. Because many different thoughts are possible in a given situation, some thoughts may be more accurate than others, and some negative emotions (or dysfunctional behaviors) may stem from these inaccurate thoughts. Cognitive restructuring is a strategy for helping people become more aware of their thoughts and beliefs in different situations and for challenging them when they are associated with strong negative feelings.

Cognitive restructuring (also referred to as rational emotive therapy as developed by Albert Ellis) has a long history dating back to the 1950s and 1960s, when it was developed primarily for the treatment of depression and anxiety (Beck et al., 1979; Ellis, 1962). Following the success of cognitive restructuring in treating these problems, numerous other applications of the technique have been developed related to substance abuse (Beck, Wright, Newman, & Liese, 1993), bipolar disorder (Basco & Rush, 2005;

TABLE 5.2. Coping Strategies for Dealing with Auditory Hallucinations

Strategies	Examples
Arousal level	
Decreasing arousal	Relaxing, deep breathing, blocking ears, closing eyes
Increasing arousal	Getting physical exercise, listening to loud and stimulating music
Behavior	
Increasing nonsocial activity	Walking, doing puzzles, reading, pursuing hobby
Increasing interpersonal contact	Initiating conversation, playing a game with someone else
Reality testing	Seeking opinions from others
Cognition	
Shifting attention	Thinking about something pleasant, listening to the radio
Fighting back	Telling voices to stop
Positive self-talk	Telling yourself, "Take it easy"; "You can handle it"
Problem solving	Asking yourself, "What is the problem?" "What else can I do about it?" "What else can I do?" etc.
Ignoring the symptom	Paying as little attention to the symptom as possible
Acceptance	Accepting that the symptom is not going to go away and deciding to get on with other goals
Prayer	Asking for help in coping from a higher power

Note. Adapted from Mueser and Gingerich (2006). Copyright 2006 by The Guilford Press. Adapted by permission.

Lam, Jones, Hayward, & Bright, 1999), dual disorders (Graham, Copello, Birchwood, Mueser, Orford, et al., 2004), and most recently, psychosis (Chadwick, Birchwood, & Trower, 1996; Fowler, Garety, & Kuipers, 1995; Kingdon & Turkington, 2004; Morrison, Renton, Dunn, Williams, & Bentall, 2004). Clinical applications of cognitive restructuring to persons with psychiatric disabilities have challenged previous assumptions that psychotherapy is not useful with this population (May, 1968), and have suggested that people with these disorders may benefit from this form of therapy.

Research

Abundant research supports the effectiveness of teaching strategies for enhancing coping as well as broad-based cognitive-behavioral therapy that includes cognitive restructuring for consumers with persistent symptoms. Multiple studies have shown that cognitive-behavioral therapy is effective for the treatment of major depression, including severe and persistent depression (DeRubeis, Gelfand, Tang, & Simons, 1999; Gloaguen, Cottraux, Cucherat, & Blackburn, 1998). In a review of coping skills enhancement, studies, Mueser et al. (2002a) reported that five controlled studies found significant benefits in terms of reduced symptom severity or distress. Even more studies have been conducted examining the effectiveness of cognitive-behavioral treatment (with an emphasis on cognitive restructuring) for persistent psychotic symptoms. Table 5.3 summarizes reviews of this literature. Inspection of this table reveals that across all reviews, there is substantial evidence supporting the effectiveness of cognitive-behavioral therapy for psychosis.

In addition, there is evidence of the effectiveness of cognitive-behavioral treatment programs aimed at both relapse prevention and coping with symptoms for bipolar disorder (Gonzalez-Pinto et al., 2004). Several controlled studies have shown the benefits of cognitive-behavioral treatment for bipolar disorder over 1- to 2-year follow-ups (Lam, Bright, Jones, Hayward, Schuck, et al., 2000; Lam, Hayward, Watkins, Wright, & Sham, 2005; Lam, Watkins, Hayward, Bright, Wright, et al., 2003; Scott, Garland, & Moorhead, 2001; Scott, Paykel, Moriss, Bentall, Kinderman, et al., 2006), with one study showing that the cost of treatment was offset by reductions in high cost services such as hospitalization (Lam, McCrone, Wright, & Kerr, 2005).

Family Collaboration and Psychoeducation

Families play an important role in the management of all chronic illnesses, including psychiatric disabilities. There are several reasons why family collaboration and psychoeducation is particularly important for helping persons with psychiatric disabilities learn how to manage their illness (Mueser & Glynn, 1999). First, consumers often live at home or spend significant amounts of time with family members, and consequently there are many opportunities for relatives to have an impact on their lives, for better or worse. Collaboration between the treatment team and family members can increase the relatives' knowledge about the consumer's mental illness and the principles of its treatment, ensuring that they support the goals of treatment as well as the consumer's own personal goals for recovery. Second, the impact of psychiatric disorders on individuals often renders them highly dependent on family members, which can lead to high levels of stress and place a burden on relatives, and pressure on consumers, which can both reduce the quality of all family members' lives and increase vulnerability to relapse and rehospitalization. To address this problem, family psychoeducation is often aimed at improving the ability of families to cope with stress and conflict and improving the overall emotional climate of

TABLE 5.3. Reviews of Cognitive-Behavioral Therapy for Psychosis

Authors	Method of review	No. of studies	Conclusions
Garety, Fowler, & Kuipers (2000)	Narrative	4	• CBT reduces psychiatric symptoms • CBT may reduce relapse rates • Better insight may predict good outcome
Gould, Mueser, Bolton, Mays, & Goff (2001)	Meta-analysis	7	• Effect size = .65 for psychotic symptoms at posttreatment • Effect size = .93 for psychotic symptoms at follow-up
Rector & Beck (2001)	Meta-analysis	7	• Large effects of CBT for both psychosis and negative symptoms • Effects of CBT are in addition to those produced by supportive therapy
Pilling, Bebbington, Kuipers, Garety, Geddes, et al. (2002b)	Meta-analysis	8	• CBT *not* more effective at posttreatment • CBT more effective at follow-up • CBT associated with lower dropout rates than standard
Tarrier & Wykes (2004)	Meta-analysis	20	• CBT more effective for consumers with chronic symptoms than for those with acute symptoms • Effect sizes for CBT lower in more methodologically rigorous studies than in less rigorous ones
Gaudiano (2005)	Narrative	16	• CBT improves symptoms in psychosis, but mechanisms of action are unknown • Effectiveness research needed on PTSD for psychosis • Most research limited to Great Britain
Zimmerman, Faurod, Trieu, & Pomini (2005)	Meta-analysis	14	• Effect size = .57 for acute psychotic episode • Effect size = .27 for chronic conditions

the family. Third, symptom relapses in psychiatric disorders often involve a loss of insight, which can naturally interfere with the ability of the individual to manage his or her psychiatric disability. Family psychoeducation teaches families (including consumers) how to recognize the early warning signs of relapse and the steps to take when such signs are detected (e.g., call the treatment team), increasing their ability to stave off full-blown relapses that can interfere with functioning and result in hospitalization.

Family psychoeducation programs typically incorporate the broad range of illness self-management components reviewed in this section in either individual or multiple-family group formats, as described in Chapter 11. As also described in Chapter 11, there is abundant evidence that family psychoeducation is effective at improving specific illness outcomes, especially relapses and rehospitalizations, with more modest effects on functional outcomes as well. For these reasons, in addition to providing family psychoeducation programs, collaboration between mental health treatment providers and family members is a common component of illness self-management programs.

Self-Help and Peer Support

As described earlier in this chapter, the consumer and self-advocacy movement played a key role in the development of illness self-management approaches for psychiatric disability. Resentment and mistrust due to traditional hierarchical and coercive treatment approaches to psychiatric disabilities led consumers to advocate for their ability to take control over their own lives, including their own treatment. Rather than looking to professionals for help, consumers were encouraged to look to one another for help and inspiration in coping with their problems and moving forward in their lives. This focus on self-reliance has been accompanied by the larger self-help movement that has spawned numerous books, DVDs, websites, and classes aimed at helping people improve all aspects of their lives, such as health, mental health, relationships, financial standing, sports, and sex. For example, within the mental health field there are numerous self-help books providing guidance for individuals and their families on how to cope with anxiety (Jeffers, 1992), depression (Burns, 1980), bipolar disorder (Miklowitz, 2002), schizophrenia (Mueser & Gingerich, 2006), posttraumatic stress disorder (Schiraldi, 2000), obsessive–compulsive disorder (Foa & Wilson, 2001), and personality disorders (Bockian, 2002; Brown, 2003).

Self-help and peer support are inextricably intertwined, and because of their very nature they have defied most rigorous scientific evaluation (i.e., people cannot be simply assigned to "self-help" or "peer support" as they might to other forms of treatment). See Chapter 17 for a more thorough discussion of this kind of support. Nevertheless, self-help and peer support are broadly accepted as valuable parts of illness self-management because they are consonant with the core theme of taking personal responsibility for one's life, including one's psychiatric disability.

STANDARDIZED ILLNESS SELF-MANAGEMENT PROGRAMS

Over the past two decades numerous programs have been developed to teach consumers how to better manage their psychiatric disabilities. In this section we describe several well-standardized and widely available programs and the research evidence supporting them.

UCLA Skills Training Modules

The Medication Management and Symptom Management modules are two of eight different skills training modules that form the Social and Independent Living Skills (SILS) program developed by Robert P. Liberman, Charles Wallace, and their colleagues at UCLA (Kopelowicz & Liberman, 1994). These modules were developed for persons with psychotic disorders with the aim of providing them with basic information about the pharmacological and psychosocial management of schizophrenia, the prevention of relapses, and coping with persistent symptoms. Other modules in the program include Basic Conversational Skills, Recreations for Leisure, Community Re-entry (for inpatients anticipating discharge to the community), Substance Abuse Management, Workplace Fundamentals, and Friendship and Intimacy.

All modules in the program are taught using the principles of social skills training (e.g., modeling, role playing, etc.) based on video demonstrations of topic areas and skills (Liberman et al., 1989b). The modules are designed to be provided in a group format, although they can also be provided individually. Each module includes a core set of materials, including an instructor's manual, participants' workbooks, a demonstration video, and fidelity and outcome measures. For the Medication Management module, teaching is organized around four topic areas: the benefits of medication, self-administration and self-monitoring of medication effects, coping with side effects, and negotiating medication issues with health providers. The Symptom Management module teaching is organized around four skill areas: identifying early warning signs of relapse and seeking early intervention, devising a relapse prevention plan, coping with persistent symptoms, and avoiding substance abuse. The duration of time needed to complete each module depends on the frequency of sessions and the level of functioning of participants, with 3–6 months of twice weekly sessions required for outpatients.

Research

A significant amount of research has been conducted on the Medication Management and Symptom Management modules, which are often provided in the context of skills training in other areas. Research on the dissemination of modules in the SILS program indicates that clinicians can implement the modules with high fidelity to the program (Wallace et al., 1992). Controlled research also shows that consumers who participate in the Medication Management and Symptom Management modules acquire and retain the targeted information and skills over 1 year, as compared with other nonskill interventions (Eckman, Wirshing, Marder, Libeman, Johnston-Cronk, et al., 1992; Wirshing, Marder, Eckman, Liberman, & Mintz, 1992).

Some controlled research also supports the effects of skills training using these modules. One study comparing intensive skills training in these modules over 6 months with occupational therapy showed significantly greater improvements in independent living skills and relief of distress for the skills training groups (Liberman, Wallace, Blackwell, Kopelowicz, Vaccaro, et al., 1998). A second controlled study showed that skills training based on these modules for 6 months, followed by 18 months of skills training in other topic areas, was associated with better social adjustment at 2 years, as compared with equally intensive supportive therapy (Marder, Wirshing, Mintz, McKenzie, Johnston, et al., 1996). Two additional controlled studies using these and other skills training modules have demonstrated the utility of involving indigenous community supporters (Tauber et al., 2000) and augmenting clinic-based training with training in the community (Glynn et al., 2002) in improving social functioning. Interestingly, across all four studies there have been no differences between groups in changes in symptom severity, relapses, or rehospitalizations. It should be noted that these studies focused on stable outpatients who were at relatively low risk for relapse.

Personal Therapy

Personal therapy is an individual psychotherapeutic approach developed by Hogarty and his colleagues (Hogarty, Kornblith, Greenwald, DiBarry, Cooley, et al., 1995) for persons with schizophrenia or schizoaffective disorder. The primary goal is the achievement and maintenance of clinical stabilization, although the therapy also strives to help people improve their psychosocial and occupational functioning. Therapy is usually initiated following a relapse or rehospitalization, hence its focus on restablization. Sessions are generally conducted about weekly for the first year and biweekly or less often for another 2 years. The program is standardized (Hogarty, 2002).

Personal therapy is divided into three phases, with specific guidelines for progressing from one phase to the next. The basic phase of personal therapy begins with the therapist engaging the consumer in treatment, establishing a therapeutic relationship (and connecting with family if involved), and developing a treatment plan. The therapist then provides psychoeducation about schizophrenia and its treatment, makes plans with the consumer to begin resuming tasks and responsibilities, and begins to help the consumer develop coping strategies for managing stress. This phase ends with social skills training to help the consumer to avoid conflict situations and to initiate positive interactions with others. Hogarty (2002) notes that the basic phase of personal therapy could stand alone as a comprehensive management approach to schizophrenia. The intermediate and advanced phases of therapy are essentially extensions of the basic phase. Further psychoeducation is provided, with refinement of the ability to recognize and cope with signs of stress, work continues on resuming tasks and roles, and additional skills are taught pertaining to social perception and social skills The advance phase continues the work of the previous phases, with additional skills taught, including use of imagery and conflict management, and further attention to social and vocational role development.

Research

Two controlled studies were conducted concurrently on personal therapy, one for consumers living with family members and another with consumers living independently (Hogarty et al., 1997a, 1997b). In the former study, consumers were randomly assigned to family psychoeducation based on the Anderson et al. (1986) model, personal therapy, supportive therapy, or personal therapy plus family psychoeducation. In the latter study consumers were assigned to either personal therapy or supportive therapy. Personal therapy was found to reduce psychotic relapses for consumers living at home, but was associated with higher relapse rates than supportive therapy for consumers living on their own. The authors interpreted the higher relapse rates among the consumers living independently to frequent housing problems and conflict with landlords in this group, mainly during the first year, and suggested that the additional stress associated with therapy may have contributed to the relapses. However, over a 3-year follow-up, personal therapy was associated with significantly greater improvements in overall symptom severity, adjustment, and work.

Illness Management and Recovery

Illness Management and Recovery (IMR) was developed with support from the Robert Wood Johnson Foundation and the Substance Abuse and Mental Health Services Administration as one of five evidence-based psychosocial implementation resource kits for psychiatric disabilities (Drake et al., 2001b; Mueser et al., 2003d). IMR was created on the basis of a comprehensive review of controlled research on illness self-management approaches (Mueser et al., 2002a). This review identified five components of illness self-management that were supported by evidence, including psychoeducation, behavioral tailoring for medication adherence, relapse prevention training, social skills training for social support, and teaching coping skills for persistent symptoms. An emphasis on establishing individual recovery goals, and pursuing these goals throughout the program, was included in the IMR program in order to motivate consumers to learn how to manage their psychiatric disabilities in pursuit of those goals (Mueser, Meyer, Penn, Clancy, Clancy, et al., 2006b; Strauss, 1989).

IMR can be delivered in either an individual or group format and generally requires 6–10 months to complete, depending on the frequency of sessions and the level of impairment of the participants (Gingerich & Mueser, 2005). The curriculum for IMR is organized into ten modules or topic areas, including:

1. Recovery strategies
2. Practical facts about schizophrenia/bipolar disorder/depression
3. Stress-vulnerability model and strategies for treatment
4. Building social support
5. Using medications effectively
6. Drug and alcohol use
7. Reducing relapses
8. Coping with stress
9. Coping with problems and persistent symptoms
10. Getting your needs met in the mental health system

Each topic is taught using a combination of educational, motivational, and cognitive-behavioral teaching strategies. The IMR program includes a series of educational handouts for consumers (one for each module), a manual for clinicians, information brochures (for consumers, family members, clinicians, policy makers), an introductory video for the program, a training video for clinicians, a fidelity scale, and outcome measures. All of these materials except the videos can be downloaded from the web at *www.mentalhealth.samhsa.gov.* An educational curriculum (module 2) has been developed for schizophrenia spectrum and mood disorders, although the rest of the curriculum is not specific to psychiatric diagnoses.

Research

Although IMR was developed on the basis of a review of evidence-based practices for illness self-management, research has just begun to yet evaluate the effectiveness of the program. One randomized controlled trial of the IMR program has recently been completed (Hasson-Ohayon, Roe, & Kravetz, in press). This study was conducted in Israel at 13 different community rehabilitation programs and involved 210 people with a psychiatric disability (84% schizophrenia) who either participated in the IMR program (delivered in groups) or received usual psychiatric services. Assessments were conducted before the IMR program and 8–11 months later. Results indicated that people who were randomized to the IMR program showed significantly greater improvements in illness self-management on the client and clinician versions of the Illness Management and Recovery Scale (Salyers, Godfrey, Mueser, & Labriola, in press), a measure of illness self-management that taps a broad range of areas targeted by the IMR program, including progress towards goals, knowledge of mental illness, medication adherence, relapse prevention plans, symptom distress, coping, social contact, involvement in structured roles, involvement in self-help, and substance abuse. People in the IMR program and those who received usual services both improved on a measure of coping with symptoms, whereas neither group changed on social support. This study provides support that the IMR program is effective at improving illness self-management skills. More research is needed to evaluate the impact of the IMR program on the course of symptoms and relapses, and community functioning. Several other controlled trials are currently under way.

Wellness Recovery and Action Plan

The Wellness Recovery and Action Plan (WRAP) was developed by Mary Ellen Copeland as a general, standardized program for helping individuals with recurring health and emotional problems to develop healthier and more rewarding lives (Copeland, 1997, 1999; Copeland & Mead, 2004). WRAP is a structured program in which an individual or group of persons is guided through developing a personal written plan for managing or reducing troubling symptoms, as well as making other desired changes in their lives. WRAP is oriented toward helping anyone with physical or mental health problems regain control and balance in his or her life, and therefore it avoids providing information about specific disorders or treatment principles. Rather, as the title suggests, the emphasis is on wellness and health.

The WRAP program is divided into seven components, each one including written plans that the consumer maintains in a workbook:

1. Creating a daily maintenance plan
2. Identifying triggers, early warning signs, and signs of potential crisis
3. Developing a crisis plan
4. Establishing a nurturing lifestyle (e.g., more healthy living)
5. Setting up a support system and self-advocating
6. Increasing self-esteem
7. Relieving tension and stress

Teaching is typically done through a combination of lecture and discussion, with time taken to complete the plans and receive advice and support. WRAP is usually provided by trained consumers, who often use their own experiences to inspire other consumers to realize that they can recover their wellness.

Research

Controlled research has not been conducted on WRAP.

Team Solutions

Team Solutions is a psychoeducational program for schizophrenia developed by the Eli Lilly Company, designed to teach consumers about the nature of the disorder and its treatment. The program is standardized and includes a video, a trainer's manual, and educational handouts and worksheets for consumers (Scheifler, 2000). Teaching can be conducted on an individual or group basis, with approximately 4 months of weekly sessions required to cover the material.

The curriculum in Team Solutions covers the following topics:

1. Understanding your illness
2. Understanding your symptoms
3. You and your treatment team
4. Recovering from schizophrenia
5. Understanding your treatment
6. Getting the best results from your treatment
7. Helping yourself prevent relapse

8. Avoiding crisis situations
9. Coping with symptoms and side effects
10. Managing crisis and emergency situations

Research

One controlled study has been conducted on the Team Solutions program (Vreeland, Minsky, Yanos, Gara, Menza, et al., 2006). This study compared the Team Solutions program with treatment as usual and included a 6-month posttreatment assessment. The results showed that consumers in Team Solutions demonstrated significant improvements in their knowledge of schizophrenia and its treatment, but there were no differences between the groups in either symptoms or community functioning.

Dialectical Behavior Therapy

Dialectical behavior therapy (DBT) is a comprehensive psychotherapeutic approach that was originally developed with a primary focus on reducing self-injurious and suicidal behavior, but is now more broadly applied to persons with borderline personality disorder (Linehan, 1993a, 1993b). *Dialectic* or *dialectics* refers to the process of resolving conflict between two apparently contradictory ideas or forces through a synthesis of the two or establishing truths on both sides, rather than attempting to prove one right and the other wrong. In DBT, dialectics are employed at the level of the therapeutic relationship by the practitioner's combined use of validation and acceptance of the consumer as he or she is, with the strategies aimed at changing behavior and achieving a better balance in the consumer's functioning. Dialectics are also used help consumers strike a balance between the "reasonable mind" and the "emotional mind" in striving to develop a "wise mind" that combines the two in an integrated fashion.

In practice, DBT involves a wide array of cognitive-behavioral techniques to improve interpersonal skills (e.g., social skills training), the self-management of negative emotions (e.g., cognitive restructuring), and practical problem solving, which are combined with mindfulness-based strategies (e.g., focusing on the present, taking a nonjudgmental stance) aimed at promoting acceptance and tolerance of the person as he or she is, including any unpleasant feelings and thoughts. DBT is usually provided using a combination of weekly individual psychotherapy and group skills training, with therapists providing DBT also participating in weekly case consultation meetings among themselves. Specific guidelines are provided for establishing a clear treatment contract between the consumer and therapist before beginning the program and for specifying the nature of and rules concerning any additional contacts (e.g., telephone calls regarding thoughts of self-injury). Although DBT was initially developed to focus on outpatients' suicidal threats or behaviors, the program has been adapted for inpatients (Bohus, Haaf, Simms, Limberger, Schmahl, et al., 2004) and persons with borderline personality disorder and substance use disorders (Linehan, Dimeff, Reynolds, Comtois, Welch, et al., 2002).

Research

In the decade following the development of DBT and the first controlled trial, it has become a widely implemented program, despite limited rigorous research on the model (Scheel, 2000). Two randomized controlled trials have been conducted comparing DBT with usual treatment services over a 1-year period in outpatients with borderline person-

PERSONAL EXAMPLE

Jerome Learns How to Manage His Illness and Get On with His Life

To address Jerome's need for improved illness self-management skills, he was engaged in the Illness Management and Recovery (IMR) program at his community mental health center. The program began with an exploration of the concept of "recovery." The clinician described to Jerome different definitions of recovery given by consumers, and encouraged him to talk about what recovery meant to him. Jerome didn't relate very much to the word *recovery*, because he had his doubts about whether he had an illness in the first place, but the conversation did lead to identifying some concrete goals that Jerome was interested in working toward, including returning to school and having some friends he could spend time with. They agreed to work toward these goals together.

Jerome's clinician then provided him with some basic information about schizophrenia, including the nature of the disorder and the common symptoms. During this discussion, Jerome made it clear that he didn't think that he had schizophrenia, and the clinician showed that she understood this and did not press him to accept the diagnosis. Jerome acknowledged that he had "nervous problems" that made him feel anxious around people and very sensitive to stimuli in his environment. The clinician showed Jerome that she understood his concerns and explained that other people also had these kinds of difficulties and that there were effective strategies for coping with them and reducing their impact on his life.

After discussing with Jerome some of the symptoms he experienced related to his "nervous problem," the clinician engaged him in a discussion about medication. She and Jerome talked about the different medications that Jerome had taken over the years and got Jerome's perspective about what taking the medications was like for him. The clinician informed Jerome that the medications could be helpful in reducing symptoms related to his nerve problems and that medications helped many people avoid hospitalization. Upon exploring this further, Jerome acknowledged that when he took his medication more regularly he felt less afraid and was less likely to be hospitalized. However, Jerome also said that he didn't like some of the side effects of the medications, including the nervous feeling that he felt inside when he took them (akathisia) and feeling lethargic. The clinician discussed common medication side effects and the importance of talking over these side effects with Jerome's doctor. The clinician role-played with Jerome how he could express his concerns with the doctor so that changes could be considered in the medications he was prescribed. Jerome agreed that this would be useful and in his next visit engaged in a discussion with his doctor, which lead to switching to a new medication with less disturbing side effects.

As Jerome became more aware of the benefits of medication and his concerns about side effects were addressed, he and his clinician began to make plans for him to resume responsibility for taking his own medication. Jerome's initial efforts to take responsibility for his medications met with limited success because he kept forgetting to take them at appropriate times. His clinician helped him incorporate taking his medications into his daily routine by teaching him to place them next to the coffeemaker so that he would be reminded to take them in the morning when he was preparing his coffee.

Although Jerome's vulnerability to relapses decreased as he began to take medication more regularly, some vulnerability continued. To reduce relapses further, Jerome's clinician helped him to develop a personal relapse prevention plan. This plan involved working with Jerome and his parents, whom he saw regularly. They first identified the unique early warning signs of relapse for Jerome and then devised a plan for responding to those signs. Jerome's early warning signs included avoiding other people and feeling "paranoid." The steps involved in Jerome's relapse prevention plan included Jerome's talking over these signs with either the clinician or his parents and scheduling a special appointment to be seen by his doctor. Jerome agreed that if other people noticed these early warning signs before he did, it would be good to have this discussion and arrange for a special meeting with the doctor. They also agreed to monitor the early warning signs on a weekly basis. Once the plan had been agreed upon, he and his clinician role-played it and Jerome's doctor was informed of the plan.

Throughout the course of teaching Jerome how to better manage his psychiatric disability, attention was also focused on helping him pursue his personal goals, including returning to school and making some friends. In the context of pursuing these goals the clinician explored with Jerome how learning how to manage his nervous problem would help him achieve his goals. With respect to returning to school, Jerome looked into taking some classes and decided to begin slowly by auditing a course at a local community college. Jerome also started going to a local consumer drop-in center, where he began to make some friends with people with more interests.

Although Jerome was pleased by being able to stay out of the hospital, he continued to be distressed by some of his symptoms. He often felt anxious and paranoid around other people and continued to occasionally hear voices that he found distracting. Jerome's clinician explained that it was not unusual for people to continue to experience some difficulties even when they were taking their medication. They then worked together to help Jerome develop coping strategies for minimizing the effects of these symptoms on his pursuing his goals. One of these strategies involved a relaxation skill that he could use when he was around other people to lower his anxiety level. Jerome also practiced refocusing his attention away from his voices and on to other things when they were bothersome. Finally, Jerome was taught how to use positive self-statements to counter the derogatory comment that the voices made about him.

Through learning illness self-management skills, Jerome became a more active participant in his own treatment and was able to take greater responsibility for managing his own care. In addition, by working collaboratively with a clinician, Jerome was able to identify personal goals and to pursue those goals while learning how to manage his illness more effectively. By combining the pursuit of personal goals with learning illness self-management, Jerome was motivated to learn these strategies and reduce the disruptive effects of the illness on his life. Finally, although Jerome did not believe that he had schizophrenia, he was able to work with his clinician to learn how to manage his disability and regain control over his life.

ality disorder, with samples sizes of 44 (Linehan, Armstrong, Suarez, Allmon, & Heard, 1991) and 58 (Verheul, Van Den Bosch, Koetter, De Ridder, Stijnen, et al., 2003). Both studies reported that consumers who received DBT had fewer instances of self-injurious (i.e., "parasuicidal") behavior, although other symptoms did not differ significantly between the groups. An additional small randomized controlled trial ($N = 20$) evaluated the effects of 6 months of DBT as compared with usual services in women veterans with borderline personality disorder (Koons, Robins, Tweed, Lynch, Gonzalez, et al., 2001) and reported significant effects favoring DBT in self-harming behavior, depression, hopelessness, and anger. In addition to applications of DBT to address self-harming behavior in borderline personality disorder, two small studies ($N = 23, 28$) have evaluated the impact of DBT in the treatment of borderline personality disorder and substance abuse (Linehan et al., 2002; Linehan, Schmidt, Dimeff, Craft, Kanter, et al., 1999). Both studies reported greater improvements in substance use for the consumers who received DBT as compared with those who received standard treatment services.

The results of research on DBT provide modest support for its effectiveness in the treatment of borderline personality disorder, especially in addressing the vexing problem of self-injurious behavior. The effects of DBT on the longer-term course of borderline personality disorder, including hospitalizations, symptom severity, and functional outcomes, remain unstudied. Further research is needed to evaluate the effects of DBT, including both studies with larger sample sizes and research conducted by independent investigators other than Linehan, who developed the intervention.

SUMMARY AND CONCLUSIONS

It is now widely accepted that consumers can play an active role in the treatment of their own psychiatric disabilities, and the teaching of illness self-management skills is crucial to accomplishing this. In addition to the improved course of mental illness that illness self-management may bring, there may be psychological benefits as well when consumers become more self-reliant in dealing with their illness and capable of handling their own affairs. Finally, improved illness self-management is important to the goals of rehabilitation and recovery, because it can minimize the disruptive effects of relapses, rehospitalizations, and persistent symptoms on people's lives.

Research on specific components of illness self-management training indicates that a combination of interventions is effective for producing various outcomes. Psychoeducation is effective at improving consumers' understanding of their psychiatric disability and its treatment, but has a limited impact on the course of illness. Behavioral tailoring is a specific strategy that is effective at improving medication adherence, although its effects on other outcomes has not been evaluated. Relapse prevention training enjoys strong empirical support, as does cognitive-behavioral therapy (CBT) for reducing distress and severity of persistent symptoms, including depression, anxiety, and psychotic symptoms. These different components of effective illness self-management have been incorporated to varying degrees into comprehensive illness management programs. In addition, many of these components are incorporated into family psychoeducation programs aimed at teaching consumers and their natural supports the rudiments of managing a psychiatric disability in collaboration with mental health professionals.

Research supports the effects of family psychoeducation on reducing relapses and rehospitalizations. In addition, research supports the individual components of illness self-management (e.g., psychoeducation, relapse prevention training, coping skills enhancement). However, the effects of comprehensive illness self-management programs on the immediate goals of illness control, and the long-term goals of improving psychosocial functioning, are less well established. More work is needed to address these important issues.

Chapter 6

Case Management

The need for case management services for persons with psychiatric disabilities emerged as a consequence of the deinstitutionalization of patients in public psychiatric hospitals. When psychiatric patients were confined to institutions, not only were their treatment needs provided for, but also all of their basic human needs. The first patients who were released generally went to live with their families. Families became the patients' de facto case managers, assisting their ill relatives in accessing the necessary services and benefits from their communities (Intagliata, Willer, & Egri, 1986). As other patients without family members available left these facilities, there was no one to assist them in navigating the complex and fragmented service systems. Furthermore, even those with families found the process of accessing the needed supports and resources exceedingly difficult, as the treatments, resources, and benefits required were in a diversity of organizations and human service systems, which necessitated information, expertise, and the wherewithal that the uninitiated frequently did not possess.

Staff at the National Institute of Mental Health (NIMH) recognized that because of the functional disabilities of the discharged population, far more than mental health treatment was essential for members of this population. They needed a range of community services and supports, including housing, medical care, and financial benefits. In the late 1970s, the Community Support Program was established at NIMH and the community support system was conceptualized to offer a model for states and local communities to plan for community-based mental health service delivery systems to ensure a comprehensive array of services to meet the diversity of needs of those discharged from psychiatric hospitals (Turner & TenHoor, 1978). Case management was designed to be the glue of the system, serving the centralized and coordinating functions of ensuring that persons with psychiatric disabilities received the services and supports that they needed when they needed them (Stroul, 1993). Consequently, case management emerged to compensate for the lack of coordination within and among numerous social and human service systems.

By the mid-1980s, Congress passed the State Comprehensive Mental Health Services Plan Act of 1986 (PL 99-660) that required states to develop a state comprehensive service plan for adults with severe mental illness in order to continue to receive their allocated federal mental health funds. One of the stipulations of these plans was that states were to make provisions for the delivery of case management services to all of those in this population who receive substantial amounts of public funds and services, and this was to be achieved by 1992. Consequently, case management continued to be a central element of a comprehensive system of care for those with psychiatric disabilities.

Recently the private sector behavioral health managed care has employed case management as a strategy to control increasing health care expenses. Case management in this context does not provide services, but rather functions as a utilization review mechanism to manage the allocation of scarce and costly resources by limiting access to services and substituting lower-cost service options for higher-cost ones, such as outpatient therapy as an alternative to hospitalization (Sledge, Astrachan, Thompson, Rakfeldt, & Leaf, 1995). This use of case management is somewhat antithetical to case management service models whose primary focus is to ensure that those with psychiatric disabilities receive the services and resources they need. This chapter focuses on case management as a service rather than as a cost containment strategy.

The chapter begins with defining case management and its functions. It then describes the various models of case management that have been employed with persons with psychiatric disabilities; discusses qualifications of case managers; describes funding mechanisms; reviews the research on the effectiveness of case management models; delineates the critical ingredients; discusses implementation and fidelity issues, and dissemination.

DEFINING CASE MANAGEMENT

Case management is a ubiquitous term that is used to describe a diversity of activities (Sledge et al., 1995). Even when clearly operationalized, the empirical referents are quite varied, as will become apparent as we describe the various case management models below (Bachrach, 1989). In the present context, *case management* is the process of accessing, coordinating, and ensuring the receipt of services to assist individuals with psychiatric disabilities to meet their multiple and complex needs in an effective and efficient manner (Intagliata, 1982; Walsh, 2000b). Solomon (1992) noted the importance of obtaining services when they are needed and for as long as they are needed in order to ensure continuity of care. Kanter (1996) indicated that case management is a practice modality that focuses on both "biological and psychological functioning, addresses the overall maintenance of the mentally ill person's physical and social environment toward goals of facilitating his or her physical survival, personal growth, community participation, and recovery from or adaptation to mental illness" (p.259). Case management is to provide a single point of accountability for assisting persons with psychiatric disabilities to receive the services they need (Rapp & Goscha, 2004). Usually case management consists of an individual case manager, but it may also include a team, as will become apparent as we discuss the various models of case management.

There are some practitioners who believe that case management is an integral component of the functions of a good therapist and that therapeutic involvement is essential to develop a comprehensive assessment of the person's needs and a subsequent plan for addressing these needs (Harris & Bergman, 1993; Lamb, 1980). Case management is generally viewed as affecting the psychiatrically disabled person's external world, but over time it may affect the person's internal abilities to cope and function in the community by teaching problem-solving and negotiating skills (Harris & Bergman, 1987). However, many of the models of case management do not include the provision of therapy, but rather the provision of supportive counseling. Similarly, the models differ in the extent to which they have a rehabilitation focus and actually employ rehabilitation technologies. Basic case management, exemplified by the broker model, merely maintains the original intent of ensuring that the client's critical needs are identified and services to address them are delivered.

Some persons with psychiatric disabilities take umbrage at the term *case management* as they feel that they are not cases to be managed and that the nature of this service is antithetical to empowerment. In their view, it is a service that creates dependency of persons with psychiatric disabilities on rehabilitation practitioners rather than independence (Everett & Nelson, 1992). But, currently, this is the widely accepted terminology in this country, whereas in other countries, such as England, the term *care management* is employed.

CASE MANAGEMENT GOALS, OBJECTIVES, AND FUNCTIONS

For persons with psychiatric disabilities, the major goals of case management are (1) to maintain contact with services; (2) to prevent decompensation of the illness in order to avoid hospitalization; (3) to reduce the length of stay when hospitalization does occur; (4) to provide rehabilitation to promote psychosocial functioning at the highest level of which the individual is capable; and, ultimately, (5) to improve the quality of life for persons with psychiatric disabilities as well as their family caregivers (Ellison et al., 1995; Sands, 2001). These goals are then translated into four basic service objectives: continuity of care, accessibility, accountability, and efficiency (Baker & Intagliata, 1992; Intagliata, 1982). These objectives are defined by these authors as follows:

- Continuity of care is the receipt of comprehensive and coordinated services at a given point in time as well as over the long term.
- Accessibility is accessing and receiving these needed services.
- Accountability is taking responsibility for ensuring the intended effect of the services provided.
- Efficiency is services being delivered when needed and in the appropriate sequence, resulting in cost-effective service provision.

These goals and objectives are then translated into numerous service functions. Regardless of the particular service model, there is a high degree of consensus as to the five basic functions performed by case managers when serving those with psychiatric disabilities. These include assessment, planning, linkage, monitoring, and advocacy (Pratt, Gill, Barrett, & Roberts, 1999; Sands, 2001). These are defined as follows:

- Assessment is the comprehensive evaluation of the strengths, deficits, problems, and needs of persons with psychiatric disabilities. This requires the gathering of information from a diversity of sources, including the individual, other treatment facilities, and significant support system members. See Chapter 4.
- Planning is the development of a service plan to meet the needs of persons with

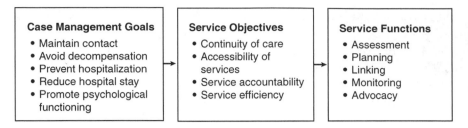

FIGURE 6.1. Goals, objectives, and service functions of case management.

psychiatric disabilities. In keeping with a recovery orientation, the individual is a partner in the development of this plan. The plan identifies the needs, specific services, resources, and supports to address these needs, and the behavioral steps to implement the plan.

• Linking is the connecting of persons with psychiatric disabilities with the services, supports, and resources needed in the implementation of the plan. For the person with a psychiatric disability this means more than making a referral to services, but also assisting the individual in accessing these services by accompanying him or her or arranging for others to help.

• Monitoring is ensuring that the services, supports, and other needed resources are received. Should obstacles in the receipt of these resources be encountered, corrective actions need to be undertaken. The progress of persons with psychiatric disabilities need to be monitored.

• Advocacy is the use of formal channels to obtain resources and services to which persons with psychiatric disabilities have a legal and ethical right, which may be denied. These persons may also be mistreated in the process of trying to obtain such services. Formal and informal strategies may have to be employed to make the necessary system changes to ensure the receipt of these supports.

These are the basic service functions provided by all case management services; various models may add on treatments and/or rehabilitation practices and technology. See Figure 6.1 for a summary of case management goals, objectives, and functions.

MODELS OF CASE MANAGEMENT

Over the years there has been a diversity of case management models developed and implemented. Currently, there are six models that have achieved prominence: (1) broker, (2) clinical, (3) strengths-based, (4) rehabilitation, (5) assertive community treatment (ACT), and (6) intensive case management (ICM) (see Table 6.1). There is some debate as to whether ACT should be categorized as a case management model, as it functions as far more than a case management program. Recognizing that other models, such as *strengths-based* and *rehabilitation* provide more than the basic functions of case management, we categorize all of these as case management, as this is consistent with much of the literature and the way most people refer to them. Each model is described, some with far more detail than others. ACT is discussed most extensively, as it is the most publicized model in terms of the scholarly literature, the most widely researched of all the models, and considered evidence-based practice. The other five models have been researched on a far more limited basis.

TABLE 6.1. Key Features of the Six Models of Case Management

Broker case management

- Basic functions: assessment, planning, linking, monitoring, and advocacy
- Mainly engages in service referrals
- High client–staff ratio
- Primarily office-based service

Clinical case management

- Basic broker functions plus clinical care
- Intermittent provision of psychotherapy
- Skill training and psychoeducation
- Environmental supports and resource acquisition

Strengths-based case management

- Identification of client's strengths
- Utilizes natural community resources
- Teaches client resource acquisition skills
- Group supervision of case managers

Rehabilitation case management

- Develop rehabilitation goal of client's choice
- Undertake functional assessment
- Provide skill training
- Teach resource acquisition skills

Assertive community treatment

- Multidisciplinary team
- Shared caseloads
- Low client–staff ratio
- Assertive outreach
- Services delivered in the community
- Time-unlimited services
- Team provides social services, rehabilitation, and psychiatric treatment to meet client's needs, including medication management

Intensive case management

- Assertive outreach
- Services delivered in the community
- Low client–staff ratio

Broker Case Management

The broker model of case management has also been referred to as generalist, traditional, or expanded broker case management and is the most basic of the models (Solomon, 1992). This was the first of the case management models to emerge in response to the deinstitutionalization movement. Case managers perform the basic tasks listed above, and for the most part do not go much beyond these functions (Intagliata, 1982). Essentially, the case manager in this model assesses the individual's needs, plans for how these needs are to be addressed, assists in linking the person with a psychiatric disability with

PERSONAL EXAMPLE

Lynn Smith Is Maintained by Broker Case Management

Lynn Smith is a 58-year-old single woman who is diagnosed with schizophrenia. She had been hospitalized until 1992 in a state hospital. Upon discharge, she moved into the family home, where she has been living since. Her father died in 1997. Her mother continued to care for Lynn in the family home, until 2½ months ago, when she fell ill and was hospitalized. Her mother subsequently died about a month ago.

Lynn has been involved with a mental health center for many years. She attends a day program there a few days a week. Lynn takes Clozaril to help with the symptoms of her schizophrenia. Every 2 weeks she goes to a lab for blood work. She also has a thyroid disorder and some digestive problems, for which she takes other medications prescribed by a family physician. She has a resource coordinator (broker case management) at the mental health center. The resource coordinator would check in with Lynn or her mother (while she was living) every 2 weeks to see how Lynn was doing. Mrs. Smith took Lynn to doctor's appointments or arranged for paratransit services, cooked, and maintained the home. If Lynn or her mother needed assistance with referrals for care or resources, they would contact the resource coordinator. Lynn was well maintained in the home and was compliant with her medication.

the range of required services, and coordinates the various service providers. Further, this model includes service monitoring to ensure the receipt of referred services and, when necessary, engages in advocacy on behalf of the person with psychiatric disabilities to obtain available services or fill gaps in services. Much of this work, and in many cases all of the work, is conducted in an office by means of referrals or phone calls, rather than in the community. These service brokers do not engage in therapy, but for the most part act as enablers, facilitators, or engagers (Mueser, Bond, Drake, & Resnick, 1998a; Sullivan & Rapp, 2002). Given these functions, broker case managers tend to have very high caseloads and to be very dependent on the existing community service system. It is evident that the case manager needs to be quite knowledgeable of the existing services available. This model requires limited training and expertise. Because of the high caseloads and consequent lower costs, this model continues to be widely used. With shrinking mental health dollars, this model continues to be widely practiced.

Given the intensive activity required to successfully engage individuals with psychiatric disabilities in services and to find and develop supports and resources, a case manager who merely engages in information sharing and referral is unlikely to be successful (Sullivan & Rapp, 2002). Further, with expanding caseloads, such case managers end up responding to crises, with limited time to be proactive in working on the assessed goals (Sullivan & Rapp, 2002). This model is often not provided in its purist form, but elements of other models are combined with these basic functions (Marshall, Gray, Lockwood, & Green, 2004). For example, supportive counseling is frequently an integral component in the provision of other functions.

Clinical Case Management

The clinical case management model posits the case manager as a clinical therapist as well as a provider of the basic functions of case management. Thus, this model incorporates the administrative functions of case management with clinical care (Kanter, 1989; Lamb, 1980; Roach, 1993; Solomon, 1998a). Clinical case managers assist clients in acquiring functional skills and in increasing their psychological growth by means of teaching various skills and problem-solving techniques and providing psychoeducation. Kanter (1989, 1996) describes clinical case managers as providing services and treatments in four service domains:

1. Initial phase—initial engagement, assessment, and planning.
2. Environmental focus—providing environmental interventions, which include linkage to services and resources, support, consultation, assistance, and advice to formal and informal members of the social network.
3. Client focus—client interventions, which include intermittent individual therapy, living skills training, and psychoeducation.
4. Client–environment focus—crisis services and monitoring.

Sullivan and Rapp (2002) note that although this model conceptually makes sense, it does not work very well in reality. Most therapists do not have the time for, or interest in, engaging in these basic broker case management activities. With the emergence of managed care, this issue has become more apparent, as clinicians are unable to assume these case management duties. This model as conceptualized requires a high level of clinical skills. Consequently, at least a master's degree in psychology, counseling, or social work is recommended.

The term *clinical case management*, as frequently used in general parlance, essentially refers to broker case management with supportive counseling. In clinical case management, as defined by this model, the case manager is a therapist who engages in psychotherapy and also carries out the case management functions. The pure clinical model is provided in practice only on a more limited basis.

Strengths-Based Case Management

Strengths-based case management was developed on the central premise that persons with psychiatric disabilities can engage in recovery and develop their full potential when given the opportunity to garner the necessary material and emotional supports needed to achieve their goals. This model has been guided from its very conception by the belief that "human behavior is largely a function of the resources available to people" (Sullivan & Rapp, 2002, p. 189). Consequently, people who are successful on their own in the community have the capability of developing their own potential and have access to needed resources to achieve their goals (Rapp, 1998b). This model focuses on the strengths or assets, rather than the deficits or problems, of the person with a psychiatric disability and utilizes an individual's natural community supports to facilitate community integration. Case managers assist those with psychiatric disabilities to identify, secure, and sustain the environmental and personal resources needed to live, work, and recreate as part of the larger community. The case manager teaches them to obtain the needed community resources for themselves. This model employs group supervision to stimulate creative brainstorming to develop strategies to acquire the necessary environmental resources and personal skills for problem resolution.

The strengths-based model is guided by six principles, which are then operationalized into a set of procedures (Rapp, 1993a). The six principles are as follows:

1. The focus is on individual strengths, rather than psychopathology.
2. The case manager's relationship with the person with a psychiatric disability is primary and essential.
3. Interventions are based on the self-determination of persons with psychiatric disabilities.
4. The community is viewed as an oasis of resources, not as a barrier.
5. Aggressive outreach is the preferred mode of intervention.
6. People with a psychiatric disability can continue to learn, grow, and change.

Rehabilitation Case Management

The rehabilitation model of case management was developed by the Boston University Psychiatric Rehabilitation Center. Within this model, case managers work with persons with psychiatric disabilities to negotiate for the services and resources they want and need and to develop the personal skills and environmental supports they need to overcome environmental and personal barriers in order to achieve their own identified goals (Farkas & Anthony, 1993). This model of case management is a combination of the functions of the broker case management model and the specific functions of psychiatric rehabilitation (Anthony, Forbess, & Cohen, 1993). The rehabilitation functions include setting an overall rehabilitation goal, conducting a functional assessment, and teaching skills needed for persons with psychiatric disabilities to function at their highest level possible in their chosen environments. The two fundamental interventions employed by the case manager are the same as those in the practice of psychiatric rehabilitation generally, providing skill training and resource acquisition. This model employs the rehabilitation technology developed by the Boston University Psychiatric Rehabilitation Center. The persons with psychiatric disabilities are active participants throughout the entire process (Anthony, Forbess, & Cohen, 1993).

Assertive Community Treatment

In the 1970s, the assertive community treatment model was created in Madison, Wisconsin, by Marx, Test, and Stein (1973) as a community-based alternative to psychiatric hospitalization. The original program was called Training in Community Living, and later the name was changed to the Program for Assertive Community Treatment (PACT). This model is now widely referred to as Assertive Community Treatment (ACT), but is also referred to as continuous care teams, full-service support, assertive outreach, and mobile treatment teams (Bond, Drake, Mueser, & Latimer, 2001b). ACT is a comprehensive system of care for persons with psychiatric disabilities, and case managers serve the coordinating function of this self-contained system of care. The intention of the program was to transfer all of the functions of a long-term psychiatric institution into the community, and, consequently, it was often called the "hospital without walls" (Stein & Test, 1980a). In the initial implementation, the staff of the hospital was actually transferred to the community as well (Test, 1998). The basic tenets of the model, as indicated by Test (1998), are the following:

- The community—not the hospital—should be the primary locus of care for persons with psychiatric disabilities, because the community is where persons with psychiatric disabilities face daily, ongoing stressors.
- Treatments and supports in the community must be comprehensive, potentially addressing all areas of life.

- Treatment and care must be flexible and highly individualized to address the vast heterogeneity of this population as well as the changing needs of the person with psychiatric disability across time.
- These comprehensive and flexible treatments and supports must be organized and delivered to reach persons with psychiatric disabilities efficiently (pp. 421–422).

This model is designed for persons who experience the most persistent and extreme symptoms of mental illness. These are individuals who have frequent episodes of symptom exacerbation and have difficulty in meeting their basic needs and keeping themselves safe. Consequently, these individuals are hard to manage. Thus, this service is reserved for those who have spent a good deal of time in psychiatric hospitals and/or living on the streets and who have problems with substance abuse and encounters with the criminal justice system (U.S. Department of Health and Human Service, 2003a).

The central feature of this model is the continuous treatment team, which is multidisciplinary. Team members have shared caseloads, whereby various team members are in frequent contact with each client served by the team. A team usually consists of a psychiatrist, a nurse, and at least two case managers. Frequently, social workers and rehabilitation counselors are team members as well. Some teams include persons with psychiatric disabilities and/or their family members (Dixon, Kraus, & Lehman, 1994; Dixon, Stewart, Kraus, Robbins, Hackman, et al., 1998). The ratio for these teams is about 1 staff member to 10 clients, but a team usually consists of 10–12 staff members serving about 120 persons with psychiatric disabilities (Phillips, Burns, Edgar, Mueser, Jenkins, et al., 2001b). Additional staff positions are contingent on the goals of the team and the nature of the population served. For example, if employment is a primary goal for many of those served by the team, then a vocational specialist is a member of the team. Or, if the team is serving a dually diagnosed population, then a specialist in substance abuse is required. With the high prevalence of substance abuse disorders among those with psychiatric disabilities today, it is common to have a team member with clinical expertise in substance abuse (Test, 1998; Bond et al., 2001b).

The ACT model goes beyond all currently existing case management models in terms of service provision, as the team is the primary provider and responsible entity for treatment, rehabilitation, and social services required by those served. This is self-contained, comprehensive program that essentially provides all services a client needs. To ensure information sharing regarding the status of each client, the team meets on a daily basis. This model provides an integrated approach to service delivery that is very much individualized to the needs of a given client. The core team provides medication, supportive therapy, problem-solving skill training, crisis intervention, and assistance with housing, finances, work rehabilitation, and anything else that is critical to living successfully in the community. The team uses assertive outreach to provide services wherever a person with psychiatric disability is located (Test, 1998; Bond et al., 2001b). The team is available 7 days a week, 24 hours a day.

Because it was found that skills taught in an exemplary program within a hospital did not generalize to community settings, ACT was designed to teach persons with psychiatric disabilities the skills needed for community living in the environment in which they were to be used (Marx et al., 1973). Services are generally provided *in vivo*, as confirmed by research by Brekke and Test (1987) on the original PACT. These researchers found that 78% of time spent with clients was on the client's own territory, whereas only 22% was spent in offices. This 80–20 split of community-to-office locations of service provision has become a rule of thumb (Bond et al., 2001b).

This program operates with a nontermination policy. If clients do not appear for appointments, they are not terminated from the service, as is sometimes the case with other models. In addition, this model was conceived of as a time-unlimited service. Recent research has indicated that this principle may be modified for those who demonstrate substantial improvement. However, a step-down transfer process should be used to ensure continuity of care, as well as the possibility of the individual's returning to ACT should this be deemed necessary (Salyers, Masterton, Fekete, Picone, & Bond, 1998).

There have been a number of variants of ACT teams developed to serve specialized populations or to add a specific service focus. Some ACT programs have smaller teams. For example, a staff of the Thresholds Bridge program has four to six members, with a caseload of 50–60 clients, and does not include all disciplines, but does consistently include a psychiatrist (Bond, McGrew, & Fekete, 1995c). Another variant is a forensic ACT team, which has been developed for community reentry or diversion from the criminal justice system (this model is discussed in Chapter 13; Solomon, 2003; Solomon & Draine, 1995e). Another enhanced model is Family-Aided Assertive Community Treatment (FACT), which adds multifamily group psychoeducation (McFarlane, Dushay, Stastny, Deakins, & Link, 1996). The specifics of multifamily groups are discussed in Chapter 11, "Family Interventions." Another variant is the use of a team composed of consumers to provide ACT (this model is discussed in Chapter 17; Paulson et al., 1999). This model has also served as a basis from which to develop other specialized services for those with psychiatric disabilities, such as supported employment, as discussed in Chapter 9 (Solomon, 1999).

More recently, there has been the development of an intervention that is referred to as In Vivo Amplified Skills Training (IVAST), which combines standard skills training with ACT (Bellack, 2004; Glynn et al., 2002). Clinic-based skill training is augmented with an In Vivo trainer who works with clients in the community, reinforcing what was learned in the clinic sessions. Liberman and his colleagues (Liberman, Blair, Glynn, Marden, Wirshing, et al., 2001) note, "IVAST supplies the missing ingredient that has proven to be an obstacle in the efforts of assertive community case managers to inculcate durable social and independent living skills to clients" (p. 109). Other compensatory interventions are being suggested to be combined with ACT, such as cognitive adaptation training. This training is based on neuropsychological, behavioral, and occupational therapy principles designed to compensate for the deficits of those with cognitive impairment in order to improve their functional adaptation. In addition, this training includes the development of environmental supports to fit the specific needs of the client (Velligan et al., 2000). For example, a program for a client who had hygiene problems was designed to obtain "special toothpaste and an extra-soft brush for his sensitive teeth [and] a large brightly colored basket on a peg at eye level for his showering supplies" (Velligan & Bow-Thomas, 2000, p. 28).

Intensive Case Management

In recognition of the lack of effectiveness of broker case management in serving heavy users of mental health services, intensive case management (ICM) emerged (Shern, Surles, & Wiazer, 1989; Solomon & Meyerson, 2003; Surles & McGurrin, 1987). This service model is sometimes referred to as assertive outreach, as it employs some of the aspects of ACT, including delivering services in the community, having low caseloads, engaging in assertive outreach, and assisting in meeting the daily needs of persons with psychiatric disabilities. Generally, this service is delivered by an individual case manager, and there are no shared caseloads. However, this is not a well-specified model. Research on the practice of ICM has found that there is no consensus on the essential ingredients of this model (Schaedle & Epstein, 2000). But, like the broker model, this model has been widely implemented, as it became apparent that individuals with psychiatric disabilities needed more than mere brokering of services, owing to their cognitive deficits. Therefore, the more assertive functions and the community service provision aspect were incorporated into a basic broker case management service (Stein, 1992). As is apparent from the common characteristics of this ICM model, ACT has greatly influenced the way in which case management is generally delivered, but most specifically with this model.

QUALIFICATIONS OF CASE MANAGERS

Case managers can be paraprofessionals, but need to be supervised by an experienced and fully credentialed person. In a national study of the practice of case management, Ellison and associates (1995) found that just over half of case managers had a bachelor's degree and about three-quarters of supervisors had a master's degree. Supervisors were also more experienced than case managers in working with persons with psychiatric disabilities, with an average of 11 years of experience. Case managers can come from a wide diversity of backgrounds, including persons with psychiatric disabilities who have been found to function effectively in the case manager role (Solomon, 2004; Solomon & Draine, 1994a, 1995a, 2001). However, case managers with limited education need training and supervision by an experienced professional and need to have access to medical professionals and other experts (Rapp & Gosha, 2004). Many of the tasks that are performed by case managers do not necessitate professional training for effective implementation, but the engagement of more qualified practitioners may result in higher-quality

---

PERSONAL EXAMPLE

Lynn Smith Revisited: More Intensive Case Management Needed

Lynn is still in the family home, as the resource coordinator has arranged for a part-time home health aide to help with general day-to-day care of Lynn and the house. However, this is a short-term solution, as Lynn cannot remain in the home. This will be difficult for Lynn, as she has lived in this home for many years and does not wish to move. At this point Lynn needs an intensive care manager to assist in finding her another housing arrangement, to help her to cope with the move, and to provide the ongoing daily management that was previously provided by her mother. Unfortunately, Lynn did not learn skills for living independently, so the type of case management services she will need will be contingent on the type of housing arrangement that is found for her. With supported independent housing, Lynn will need intensive case management to help her access resources and supports, to maintain her in her home, and to teach her skills of daily living. As long as Lynn adjusts to her new living arrangement and remains compliant with medication, she is not likely to need an ACT team. Should Lynn be placed in a community residential rehabilitation facility, she will likely need only a broker case management service, as in her previous situation.

services (Johnson & Rubin, 1983). Furthermore, professionals do not like to engage in the types of activities that are often required of case managers, as they do not feel that this enables them to use their professional training and skills (Solomon, 1998a). Research on ACT programs has also found that the only practitioners whose discipline was related to positive outcomes were nurses (McGrew, Bond, Dietzen, & Saylers, et al., 1994).

In a commentary on a study of the cost-effectiveness of intensive versus standard case management, Gournay and Thornicroft (2000) voiced concern regarding the possible insufficient training provided to intensive case managers and attributed the lack of positive outcomes to this issue. They then suggested that studies of training to assess "skill acquisition and knowledge gain" are now needed, and concluded: "Although randomized controlled trials of training interventions will be costly, the price of not knowing whether training makes a difference is much greater" (p. 371). A study by Morrison and his colleagues (Morrison, Meehan, Gaskill, Lunney, & Collings, 2000) did find that training case mangers in assessment and management of side effects of medication helped to reduce the side effects for persons with psychiatric disabilities and enabled the case managers to teach these clients strategies for dealing with unwanted side effects.

Some states have instituted credentialing of case managers, and some state and local offices of mental health require a limited amount of orientation and continued training thereafter for case managers. Although case managers need not be professionals, they clearly need some requisite knowledge of severe psychiatric disorders, community resources, psychiatric medications, and managing psychiatric crises. The clinical model of case management requires professional training such as a master's degree in social work, counseling, or psychology, given that these case managers engage in psychotherapy. Further, a survey of case managers in Oregon found that the perceived lack of specialized training in psychiatric rehabilitation was related to job dissatisfaction (Hromco, Lyons, & Nikkel, 1995).

FUNDING OF CASE MANAGEMENT

Case management services are frequently funded through Medicaid. ACT is also funded under the Medicaid rehabilitative services or targeted case management categories (Phillips et al., 2001b). Reimbursement under Medicaid does not always cover all case management activities, such as failed attempts to contact a client. Some case management activities may be funded from other revenue sources, such as substance abuse or housing funds (Phillips et al., 2001b). State or local mental health dollars may also be used to pay for portions of these services. ACT is particularly difficult to fund, as the complexity of the service makes it reimbursable across various service funding categories. The way in which case management services are funded differs by state, as well as locally.

EFFECTIVENESS/COST-EFFECTIVENESS OF CASE MANAGEMENT

To address the question of whether case management is *effective* is extremely difficult to answer, given the various ways in which this term is used and the diversity of models. It is easiest to address this question when comparable models of case management are assessed (Holloway, Oliver, Collins, & Carson, 1995). Some reviews have focused on specific models, such as the strengths-based model and ACT, whereas others are more comprehensive, focusing on a diversity of models. The assessment here focuses on more recent published reviews from 1995 to the present (see Table 6.2), although there were a number published earlier (e.g., Chamberlain & Rapp, 1991; Holloway, 1991; Olfson, 1990; Rubin, 1992; Solomon, 1992). These reviews have been both narrative and statistical. Some have limited the studies to those that employed a randomized design or quasi-experimental designs.

Much of the more rigorous research has been conducted on ACT, given that it is a more highly specified model. There is a great deal of consistency with regard to the outcomes reported for ACT, regardless of the type of review conducted. ACT has a greater likelihood of keeping persons with psychiatric disabilities engaged in services, increasing housing stability, reducing hospital admission and length of hospitalization when a client is hospitalized, and promoting high client and family satisfaction. A few reviews have concluded that there is improvement in symptomatology and quality of life, but most reviews find little effect of ACT on social functioning. Reviewers have noted that when there is greater fidelity to the original intervention, the outcomes are better (Bond et al., 2001b; Scott & Dixon, 1995). Some reviewers have questioned whether increased adherence to medication may produce the reduction in hospitalizations, but surprisingly few studies have assessed medication adherence (Baronet & Gerber, 1998; Burns & Santos, 1995; Holloway et al., 1995; Ziguras & Stuart, 2000). Part of the reason for not assessing medication adherence is the difficulty in being able to assess it reliably with easy-to-administer self-report measures, as opposed to more costly, complex, and accurate procedures, such as pill counts. This lack of assessment of medication compliance is a concern, as some critiques of ACT indicate that the positive outcomes are due to this factor. Reviewers have also commented on the fact that for ACT to achieve specific desired outcomes such as increased employment, reduced substance abuse, and reduced homelessness, the intervention has to be directly targeted at these outcomes (Burns & Santos, 1995). ACT is being widely adapted for special populations, but there is limited research on the effectiveness of these adaptations.

In regard to those reviews that were able to assess the cost of ACT, they noted a reduction in cost, which was attributed to a reduction in hospitalization, a very costly service among the states. Wolff and her colleagues' (Wolff, Helminiak, Morse, Caslyn, Klinkenberg, et al., 1997) evaluation of the cost-effectiveness of three approaches to case management for homeless clients with mental illness found that ACT had better outcomes at no greater cost, thus concluding that ACT is more-cost effective than brokered case management. Latimer (1999) conducted an economic review of the impact of ACT and found that regardless of the approach to cost assessment, ACT seems to result in lower costs. But Latimer cautioned that as systems come to rely less on hospitals, the advantages of ACT, with its reductions in hospitalizations, will be harder to achieve and the justification for implementing ACT will more likely be based on clinical benefits. This is consistent with the suggestion by Marshall and Lockwood (1999), that ACT should be reserved for heavy service users.

ACT has achieved the status of evidenced-based practice for persons with psychiatric disabilities, as based on the consistent positive outcomes from rigorously designed studies. This is one of only five psychosocial interventions for persons with psychiatric disabilities to achieve this status. However, it is also recognized that this is a costly intervention that should be reserved for the most vulnerable of the population with psychiatric disabilities.

The reviews that have specifically focused on case management, excluding ACT, have come to very different conclusions than those arrived at for ACT. These reviews have usually focused on broker or intensive case management. Like ACT, these types of

TABLE 6.2. Reviews of Case Management Models, 1995–2004

Reviewers	Type of review	Case management type	No. of studies	Inclusion criteria	Outcomes
Burns & Santos (1995)	Narrative	ACT	8	Articles 1990–1994 reporting results of randomized controlled trials	Fewer days hospitalization; improved clinical outcomes; high rates of clients remaining in treatment; high rates of client and family satisfaction
Bond, Drake, Mueser, & Latimer (2001b)	Narrative	ACT	25	Randomized controlled trials	Reduced hospital use; increased housing stability; moderately improved symptoms and subjective quality of life
Baronet & Gerber (1998)	Narrative	ACT	22	No specifics	Decreased number of hospitalizations; decreased length of hospital stay; increased medication adherence; increased involvement with mental health treatment; improved symptomatology; client and family more satisfied; improved residential stability; cost less because of reduced hospitalization
Baronet & Gerber (1998)	Narrative	CM and ICM	25	No specifics	Tendency to increase use of mental health services; increased level of social functioning; increased hospital use
Bedell, Cohen, & Sullivan (2000)	Narrative	Full service, broker, and hybrid (ICM, rehabilitation, strengths, and clinical)	8 reviews	Reviews of CM	Full service increased service retention; full service reduced hospitalizations; full service and ICM, modest cost savings; full service increased satisfaction; broker model, increased cost
Holloway, Oliver, Collins, & Carson (1995)	Narrative	All CM models	23	Outcome studies, all designs	Decrease in hospital use and length of stay—attributed to ACT; CM may increase use of other services; satisfaction with CM; some improvement in quality of life; social functioning mixed; no increase in family burden; improved social network/relationships; cost varied—less for ACT

150

Study	Type	Model	N	Methods	Findings
Scott & Dixon (1995)	Narrative	ACT, CM, and ICM	22	ACTs—faithful to model; Randomized controlled trials and quasi-experimental	ACT reduced rate and duration of hospitalizations; ACT less costly; ACT reduced symptomatology; improved social functioning, promoted residential stability, and independent living. ICM suggested reduce hospitalization; ICM, broker, rehabilitation increased use of other mental health services
Mueser, Bond, Drake, & Resnick (1998a)	Narrative	ACT, ICM, broker, strengths-based, and rehabilitation	75	Assessed at baseline and follow-up for two groups	ACT and ICM improved housing stability, reduced time in hospital; moderate effect on symptomatology and quality of life, withdrawal deterioration of gains, some evidence for client and family satisfaction; broker increased rates of hospitalization; ACT cost savings—effected by context
Sullivan & Rapp (2002)	Narrative	Strengths-based	8	All studies of strengths-based model	Decreased hospitalization; two studies found reduced symptoms; improved independent living, educational, vocational functioning, leisure time activities
Simmonds, Coid, Philip, Marriott, & Tyrer (2001)	Meta-analysis	Multidisciplinary CMH teams—ICM-type teams	5	Randomized controlled trials with standard care control	Fewer deaths, including those by suicide; fewer dropouts; shorter duration of hospital stay; lower cost of care
Herdelin & Scott (1999)	Meta-analysis	PACT	19	Randomized controlled trials comparison standard inpatient/outpatient treatment; excludes studies focused on specific diagnoses	Fewer hospitalizations; shorter hospital stay; higher social functioning; lower symptomatology; greater client satisfaction; lower cost, but limited to those with reduced hospitalization
Marshall, Gray, Lockwood, & Green (2004)	Meta-analysis	CM—broker, strengths-based, clinical	11	Randomized controlled trials—high-quality methods, standardized measures, less than 50% attrition	Retention in mental health treatment; trend toward higher mortality; higher hospitalization; tentative increase in hospital stay; tentative more compliance with medication; cost—increase cost for providers, but may reduce societal costs

(continued)

TABLE 6.2. (continued)

Reviewers	Type of review	Case management type	No. of studies	Inclusion criteria	Outcomes
Marshall & Lockwood (1999)	Meta-analysis	ACT versus standard care	17	Randomized controlled trials	More days in stable housing—living independently and fewer days homeless; less likely to be unemployed; less likely to be hospitalized; shorter hospital stay. Client more satisfied; less costly, but cost consideration does not favor ACT
Marshall & Lockwood (1999)	Meta-analysis	ACT versus hospital-based rehabilitation	3	Randomized controlled trials	Less likely to be hospitalized; more likely living independently
Marshall & Lockwood (1999)	Meta-analysis	ACT versus CM	9	Randomized controlled trials	Shorter hospital stay; less costly, ACT no clear-cut advantage
Gorey, Leslie, Morris, Carruthers, Lindsay, et al. (1998)	Meta-analysis	PACT (full support)	24	No specifics	Prevention of hospitalization; functioning better, quality of life better, cost less
Marshall & Creed (2000)	Meta-analysis	ICM	6	No specifics	Increase in contact with clients; increase in hospital admissions; increase in cost
Ziguras & Stuart (2000)	Meta-analysis	ACT and clinical versus usual treatment; ACT versus clinical	44	Randomized controlled trials and quasi-experimental	ACT and clinical vs. standard treatment—clients admitted more frequently to hospital; shorter hospital stay; smaller proportion of clients admitted to hospital; more contacts with mental health and other services; lower dropout rate from mental health treatment; greater client and family satisfaction with care; less family burden; lower cost ACT vs. clinical—ACT fewer hospital admissions and smaller proportion of clients admitted to hospitals; clinical—greater number of contacts with mental health services
Bond, McGrew, & Fekete (1995c)	Meta-analysis	ICM (Assertive Outreach)	9	Experimental, quasi-experimental, pre–post	Retention rate higher; fewer hospitalizations; shorter hospital stay

case management result in increased likelihood of clients staying in contact with services, but in contrast to ACT, clients are more likely to be admitted to a hospital and to have a longer duration of hospital stay (Baronet & Gerber, 1998; Marshall et al., 2004; Marshall & Creed, 2000) or increased use of mental health services (Scott & Dixon, 1995). However, given that these are not full support models and they do refer clients to other services, increased use of mental health outpatient services is not an unexpected outcome. Sullivan and Rapp (2002) conducted a review of strength-based case management and found a decrease in hospitalization and moderate improvement in some areas of social functioning, such as independent living and leisure time use.

Some of the reviewers point to other factors than the case management service per se that may well affect outcomes. For example, the environmental context in which case management is embedded in terms of service and resource availability is extremely important to most models of case management other than ACT (Mueser et al., 1998a; Ziguras & Stuart, 2000). But even ACT, to some extent, relies on the system in terms of housing and hospital bed availability. Moreover, case management may not be equally effective for all persons with psychiatric disabilities; some benefit whereas others may not (Ziguras & Stuart, 2000).

A cost-effectiveness study assessed the outcomes and costs of intensive case management (ICM) as compared with routine case management, employing a randomized design. The major distinction between the two services was a caseload differential, 8–10 cases as compared with 20–40. The investigators found that ICM clients were more likely to remain in treatment and to show clinically significant improvement in functioning. The cost-effectiveness ratio indicated an additional cost of $27,766 per year for one additional client served in ICM. However, these investigators indicated that further research was necessary to determine if this expenditure was a worthwhile use of mental health resources (Johnson, Salkeld, Sanderson, Issakidis, Teesson, & Buhrich, 1998).

The expertise, training, and attitudes of case managers may also influence client outcomes. A few recent studies have found that case managers can also have high expressed emotion (EE)—that is, being overcritical and hostile toward a client (EE is discussed more fully in Chapter 11)—and that high EE does result in poorer outcomes (Oliver & Kuipers, 1996; Tattan & Tarrier, 2000). On a more positive side, a recent review of the research on the therapeutic alliance in case management found encouraging evidence that the strength of a positive alliance is associated with improved outcomes. These reviewers noted that the research on the therapeutic alliance within case management is rather sparse and requires further examination. The reviewers concluded that promoting partnership between persons with psychiatric disabilities and case managers maybe a powerful strategy for helping clients to manage their illness and to optimize their strengths (Howgego, Yellowlees, Owen, Meldrum, & Dark, 2003).

ACTIVE INGREDIENTS OF EFFECTIVE CASE MANAGEMENT

Rapp and Goscha (2004) undertook a review of effective case management services to determine the active ingredients in case management, specifically, those elements that produce positive outcomes for persons with psychiatric disabilities. Included in the review were 21 randomized or quasi-experimental design studies of ACT and strengths-based case management models. Table 6.3 lists the active ingredients of effective case management. These ingredients were determined by evidence from at least six published studies employing an experimental and/or quasi-experimental design. It is evident from

TABLE 6.3. Active Ingredients of Effective Case Management

- Case managers should deliver as much of the help or services as possible, rather than making referrals to multiple formal services.
- Natural community resources are the primary partners.
- Case management is delivered primarily in the community.
- Individual and team case management work well.
- Case managers have primary responsibility for delivering treatment, rehabilitation, and support services.
- Case managers can be paraprofessionals. Supervisors should be experienced and fully credentialed.
- Caseload size should be small enough to allow for a relatively high frequency of contact.
- Case management service should be time-unlimited (if necessary).
- Clients need access to familiar persons 24 hours a day, 7 days a week.
- Case managers should foster choice on the part of clients.

Note. Data from Rapp and Goscha (2004).

this review that case management that delivers and maintains primary responsibility for the client's rehabilitation, treatment, and support, utilizes the natural community rather than mental health services, and delivers these services wherever the person with psychiatric disability is, have better outcomes. Further, the manner in which these services are delivered, that is, are individualized, include assertive outreach, address a broad diversity of life domains, and have small caseloads, is the key ingredient necessary for producing positive outcomes. No study found positive effects when caseloads exceeded 20:1 client-to-staff ratios. Moreover, given the lifelong cyclical nature of psychiatric disabilities, these services need to be time-unlimited. Although short-term gains can be attained with case management of limited duration, research has found that these gains do not seem to be sustainable on a long-term basis. Again, given the cyclical nature of psychiatric illnesses, persons with psychiatric disabilities need emergency service availability 24 hours a day, 7 days a week. These reviewers also found a diversity of research indicating that an emphasis on choice resulted in enhanced outcomes.

This assessment also puts forth the pros and cons of individual and team case management. The advantages of a team approach are reduced burnout, increased availability of practitioners who are familiar with the client, and greater creativity in service planning; its disadvantages are that it is human-resource-intensive, time-consuming, and inefficient because of the extensive meetings required, and finally, that it does not designate a specifically responsible practitioner. Further, in rural areas the use of teams can be impractical, as meeting on a daily basis is not feasible and case managers may have to travel long distances to contact their clients. The advantages of individual case management are a single point of accountability, greater efficiency, greater clarity of tasks to be performed, and only one practitioner for the client to relate to, rather than a team. Consequently, Rapp and Goscha (2004) concluded that both individual and team structures can produce positive outcomes.

Other researchers have assessed the characteristics of ACT programs that commonly produce the most effective outcomes for persons with psychiatric disabilities, as compared with an alternative. Phillips and her colleagues (2001b) concluded that these attributes were a "team approach, *in vivo* services, assertive engagement, a small caseload, and explicit admission criteria" (p. 775). Three of these five attributes were consistent with those determined by Rapp and Goscha (2004) for case management generally. However, much of the evidence for the Rapp and Goscha assessment was derived from research on ACT.

CONCERNS REGARDING CASE MANAGEMENT

A number of criticisms have been leveled at case management in general, with some being directed specifically at ACT. Stein (1992) directed his criticisms not at case managers, but at the expectations of mental health systems regarding broker-type case management models, including ICM. Unlike ACT, most of these models rely on referral to available resources in their communities, which in some situations may include referrals within the case manager's own agency. Unfortunately, many of the needed services are unavailable and those that do exist do not necessarily coordinate with other services. To rectify this situation, the assumption has been that the case manager could fill these gaps by providing the clinical services needed. But Stein (1992) believes that expecting case managers with high caseloads and limited clinical expertise to remedy these problems for persons with psychiatric disabilities, who often have complex problems, is unrealistic. A corrective action proposed in some instances has been the utilization of a team of case managers, as this is thought to help to reduce the burnout problem encountered by case managers serving this often difficult population, by virtue of sharing caseload responsibility. Research by Boyer and Bond (1999) did find that ACT programs were protective against burnout. However, Stein (1992) notes that a team of case managers does not possess the diversity of expertise necessary to serve this population, nor do they have the time available to respond to immediate needs and crises. Consequently, Stein proposed ACT as the means to remedy these system deficiencies in serving this highly vulnerable population. Similarly, Marshall and his colleagues (2004), in their review of the outcomes of case management, criticized broker case management for increasing the rate and duration of hospitalizations and therefore promoted ACT as the means to correct these poor outcomes.

Specifically, there have been critics of ACT who believe that this model is too coercive and paternalistic, creating dependency as opposed to independence (Diamond, 1996; Gomory, 1999, 2001; Phillips et al., 2001b). Diamond noted, "In the early stages, of PACT, consumer empowerment was not a serious consideration . . . it was designed to 'do' for the client what the client could not do for himself or herself." (pp. 53–54). In response to these criticisms, Test and Stein (2001) asserted that ACT was not, and is not currently based on a coercive approach. If anything, it was designed with the idea that persons with psychiatric disabilities could live in the community, which was not a prevalent conception at the time of its development.

One study that was designed to assess coercive strategies within an ACT program found that case managers engaged in a diversity of limit-setting techniques. Therapeutic limit setting in this study was defined as "activities by the treatment provider to pressure a client to change behavior that is disturbing, dangerous or destructive or engage further in treatment" (Neale & Rosenheck, 2000, p. 409). Case managers generally relied on "verbal strategies rather than coercive alternatives" (p. 504). For example, they used involuntary hospitalization and other external authorities with less than 5% of their clients. In a more recent study, the same researchers (Rosenheck & Neale, 2004) found that clients of an ACT program who were exposed to limit-setting interventions had poorer outcomes than those who were not exposed to the same strategies. It should be noted that limit-setting strategies may well be employed in other case management models, and may possibly be employed to a greater extent in other models in which there is a lack of rehabilitation options (Solomon & Draine, 1995e). The employment of these strategies probably has to do with the nature of the population, the expertise of the provider, and the available treatment options, rather than the model of case management per se.

Although there has been limited research on the satisfaction of ACT, generally consumers and families have been more satisfied with this service model than with other interventions (Gerber & Prince, 1999; Phillips et al., 2001b). A recent study assessing the perspectives of consumers regarding satisfaction with ACT found individuals served by its teams to be reasonably satisfied, although they did express some concerns. The area that received the most negative comments was the team approach. Some clients did not like relating to so many people, did not feel that all of the providers knew them, and found it cumbersome dealing with so many staff persons. Clients also disliked the intrusive, controlling nature of ACT and did not think that they needed to be visited so frequently. On the flip side, positive remarks were made about the availability of the team and the home visits (Redko, Durbin, Wasylenki, & Krupa, 2004). A narrative review on continuity of care by Crawford and his colleagues (Crawford, deJonge, Freeman, & Weaver, 2004) concluded that although the team approach has been emphasized in serving individuals with psychiatric disabilities, research suggests that this population values continuity of care from the same single provider. Similarly, McGrew, Wilson, and Bond (1996) found that clients served by ACT teams valued staff availability and the alliance with their case managers. Consistent with these findings, Krupa and colleagues (Krupa, Eastbrook, Hern, Lee, North, et al., 2005) found that clients valued one primary relationship with a team member; for some, it was the only positive helping relationship in their lives. But the importance to persons with psychiatric disabilities of having someone there for them, who listens and understands them, has been noted with case management models other than ACT (Goering & Stylianos, 1988).

PRACTICE GUIDELINES/BEST PRACTICES

Professional organizations and expert consensus panels have developed practice guidelines for persons with severe and persistent mental illness, most especially for persons diagnosed with schizophrenia. Consistent with the fact that ACT is recognized as an evidence-based practice, all have acknowledged the essential need for case management; and when endorsing a particular service model of case management, ACT has been the model of choice based on the research evidence (American Psychiatric Association, 1997; McEvoy, Scheifler, & Frances, 1999).

Government-sponsored practice guidelines/ best practices have also been issued that have related to case management. Most recently, the President's New Freedom Commission on Mental Health (2003) promoted the delivery of ACT as one of the evidence-based practices, noting that this, as well as other evidenced practices, are available only on a limited basis. Therefore, many who could benefit from ACT are not receiving it. In 1992, the Agency for Health Care Policy and Research and the National Institute of Mental Health funded the Schizophrenia Patient Outcomes Research Team (PORT) to assess the existing scientific evidence in order to develop and disseminate recommendations for the treatment of persons with schizophrenia. The recommendations were developed based on an exhaustive review of the literature and experts' rating of draft recommendations. The PORT recommendation related to case management stated that "systems of care serving persons with schizophrenia who are high service users should include assertive case management (ACM) and assertive community treatment (ACT) programs" (Lehman et al., 1998a, p. 9). Given that scientific advances have occurred since 1998, an update of the PORT treatment recommendations has recently been issued (Lehman et al., 2004). The recommendation related to case management has been modified to be more limited in service scope and targeted to those with specific characteristics. They have narrowed the recommendation to ACT and have specified that receiving this intervention should be reserved for individuals who are at high risk for repeated hospitalizations, have difficulty remaining in traditional services, or were recently homeless (Lehman et al., 2004, p. 202). This is consistent with the recent conclusion by Len Stein, one of the originators of PACT, and Gary Bond, principal researcher of ACT, that ACT needs to be available for the 10–20% heaviest service users (Rapp & Goscha, 2004).

In 1997, the National Association of Case Management (NACM) and the Community Support Program of the Center for Mental Health Services of Substance Abuse and Mental Health Services Administration issued case management practice guidelines for adults with severe and persistent mental illness (Hodge & Giesler, 1997). This document did not endorse a particular model of case management. The document defines case management, specifies the functions and critical ingredients of case management, and defines three levels of intensity of case management. The guidelines stress greatly a partnership approach. The definition of case management used is

> a practice in which the service recipient is a *partner*, to the greatest extent possible, in assessing needs, obtaining services, treatments and supports, and in preventing and managing crisis. The focus of the *partnership* is recovery and self management of mental illness and life. The individual and the practitioner plan, coordinate, monitor, adjust, and advocate for services and supports directed toward the achievement of the individual's personal goals for community living. (p. 22, Hodge & Giesler, 1997, emphasis added)

The critical elements noted in the NACM guidelines are coordination; consumer choice; determining strengths and preferences; comprehensive, outcome-oriented service planning; collaboration with psychiatrists and other service providers; continuity of care; and family kindred support. Because the document contained a limited review of the research literature, these guidelines emerged more from an ideology of consumer choice and empowerment (in the recent assessment of critical ingredients of case management by Rapp and Goscha (2004), they document the evidence base for this) and practice wisdom, than from science. This document is important in that it offers direction for its membership, largely practicing case managers who likely are delivering broker or modified broker and intensive case management, rather than ACT.

IMPLEMENTATION ISSUES IN CASE MANAGEMENT

Implementation issues in case management relate to the extent to which evidence-based practice or practice guidelines are being implemented and the extent to which the evidence-based practice model, which in this instance is ACT, is being faithfully implemented. With regard to the first issue, Lehman and colleagues (1998b) conducted a study to assess the extent to which usual care conforms to PORT recommendations. These investigators were unable to determine the extent to which clients in their survey were in programs that met the formal criteria of ACT. However, these researchers were able to determine whether the client received case management services from a community-based team, was seen at least weekly, and received help in at least four of seven life domains. They found that no more than 10% of clients were receiving services that met these criteria very broadly. If these were ACT programs, this figure is consistent with the estimated 10–20% needing ACT stated by Stein and Bond, assuming that these are individuals meeting the criterion of being heavy users.

In regard to the faithfulness of implementation or program fidelity, in the arena of case management, as previously noted, only the ACT model is well specified enough to allow assessment of fidelity to the model. Only ACT has a manual that specifies the model and how to go about implementing the program. The only other case management model that comes close to having a manual is the strengths-based model, which has a textbook on the strengths-based approach that explicates this approach for a number of populations in a diversity of situations, beyond the provision of case management for persons with psychiatric disabilities per se (Rapp, 1998b).

The National Alliance for the Mentally Ill (NAMI) has sponsored the development of a manual, *The Pact Model of Community-Based Treatment for Persons with Severe and Persistent Mental Illnesses: A Manual for PACT Start-up* (1999), and an organization to provide technical assistance in the development of ACT teams, the Assertive Community Treatment (ACT) Technical Assistance Center. This technical assistance center received funding from a federal agency, the Substance Abuse and Mental Health Services Administration. This is the first time that NAMI has not only endorsed, but also promoted a specific psychosocial intervention. This support is based on the fact that ACT, with its comprehensiveness and assertive outreach, offers families a feeling of having a safety net (Burns & Santos, 1995). In 2003, Allness revised this manual to ensure that ACT teams meet the standards of ACT; the document is entitled the *National Program Standards for ACT Teams*. Meeting standards is essential to attain the positive outcomes that have been achieved in the experimental studies (McHugo et al., 1999; Fekete, Bond, McDonel, Salyers, Chen, et al., 1998).

Recently, the Commission for Accreditation of Rehabilitation Facilities has issued a manual that includes criteria for ACT programs (CARF, 2000). These standards are similar to guidelines for a fidelity assessment (Bond, Williams, Evans, Saylers, Hea-Won, et al., 2000b). To date, only ACT has a fidelity assessment measure. In fact, it has three measures. These scales rate the presence or absence of, or the degree to which specific ACT features are present in the program, such as inclusion of a nurse on the team; inclusion of a no-dropout policy; program engages and retains persons with psychiatric disabilities at a mutually satisfactory level (McGrew et al., 1994; Teague, Drake, & Ackerson, 1995). A draft ACT implementation package disseminated by the federal government is currently being pilot tested (U.S. Department of Health and Human Services, 2003a). Such material will help to implement this evidence-based practice in the routine mental health care system and to ensure that the program is adherent to the model (Mueser et al., 2003d).

DISSEMINATION OF CASE MANAGEMENT

As other countries have deinstitutionalized, they have also moved toward providing case management services. Of all of the case management models, given its stature as an evidence-based practice, ACT has been most widely disseminated. The goal of NAMI, with the PACT manual and the technical assistance center, is for every community in the

United States to have an ACT team. Canada has implemented some ACT programs, and some provinces have plans for further dissemination (Bond et al., 2001b). Australia and England have also implemented ACT, and England has debated the inclusion of ACT standards in its national standards for case management (Tyrer, 1998). Japan is about to begin deinstitutionalization, and the government is currently sponsoring the implementation of an experimental ACT program (Oshima, Cho, & Takahashi, 2004). In the United States there are a number of states and locales that have ACT training and technical assistance centers, such as the ACT Center of Indiana.

SUMMARY AND CONCLUSIONS

It is evident from this review that case management remains the essential service element for helping to maintain persons with psychiatric disabilities in the community, and the more rehabilitative models, particularly ACT programs, help persons to develop their own skills in order to be more independent and to grow and change in productive ways. It is not surprising that ACT results in more positive outcomes than other case management models, given its comprehensive service program. ACT clearly goes beyond the delivery of case management services. Although this model has achieved evidenced-based practice status, it has some deficits. Recent supplemental interventions, such as IVAST, have the potential to improve outcomes in the domain of social functioning and other outcomes of importance to consumers. Just as research has found that to obtain improvements in specific outcomes, ACT programs need to be targeted to these outcomes; so too must ACT be targeted at improving social functioning. The design of ACT makes good clinical sense for those with psychiatric disabilities and, consequently, has been the building block for other interventions for this population, such as supported housing, supported employment, and dual-diagnosis programs (Solomon, 1999).

ACT is not for all persons with psychiatric disabilities, but should be reserved for those who are most difficult to manage. This, then, offers a challenge to psychiatric rehabilitation practitioners and researchers to improve the effectiveness of the other case management models. It should be recognized that an intervention that emphasizes monitoring, as does the broker model, will, for example, observe psychotic deterioration. However, without rehabilitative interventions to change behaviors that could conceivably prevent such an exacerbation of the illness, the case manager is left with few options other than to hospitalize a client when a crisis arises.

As evident in the case study of Lynn, there is need for a diversity of case management service models, and the appropriate model for a given individual may change as circumstances change. For those case management models that are dependent on the service system or on aging parents to function as de facto case managers, there needs to be a refocus from case management supporting the service system, to the service system having the available services and resources to support case management as well as families. There is also a need for agency support of case managers, as research has found that a lack of perceived organizational support for case management leads to job stress (Gellis, Kim, & Hwang, 2004). Case management is a highly stressful job that requires a supportive environment to retain well-qualified case managers. With high turnover rates of case managers, as is the situation in many places, the establishment of positive working relationships between case managers and clients becomes attenuated.

Chapter 7

Medications and Psychiatric Rehabilitation

Medication use is a cornerstone of effective treatment for acute episodes of severe mental illness and for the prevention of relapses as well. For a variety of reasons, however, people with mental illness often avoid medications or do not use them effectively. In this chapter, we discuss how psychosocial interventions can help people use their medications effectively.

The example below describes the typical medication management dilemma for many people with severe mental illness. Mental health practitioners believe that "medication compliance" is absolutely essential and encourage people to use their medications as prescribed. Yet clients themselves often question the need for medications, perceive a mixed picture of benefits and negative effects related to medications, get information from many sources, quietly experiment with their medications, and make decisions on their own about how and when to take them. In this chapter, we review the history and current status of medications for major psychiatric illnesses, the concept of nonconcordance, and the conceptual shift from emphasizing compliance to emphasizing a working alliance and illness self-management. We also suggest several roles for psychiatric rehabilitation staff members.

THE EFFICACY OF MEDICATIONS

The modern era of psychotropic medications began in the 1940s with the accidental discoveries that a compound called chlorpromazine quelled the frightening voices and paranoid ideas of many people with schizophrenia and that a common element, lithium, muted the wild cycles of mood and energy of many people with manic–depressive illness.

PERSONAL EXAMPLE

John Johnson Uses Medicines Inconsistently

John Johnson is a 24-year-old, single African American male with a diagnosis of schizophrenia. He has had two psychotic episodes and hospitalizations, but none in the past year. He is struggling to find a job and maintain his apartment and girlfriend. He is prescribed one of the relatively new antipsychotic medications, but he has concerns about weight gain and sexual problems, both of which he has definitely experienced. John is also worried about diabetes and heart disease, which he has heard may be caused by medications. His social worker, employment specialist, nurse, and doctor have all emphasized repeatedly that he needs to stay on his medication to avoid another episode of illness and hospitalization. They frequently ask him if he is still taking his medication. Yet he hears different stories from his family members and from friends at the mental health center, most of whom do not take their medications as prescribed. He is worried about the long-term side effects as well as the current problems he is experiencing related to medication. He frequently skips doses and sometimes goes for days or weeks without taking the medication; he feels better when not using it. John has been advised by friends and has learned from experience not to tell his care providers when he skips medications.

Since that time, there has been a steady proliferation of medications for the major psychiatric disorders of schizophrenia, bipolar disorder (manic–depressive illness), and depression (Mellman, Miller, Weissman, Crismon, Essock, et al., 2001). Today there are several different types, or classes, of medications for each disorder and numerous specific medications within each class; most of these are summarized in Table 7.1. Further, several professional organizations and research groups have developed medication algorithms, which offer step-by-step approaches to the pharmacological treatment of specific disorders based on a combination of scientific evidence and a consensus of expert clinical judgment (e.g., American Psychiatric Association: *www.psychiatryonline.com/resourceTOC.aspx?resourceID=4*; Texas Medication Algorithm Project: *www.dshs.state.tx.us/mhprograms/TIMA.shtm*).

The fundamental point here is that numerous effective medications are now available to alleviate the symptoms of severe mental illnesses of all types (U.S. Surgeon General, 1999; New Freedom Commission on Mental Health, 2003). Evidence on this point is incontrovertible. To be marketed in the United States, medications must be approved by the Food and Drug Administration (FDA). Pharmaceutical companies are required to demonstrate basic safety and efficacy in placebo-controlled trials before they receive a license to market a medication. FDA approval requires that a medication be more efficacious than placebo for a specific condition in at least two independent randomized controlled trials. Placebo controls are used to ensure that the medications, rather than expectations, temporal factors, or the natural course of an illness, account for the improvements. These controlled studies show that people with schizophrenia, bipolar disorder, or major depression respond to a variety of specific medications during acute episodes of illness and that they are less likely to suffer additional episodes of illness if they continue to take the medications (Mellman et al., 2001).

Because FDA approval studies focus on a medication's optimal benefits when used under ideal circumstances, they establish "efficacy" rather than "effectiveness." Medica-

TABLE 7.1. Common Medications for Depression, Psychosis, and Bipolar Disorder

A. *Antidepressants*, which relieve biological (e.g., insomnia and low energy) and psychological (e.g., low mood and hopelessness) symptoms of depression.

  1. *Tricyclic and tetracyclic medications*: amitriptyline (Elavil), clomipramine (Anafranil), desipramine (Norpramin, Pertofrane), doxepin (Adapin, Sinequan), imipramine (Tofranil, Janimine, Sk-Pramine), nortriptyline (Aventyl, Pamelor), protriptyline (Vivactil), trimipramine (Surmontil), amoxapine (Asendin), maprotiline (Ludiomil).
  2. *Monoamine oxidase inhibitors*: phenelzine (Nardil), selegiline (Eldepryl), tranylcypromine (Parnate), isocarboxazid (Marplan).
  3. *Selective serotonin reuptake inhibitors*: citralopram (Celexa), fluoxetine (Prozac), fluvoxamine (Luvox), paroxetine (Paxil), sertraline (Zoloft).
  4. *Other common antidepressants*: nefazodone (Serzone), trazodone (Desyrel), bupropion (Wellbutrin), venlafaxine (Effexor), mirtazepine (Remeron).

B. *Antipsychotics*, which relieve the positive symptoms of psychosis, such as paranoia, hallucinations, and delusions.

  1. *Conventional ("typical") antipsychotics*: chlorpromazine (Thorazine), chlorprothixene (Taractan), droperidol (Inapsine), fluphenazine (Permitil, Prolixin), haloperidol (Haldol), mesoridazine (Serentil), molindone (Moban), perphenazine (Trilafon), pimozide (Orap), prochlorperazine (Compazine), thioridazine (Mellaril), thiothixene (Navane), trifluoperazine (Stelazine).
  2. *Newer ("atypical") antipsychotics*: aripiprazole (Abilify), clozapine (Clozaril), olanzapine (Zyprexa), risperidone (Risperdal), ziprasidone (Geodon).

C. *Mood stabilizers*, which control symptoms of bipolar disorder (mania and depression): lithium carbonate (Eskalith, Lithane, Lithotabs, Eskalith CR, Lithobid), lithium citrate (Cibalith-S), carbamazepine (Tegretol), valproic acid (Depakene, Depakote), lamotrigine (Lamictal), gabapentin (Neurontin).

Note. Generic names of medications are in lowercase; trade names are in upper- and lowercase, in parentheses.

tions are considered efficacious after they are tested with homogeneous clients (e.g., those without co-occurring conditions) who take their medications as prescribed under carefully controlled conditions (e.g., in a university hospital with specific protocols used by prescribing doctors). As we discuss below, *effectiveness* refers to use under real-world conditions. To get a rough idea of the magnitude of the efficacy of current medications, consider that about 70% of people with symptoms of major depression respond to an efficacious antidepressant, as compared with about 40% in a control group who respond to placebo. Similarly, in 1 year of follow-up about twice as many people with schizophrenia experience a psychotic relapse if they are taking a placebo (70%), as compared with those taking an antipsychotic medication (35%). These figures vary from study to study and in regard to specific medications and situations, but the findings often show a ratio in the range of 2:1 to 3:2 for medication versus placebo.

A second key point is that medications of a specific class, such as antipsychotic medications or antidepressant medications, often have approximately similar efficacy. All antipsychotic medications, for example, have remarkably similar efficacy, with the single exception of clozapine, which has greater efficacy but also has dangerous side effects and is therefore not considered a front-line medication.

A third key point regarding efficacy is that the medications in a particular class may differ markedly from one another in terms of side effects. See Table 7.2. Among antipsy-

TABLE 7.2. Common Medication Side Effects

Tricyclic and tetracyclic antidepressants

- *Anticholinergic*: dry mouth, constipation, urinary hesitance, esophageal reflux.
- *Cardiovascular*: orthostatic hypotension, palpitations, conduction slowing, hypertension.
- *Central nervous system*: tremor, sedation, stimulation, myoclonic twitches, seizure, extrapyramidal symptoms.
- *Other*: perspiration, weight gain, sexual dysfunction, impotence.

Monoamine oxidase inhibitor antidepressants

- Orthostatic hypotension, hypertensive crises (interactions with foods or medications), hyperpyrexic reactions, sexual dysfunction, insomnia, sedation, stimulation, muscle cramps, urinary hesitancy, constipation, dry mouth, weight gain, myoclonic twitches.

Selective serotonin reuptake inhibitor antidepressants

- *Gastrointestinal*: nausea, dyspepsia, diarrhea, emesis, cramping.
- *Neurological*: insomnia, jitteriness, agitation, restlessness, headache, tremor.
- *Autonomic*: excessive perspiration, sexual dysfunction: decreased libido, delayed orgasm.

Conventional ("typical") antipsychotics

- *Wakefulness*: sedation, fatigue.
- *Cardiovascular*: postural hypotension.
- *Endocrine*: increased prolactin (with breast enlargement and milk production).
- *Skin*: allergic skin rashes, pigmentation, skin photosensitivity.
- *Neurological*: dystonia (severe muscle spasms), pseudoparkinsonism (tremor, muscle stiffness, rigidity, stooped posture, mask-like face), akinesia (reduction in spontaneous movements), akathisia (internal restlessness), tardive dyskinesia (involuntary movements, often in mouth, tongue, or fingers).

Newer ("atypical") antipsychotics

- Sedation, hypersalivation, constipation, dry mouth, obesity, metabolic changes (lipids and glucose), Type II diabetes mellitus, pseudoparkinsonism at higher doses, agranulocytosis (sudden drop in white blood cells affecting about 1% of clients on clozapine).

Mood stabilizers

- *Neurological*: tremor, ataxia (balance problems), sedation.
- *Gastrointestinal*: dyspepsia, weight gain, diarrhea.
- *Skin*: rash, hair loss.
- *Cardiovascular*: arrhythmia.
- *Hematological*: low blood counts.
- *Endocrine*: hypothyroidism.

chotic medications, for example, some are more likely to produce weight gain, changes in glucose and lipid metabolism, and diabetes, whereas others are more likely to produce neurological side effects such as restlessness (akathisia), muscle spasms (dyskinesias), and persistent movement disorders (tardive dyskinesia). Similarly, medications for depression and for bipolar disorder tend to have comparable efficacy but different side effects.

A fourth point from the research shows that medications are effective when used properly for about 70% of clients. For the other 30%, the scientific information becomes thin. There are relatively few studies of specific medications for people who do not respond to an initial medication, and there are even fewer studies of the combinations of medications (called coprescription or polypharmacy) that are now commonly used with people who are nonresponders or incomplete responders. The good news regarding polypharmacy is that prescribers and clients now have higher expectations and are willing to experiment with combinations of medications to obtain more complete symptom control. The bad news is that there is little scientific evidence on these combinations, some of which may be dangerous in terms of cumulative side effects.

The characteristics of specific medications, dosages, efficacy, and side effects for specific conditions are important but beyond the scope of this chapter. Further, specific guidelines would be out of date by the time they appear in print because they are being updated continuously. Finding current information on specific medications and guidelines for use nonetheless represents a critical, everyday task for mental health and psychiatric rehabilitation practitioners. Information can be obtained from several widely available sources that we do not recommend. This includes information from the pharmaceutical industry, the *Physicians' Desk Reference* (2005), and an unstructured search via the Internet. Mental health and rehabilitation staff should avoid information from pharmaceutical companies and should advise their clients to do so as well. This type of information represents advertising disguised as education. It tends to be biased and is sometimes seriously misleading. Many people consult the *Physicians' Desk Reference*, but it is not particularly useful because the writing is dense and the information includes a comprehensive list of every possible side effect that has been reported, rather than a realistic perspective on side effects. Using the World Wide Web can also be problematic and misleading because the rapidly proliferating health information sites are not regulated and screened for accuracy. Thus, although the Internet has become a source of vast amounts of medical information, much of it is anecdotal and misleading.

Where, then, does one find accessible, useful, accurate, and unbiased information? The American Psychiatric Association publishes several excellent textbooks on psychiatric medications, and several of these contain simple tables of information that can be shared with clients and family members (e.g., Schatzberg et al., 2007). A simpler text for nonmedical personnel is Diamond's (1998) *Instant Pharmacology*. The difficulty with all printed texts, however, is that they tend to be a few years out of date, depending on when they were written and published. Because information on psychopharmacology changes rapidly, its being 2 or 3 years out of date can be critical. Experts therefore recommend accessing current information via specific resources screened for scientific accuracy on the World Wide Web (Slawson & Shaughnessy, 2005).

There are several useful resources on the web. First, there are textbooks, such as eMedicine (*www.emedicine.com*), which are updated daily and are therefore much more current than printed texts. Second, a reliable source of pharmacological information on the Internet is Clinical Pharmacology Online (see *cp.gsm.com/* and click on "about clinical pharmacology"). Epocrates online (*www2.epocrates.com/products/online/*) is a free resource and offers similar information. Third, MedlinePLUS (*medlineplus.gov/*), which is from the National Library of Medicine, offers an excellent site for consumers because it includes a consumer-focused drug database and disease-specific information. Fourth, the Centers for Education and Research on Therapeutics (*www.cert.hhs.gov/index.html*) conducts research and provides education on medications, medical devices, and biological products. The program is administered by the Agency for Healthcare Research and Quality, in conjunction with the FDA. Fifth, the Texas Medication Algorithm Project (Miller, Chiles, Chiles, Crismon, Rush, et al., 1999) has produced practical guidelines for medication management decisions related to schizophrenia, bipolar disorder, and depression (*www.dshs.state.tx.us/mhprograms/TIMA.shtm*). These guidelines emphasize client education and shared decision making (see below) and are updated as major new studies emerge.

THE EFFECTIVENESS OF MEDICATIONS

Given that psychotropic medications are about 70% efficacious under optimal conditions, how "effective" are they under routine conditions? *Effectiveness* refers to how medications work in real-world situations, as compared with their efficacy under highly controlled and relatively ideal conditions. The question is, how effective are these medications when used by clients who have complicated co-occurring conditions, such as substance abuse, when prescribed by practitioners who may be inexpert in using medications and have limited time to answer questions and develop a relationship with their clients, and when used in routine settings where many additional factors, such as insurance limitations and poverty, affect use?

The simple answer is that medications are considerably less effective in real-world situations owing to all of these factors. How much less effective? At a recent National Institutes of Health workshop on medication trials, the point was repeatedly made that in the real world medications have only "small" effects, approximately .2 (NIAAA/NIDA/NIHM, 2006). Consider this realistic but discouraging estimate: If only 30% of people with schizophrenia who are in outpatient treatment are prescribed a correct medication at a correct dose (Lehman et al., 1998b), and if only 50% of those with a correct prescription actually use the medication in an appropriate fashion (Fenton et al., 1997), an expected effectiveness level would be 15%, assuming that all who appropriately use the correct medication at the correct dose are good responders. Our task is to understand real-world effectiveness better so that we can help our clients to use medications and manage their illnesses effectively.

Realistic Limitations of Medications

Lack of Efficacy

Remember that even under the best of efficacy conditions, many people, typically about 30% of those prescribed any specific medication, do not respond, for reasons that are poorly understood but probably have to do with differences in underlying biology. This means that when these clients take the medications as prescribed, they get limited or no benefit, but they are still likely to incur side effects. Further, medication nonresponsiveness may occur immediately or may develop over time because the medication loses its efficacy, again for reasons that are poorly understood but probably have to do with changes in biological homeostasis. Because of medication nonresponsiveness, many relapses occur even when people are conscientiously using their medications. Weiden and Olfson (1995) estimated that approximately 60% of relapses among people with schizophrenia occur because of medication nonresponsiveness, and approximately 40% are related to not using the medications properly. With the new antidepressant medications, called selective serotonin reuptake inhibitors (SSRIs), it is well known that efficacy deteriorates over time, leading to symptom recurrences and the need to increase the dose or change the medication.

Prescribing Errors

Medications of any type are unlikely to be effective unless they are prescribed correctly. The prescribing practitioner must make the correct diagnosis, prescribe an appropriate medication, and titrate the medication to the effective dosage range in relation to monitoring the client's symptoms and side effects. If any one of these steps fails, medication effectiveness declines substantially. Unfortunately, the evidence suggests that the process often goes awry. For example, in the Schizophrenia Patient Outcome Research Team (PORT) studies, Lehman and colleagues (1998b) found that only 29% of outpatients with a diagnosis of schizophrenia in two large state mental health systems were receiving an appropriate medication at an appropriate dose. In other words, even if we assume that the diagnoses of schizophrenia were made correctly, more than two-thirds of the clients were on an incorrect medication or an incorrect dose! This is an astounding finding to those who are unfamiliar with the enormous gap between scientific evidence and actual medical practice; it should remind us that we are all responsible for helping to reduce medical errors. An important development in recent years is the use of nurse care coordinators, electronic decision support systems, and other quality improvement mechanisms that increase the quality of medication management (Trivedi, Kern, Grannemann, Altshuler, & Sunderajan, 2004; Young, Mintz, Cohen, & Chinman, 2004).

Side Effects

A central problem in prescribing and using psychotropic medications is that side effects interfere with tolerability. Side effects can be more or less severe in terms of subjective distress, physical changes, and long-term medical problems. Many side effects are merely annoying, but others are medically dangerous. All are important. Van Putten (1974) found many years ago that early subjective response to medications, often due to subtle side effects, predicted that clients would not use the medications over time. Yet practitioners often fail to pay attention to early subjective response. Other side effects that are not so subtle may also lead to discontinuation. For example, many clients understandably do not want to take medications that cause them to drool, to gain 30 pounds, to become sexually impotent, or to feel mentally dulled.

Although newer medications are often marketed as safer than earlier medications, medically serious side effects continue to be a problem. The first generation of antipsychotic medications, often called "typicals," are prone to cause long-term neurological side effects, called tardive dyskinesia, that can be disfiguring or disabling. The newer antipsychotic medications, often called "atypicals," are less prone to cause tardive dyskinesia, but are now known to produce other medically serious side effects, such as obesity, metabolic changes, diabetes, and blood abnormalities. A high percentage of medications are on the market for only a few years before they are withdrawn or before dangerous side effects related to long-term use become apparent. The recent history with atypical antipsychotics illustrates this point (Marder, Essock, & Miller, 2004). The atypical antipsychotic medications were marketed aggressively, with advertising campaigns announcing that they were more effective and had fewer side effects than typical antipsychotics. Yet the claims of greater effectiveness have not been substantiated (Lieberman, Stroup, & McEvoy, 2005), and serious side effects continue to become more apparent as these medications are used widely (Marder et al., 2004). As a result, some of these medications have already been taken off the formularies in many states.

Nonconcordance of Perspectives

Because of side effects and other issues, people with mental illness are often reluctant to use medications as prescribed for long periods of time (Fenton et al., 1997). This finding, which is sometimes called noncompliance or nonadherence, describes the realistic medication use pattern for a majority of people with other long-term illnesses, such as asthma, hypertension, and diabetes (McLellan, Lewis, O'Brien, & Kleber, 2000), as well as for people with long-term mental illnesses (Fenton et al., 1997). Because the terms *noncompliance* and *nonadherence* imply an authoritative prescriber and a passive client (see the section below on shared decision making), we prefer the term *nonconcordance*, which implies a lack of agreement between collaborators. Nonconcordance can occur as a result of different perspectives. The prescriber uses his or her best judgment to find the right medication and dose, and the client simultaneously uses his or her best efforts to find the optimal way to manage an illness. Their approaches to illness management can differ, which is termed *nonconcordance* (Deegan, 2005).

The rate of medication nonconcordance is clearly very high, probably 50% or greater, depending on the time frame and on how nonconcordance is defined and assessed (Byerly, Fisher, & Rush, 2002; Dolder, Larco, & Dunn, 2002; Gilmer, Dolder, Lacro, Folsom, Lindamer, et al., 2004; Weiss, Smith, Hull, Piper, & Huppert, 2002). Partial use of medications is probably the typical pattern for most people with mental illness (Fenton et al., 1997), but many people discontinue medications completely and others overuse their medications. Those who discontinue completely are at increased risk (at least double) for hospitalizations, emergencies, treatment dropouts, and homelessness (Olfson, Mechanic, Hansell, Boyer, Walkup, et al., 2000). Those who overuse may be at even greater risk for hospitalization (Gilmer et al., 2004), perhaps because they are not responding to their current medications. Those who overuse medications are also at risk for developing medication abuse if they are prescribed a medication, such as a benzodiazepine, with addictive potential (Weiss et al., 2002).

Nonconcordance has been studied extensively and appears to be related to numerous personal, environmental, and practitioner factors (Breen & Thornhill, 1998; Fenton et al., 1997; Kamali, Kelly, Gervin, Browne, Larkin, et al., 2001; Liraud & Verdoux, 2001; Warner, Taylor, Wright, Sloat, Springett, et al., 1994). Most of the demographic and clinical factors that have been identified are inconsistent from study to study (Fenton et al., 1997). The four most consistent factors, in terms of frequency, are co-occurring substance abuse, medication side effects, quality of relationship between the client and the practitioner, and practical problems involved in using medications effectively. Each of these has important clinical implications.

Substance Abuse

Substance abuse is clearly an enormous factor in reducing people's ability to use medications effectively (Drake & Wallach, 1989; Olfson et al., 2000; Owen, Fischer, Booth, & Cuffel, 1996). For example, Owen and colleagues (1996) found that people who were abusing drugs were eight times as likely to experience medication nonconcordance as those without substance abuse. People stop using their medications when they are using alcohol and other drugs for several reasons, such as fear of interactions, decreased euphoria in response to the drugs of abuse, and interference with usual routines. The reality of interactions is that some medications do present potentially dangerous combinations with drugs of abuse (e.g., alcohol and benzodiazepines), but most do not (e.g., alcohol and antipsychotic medications). People with mental illness therefore need better information about interactions, as well as effective treatment for co-occurring substance use disorders.

Medication Side Effects

As discussed above, side effects, both medically serious and annoying types, lead people to discontinue medications (Breen & Thornhill, 1998; Ruscher, deWit, & Mazmanian, 1997; Warner et al., 1994; Weiss, Greenfield, Najavits, Soto, Wyner, et al., 1998). Thus, it is critically important that practitioners offer good education, careful monitoring, and options for changing medications when side effects occur. It is important to be aware that some side effects (e.g., a subtle tremor that interferes with work function) are apparent to clients and rehabilitation specialists before they are recognized by doctors. Thus, a broader base of responsibility for medication management, including people taking the medications themselves and all of their staff contacts, seems warranted.

Treatment Alliance

In many studies, the quality of the relationship between client and prescriber is identified as the most important problem in medication nonconcordance (Breen & Thornhill, 1998; Frank & Gunderson, 1990; Holzinger, Loffler, Muller, Priebe, & Angermeyer, 2002; Marder, Mebane, & Chien, 1983; Nelson, Gold, Huchinson, & Benezra, 1975; Olfson et al., 2000). Clients themselves emphasize this point strongly (Schneider, Scissons, Arney, Benson, Derry, et al., 2004). Finding the optimal medication and dose is a highly individualized process and may require several collaborative experiments over time. This can occur only in the context of a trusting relationship. Though denial or lack of awareness of illness is often raised as an issue in medication nonconcordance, such issues are often resolved by developing a trusting relationship (Diamond, 1998).

Practical Issues

Clients themselves often report that they intend to use medications but encounter a variety of practical problems, such as lack of family support, insurance and financial barriers, forgetting, unstable living situations, and poor access to prescribers, which interfere with their intentions over time (Fenton et al., 1997; Olfson et al., 2000; Sellwood, Tarrier, Quinn, & Barrowclough, 2003). People with mental illness also often have cognitive difficulties that make learning, attention, and problem solving more difficult. Educational materials and compensatory supports need to address the range of barriers with practical solutions (Velligan et al., 2000).

INTERVENTIONS TO IMPROVE ADHERENCE

Given the well-recognized finding that people with long-term illnesses (of all types, not just mental illness) have difficulty in sustaining regular medication use, many interventions have been developed to improve adherence to medication regimens by changing knowledge, attitudes, and behaviors. These include educational interventions to increase the client's knowledge regarding medication, motivational interventions to improve the client's attitude toward taking medications regularly, behavioral interventions to help with the practical issues of remembering to use a medication regularly, and coercive interventions designed to ensure compliance by, for example, requiring an injection each month (Mueser et al., 2002a; Swartz, Swanson, Wagner, Burns & Hiday, 2001; Zygmunt et al., 2000).

Interventions to improve adherence are often but not always effective (Mueser et al., 2002a; Zygmunt et al., 2000). More effective interventions tend to be those that focus on concrete problem solving, motivation, and practical behaviors (Zygmunt et al., 2000) and that emphasize cognitive-behavioral skills and behavioral tailoring (Mueser et al., 2002a). Behavioral tailoring, perhaps the most effective approach, involves simplifying medication strategies and using routine habits to change behavior (Velligan et al., 2000). For example, taking medications once a day rather than twice a day and pairing medication use with brushing one's teeth by placing the medication container next to one's toothbrush are often helpful. Effective interventions emphasize helping the client to take responsibility for managing medications by using cognitive, behavioral, or environmental coping strategies that are similar to strategies found useful in helping people to manage other long-term illnesses.

There is little evidence that using more coercive interventions, such as changing to depot medications (injections) or invoking court orders to force people to take medications, result in better concordance or better outcomes over time (Fenton et al., 1997). Typically, people who are forced to use medications reject them as soon as they have a choice.

In the compliance paradigm, the doctor's role is to make the correct diagnosis, prescribe the correct medication at the correct dosage, and monitor and manage side effects; the client's role is to follow advice, report side effects, and "comply" with the prescriptions. However, many current interventions shift toward a paradigm of equal partnership, termed *shared decision making*.

EVIDENCE-BASED MEDICINE AND SHARED DECISION MAKING

Over the last century or more, American medicine has moved steadily away from the "eminence-based" model of care, which relied on the clinical experience of practitioners, to the "evidence-based" model of care, which relies on scientific research (Sackett, Richardson, Rosenberg, & Haynes, 1997). Early in the 20th century, this movement shifted the field away from miasmas, humors, and other nonscientific models to understanding disease and healing on the basis of scientific studies of bacteria, viruses, wound healing, epidemiology, and so forth. Within the scientific paradigm of evidence-based medicine, it rapidly became apparent that the client played an active role in responding to, coping with, and overcoming illness (Balint, 1957; Engel, 1960). A client-centered approach emphasizes the individual's personal experience of illness, personal values regarding autonomy, treatments, and outcomes, preferences for active involvement in medical decision making, and responsibility for managing his or her illness (Barofsky, 1978; Laine & Davidoff, 1996; Levenstein, McCracken, McWhinney, Stewart, & Brown, 1986).

Evidence-based medicine assumes that the client is an expert regarding his or her own experiences, values, and preferences for treatments, risks, and outcomes (Guyatt & Rennie, 2002; Strous, Richardson, Glasziou, & Haynes, 2005). The current paradigm of shared decision making prescribes a complementary relationship in which the practitioner provides scientific information and the client provides his or her preferences and makes choices. Mental health, like other areas of medicine, is moving toward evidence-based medicine (Drake et al., 2003c) and shared decision making (Adams & Drake, 2006).

MEDICATION MANAGEMENT AND SHARED DECISION MAKING

How does shared decision making affect medication management? The practitioner's role shifts fundamentally away from being the authoritative decision maker who expects compliance, to a collaborative partner who helps the client learn to manage his or her own illness, in a manner that is consonant with the client's own values, preferences, and goals, by providing the most current scientific information, by answering questions and offering choices, by participating in a true partnership in which the client's choices are honored, and by creating an environment of trust in which honesty, choice, experimentation, and individual responsibility can thrive (Deegan & Drake, 2006). Shifting to a collaborative approach to medication management has an extensive tradition in psychiatry (Corrigan et al., 1990; Diamond, 1983, 1998; Eisenthal, Emery, & Lazare, 1979; Frank & Gunderson, 1990).

To participate in shared decision making, clients need better education, better activation and empowerment to express their preferences, better decision supports to help them to clarify values and resolve ambivalence, and an environment of trust in which they can be straightforward with practitioners about how, when, and why they choose to use or not use medications. It is remarkable that computerized and multimedia decision supports, which help clients to understand illnesses, treatments, and side effects, to clarify their values, and to make choices, are available in most of medicine but nearly absent in mental health (O'Conner, Rostom, & Fiset, 1999).

In the current paradigm, rather than insisting on compliance with medication or any other treatment, practitioners emphasize helping people learn to manage their own illnesses. Clients may learn to use numerous coping strategies: diet, exercise, sleep hygiene, relaxation, work, relationships, hobbies, and so forth. They also address common barriers, such as stress, lack of meaningful activities, substance abuse, lack of accurate information, lack of trusting relationships with caregivers, fears of coercive interventions, learning difficulties, practical problems, and other difficulties. Thus, using medications effectively becomes part of a larger package of illness self-management (Mueser et al., 2002), personal medicine (Deegan & Drake, 2006), or wellness recovery (Copeland, 2001). Helping people learn to use medications effectively involves activating both parties. Clients need to understand medications and choices, to communicate preferences and reactions to medications, to identify barriers and practical needs, and to take responsibility; practitioners need to present information clearly, to enhance the therapeutic alliance, to offer and honor choices, and to recognize clearly that the client is in charge.

Several objections to shared decision making have emerged, and these need to be addressed in a straightforward, ethical, and empirical way. For example, some mental health professionals believe that problems with effective medication use are due to cognitive incompetence (Amador et al., 1991). This view was contradicted by the recent CATIE schizophrenia trial, in which only 5 prospective clients (of more than 1,400) were screened out due to inadequate decision-making capacity (Stroup, Appelbaum, Swartz, Patel, Davis, et al., 2005). Nonetheless, competence to make decisions and other issues need to be investigated scientifically to identify conditions, states, or circumstances (other than poor care) that should limit our ethical commitment to the client's autonomy. In such cases, we need to develop interventions that help to overcome barriers. For example, efforts to address practical aids to using medications effectively (Velligan et al., 2000), to offer advance directives to those who may experience temporary decisional incapacity (Swartz et al., 2001), and to address cognitive skills to overcome problem-solving difficulties (Stroup et al., 2005) may all have a legitimate place in helping people learn to manage their own illnesses.

ROLES FOR PSYCHIATRIC REHABILITATION PRACTITIONERS

Several roles have been suggested for nonmedical staff to help with medication management—for example, in education, monitoring, teaching problem-solving skills, and behavioral tailoring (Bentley, Rosenson, & Zito, 1990; Diamond, 1998). We recommend that psychiatric rehabilitation practitioners take a broader role in helping people learn to manage their illnesses by following these guidelines.

First, substance abuse is a potent issue that supercedes medication management per se. Substance abuse independently predicts relapse and hospitalization, interferes with the effectiveness of medications, and undermines people's ability to use their medications effectively. Helping people to recover from substance abuse is of paramount importance. As described in Chapter 15, addressing substance abuse involves rehabilitation practitioners in an integrated approach to screening, assessment, treatment planning, interventions, and follow-up.

Second, the most important factor in helping people learn to use medications effectively is establishing a trusting, collaborative relationship, or therapeutic alliance. People need to have a medication prescriber who understands how difficult it is to take medications for any long-term illness, who pays close attention to subjective responses and side effects related to medications, who provides education and answers questions, and who is willing to help them experiment with different medications and doses in order to find an optimal regimen. Given the current constraints on physicians' time, developing a working alliance can be challenging at best. Rehabilitation practitioners can advocate for the client, help to gather educational materials, help the client to understand medications and report concerns, and help the prescriber to understand the client's experiences with illness, medications, and side effects. The therapeutic alliance often requires a team effort.

Third, as a corollary of the second point, both clients and prescribers can be encouraged to participate in shared decision making. Prescribers need to understand that their role is to provide information, answer questions, offer choices, and help people to find optimal interventions. Clients need to be prepared to learn about medications, ask questions, report experiences, make choices, and take responsibility. Many participants on both sides will need education, discussion, motivational interventions, and practice to fulfill these roles. Rehabilitation practitioners can encourage shared decision making at all levels: changing attitudes, planning for implementation, adopting information systems that include decision support systems, discussions in team meetings, and individual meetings with clients and/or families.

Fourth, rehabilitation practitioners can also help clients to overcome practical problems in the process of using medications effectively. Medication tailoring, skills training, and other practical problem-solving approaches need to be highly individualized. People with greater cognitive impairments need more intense help and perhaps different learning approaches. Each person can adopt a system of using medications that works for him or her.

Fifth, using medications effectively needs to be seen in the context of individual responsibility for illness self-management. Many factors, not just substance abuse, affect an individual's ability to cope with a mental disorder. These include (but are not limited to) sleep hygiene, healthy diet, regular exercise, stress management, routine health care, social supports, and hope. A rehabilitation team can be optimally useful by helping people to reclaim hope, take personal responsibility, and attend to illness management in a more comprehensive sense.

Finally, all of these approaches to helping people assist them in managing their own illnesses, which minimizes the need for coerciveness. Fear of involuntary interventions can undermine or negate each step. Mental health providers can eschew coercive treatments to the greatest extent possible under the law. Avoiding coercive interventions can be discussed often between staff members and clients, temporary decisional incapacity can be planned for by using advanced directives, and coerciveness can be relegated largely to the legal system. In the event of a dangerous emergency, help can be provided in the form and sequence that the individual has specified ahead of time, and trusted providers can be involved in the manner that the individual has specified. Illness self-management is fundamentally built on a trusting relationship.

In contrast to the example at the beginning of this chapter, the example below reveals some of the benefits of using shared decision making and a broader approach to illness management. It should be obvious that Carlos and his team will make it through a crisis and continue to pursue recovery more easily than John and his mental health providers.

SUMMARY AND CONCLUSIONS

Learning to use medications effectively is part of most people's recovery process. However, doing so is not easy. It requires learning about medications in the broader context of taking responsibility for managing one's own illness. For most people, it also involves education, experimentation, and, perhaps most important, a trusting relationship with a prescriber. Psychiatric rehabilitation staff can facilitate this process in many ways, such as providing education and helping the person to communicate effectively and build a trusting relationship with a prescriber, overcome substance abuse, and develop personal strategies for using medications effectively.

PERSONAL EXAMPLE

Carlos Ramirez Learns to Manage His Illness

Carlos Ramirez is a 29-year-old, single Hispanic American male with a diagnosis of schizophrenia. He has had several episodes and hospitalizations, but none in the past year. The rehabilitation team has helped him to maintain his job, apartment, and relationship with his girlfriend. After trying several typical and atypical antipsychotic medications and experiencing a variety of distressing side effects, he and his medical team have found a medication combination with dosages that he is able to tolerate. He and his girlfriend are both well informed about his illness and use a variety of coping strategies. She helps him attend to stress, sleep, diet, exercise, job, and medications. They both feel fortunate to work with a mental health and rehabilitation team that helps them learn about illness management, experiment with different medications, and maintain employment. They continue to ask questions as they acquire new information from friends and the media, but they know they can count on the team to help them find accurate answers.

Chapter 8

Housing

PERSONAL EXAMPLE

Where Should Agnes Stone Live?

Agnes Stone was a 56-year-old woman who had been hospitalized dozens of times for the symptoms of schizophrenia. Housing had always been an issue for her, having been evicted several times from facilities throughout the city, sometimes for nonpayment of rent. Soon after joining the Thresholds Bridge program (a Chicago ACT team), she moved from an intermediate care facility to an efficiency apartment in a large, run-down building on the near North Side. Over a 1-year period after joining the Bridge, she broke her pattern and avoided rehospitalization except for a brief stay at a private hospital.

This is not to say she was symptom-free, quite the contrary. Even though she received twice-weekly Bridge visits and 15-minute sessions every other week with an unusually empathic psychiatrist, Agnes functioned at marginal levels in all areas of her life and displayed a wide range of bizarre behaviors. Bridge workers helped her keep her apartment in some semblance of order—her housekeeping was atrocious. They helped with routine activities, such as budgeting her money and keeping psychiatrist appointments, and they made friendly suggestions regarding her diet.

Agnes's dress was unusual. In the heat of summer, she sported duck-hunting boots, a miniskirt, and an old gray sweatshirt, and one cheek was decorated with a half-inch mascara "beauty mark." Her thought disorder intruded on her everyday life in countless ways. She conducted animated discussions with herself in public; she barricaded her closet door to prevent a snake from slithering into her apartment; she insisted that an acquaintance call her Clark Gable, because she was actually a man. Fortunately, her building housed an assortment of "characters," some as picturesque as Agnes. They included her landlady, who was tolerant of Agnes's behavior, which was one key to Agnes's residential stability (adapted from Witheridge, Dincin, & Appleby, 1982).

Housing has a central role in psychiatric rehabilitation, both as an *outcome*—a universal personal goal, and an *input*—a set of factors influencing the psychiatric rehabilitation process (Newman, 2001b). The importance of housing as a valued outcome is self-evident, from the perspective of both society and the individual. Regarding the societal/research perspective, community tenure—that is, living in the community and not on the streets or in an institution—is perhaps the single most common and face valid indicator of successful community adjustment. At the individual level, having a decent, safe place to live, including both the physical and social environment, is basic to life satisfaction.

In regard to housing as an *input*, one popular hypothesis has been that type of living arrangements influences other domains of living, including social integration (Wong & Solomon, 2002) and clinical and role functioning outcomes (Newman, 2001a, 2001b). One application of this conceptualization is that adequate housing may be a precondition for successful psychiatric rehabilitation (Carling, 1993). Put another way, unsatisfactory housing undermines the pursuit of other recovery goals (Alverson, Alverson, & Drake, 2000). The absence of stable housing makes it difficult to concentrate on even simple life tasks, as evidenced by many people in the familiar experience of disorientation after moving to a new community before securing a place to live. This impact is most apparent for individuals who are homeless (Tsemberis & Asmussen, 1999) or hospitalized without a permanent home (Witheridge, 1990). Residential instability is a major risk factor for rehospitalization (Appleby & Desai, 1987) and other adverse outcomes such as victimization. The lack of supports for unstably housed consumers may prevent them from having their illness managed effectively or having other basic needs met. Moreover, the inappropriate behavior of unstably housed people is more likely to be in the public eye, which may make them targets for involuntary hospitalizations. Beyond having a place to live, the *nature* of the living arrangements can help or hinder the recovery process. For example, an emotionally charged living environment is contrary to emotional well-being (Brown, Birley, & Wing, 1972).

Housing has a third role in psychiatric rehabilitation; that is, it has often been viewed as a *treatment/rehabilitation setting* (Budson, 1978; Dincin, 1988). The rationale for creating residential rehabilitation programs is straightforward: Many consumers lack the skills needed for successful independent living, and a program designed to systematically teach these skills may prepare them to live on their own. Within the psychiatric rehabilitation field there has been a spirited debate for more than two decades on whether residential rehabilitation programs should be promoted, or whether housing should be conceptualized as distinct and separate from rehabilitation (Carling, 1988; Dincin, 1988).

Despite its central role in the rehabilitation process for consumers, housing has not been given the priority it warrants, by either mental health planners or researchers (Dincin, 1988; Newman, 2001b). Housing issues are enormously complex. Many basic issues remain unresolved, including who should be responsible for providing housing for people with severe mental illness (SMI), how to secure financing, and which housing models should be promoted. Other issues include poverty, availability of housing, safety, financing, community acceptance, and consumer choice (Carling, 1995). These issues are discussed below.

A TYPOLOGY OF RESIDENTIAL ARRANGEMENTS

The terminology in the residential literature is confusing and contradictory. In Table 8.1 we present a typology of living arrangements adapted from Press, Marty, and Rapp (2003). It is organized loosely along the dimension of supervision/independence, although

TABLE 8.1. A Typology of Residential Arrangements

Homelessness

Homelessness includes several gradations (Drake, McHugo, & Biesanz, 1995; McHugo et al., 2005; McKinney Act, 1987):
- *Literally homeless.* "An individual who lacks a fixed, regular, and adequate nighttime residence" (McKinney Act, 1987).
- *Marginally homeless.* Individuals living in temporary settings such as emergency shelters or who "double up" with other households, because they have nowhere else to go.
- *Functionally homeless.* Individuals living in "temporary and institution settings that are preceded by literally homelessness" (McHugo et al., 2005, p. 973).

Institutions/custodial care
- *State psychiatric hospitals.* State-operated facilities whose primary function is the treatment of mental disorders.
- *Private psychiatric hospitals.* Private hospitals whose primary function is the treatment of mental disorders. Inpatient units operated by community mental health centers are included here.
- *General hospital psychiatric wards.* Psychiatric wards located in general medical centers providing short-term, acute crisis care.
- *Substance abuse hospitalization.* Hospital wards with a primary function of treatment of substance disorders.
- *Nursing homes or intermediate care facilities.* Facilities responsible for medical and physical care of consumers and licensed as such by the state (Shadish & Bootzin, 1981).
- *Correctional facilities.* Jails, prisons, and other correctional facilities.
- *Licensed board-and-care facilities.* "Non-medical community-based facilities that provide at least two meals a day and/or routine protective oversight to one or more residents with limitations in two or more daily living activities. There is enormous variation among these facilities in size, resident mix, daily charges and services. Similarly, the amount, type and extent of board and care regulation varies greatly at the State level" (ASPE Research Notes, 1993). California is one state with an extensive network of board-and-care facilities (Lindamer et al., 2003; Segal & Aviram, 1978). Licensed board-and-care facilities are distinguished from unlicensed boarding homes, described below.
- *Living with others who provide substantial care*
  - *Adult foster care.* Housing provided by a family funded by a government program (e.g., state mental health authority or Veterans Administration), in which a consumer is living in a single-family dwelling with a nonrelative who provides "substantial care," including a majority of the following functions: monitoring medication, transportation, cooking, cleaning, making restrictions on leaving the home, and/or money management.
  - *Living with relatives (heavily dependent for personal care and control).* A key criterion for classifying a consumer in this category is the assumption that if the family were not involved, the person would be living in a more restrictive setting. The same caretaking criteria used for adult foster care are considered in making this classification.

Crisis housing as an alternative to hospitalization
- Structured, supervised group living arrangements provided as a short-term alternative to psychiatric hospitalization. Length of stay is typically limited to about 90 days (Stroul, 1988).
- Housing alternatives to hospitalization are addressed on an individualized basis, using community lodging (e.g., hotels) (Bond et al., 1989).

(continued)

TABLE 8.1. (continued)

Semi-independent setting

- *Group home.* A residence supervised by staff members who assist residents in completing chores essential to independent living (e.g., shopping, meal preparation, laundry). Typically, group homes have live-in staff members. Group homes may be time-limited or permanent residences (Golomb & Kocsis, 1988; Winerip, 1994).
- *Fairweather lodge.* A self-governing communal living arrangement in which residents share household duties and often work together on mobile work crews (Krepp, 2000).
- *Boarding home.* A facility that provides meals and lodging, but it is not seen as an extension of a mental health or psychiatric rehabilitation agency, nor is it staffed with mental health personnel, and residents generally have autonomy to come and go.
- *Supervised housing program.* Housing sponsored by a provider agency in which consumers live mostly independently. Criteria for this category pertain to the degree of control the provider agency staff members have over key aspects of the living arrangements. Indicators include (1) the provider agency signs the lease, (2) the provider agency has keys to the residence, (3) the provider agency provides on-site day or evening staff coverage, and (4) the provider agency mandates consumers to participate in mental health services, such as a medication clinic or day program as a condition for tenancy. When assistance is limited to case management support and/or financial aid, this setting is not classified as supervised housing.

Independent living

- *Independent living.* This category includes housing in the open rental market as well as subsidized housing. Independent living includes a wide range of housing arrangements, including single-room occupancy (SRO) hotels. Independent living includes shared housing for reasons not related to mental illness (e.g., personal choice related to cultural and/or financial considerations). Consumers living with others are considered to be living independently if they perform daily living functions without the supervision of a family member or case manager, even if they receive intensive case management.
- *Agency-sponsored scattered-site housing program.* Residents live in apartments secured by a social service agency, which provides ongoing case management support, but the supervisory role in daily living functioning is limited. "Scattered-site" refers to the proximity of housing; if all residences are clustered within a single apartment complex, this would not be scattered-site housing and may fit more closely with the category of supervised housing.

other pertinent dimensions include expected duration of stay and housing management type (e.g., is the residence part of a housing program operated by either a provider organization or private housing corporation?). In this chapter we refer to *provider agency* as a general term to include community mental health centers, psychiatric rehabilitation centers, and other not-for-profit agencies that are recognized by state mental health authorities as vendors of mental health/rehabilitation services.

WHERE DO CONSUMERS LIVE?

There is no reliable national information on living arrangements for people with SMI (Kuntz, 1995). In fact, in testimony to Congress in 1986, the director of the National Institute of Mental Health admitted to having no data on the whereabouts of more than half of the people with schizophrenia in the United States (Torrey, 1988). No national housing surveys have been conducted, and existing surveys on limited samples are dated. Even if there were resources to conduct such a survey, precise epidemiological estimates would be hampered by definitional problems (i.e., defining housing status and mental illness) and the difficulty in locating transient populations. Finally, living arrangements vary according to community. For example, urban and rural housing options are very different.

A general picture of modal living arrangements comes from several sources. Torrey (2001) made rough estimates on where individuals with schizophrenia live, as shown in Figure 8.1. He estimated that 34% were living independently, 25% with family, 18% in custodial and supervised housing (i.e., semi-independent living and board-and-care), 8% in nursing homes, 6% in correctional facilities, 5% in psychiatric hospitals, and 5% in shelters or on the streets. Another source is a 1999 San Diego survey of nearly 5,000 consumers served by the public mental health system who were not living in institutions (Lindamer, Bailey, Hawthorne, Folsom, Gilmer, et al., 2003). This survey found that 57% were living independently, 14% with family, 20% in assisted living facilities (i.e., board-and-care), and 10% were homeless. Tanzman (1993) summarized 26 state and city/county surveys, conducted between 1986 and 1992, spanning all sections of the United States. Most of these surveys used convenience samples. The three most common living arrangements and the range of proportions were as follows: living independently (35–50%), living with family (15–35%), and living in boarding homes (0–35%). More recently, a survey conducted by the National Alliance on Mental Illness (NAMI) reported that 31% of consumers lived alone and 9% lived in supervised community residences (Hall et al., 2003). Also informing our understanding of where individuals with SMI live are snapshots from longitudinal studies. For example, in a 1-year follow-up of a multisite sample of more than 5,000 homeless people with mental illness receiving case management and housing assistance, 37% were living independently, 42% were "dependently

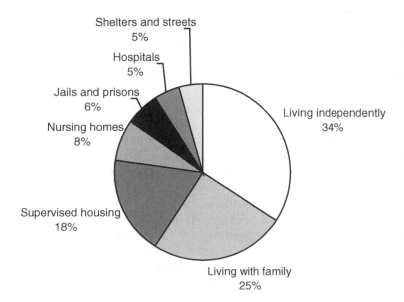

FIGURE 8.1. Living arrangements for people with schizophrenia in the United States. Data from Torrey (2001).

housed," 10% were in an institution, and 11% were homeless (Mares & Rosenheck, 2004).

Two national surveys found a significant decline in the number of nursing homes residents with schizophrenia from about 140,000 in 1985 to about 100,000 in 1995 (Mechanic & McAlpine, 2000). Comorbid conditions, especially dementia, make it difficult to obtain meaningful estimates of severe mental illness in this setting.

Estimates of the rate of SMI among the homeless population vary, but one source suggests that 5% of an estimated 4 million people who have an SMI are homeless at any given point in time (Federal Task Force on Homelessness and Severe Mental Illness, 1992). Others have estimated a prevalence rate between 6 and 16% for SMI in correctional facilities in the United States (Ditton, 1999; Lamb & Weinberger, 1998; Teplin, 1990; Teplin et al., 1996).

FACTORS INFLUENCING WHERE CONSUMERS LIVE

Poverty

Most people with SMI live in poverty most of the time (Draine, Salzer, Culhane, & Hadley, 2002). The main source of income for most of these consumers is a monthly check from Supplemental Security Income (SSI) and/or Social Security Disability Insurance (SSDI). The continuity of these payments can be interrupted for any of a number of reasons, sometimes capriciously. More than two-thirds of consumers with severe psychiatric disabilities are almost entirely dependent on Social Security programs for income support (U.S. General Accounting Office, 1996). Thus, for the majority of those with SMI, except for a fortunate small minority with access to housing subsidies or special programs, housing options are severely limited. A national study of housing affordability concluded that a person whose sole source of income was SSI would be required to pay, on average, 66% of his or her income in order to rent an efficiency apartment (McCabe, Edgar, Mancuso, King, Ross, et al., 1993). A more recent analysis concluded, "On average, rental of a modest, one bedroom apartment costs 98% of year 2000 SSI benefits" (Cook, 2002). These levels far exceed the U.S. Department of Housing and Urban Development (HUD) suggested guideline of allocating no more than 30% of income to housing expenses. It even exceeds the more liberal 50% guideline suggested by NAMI (Sperling, 2005). The disparity between SSI income and housing costs is exacerbated in large cities, where most consumers with SMI live, forcing many to live in substandard housing (Levstek & Bond, 1993).

Living close to the poverty line means that consumers are vulnerable to homelessness. Financial problems are especially evident in consumers addicted to drugs, who typically spend half or more of their disability income on drugs (Shaner, Eckman, Roberts, Wilkins, Tucker, et al., 1995). In these circumstances, it is not difficult to understand why many are homeless or frequently institutionalized.

Estimates of the prevalence of SMI among homeless people vary widely, depending upon sampling method, criteria for mental illness, and criteria for homelessness (Draine et al., 2002; Robertson, 1992). A 1996 national survey of 2,974 homeless persons found that 56% met a broad definition of lifetime mental illness, and 22% met a narrow definition (i.e., meeting diagnostic criteria and a history of psychiatric hospitalization) (Mojtabai, 2005). A meta-analysis of the more rigorous studies of homelessness concluded that the rate of severe mental disorders in homeless people was between 18 and 22% (Lehman & Cordray, 1993).

Availability of Housing

Starting in 1937, the federal government began subsidizing housing in the form of funds to construct public housing and income subsidies to allow people to rent in the open housing market (Youmans, 1992). More than 1.4 million housing units were constructed in cities and 450,000 in rural areas (Youmans, 1992). The surge in homelessness in the 1980s has been attributed to many factors, including policies initiated by the Reagan administration to make huge cuts in federal housing subsidies for low-income groups (Youmans, 1992) and the "gentrification" of inner cities, whereby inexpensive hotels and apartment buildings were torn down and replaced with upscale housing (Carling, 1990).

Safety

Unfortunately, in many communities, affordable housing for individuals living on SSI is found mainly in unsafe neighborhoods. Crime, drug activity, and urban decay compromise the quality of life, especially for people with SMI, who are often targets of exploitation.

Financing

To bridge the gap between housing costs and consumers' limited budgets, a variety of approaches to subsidized housing have been used. For example, nursing home residents have their housing costs covered through a combination of the residents' income and Medicare. Nursing homes typically receive all of a resident's income, save for a paltry allowance (e.g., $25/month). Obviously, this arrangement serves as a powerful disincentive to seeking paid employment, because earnings go directly to the institution.

Carling (1994) describes three broad strategies to financing housing: offering access to existing housing, preserving existing housing, and developing new affordable housing. These approaches often involve the use of subsidies, which can be directed to individual consumers in the form of individual vouchers or to housing developments as a whole. Sources of subsidies include federal, state, local, and private entities (Dincin, 1988). Sometimes the focus of housing development has been aimed at people with SMI, in other cases it has been more broadly aimed at people with disabilities, and still other strategies have been aimed at the homeless population (Hopper & Barrow, 2003).

A variety of public and private organizations within and outside the mental health and psychiatric rehabilitation systems provide housing. Thresholds in Chicago is one of many psychiatric rehabilitation agencies (and other types of provider agencies) providing housing to mental health consumers. Examples of private housing corporations serving homeless people include the Corporation for Supportive Housing in Oakland, California, and the 1260 Housing Development Corporation in Philadelphia.

The development of housing programs requires persistence, overcoming community resistance, and knowledge of endless regulations (Dincin, 1988; Winerip, 1994). Operating a housing program is also a *business*, which requires a somewhat different set of skills than managing a psychiatric rehabilitation program. An ongoing debate concerns where the locus of responsibility for developing and managing housing programs should reside (e.g., in public housing authorities or in the mental health system). One multicity project concluded that although the development of housing for people with SMI involved greater management attention than conventional housing, in most ways it resembled the development of market-rate housing for any low-income tenants (Harkness, Newman, Galster, & Reschovsky, 2004).

Regarding individual subsidies, HUD began a voucher program in 1983 known as "Section 8," which provides a monthly rent subsidy to eligible low-rent tenants and reimburses landlords the difference between the actual rent and what the tenant can afford (defined as 30% of income) (Youmans, 1992). Unfortunately, the waiting period to obtain such a voucher can be lengthy. Moreover, consumers with an arrest record may be ineligible for public housing.

Community Acceptance

The phenomenon of discrimination against consumers with SMI is most dramatic in the development of group homes (Dincin, 1988; Winerip, 1994). *NIMBY* (Not in My Back Yard) refers to the attitude expressed by homeowners who give lip service to the view that individuals with mental illness should not be discriminated against, while contending that group homes should not be located in *their* neighborhoods. A common belief is that the presence of group homes drives down property values. In fact, a review of 40 studies assessing the impact of group homes has suggested otherwise (CRISP, 1986). Community opposition is usually greatest prior to the establishment of a group home, typically dissipating about 6 months after the residents have moved in (Dincin, 1988).

Community acceptance appears to be influenced by community characteristics, with "diverse-disorganized" communities appearing to be most welcoming (Newman, 2001a). In their study of board-and-care homes, Segal and Aviram (1978) examined "external social integration" defined by indicators such as access to goods, services, and social contacts and whether consumers used community resources apart from facility sponsorship. They found that conservative, middle-class neighborhoods were extremely negative in their reactions to individuals with mental illness living in their midst, whereas liberal, nontraditional communities were the most accepting. They also found that many consumers preferred to live in commercially zoned, relatively transient areas, because of the anonymity and de facto community tolerance of mental illness.

Consumer Preferences

A critical consideration in housing decisions is where each individual would like to live, with respect to type of housing, location, degree of autonomy, and other factors. Based on a nonrandom sample of more than 4,000 consumers receiving public mental health services, Tanzman (1993) found that about 70% of consumers indicated that the preferred housing arrangement was for a person to live in his or her own house or apartment. Group homes and single-room-occupancy hotels were consistently among the least popular options. One study found that 81% of consumers preferred not to live with other consumers (Wong, 2005). Numerous other surveys have found similar patterns of consumer preferences; in contrast, clinicians and family members often think that living in a group home would be better, especially for clients recently discharged from a hospital (Holley, Hodges, & Jeffers, 1998; Minsky, Gubman, & Duffy, 1995; Schutt, Weinstein, & Penk, 2005).

Consumers who obtain housing consistent with their preferences have greater residential stability and greater satisfaction with housing (Newman, 2001a, 2001b). Shared decision making with attention to consumer preferences is an evidence-based principle of psychiatric rehabilitation (Drake, Merrens, & Lynde, 2005a); this principle is also relevant in other life domains, such as employment (Becker et al., 1996).

HOUSING MODELS

Broadly speaking, three housing paradigms have dominated the thinking in the psychiatric rehabilitation field: the *custodial care* paradigm, the *residential treatment* paradigm, and the *supported housing* paradigm (Parkinson, Nelson, & Horgan, 1999). Two versions of the residential treatment paradigm are the housing *continuum* and the housing *array*. In practice, approaches to housing are typically more loosely implemented than theoretical descriptions would suggest, and hybrid approaches are common (McHugo, Bebout, Harris, Cleghorn, Herring, et al., 2005).

Custodial Care

Custodial care refers to residences in which in-house staff members provide care services (meals, cleaning, and medication) (Parkinson et al., 1999). Custodial housing aims at maintenance; there is no intention of rehabilitation. Examples include nursing homes and licensed board-and-care homes. Most custodial care facilities operate as for-profit businesses. A 1991 national survey conducted by the U.S. Census Bureau identified 28,188 licensed board-and-care homes nationwide (ASPE Research Notes, 1993), of which 64% were operated on a for-profit basis. However, only a small percentage (14%) in this survey served people with mental illness.

Custodial care is intended for the segment of the population of those with SMI unable to live independently because of medical or psychiatric impairments. Studies show that, as compared with consumers who are living more independently, consumers living in custodial housing typically have poorer independent living skills, more psychiatric symptoms, and a more extensive history of psychiatric hospitalizations (Parkinson et al., 1999).

Criticisms of Custodial Care

Custodial care is demoralizing and fosters dependency (Parkinson et al., 1999). The quality of life is often poor in such facilities (Segal & Aviram, 1978; Shadish & Bootzin, 1981). The living environments in such facilities have the oppressive and stultifying characteristics of institutional living, which clearly do not promote recovery. Although most psychiatric rehabilitation practitioners would not endorse custodial care as a desirable housing option, it is the de facto housing option for as many as one-quarter of the population with SMI (Goldman, 1984).

Housing Continuum Model

The fundamental assumption in the housing continuum model is that rehabilitation can and should occur within the residential setting. The model includes these elements (Ridgway & Zipple, 1990):

- There are a series of residential settings, varying in their provision of service, staff supervision, and restrictiveness.
- As they improve, program participants are expected to move sequentially through the continuum, eventually graduating to independent living. Some transitional housing programs stipulate a maximum amount of time a resident can remain in a particular residence.

- Within each setting, participants are similar in level of functioning.
- Attendance in day treatment or other provider agency programs is often a requirement of residency in supervised group homes.
- A participant who decompensates and returns to the hospital starts over and recycles through the continuum.

The housing continuum model originated in the early days of deinstitutionalization, when the transition from the hospital to the community was viewed as best accomplished through a series of gradual steps, during which an inpatient progressed from a residence on the grounds of the hospital property (a "quarterway house") to a structured, supervised home in the community (a halfway house), and eventually to independent living. Although the concept of the halfway house continues to be popular in the corrections and substance abuse treatment fields, this terminology has fallen out of favor in the mental health field. The term *transitional group home* is now more common, and transitional housing remains a central element in the continuum model. Although psychiatric hospitals originally operated most transitional housing programs, today most are operated by community mental health centers (CMHCs) or psychiatric rehabilitation agencies, although they are sometimes run by nonprofit organizations operating independently of the mental health system (Randolph, Ridgway, Sanford, Simoneau, & Carling, 1988). More recently, the housing continuum model has also been adopted for homeless people, who are often first housed in shelters on a temporary basis before "earning" the right to more permanent housing.

In addition to rehabilitation, a critical function of structured group homes is *protection*. Drug dealers and others often victimize consumers, especially those with severe cognitive impairments, leading to homelessness, incarceration, and other unfortunate outcomes (Sells, Rowe, Fisk, & Davidson, 2003). Group homes can provide a safe haven.

A contemporary example of the continuum model is New York City's service system for homeless individuals with mental illness (Tsemberis & Eisenberg, 2000). This model begins with outreach, encouraging consumers to accept a referral to a low-demand shelter, where they may be assessed for their readiness for permanent housing.

Criticisms of the Continuum Model

Although the linear continuum model was the dominant housing paradigm in the United States from the 1960s until the mid-1980s (Ridgway & Zipple, 1990), it has fallen out of favor. In reality, the continuum model has always been more of a conceptual model than a practical guide to operating a residential treatment program. Few mental health systems have ever actually invested sufficient resources in housing to the extent necessary to implement this paradigm properly or to serve more than a tiny segment of the total consumer population. Even at the paradigm's apex of influence, fewer than 5% of consumers actually received services approximating the continuum model (Randolph et al., 1988).

Starting in the mid-1980s, Paul Carling and others constructed a forceful critique of the linear continuum model (Carling, 1988, 1990, 1993, 1994, 1995). Criticisms included the following: (1) Group homes are often incompatible with consumer preferences. Most consumers want to live independently. (2) It is difficult in a group setting to provide *individualized* treatment and rehabilitation. Yet individualization is a fundamental principle of evidence-based psychiatric rehabilitation (Rapp & Goscha, 2005). (3) A related point is that the skills needed to adjust to group living are different from the skills needed to live independently (Stein & Test, 1980a). (4) The continuum model requires consumers to prepare continuously for the next environment. Yet transitions are often stressful, artificially timed, and contrary to consumer preferences. Designing a housing program based on multiple transitions does not take into account the findings that consumers find it difficult to adjust to new environments (Stein & Test, 1980a). (5) Housing programs become preoccupied with facility issues (rules, staffing, keeping placements filled, etc.), not on developing the skills and supports needed to live independently. (6) Housing programs often fail to provide the last step in the continuum—stable, affordable, housing. Consequently, consumers become "stuck" in group housing. (7) Transitional housing programs may require fixed lengths of stay that are not suited to the needs of everyone. Because the trajectories of psychiatric illnesses are idiosyncratic and nonlinear (Strauss, Hafez, Lieberman, & Harding, 1985), the requirements for specific lengths of stay are often artificial.

Housing Array

The *housing array* approach is based on the assumption that the population with SMI is heterogeneous and housing needs are diverse (Dincin, 1988; Fields, 1990). The housing array and housing continuum models incorporate similar types of housing alternatives. Like the housing continuum model, the housing array model assumes that some consumers (although not all) need training in independent living skills and that various levels of support and assistance should be tailored to the needs, competencies, and preferences of individual consumers. However, in contrast to the stepwise progression assumed in the housing continuum model, the housing array approach is more flexible. A housing array does not imply any set sequence, and residents are not required to transition through various housing options. For example, permanent residence in a group home is one option within this model. In addition, the housing array model assumes that some consumers simply need a place to live without the requirements for a rehabilitative residential environment.

Group homes are often viewed as a best fit for consumers lacking basic independent living skills (e.g., shopping, cooking, and cleaning). Group homes also offer a built-in community, which can serve as an antidote to the sparse social networks of consumers (Pescosolido, Wright, & Lutfey, 1999). Special needs groups, such as consumers who are deaf and mentally ill, may benefit from congregate living, given the isolating features of their illness (Dincin, 1988). Supervised group homes also have been widely used for consumers with co-occurring substance use disorders (Brunette, Mueser, & Drake, 2004a).

Analogous to dormitory living in colleges, group homes for young adults with mental illness have been offered as a transitional step as they leave their families of origin (Dincin, 1995a). Dincin (1995a) has suggested that "emancipation" or "constructive separation" from the family (while maintaining a strong alliance with the family) is often the best course of action in the recovery process for young adults, especially those who are overdependent on parents.

In addition to group homes, agency-sponsored scattered-site apartment programs are a common element in a housing array. Often, provider agencies become involved in developing housing programs by default; without such efforts, consumers may lack viable housing options (Dincin, 1988).

The housing array approach gained popularity in the United States during the 1980s. During this period CMHCs greatly increased their role in community-based residential programs. A 1987 survey funded by the National Institute of Mental Health (NIMH) identified 647 mental health organizations providing residential services, totaling more than 24,000 beds (Randolph et al., 1988). These residential programs offered a range of housing options: group homes, cooperative apartments, and scattered-site apartments (Randolph et al., 1988). Although unavailable in most states, the Fairweather lodge (described in Chapter 3) continues to be part of the housing array in some states (e.g., Michigan, Minnesota, Texas, Arkansas, and New York). Modest program evaluations continue to show reduced hospitalization and other positive outcomes for lodge residents (Krepp, 2000). The rationale for Fairweather lodges and similar housing rests on the assumption that a subgroup of the population with mental illness thrives in communal living.

The intent in the housing array approach is to match the level of support and structure with the level of client need. In support of the matching hypothesis, some observers have noted that residents in supervised group living appear to be a different population than those living independently (Fields, 1990). Some research supports this contention (Fakhoury, Murray, Shepherd, & Priebe, 2002; Lipton, Siegel, Hannigan, Samuels, & Baker, 2000).

Criticisms of the Housing Array Model

Some, but not all, of the criticisms of the housing continuum model also apply to the housing array model. Two main drawbacks to supervised housing are that many consumers prefer not to live in such facilities and that the clinical decision process for determining who needs supervised housing is not evidence-based. Too often, the development of group homes has been a reflexive response to deinstitutionalization. For example, when Indiana closed a state hospital in 1994, the general response by community providers was to develop a network of group homes (McGrew, Wright, Pescosolido, & McDonel, 1999). Little planning was given to other aspects of the closing, such as provision of intensive case management.

The challenges involved in operating a group home are formidable (Budson, 1978; Dincin, 1988; Lamb, 1976; Winerip, 1994). Securing financing for housing programs requires determination and creativity. Zoning laws and community resistance are major challenges in planning the location of a new facility. Continued financial viability requires that group homes remain filled, which implies a recruiting dynamic ("We must keep this building full") that may be at cross-purposes to individual consumer needs. Beyond financing and community acceptance, the numerous headaches involved in running a group home include building maintenance, hiring staff, and managing the residence. Group homes are frequently staffed by underpaid and untrained individuals who may not be well versed in psychiatric rehabilitation principles. Staff positions in group homes are notoriously high-burnout, high-turnover positions (Bond, Witheridge, Wasmer, Dincin, McRae, et al., 1989; Winerip, 1994), creating further challenges. Managing a group home involves setting policies regarding substance abuse, assaultive behavior, property damage, refusal to take medications as prescribed, suicidal behavior, and medical illnesses. Defining rules that foster autonomy while protecting the rights of the group is a balancing act.

Supported Housing

Supported housing is defined simply as helping consumers achieve independent living in housing arrangements of their choice, while providing adequate case management support matching individual needs. Ridgway and Rapp (1997) identified the critical ingredients of supported housing, which fall into two categories: housing assistance and intensive case management, as shown in Table 8.2. With its emphasis on normalization, individualization, and intensive support, the philosophy of supported housing is highly compatible with the assertive community treatment (ACT) model. Thus, it is not surprising that ACT and supported housing are often offered together (Witheridge, 1990). The one key difference is that supported housing is intended for a broader spectrum of the population of those with SMI than is ACT. In other words, although supported housing is an appropriate option for most ACT consumers, it is also appropriate for consumers who do not need the level of intensity ACT teams provide.

Supported housing has many roots. First defined in the 1980s, it originated in the work of mental health advocates who championed normal housing in the community as an alternative to clinically managed treatment programs. They saw supported housing as a "paradigm shift" from the linear continuum model, as shown in Table 8.3 (Ridgway & Zipple, 1990). Advocates included those from the consumer movement who noted the dehumanizing and paternalistic attitudes common in residential treatment programs (Howie the Harp, 1990). The surge of homelessness in the 1980s gave further impetus to the supported housing movement. As described by Hopper and Barrow (2003), two distinct traditions within the supported housing movement are "integrated housing development" (the perspective of mental health advocates) and "housing as housing" (the perspective of housing advocates). Advocates for homeless people have viewed housing issues through the broader perspective of the needs of all individuals living on the margins of society. They have generally seen their role as community *building*, rather than as finding housing in normalized settings. To contrast the strategies, then, the integrated housing development approach searches for affordable housing within existing stock, whereas the housing-as-housing approach is more likely to develop new housing (through purchasing housing, rehabilitating existing buildings, or constructing new residences). Still another variant of supported housing is suggested in the independent living movement, in which consumer self-help is viewed as an alternative to professional support (Pratt, Gill, Barrett, & Roberts, 2006).

TABLE 8.2. Critical Components of Supported Housing

Housing assistance

- Rental subsidies are provided.
- Consumer choices are honored (e.g., where they live and with whom).
- Assistance is provided in obtaining and establishing a home.
- Consumers control personal space and have typical tenant roles and responsibilities.

Intensive case management

- Staff to client ratios are about 1:10.
- Case management contact with clients is frequent (up to several times a week), individualized to client need, and clients have ready access to crisis services.
- Most services and support are provided directly by the case manager, not brokered.
- Case management is mostly provided in home and community settings, and services tailored to each individual.
- Programs have explicit goals to increase residential stability, reduce homelessness and hospitalization, improve quality of life, and increase access to affordable housing.

Note. Based on Ridgway and Rapp (1997).

TABLE 8.3. Elements of the Supported Housing Paradigm Shift

New paradigm	Old paradigm
A home	Residential treatment setting
Choice	Placement
Normal roles	Client role
Client control	Staff control
Social integration	Grouping by disability
In vivo learning in permanent settings	Transitional preparatory setting
Individualized flexible services and supports	Standardized levels of service
Most facilitative environment	Least restrictive environment
Goal: Independent living with ongoing support	Goal: Independence from mental health system

Note. Based on Ridgway and Zipple (1990).

Several states, such as Ohio and Texas, have had statewide initiatives for adopting supported housing. One reason may be that supported housing is less expensive than residential treatment (Hogan, 1999).

Beyond the broad characterization of supported housing and its contrast with the continuum model, many specific variants have been developed. One of these is the *Pathways to Housing* program in New York City for individuals who are homeless and mentally ill (Tsemberis & Asmussen, 1999; Tsemberis & Eisenberg, 2000; Tsemberis, Gulcur, & Nakae, 2004). This program holds the value that housing is a basic human right. Therefore, unlike traditional programs, Pathways does not make housing assistance contingent on consumers' agreeing to sobriety or treatment compliance or other such conditions. Consumers are provided immediate assistance in locating and securing permanent housing in the open market. Most often, the consumer holds the lease on his or her apartment, although Pathways serves as representative payee for disability income (that is, monthly Social Security checks), ensuring that the rent is paid. Most residents receive rent subsidies from a variety of governmental sources. Pathways has also adopted a *harm reduction* philosophy (described in Chapter 15), which states that abstinence is not a prerequisite for assistance, and residents are encouraged to pursue less harmful behaviors even while refusing to abstain. The Pathways program provides intensive case management services based on the ACT model, but it allows clients to determine the type and intensity of services or even to refuse most services, although consumers are required to maintain two case management contacts per month. Pathways to Housing has now been replicated in Washington, D.C., and six other cities.

Criticisms of Supported Housing

Critics have challenged the contention held by some supported housing proponents, that it is applicable to the entire population with SMI. As discussed in the previous section, the alternative view is that some subpopulations, and some consumers during initial stages of their recovery, may benefit from a more structured approach. A second major criticism of supported housing concerns social isolation, which is a commonly reported disadvantage for consumers living independently in the community (Delespaul & deVries,

1987; Fakhoury et al., 2002; Krupa, McLean, Eastabrook, Bonham, & Baksh, 2003; Parkinson et al., 1999). Although supported housing is based on the value of community integration, achieving external integration is not easily achieved, and many consumers stayed confined in their apartments with little contact with community residents. A third criticism of supported housing is that it sometimes does not take into account the economic realities of a community. Safe, affordable, attractive housing may not be available in the open rental market. It is, in fact, the absence of appropriate housing that leads some advocates to propose the development of agency-run housing programs (including scattered-site housing that can be operated as supported housing) (Dincin, 1988).

Crisis Housing

The episodic nature of mental illness suggests the need for crisis services. In particular, psychiatric crises often involve housing issues. Having no place to live is often a contributing reason for seeking help in a psychiatric emergency room (Bond et al., 1989). Finding and keeping housing is a recurring challenge for many consumers, especially in metropolitan areas. Aside from financial problems, some consumers are evicted from residences because of behavioral problems. Thus, crisis housing is a pragmatic alternative to psychiatric hospitalization when the underlying reason for seeking psychiatric admission is housing instability. Crisis residential programs always have exclusion criteria to screen out individuals who legitimately need hospitalization. Typical screening criteria are "likelihood of homicidal, assaultive, suicidal, or self-destructive behavior, and impairments so severe as to preclude self-care in a community setting [and] individuals requiring medical attention needed for a physical condition and those with a primary diagnosis of substance abuse" (Bond et al., 1989, p. 179).

Stroul (1988) distinguished two types of crisis residential services: individual and group. The *individual* approach, exemplified by the Southwest Denver foster care program, places one or two clients at a time in foster homes (Polak & Kirby, 1976). Another variant on the individual approach is the use of generic community lodging—for example, placing crisis clients in single-room occupancy hotels and other inexpensive lodging, supplementing this with intensive case management (Bond et al., 1989; Cohen, Sichel, & Berger, 1977). The *group* approach typically involves licensed crisis residential facilities designated expressly for this purpose (Hawthorne, Green, Lohr, Hough, & Smith, 1999). Program evaluations of both types of crisis housing approaches have generally supported the hypothesis that crisis housing is a viable alternative to hospitalization for a sizeable proportion of those presenting for admission. Though few long-term studies of crisis housing have been reported, the short-term findings are favorable, particularly in regard to averting hospitalization. Cost analyses suggest that crisis housing is less expensive than hospitalization.

RESEARCH ON HOUSING MODELS

Among the reviews of the housing literature are three early reviews (Cometa et al., 1979; Nelson & Smith Fowler, 1987; Rog & Raush, 1975) and seven completed in the last decade (Eichler, Gowdy, & Etzel-Wise, 2004; Fakhoury et al., 2002; Newman, 2001b; Ogilvie, 1997; Parkinson et al., 1999; Ridgway & Rapp, 1997; Rog, 2004). All reviewers agree that housing research has been methodologically weak and usually not based on a conceptual framework. Most studies lack clear definitions of terms and few have employed fidelity scales, although recently a fidelity scale for supported housing has been developed (Rog, 2004). Another glaring shortcoming has been that researchers have failed to agree on a set of standard housing outcome measures. Newman (2001a, 2001b) has clarified one source of confusion in the literature, namely, that housing can be conceptualized as both an *input* and an *outcome*. Specifically, conceptualizing housing as an outcome, some research has been directed at identifying predictors of success in housing, as defined by residential stability, satisfaction with housing, and community integration (Wong & Solomon, 2002). Research seeking to understand housing as an input has sought to demonstrate the consequences of providing consumers with specified housing assistance and to examine typical psychiatric rehabilitation outcomes (e.g., community tenure, functional and clinical outcomes). In some studies this distinction is blurred, so it can be said that a study is examining housing as both an input and an outcome. A final criticism of the housing literature is that much of it is nonexperimental, precluding strong conclusions.

Although we have identified four conceptually distinct housing paradigms (custodial care, housing continuum, housing array, and supported housing), the research literature is not organized in this fashion. Except for supported housing, the literature does not include many direct tests of these paradigms. In fact, we are not aware of a single study that has systematically evaluated a comprehensive housing continuum approach, as defined above. Similarly, the housing array model has not been systematically studied. Therefore, we have organized the research on housing according to the following categories: custodial housing, supervised group homes, and supported housing. Next, we include a section examining studies that compare two housing models, typically supported housing versus a hybrid of the housing continuum/array. A final section summarizes two general reviews of the housing literature.

Custodial Care

Very little research has examined custodial care. In a Canadian review, Parkinson et al. (1999) concluded that the physical environment of custodial housing was often unpleasant (e.g., foul odor, poor lighting, worn-out furniture). The authors found no studies with positive outcomes from custodial housing. One 10-year follow-up of board-and-care residents suggested deterioration in health, symptoms, and independent social functioning and family contact (Segal & Kotler, 1993). Despite the dearth of research, it seems safe to conclude that the custodial model is not compatible with recovery.

Supervised Group Housing

Numerous program evaluations of transitional housing programs were completed in the 1960s and 1970s. Based on 26 program evaluations, one early review of the halfway house literature optimistically concluded that it was effective in reducing hospitalizations and that approximately 80% of halfway house residents "adjusted to community living" (Rog & Raush, 1975, p. 155). A subsequent review encompassing 109 halfway house studies was far less enthusiastic, noting that major methodological deficiencies in the literature precluded any rigorous conclusions (Cometa et al., 1979).

A more recent review examined the impact of group housing without distinguishing between transitional and permanent living arrangements. Drawing on studies conducted in Canada, the United Kingdom, and the United States, Nelson and his colleagues

(Nelson, Hall, & Walsh-Bowers, 1998; Parkinson et al., 1999) reached optimistic conclusions regarding the effects of group housing, which included "increased participation, self-respect, self-concept, independent functioning, social support, and involvement in leisure activities, as well as decreased medication use and treatment use" (Parkinson et al., 1999, p. 156).

Supervised group living programs vary widely in their program philosophies. One area with sharp differences in program philosophy is in the treatment of co-occurring mental illness and substance use disorders. A review of 10 controlled studies found that programs that integrated treatment for mental illness and substance abuse and that had less rigid admission criteria and rules forbidding abstinence had better outcomes (Brunette et al., 2004a). Consumers who remained in these residential programs longer had better outcomes. The authors also tentatively concluded that long-term programs might be more effective than short-term programs.

Some research has examined factors influencing outcomes within group homes. A greater number of residents in a facility was correlated with poorer outcomes in an early study (Linn, 1981), and further studies have supported this conclusion (Newman, 2001a). Staff attitudes reflecting hostility and criticality have also been found to adversely affect consumer outcomes (Fakhoury et al., 2002). Conversely, housing arrangements that approximate "a small family-living arrangement with an atmosphere characterized by mutual support and expectations for responsible behavior . . . [and providing] privacy, dignity, and autonomy" have been postulated to promote greater external and internal integration (Nelson & Smith Fowler, 1987, p. 83). Some correlational evidence supports this contention.

In summary, it is not meaningful to ask whether supervised group housing is or is not an effective model. The effectiveness of supervised group residences likely depends on many factors, including staff competence, integration with mental health services, program philosophy, program environment, and number of residents. In addition, although it has not been well studied, it has been hypothesized that group housing is an important option for some subgroups within the population of those with SMI (e.g., individuals who are deaf and mentally ill, young adults, individuals with co-occurring mental illness and substance use disorders).

Supported Housing

The largest sources of information about the impact of supported housing are three large multisite demonstration projects, two of them aimed at a population of mentally ill homeless people (Mares & Rosenheck, 2004; Newman & Ridgely, 1994; Shern, Felton, Hough, Lehman, Goldfinger, et al., 1997). Although these projects did not prescribe a specific housing model, all generally followed supported housing principles. In fact, the individual sites in these projects differed widely in their approaches, although all provided intensive case management and assistance in finding housing.

The first of these was the Robert Wood Johnson Nine-Cities Project (Newman & Ridgely, 1994). The general purpose of this project was to improve the organization of mental health services in nine cities, primarily through better coordination of services among different federal, state, and local agencies. Participants were clients in the local mental health systems.

The second multisite project was known as the Second Round McKinney Program (Center for Mental Health Services, 1994; Shern et al., 1997). The project evaluated outcomes for 896 homeless mentally ill adults at five demonstration sites receiving housing and rehabilitation services. At follow-up (1–2 years postadmission), 78% of consumers in the active treatment conditions were stably housed.

The third multisite project was also a homeless outreach study known as the Access to Community Care and Effective Services and Supports (ACCESS) program (Rosenheck, Lam, Morrissey, Calloway, Stolar, et al., 2002). A total of 5,325 clients were enrolled in this project. At 1-year follow-up, 37% were independently housed, and 11% were homeless, 10% were living in an institution, and the remaining 42% were unstably housed (Mares & Rosenheck, 2004).

These projects documented the feasibility of supported housing approaches for consumers with SMI. Their longitudinal results demonstrated that housing outcomes generally were much better at follow-up than at program admission. However, the findings varied dramatically between the three projects and from site to site within each project, depending on admission criteria and housing options, making generalizations difficult. Moreover, with only a couple of exceptions, none of the study sites provided rigorous comparisons to specific alternative housing models (e.g., exemplars from the housing continuum or housing array). Nor did the individual projects share a common set of specific operating principles; therefore, it is difficult gauge the critical ingredients of these housing approaches that led to better outcomes. A final limitation to these multisite projects was that many sites screened out high-risk clients, therefore limiting the generalizability of the findings.

We found five recent reviews of the supported housing literature (Eichler, Gowdy, & Etzel-Wise, 2004; Ogilvie, 1997; Parkinson et al., 1999; Ridgway & Rapp, 1997; Rog, 2004). Although the sets of studies reviewed by these authors varied considerably, all reached favorable conclusions regarding supported housing despite methodological limitations in the supported housing research.

Oglivie (1997) examined a handful of descriptive pre–post studies of supported housing. Her overall conclusions were cautious but generally positive. The heterogeneity of the outcomes used in these studies made it difficult to draw firm conclusions. Examples of the outcomes reported included reduced hospitalization, improved social networks, and greater life satisfaction. Similarly, Parkinson et al. (1999) concluded that supported housing increased residential stability and independent living, while reducing psychiatric hospitalizations.

On the basis of their review of 14 mostly uncontrolled studies of supported housing, Ridgway and Rapp (1997) concluded that supported housing (1) is successful for people who are severely psychiatrically disabled, homeless for extended periods of time, and/or profoundly disaffiliated from the mental health system; (2) helps people achieve residential stability, (3) reduces homelessness, (4) reduces hospitalization, and (5) may help reduce psychiatric symptoms, increase social and personal functioning, improve physical health, and improve quality of life. They also concluded that perceived choice in housing was related to residential stability.

In contrast to earlier reviews, Rog (2004)'s review limited its focus to relatively rigorous evaluations. She included 15 evaluations (5 randomized controlled trials [RCTs], 9 quasi-experimental studies, and 1 longitudinal study) published between 1988 and 2002. Although housing models differed across studies, all shared these characteristics: community based, housing assistance provided independently of mental health services, and consumer choice in services. Rog (2004) concluded that, as compared with usual services, supported housing increased housing stability, reduced homelessness, and reduced hospitalization. However, she found only "limited evidence of greater impact of supported

---

PERSONAL EXAMPLE

Ed Kimball Needs Help in Housing

A 19-year-old college student, Ed, was relieved to be accepted into Highland Group Home after a 6-month wait, allowing him to be discharged from the state psychiatric hospital where he had been diagnosed with schizophrenia. He had been advised by the hospital staff not to return to live with his parents. He had flunked out of college, so an immediate reinstatement there was not a viable option. Ed had had conflicts with his roommates at college, and thus was apprehensive when he was assigned a roommate at Highland. He had gotten heavily into the drinking scene at college and was unsure how the house rules forbidding any alcohol on the premises would work for him. Overall, he resented the rules for the group home, although after the oppressive institutional living of the hospital, the group home was a welcome change. The residential staff include three house managers, two of whom he was friendly with, but one with whom he did not get along. Ed did not like the rules requiring him to go to day treatment every day, to take his medications (which made him gain weight), and he did not like clean up or the other chores. From the first day, Ed was eager to move out.

---

housing over alternatives" (p. 338), meaning that these findings may not generalize when compared with active housing alternatives. In fact, "usual services" typically implies fragmented and understaffed systems of care.

A subsequent review by Eichler et al. (2004) included a computerized literature search for additional studies beyond those included in the Rog (2004) and Ridgway and Rapp (1997) reviews. However, they found no more recent published studies to add to these two reviews. Eichler et al. (2004) identified four shortcomings in the literature not highlighted by prior reviews: (1) the limited generalizability of most experimental and quasi-experimental studies of supported housing, most of which have evaluated programs serving urban homeless populations, (2) in most cases, a poor choice of the major dependent variable (most researchers have measured residential stability rather than stable independent living), (3) the lack of inquiry into the specifics of direct practice interactions between case managers and consumers, and (4) the absence of information on the lived experiences of consumers in supported housing. The reason for focusing on stable independent living is that residential stability is too global a construct; it masks differences between supervised and independent living regarding the many freedoms independent living brings.

Housing Assistance versus Case Management

An important question that has received only modest research attention concerns the relative importance of the two major components of supported housing: housing assistance and case management support.

The most rigorous study to examine this set of questions was conducted by Hurlburt, Hough, and Wood (1996). Homeless clients with mental illness were randomly assigned to four conditions. Half of those in the sample had ready access to Section 8 rent subsidy certificates, whereas the others did not. Within each of these two experimental groups, half were randomly assigned to receive comprehensive case management services, and half received more brokered case management. The study found a strong advantage for consumers who had access to Section 8 housing certificates in achieving independent housing, but intensity of case management did not show any experimental differences. Substance abuse also had a significant influence on outcome.

A quasi-experimental study addressing the issue of guaranteed access to housing compared two homeless programs. One was a comprehensive approach offering guaranteed access to housing, as well as housing support services and case management, and the other also provided intensive case management, but no guaranteed housing (Clark & Rich, 2003). The comprehensive approach found housing for consumers either in individual apartments owned and managed by the provider agency or in the open market. The authors found no differences between programs for consumers with low- or moderate-intensity psychiatric symptoms and few substance abuse problems; however, the comprehensive housing approach had better housing outcomes for consumers with severe symptoms and frequent substance use.

A third study, a small qualitative study of 22 "difficult-to-serve" consumers, although not systematically evaluating the access to housing subsidies, provides important contrasting conclusions (Eichler et al., 2004). Based on interviews with consumers, case managers, and family members, the authors concluded that intensive case management was the most important component in supported housing.

Summary of Supported Housing Research

Supported housing has one major advantage over congregate housing approaches: Most consumers prefer to live on their own. For a majority of consumers, supported housing is feasible and can lead to stable living arrangements and reduced vulnerability to hospitalization, provided it is accompanied by competent clinical case management. The clinical, social, and functional outcomes of supported housing are not as well established. The three main limitations of supported housing are the lack of feasibility in some communities, the potential unsuitability of supported housing for some subgroups, and the problems of isolation that may follow from living independently.

Direct Comparisons between Supported Housing and Residential Treatment Approaches

An RCT comparing the impact of individual residential placements with supervised group housing approaches for homeless persons with mental illness found modest differences favoring the group approach regarding the reduction of homelessness (Goldfinger, Schutt, Tolomiczenko, Seidman, Penk, et al., 1999). However, the findings on other outcomes were mixed. In addition, the residential group approach was an idiosyncratic program model described as "evolving households," making generalizations from this study tenuous.

Another RCT compared two housing programs for homeless individuals with SMI: a "housing first" supported housing approach (immediate housing without treatment prerequisites) and a housing continuum approach in which housing was contingent on treatment and sobriety (Tsemberis et al., 2004). Consumers in the supported housing condition had significantly better housing outcomes (being housed sooner, remaining stably housed more consistently, and experiencing more choice in housing). There were no differences in substance use.

A recent RCT compared two housing approaches for consumers with co-occurring mental illness and substance use disorders (McHugo et al., 2005). This study compared an "integrated approach," corresponding roughly to the housing array model (with supervised living as one of the options), with a "parallel approach," corresponding roughly to supported housing. Consumers in the integrated condition spent less time homeless and had less severe psychiatric symptoms during the follow-up period, which the authors attributed to the closer integration of the clinical and housing services.

SUMMARY AND CONCLUSIONS

It is remarkable that a half-century after the inception of deinstitutionalization, few evidence-based principles can be stated in the area of housing, despite its acknowledged central role in the psychiatric rehabilitation process. We can confidently say that housing is in fact crucial to the recovery process. Primarily on the basis of correlational evidence, we can also fairly confidently say that custodial housing is an undesirable destination with its insidious long-term effects on morale and well-being. Assistance in finding safe and affordable permanent housing that is consistent with consumer preferences leads to better consumer outcomes—most notably, reduction of homelessness and hospitalization. Consumer choice appears to be a critical ingredient in successful housing. Ongoing support, in the form of competent clinical case management congruent with ACT principles (Rapp & Goscha, 2004), appears to be an essential ingredient of all effective housing approaches. In fact, it is hard to disentangle the effects of case management and housing supports. Consumer characteristics, particularly substance use, have important influences on housing outcomes and are important considerations in deciding where people live. Although not yet empirically established, there may be certain consumer subgroups who benefit from supervised housing during certain stages of their recovery process.

There are several reasons that research has not advanced quickly in this field. The first concerns the formidable challenges of orchestrating a true field experiment to answer the housing question. Housing is the quintessential real-world intervention; confounding variables include changes in the housing market, new funding opportunities, the economy, and racism, to name a few. A second set of issues concerns ethical issues posed by randomized designs. Because lodging is a basic human need, providers often voice the concern that withholding housing, even temporarily, is unethical. As a practical matter, complications in randomization occur when a consumer needs housing and an appropriate residence is available. In these circumstances, providers are inclined to override the research design and make a placement. Conversely, many providers are reluctant to place discharged patients directly from the hospital into independent housing, further limiting the source of research referrals for a randomized study (Eichler et al., 2004).

Another challenge in conducting housing studies is separating the effects of case management from the "pure" effects of housing assistance. All of the housing models described above involve extensive psychosocial rehabilitation interventions, including skills training and direct support. ACT has been shown to improve housing outcomes (Bond et al., 2001b), but the ACT model includes housing assistance as a key component, so that the impact of ACT sans housing assistance has not been directly examined (and many would argue that an ACT program that brokered housing assistance would not be a fair test of ACT). Although the Hurlburt et al. (1996) study suggested that intensive case management had no additional impact on housing success above access to affordable housing through Section 8 subsidies, this was not a direct test of the ACT model. More research is needed on the specific psychosocial interventions (e.g., engagement, money management) accompanying the access to housing that lead to better outcomes.

As is true for evaluations of other psychiatric rehabilitation practices, another critical issue concerns what the housing intervention is being compared with. Is the housing program being compared with "usual services"? If a housing program for homeless people is compared with usual services, it is often a very weak comparison that sets a low bar for success. Only a handful of studies have attempted to compare specific housing models with each other.

Integration between mental health treatment and housing services has not been systematically scrutinized, although one study concluded that integration was a critical ingredient of an effective housing program (McHugo et al., 2005). Given the evidence-based principle of integration of services empirically validated in other domains (e.g., employment and mental health treatment, substance abuse treatment and mental health treatment), it seems critical that this feature be more fully examined in future housing studies.

The literature also suggests that specific features of housing arrangements and neighborhood characteristics may also be facilitative of better housing outcomes. In congregate living situations, the number of residents seems to matter, with a smaller number of residents being the better arrangement. Housing located in tolerant neighborhoods facilitates social integration, although social integration remains one of the significant challenges in the psychiatric rehabilitation field. For consumers who live in supervised settings, caretaker attitudes are important. Residential staff who are recovery oriented facilitate better outcomes. Conversely, providers who display high expressed emotion have deleterious effects on residents.

Causal links between housing outcomes and mental health and psychosocial outcomes must be regarded at this point as hypotheses and not as well-validated findings. Large-scale longitudinal studies using advanced statistical models may help to promote our understanding in this area. For example, the effects of different approaches to housing on the increasing problem of incarceration of people with severe mental illness are largely unknown.

There is some evidence, specifically regarding consumers with dual disorders, suggesting that a residential treatment approach may be the recommended approach for some subgroups, but more research is clearly needed. In this regard, the housing area stands in contrast to the employment area, where the current evidence has converged on a single rehabilitation model that appears to be the recommended model for all subgroups.

Although more controlled research has been conducted on supported housing than on any other housing approach, the evidence for its effectiveness as a specific model defined by a fidelity scale has not yet been established. Certainly, it is safe to say that providing supported housing (or any form of housing assistance) will yield better housing outcomes than the neglectful nonsystem of care that is the status quo in some places.

Chapter 9

Employment and Education

Adult role functioning constitutes the traditional domain of psychiatric rehabilitation. The President's New Freedom Commission on Mental Health Report, *Achieving the Promise*, reinforces the centrality of adult role functioning by stating that the primary goal of the mental health system is to help people with mental illnesses in "living, working, learning, and participating fully in the community" (New Freedom Commission on Mental Health, 2003, p. 1). In this chapter we review current research on helping people with mental illness to succeed in employment and education. We begin with employment because the research base on vocational services is more extensive and because current approaches to supported education are an extension of validated models of supported employment.

Most of the approaches that we now include under the rubric of "traditional vocational services" were train-and-place models. That is, they relied on extensive assessments, prolonged counseling or training, stepwise supervised or sheltered experiences, and judgments by professionals as to when people were ready for competitive employment and what they were ready to do. (See example below.) Reviews of the vocational rehabilitation literature prior to the development of supported employment consistently found little evidence for the utility of any of these approaches (Bond, 1992; Bond, Drake, Becker, & Mueser, 1999; Lehman, 1995).

SUPPORTED EMPLOYMENT

Over the past 15 years supported employment has emerged as an evidence-based approach to vocational services (Becker & Drake, 2003; Bond, 2004; Becker & Bond, 2002; Lehman et al., 2004). Supported employment has rapidly displaced or been incor-

PERSONAL EXAMPLE

Martha Simpson Gets Unneeded Training

Martha was a 54-year-old divorced woman with a long and turbulent history of bipolar disorder. She had worked extensively though intermittently as a secretary between episodes of illness over many years and desired to return to secretarial work after leaving the hospital. Her mental health team referred her to a local psychosocial rehabilitation program. After a 6-week assessment process that included many interviews, paper-and-pencil tests of interests and personality, and a lengthy evaluation of her work skills in different areas, she was placed in the kitchen unit of the rehabilitation center. Though kitchen work was not her goal, Martha was told that this experience would help to ensure that her work habits, grooming, and social skills were ready for returning to competitive employment. She went along with cooking for the day program, which seemed to her like "playing house," for another month. The final straw was struggling to learn to use a modern potato peeler. After several demonstrations by a young rehabilitation worker, Martha picked up a knife and showed the staff person how she had been peeling potatoes for decades. After this incident, Martha left the day program and found a secretarial job on her own. She struggled to keep this job because she had no follow-along supports.

porated into other approaches. Although states have had variable success with implementation, nearly every state includes supported employment as part of its state plan (Ganju, 2004). Traditional rehabilitation programs, such as psychosocial clubhouses, psychosocial rehabilitation programs, housing programs, and others, now provide supported employment. This shift presents a remarkable example—rare in the field of mental health—of how research can rapidly transform standards of care and actual practice. The historical perspective on these changes in vocational services is discussed in Chapter 3.

Supported employment fundamentally shifts vocational rehabilitation from a train-and-place to a place-and-train orientation. In other words, the goal is to help clients find jobs they are interested in as quickly as possible and to provide the training and supports they need in order to succeed on the job. Stepwise approaches, such as extensive preemployment assessment, training, and practice, are eschewed in favor of real-world experience.

Although several approaches to supported employment for psychiatric rehabilitation emerged in the late 1980s, standardization has evolved as research has clarified several evidence-based principles (Bond, 2004; Becker & Bond, 2002). In addition to the train-and-place approach, the principles focus on empowering clients to make decisions, to search for jobs of their choice directly (without delays for prolonged assessment and training), and to count on service providers to support them by integrating mental health and vocational services and making them available for as long as they are needed. Table 9.1 describes seven evidence-based principles. These principles are consistently incorporated into current models of supported employment, and several studies show that fidelity to these principles at the program level is associated with better competitive employment outcomes (Becker et al., 2001b; Becker, Xie, McHugo, Halliday, & Martinez, 2006; Cook, Lehman, Drake, McFarlane, Gold, et al., 2005).

The basic model of evidence-based supported employment (Becker & Drake, 2003; Becker & Bond, 2002) proceeds as follows. Helping people achieve their employment

TABLE 9.1. Principles of Evidence-Based Supported Employment

1. *Zero exclusion.* Rather than professionals making decisions about readiness, clients themselves should make such decisions. The policy of zero exclusion reflects federal guidelines, the ethical principle of autonomy, the philosophical commitment to client-centeredness, and empirical findings.

2. *Integration of vocational and mental health services.* Complete collaboration between vocational rehabilitation and mental health at all levels would be ideal. At the national level, collaboration would involve the Social Security Administration, the Centers for Medicaid and Medicare Services, the Department of Rehabilitation Services Administration, the Department of Labor, the National Institutes of Health, the Substance Abuse and Mental Health Services Administration, and other relevant federal organizations. At the state level, the Departments of Vocational Rehabilitation and Mental Health are to cooperate on all policies, funding decisions, and organizational issues. At the local level, mental health and vocational staff should work together on multidisciplinary teams. The services should appear seamless to clients.

3. *Benefits counseling.* In order to make good decisions about vocational goals and pursuits, people need to have an accurate understanding of their benefits, including Social Security payments, health insurance, housing assistance, food assistance, and so forth. Professional benefits counseling services are often provided through the Department of Vocational Rehabilitation.

4. *Client preferences.* Vocational goals, supports, and timing should be highly individualized according to the client's preferences, not the professional's judgments. The client is likely to have preferences regarding type of work, work setting, hours, other job features, and disclosure of mental illness. This principle eliminates group placements, generic placements, and professional choices in favor of jobs that reflect the specific preferences of the individual clients.

5. *Rapid job search.* Assessment is minimized in favor of rapidly helping the client to pursue a job that he or she chooses. For clients who have no preference, perhaps because of lack of prior work experience, the job search itself becomes a way to learn about various jobs.

6. *Follow-along supports.* Services to help ensure vocational success are individually tailored, again according to client preferences, and provided as needed without time limits. Follow-along services can include on-site and/or off-site supports to the worker and to the employer. These services are available as needed for as long as the client requests them, including help in ending a job or finding a new job.

7. *Team-based services.* Supported employment services are most effective and efficient when they are provided by a multidisciplinary team that works with the client closely to identify a vocational plan, find a job, and help ensure success on the job. The team typically includes members with expertise in several relevant areas, such as work, benefits, mental health, substance abuse, housing, and medical illness.

goals needs to become a fundamental feature of mental health care as well as vocational rehabilitation services. To accomplish this most effectively, mental health and vocational rehabilitations systems need to be integrated and collaborative at all levels. Although this rarely happens at the federal level, many state and local systems have adopted this type of collaborative partnership (Drake, Becker, Goldman, & Martinez, 2006a). At the state level, the two departments collaborate on all efforts related to helping people with severe mental disorders attain and succeed in employment, which include setting policies, financing, training, oversight, creating positions, and so forth. At the local level, vocational rehabilitation counselors join mental health teams to ensure that services are individually tailored and take advantage of the expertise and resources of both agencies.

Within the agencies providing supported employment, vocational services and goals become completely integrated with traditional mental health services and goals. In most situations, this is accomplished by having employment specialists join multidisciplinary teams. Employment becomes part of the initial assessment, the treatment plan, the service delivery package, and the outcomes review process for every client who has a vocational goal. Research shows that in most settings about 75% of persons with mental illness want to work (McQuilken, Zahniser, Novak, Starks, Olmos, et al., 2003; Mueser, Salyers, & Mueser, 2001a; Rogers, Walsh, Masotta, & Danley, 1991b).

In practice, all clients in a mental health center or other service setting should be screened for vocational interests, and those with an interest in employment should be immediately connected with an employment specialist and other practitioners on a multidisciplinary team that incorporates employment into the overall plan. Typically, an employment specialist can actively work with about 18–20 clients at one time. Thus, the number of employment specialists on a team is determined by the total number of clients with an employment goal. A typical team may include case managers, a substance abuse specialist, a nurse, a psychiatrist, and an employment specialist. Ideally, a counselor from the state vocational rehabilitation agency would meet with the team weekly and provide benefits counseling, as well as linkage with funding and services.

This approach seeks to provide *individualized care*, which means that the person's overall goals, strengths, difficulties, and situation are taken into account throughout the process. For example, in helping a client to select a potential job, the team may consider with the client details like past work experiences, preferences for job type and hours, amount of stimulation and support in the work environment, how to handle benefits and insurance, and supports off the job site. This effort involves the entire team. The psychiatrist may have to adjust medications, the benefits counselor may need to go over details regarding insurance and social security payments, the case manager may need to reassure the family about the client's work, and the employment specialist may need to help the client to identify potential job sites and prepare for an interview.

To ensure that services are client-centered, everything begins with the client's goals. Practitioners work within a model of shared decision making, which means that they try to provide the client with the information needed to make informed choices and to honor the client's choices. Therefore, when to seek employment, what kind of job to seek, whether and how much information to disclose to employers, how to arrange interviews, and so forth should be consistent with the client's preferences. The same is true for mental health services.

Once a person has obtained a job of choice, the plan changes to emphasize the supports that will enhance the likelihood of success. The entire team is involved. Support may mean, for example, that the employment specialist visits the job site weekly to check in with the worker and the employer, that the psychiatrist monitors and changes medications to accord with the client's new sleep cycle, and that the client attends a substance abuse support group in the evening. Supports are diverse and change over time. Again, the client directs this process through discussing and choosing specific services.

Support includes help with ending a job and moving on to another job or an educational experience. The team may need to be involved in helping the client to understand all aspects of a decision to end a job, in practicing an exit interview with the employer, and in searching for a new job. The assumption here is that learning to become a steady worker and developing a sense of career is a longitudinal process and, for most of us, involves trying a number of jobs.

Research Evidence on Supported Employment

The research on employment services addresses several important topics. In this section we summarize the findings related to efficacy, effectiveness, generalizability, nonvocational outcomes, implementation, dissemination, and costs. We also address concerns and future directions.

Efficacy

Research clearly demonstrates the efficacy of supported employment for individuals with severe mental illness. The published and publicly reported research includes (1) six quasi-experimental studies, involving five conversions from day rehabilitation programs to supported employment (Bailey, Ricketts, Becker, Xie, & Drake, 1998; Becker, Bond, McCarthy, Thompson, Xie, et al., 2001a; Drake, Becker, Biesanz, Torrey, McHugo, et al., 1994; Drake, Becker, Biesanz, Wyzik, & Torrey, 1996a; Gold & Marrone, 1998) and one conversion from a sheltered workshop to supported employment (Oldman, Thomson, Calsaferri, Luke, & Bond, 2005), and (2) 13 randomized controlled trials (RCTs) that compared supported employment with other approaches (Bond, Dietzen, McGrew, & Miller, 1995a; Bond, 2004b; Drake, McHugo, Becker, Anthony, & Clark, 1996b; Chandler, Meisel, Hu, McGowen, & Madison, 1997; Gervey & Bedell, 1994; Gold, Meisler, Carnemolla, Williams, et al., 2006; Latimer, LeComte, Becker, Drake, DuClos, et al., 2006; Lehman, Goldberg, Dixon, McNary, Postrado, et al., 2002; McFarlane, Stastny, & Deakins, 1995; Mueser, Clark, Haines, Drake, McHugo, et al., 2004a; Twamley, Bartels, & Becker, 2004; Wong, Chiu, B. Tang, Chiu, & J. Tang, 2005). The comparison groups were diverse. Two studies used a comparison group receiving a brokered form of supported employment (i.e., freestanding rehabilitation programs providing a version of supported employment lacking integration of mental health treatment and employment services) (Drake et al., 1996b; Mueser et al., 2004a). In two studies the comparison group consisted of clients in a psychosocial rehabilitation program (Lehman et al., 2002; Mueser et al., 2004a). In three studies the comparison group consisted of those in sheltered workshops (Drake, Becker, Clark, & Mueser, 1999a; Gervey & Bedell, 1994; Gold et al., 2006). One study compared rapid job search supported employment to a condition in which consumers received prevocational training prior to referral to supported employment (Bond et al., 1995a). The final two studies compared supported employment to referral to the state–federal vocational rehabilitation (VR) program (Chandler et al., 1997; McFarlane et al., 1995).

In every one of these 13 RCTs, summarized in Figure 9.1, individuals were significantly more likely to achieve competitive employment through a supported employment program than through alternative programs. In 8 of the 13 RCTs, the supported employ-

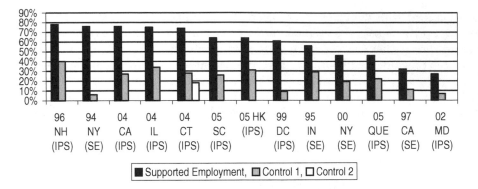

FIGURE 9.1. Competitive employment rates in 13 randomized controlled trials of supported employment. Studies are labeled by year of publication/presentation and state (province) where completed. Studies labeled IPS refer to studies that were monitored using an IPS fidelity scale. The studies and the follow-up periods are: 96 NH (14)—18 months; 94 NY (8)—12 months; 04 CA (18)—12 months; 04 IL (7)—24 months; 04 CT (17)—24 months; 05 SC (9)—24 months; 99 DC (13)—18 months; 95 IN (11)—12 months; 00 NY (16)—18 months; 05 QUE (10)—12 months; 97 CA (12)—36 months; 02 MD (15)—24 months.

ment program met high standards of fidelity to the individual placement and support (IPS) model (systematic monitoring with fidelity scale); in these 8 studies, an average of 63% of supported employment participants attained at least one competitive job, as compared with 23% of participants in other vocational services; the effect size for this difference is .84. In the 4 "pre-IPS" studies, which followed similar principles of IPS before the manual, 53% of supported employment participants attained competitive jobs, as compared with 16% of controls, yielding a nearly identical effect size of .82. The increased employment rates for both experimental and control groups in the latter set of studies are probably a result of three factors: better implemented supported employment programs, stronger alternative program models, and longer follow-up periods.

In addition to being much more successful in helping clients to obtain competitive jobs, supported employment also helps those who obtain work to obtain it faster. Across six of the recent studies reporting days to first job (Bond, 2004b; Drake et al., 1999b; Gold et al., 2006; Latimer et al., 2006; Lehman et al., 2002; Mueser et al., 2004a), the average number of days to first competitive job was 143 days for 305 supported employment clients versus 234 days for 129 control clients. In other words, not only did more clients get jobs, but they also obtained their first jobs an average of 3 months sooner. Incidentally, a common misconception is that supported employment is a rapid job *placement* model. In fact, supported employment is better described as a rapid job *search* model. In other words, the search for work begins soon after program entry, even though not everyone will obtain work immediately.

Supported employment clients also work twice as many weeks annually as do controls. We examined six studies with variable follow-up periods, converting weeks worked for the follow-up period to an annual rate (Bond, 2004b; Drake et al., 1999b; Gold et al., 2006; Latimer et al., 2006; Lehman et al., 2002; Mueser et al., 2004a). A total of 562 supported employment clients averaged 11.4 weeks of work per year, more than twice the average of 4.6 weeks per year for 566 controls.

Job satisfaction generally has not differed between clients enrolled in supported employment and those enrolled in alternative programs, but one recent study did find differences in initial job satisfaction favoring supported employment (Bond, 2004b).

Effectiveness

The standard distinction between efficacy and effectiveness research entails the change from highly controlled research situations, usually involving homogeneous clients without co-occurring conditions, university clinics, highly trained research clinicians, closely monitored interventions, and unusually generous resources, to real-world conditions, which typically include heterogeneous and complicated clients, routine clinics and clinicians, unmonitored interventions, and scarce resources (Wells, 1999). According to these criteria, the existing studies of supported employment (reviewed above) combine efficacy and effectiveness methods. Most of the participating clients were routine clients with a range of complicating conditions. In nearly all of the RCTs, clients self-selected for interest in employment, which offers ecological validity inasmuch as vocational services are usually not offered to clients without interest in employment. However, the day treatment conversion studies described above included clients who did not have work goals, yet many obtained jobs, suggesting that interest in work may be influenced by program philosophy. Nearly all of the studies utilized real-world clinics and clinicians. Because of the research projects, clinicians were trained, supervised, and monitored more extensively than in routine care, and research typically added extra resources and other artificial constraints.

Thus, to a large extent, supported employment research has been conducted using rigorous experimental methods in real-world settings with real-world clients and practitioners. Skipping over some of the earlier stages of intervention development (Rounsaville, Carroll, & Onken, 2001), which often involve highly artificial conditions that do not transfer to real-world conditions, may be one reason that supported employment has been developed, empirically validated, and shown to be effective in different settings so rapidly.

Generalizability

The evidence indicates that the effects of supported employment are quite robust across many types of clients and settings. All studies of supported employment show similar results for women and men. Individual studies show excellent results for African American clients (Bond, 2004b; Drake et al., 1999b), Hispanic American clients (Mueser et al., 2004a), rural clients (Drake et al., 1996a), older clients (Twamley et al., 2004), French Canadian clients (Latimer et al., 2006), Asian clients (Wong et al., 2005), and clients with co-occurring substance use disorders (Drake et al., 1999b). The exception appears to be clients who do not have vocational goals (Lehman et al., 2002). Preliminary findings from a current study of young clients experiencing a first episode of schizophrenia also indicate excellent employment outcomes at 6 and 18 months (Nuechterlein, Subotnik, Ventura, Gitlin, Green, et al., 2005). Similar findings have been reported in the United Kingdom (Rinaldi, McNeil, Firn, Koletsi, Perkins, et al., 2004).

Whether supported employment will be effective in other countries with different cultures, economic systems, work force issues, and health care issues remains to be seen. The current studies have largely been conducted in several regions of the United States, though recent RCTs in Montreal (Latimer et al., 2006) and Hong Kong (Wong et al., 2005) show similar results. A current study in six diverse European countries (Burns, Catty, Becker, Drake, Fioritti, et al., in press) may shed further light on generalizability. Because supported employment was developed in the U.S. economic, social, and health care context, one might expect that the intervention, as well as local labor regulations, insurance laws, and cultural beliefs regarding recovery, may have to be altered in other countries to produce similar employment benefits.

Nonvocational Outcomes

What effect does supported employment have on nonvocational outcomes, such as illness management, psychological health, relationships, and quality of life? In some sense, this is an inappropriate question because, in theory, it is employment itself, not supported employment services per se, that should lead to nonvocational benefits. Because it is complicated and ethically problematic to assign interested volunteers randomly to competitive work versus no work, the question regarding nonvocational outcomes inevitably leads to correlational analyses, with all the inherent problems of nonequivalence. Nevertheless, several conclusions can be drawn from the existing literature.

First, as drawn from dozens of studies, there are no known adverse effects of exposing people to supported employment or to employment itself. The studies of conversions of day treatment described above support this finding by showing an absence of the negative outcomes often predicted (Torrey, Clark, Becker, Wyzik, & Drake, 1997). This finding is important because many mental health professionals were trained in the stress-diathesis model of mental illness (Zubin & Spring, 1977), which was often the justification for providing low expectations, paternalistic environments, and slow, stepwise approaches to rehabilitation (Bond, 1992). The stress-diathesis model undoubtedly has much validity, but many mental health clients have pointed out—and population studies have confirmed—that unemployment can be much more stressful than employment (Ralph, 2000; Rogers, 1995; Steele and Berman, 2001; Warr, 1987).

Second, correlational studies consistently show that employment is associated with nonvocational gains (Arns & Linney, 1993, 1995; Bond, Resnick, Drake, Xie, McHugo, Bebout, et al., 2001c; Fabian, 1989, 1992; Mueser, Becker, Torrey, Xie, Bond, et al., 1997a; Van Dongen, 1996, 1998). Improvements associated with employment are typically stronger in the areas of psychological health (e.g., self-esteem) and quality of life (e.g., financial support) than in areas of illness management (e.g., symptom control). Perhaps the most elegant study of this type is a case-control comparison by Bond et al. (2001c). In this study, clients who were equivalent in other characteristics were selected because of working substantially in competitive versus sheltered settings as a result of random assignment to supported employment versus other vocational services. Outcomes showed that the group in competitive employment fared better in terms of higher rates of improvement in symptoms, greater satisfaction with vocational services, leisure, and finances, and higher self-esteem, as compared with those in a combined minimal/no work group. The sheltered work group showed no such advantage.

Third, long-term follow-up studies, which we describe below, indicate that people with mental illnesses themselves perceive numerous benefits related to supported employment and competitive jobs.

In sum, although experimental evidence is lacking, studies of various kinds tend to confirm first-person accounts that for years have indicated that employment is an essential component of recovery for many people with mental illnesses. The primary benefits of working appear to be better income, better psychological health, and improved quality of life, but people with mental illnesses themselves often argue that the benefits of working extend to illness management as well.

Implementation

Because the implementation of supported employment has now been accompanied by research scrutiny in dozens of programs, guidelines for implementation are clearer for this intervention than for many others (Becker & Bond, 2002; Bond, Becker, Drake, Rapp, Meisler, et al., 2001a; Drake et al., 2006a; Torrey et al., 2003). The utility of these guidelines has also been confirmed, though not yet reported, in the National Evidence-Based Practices Project (Torrey et al., 2001). Current guidelines include several principles: Supported employment is best implemented by starting with voluntary programs, so that early adopters can be models and training sites for other programs later; total collaboration of the departments of mental health and vocational rehabilitation at the state and local levels; building consensus with all stakeholders (state authorities, local administrators, practitioners, and persons with mental illnesses), so that support and sustainability become part of implementation; and attending to the relevant tasks, such as adopting a new philosophy, training staff, changing medical records, and billing, during each of the three phases of preparation, implementation, and maintenance. Table 9.2 describes the current guidelines by phase.

Dissemination

Several studies show that supported employment can be implemented broadly in routine practice settings. Indeed, one of the strengths of supported employment is its transportability; with a minimum of training and supervision, rehabilitation practitioners can join with routine mental health teams and learn the specific skills necessary to implement supported employment with good fidelity. In both the National Evidence-Based Practices Project (Torrey et al., 2001) and the Johnson & Johnson–Dartmouth Community Mental Health Program (Drake et al., 2006a), evidence-based supported employment was implemented in a variety of routine practice settings, with results that were roughly comparable to those found in research studies. The primary barriers to dissemination and adoption are funding, the traditional separation of vocational rehabilitation and mental health services, and failure in some settings to adopt a recovery-oriented ideology. All of these barriers have been overcome in the above demonstrations without enormous external resources and have generally led to an expansion of supported employment programs in each state or region.

Concerns

Several concerns about supported employment have been raised. The most serious have to do with length of job tenure, long-term career trajectories, and costs.

JOB TENURE

A common concern regarding supported employment is that job tenure is relatively brief. In six recent RCTs (Drake et al., 1996a; Lehman et al., 2002; Mueser et al., 2004a; Bond, 2004b; Latimer et al., 2006; Gold et al., 2006), supported employment clients who

TABLE 9.2. Guidelines for Implementing Supported Employment

Preparatory phase (6–12 months)

1. Address the collaboration between mental health and vocational rehabilitation at the state and local levels. This typically includes planning, funding, supervising, training, and other functions at the state level. Locally, integrated interventions require regular personal contact as a team.

2. Start with interested programs. Early adopters have a better chance of success and can provide models, training sites, supervisors, and peer pressure for other programs.

3. Plan for implementation locally (financing, structure of teams, training, supervision, records). The local problems of implementation are often unique to sites, and problem solving must be done at the local level.

4. Involve all stakeholders, including clients, families, practitioners, and administrators. To make changes that will be solid and sustainable, problems will need to be solved and plans made by each of these groups.

Implementation phase (6–12 months)

5. Train teams (employment specialist and mental health practitioners) for at least 1 year via regular supervision. Practitioners change their behaviors by seeing and hearing about a new approach and then having an opportunity to try new behaviors with their own clients and with regular supervision. It takes 6–12 months for practitioners to develop new skills and feel comfortable in applying them routinely.

6. Use an external trainer/supervisor initially if there is not a local supported employment expert. Supervision is often provided by telephone conference calls with the team. The external supervisor says less and slowly backs out of the process as the local supervisor develops proficiency and takes over.

7. Allow local teams to solve local problems. Many of the problems that arise are idiosyncratic to the local program, economy, health care environment, population, and so on. Problem solving must rely on local experts.

8. Assess fidelity and outcomes regularly and independently (outside the team). To be predictive of outcomes and reflect principles of supported employment accurately, fidelity assessment must be done by someone who is independent of the local team. This usually starts with an outside expert or trainer, but can be shifted to local quality assurance procedures over time. If outcomes are consistently meeting benchmarks, ongoing fidelity assessment is unnecessary.

Sustaining phase (continuous following high-fidelity implementation)

9. Value, measure, and track employment outcomes. The most important outcome is individual, satisfying, and lasting employment for people who want to work. Programs must monitor employment outcomes to ensure that they stay on course.

10. Renew consultation and training if employment outcomes are not satisfactory. If employment outcomes decrease over time, a consultation, perhaps based on fidelity assessment, is indicated.

11. Plan to incorporate new evidence-based components. Evidence-based practices, by definition, are based on current best evidence and will change. Programs will therefore need to be updated by emerging research on a regular basis. This change should be part of staff expectations.

12. Ensure that local teams continue to solve local problems. Over time, idiosyncratic problems occur in each program, and local experts from multiple stakeholder groups need to be empowered to solve these problems.

obtained work were employed for about the same length of time as those enrolled in alternative programs, with the average job tenure on longest job 21.3 weeks for supported employment clients, as compared with 17.3 weeks for those in other programs. In each of these studies, some clients were still employed at follow-up, resulting in an underestimate of actual job tenure. Nevertheless, the evidence shows that tenure in initial jobs is relatively short.

The counterargument is that short first job tenure is not necessarily a negative outcome; new workers can be expected to try different jobs while they are learning what working is like, what specific jobs are like, what kinds of work they enjoy, what their skills are, and so forth. These are normal and appropriate steps in the process of becoming a steady worker and developing a career. Success ultimately entails the development of long-term, satisfying jobs that people consider careers, not the length of a first job. In other words, supported employment aims to help people attain a positive and satisfying longitudinal vocational trajectory.

LONG-TERM EMPLOYMENT TRAJECTORIES

The long-term evidence on supported employment is just emerging, but three recent studies indicate that clients who have access to supported employment services over a number of years do work more over time and do acquire long-term, satisfying jobs (Salyers, Becker, Drake, Torrey, & Wyzik, 2004a; Becker, Whitley, Bailey, & Drake, 2007; Drake, McHugo, Xie, Fox, Packard, et al., 2006). Salyers et al. (2004a) followed a small cohort of clients exposed to supported employment over 10 years, following the closure of a day treatment program, and found that 33% of the clients worked substantially over time. Moreover, their jobs at 10-year follow-up tended to be long-term and competitive, and the clients attributed gains in several other areas, including hope, self-esteem, and substance abuse, to their success in employment. Becker et al. (2007) recently completed an 8–12-year follow-up of clients who had participated in earlier studies of supported employment and found even more impressive results, including a remarkable 75% rate of substantial employment and reports of nonvocational improvements attributed to working, similar to results of the Salyers et al. (2004a) study. The amazingly high rate of employment over time was probably related to the fact that all of these clients originally signed up for supported employment studies. Drake et al. (2006b) followed clients in the New Hampshire Dual Diagnosis Study for 10 years and found a steady increase in competitive employment, from 7% to more than 40%. This outcome was unexpected, because the participants in this study were selected for co-occurring substance abuse and high instability rather than for vocational interest. Nonetheless, employment was clearly a major part of recovery for many.

COSTS

Another concern regarding supported employment has been its cost and cost-effectiveness. Latimer (2001) reviewed the research from eight sets of studies (some databases were used in multiple evaluations) and concluded that the supported employment programs were no more expensive than the alternative approaches, such as day treatment or sheltered employment, but did not produce substantial cost offsets, at least over the short term. This suggests that providing supported employment programs may increase costs relative to providing no vocational services and be cost neutral relative to alternative vocational or rehabilitation approaches.

A problem with the studies reviewed by Latimer is that the constraints of controlled research often distort cost estimates that would obtain under routine program conditions. Evidence on the costs of routine supported employment programs comes from a study of seven real-world programs operating with high fidelity to the IPS model (Latimer, Bush, Becker, Drake, & Bond, 2004). Costs per "full-year-equivalent client," which means the average costs of 1 year of continuous supported employment (SE) services per slot, were approximately $2,500 per year. Because some clients change their minds about pursuing employment and others obtain jobs and require little or no follow-up support, in both cases opening slots for new clients, the costs per actual client served were considerably more modest.

Another problem with the current economic research is the short-term perspective. If people increase their time working and their independence from the mental health system over time, as suggested by the long-term follow-ups, the true economic impact of supported employment must be considered over decades, not 1 or 2 years. Over the long run, attachment to a job and immersion into a job-related employment culture may improve health outcomes and reduce long-term public welfare dependency by, for example, reducing the use of illegal and legal substances, increasing activity levels, and increasing social contacts with family and friends. Even marginal improvements in health and functioning could have substantial cost impacts, because of the high cost of treating chronic conditions and nursing home care. However, the longer-term economic effects of supported employment programs have not been addressed, owing to the unavailability of long-term data.

It is truly remarkable that the health-care system should demand that supported employment produce cost offsets. The overall costs are very modest in relation to those of other mental health interventions, especially considering the evidence showing that it results in such robust benefits. Perhaps the underlying issue is that because supported employment is a nontraditional service that combines mental health and vocational rehabilitation resources, policy makers have not yet decided how it should be financed.

Current Challenges

Current challenges include increasing access to supported employment nationally, improving outcomes among participants who do not become steady workers, and enhancing outcomes among those who do become steady workers but are limited in their career development trajectories. We next address current efforts in relation to these three issues.

ACCESS

The central issue regarding access is, of course, that vocational rehabilitation of all kinds, and especially evidence-based supported employment, is grossly underfunded in the United States (Wehman & Moon, 1988). Because of limited funding, only 5–7% of eligible disabled persons receive vocational rehabilitation services (General Accounting Office, 1993). Moreover, people with psychiatric disabilities encounter additional barriers in accessing vocational services (Andrews, Barker, Pittman, Mars, Struening, et al., 1992; Marshak, Bostick, & Turton, 1990), and much of the funding goes to prolonged and non-evidence-based assessments, evaluations, and training (Noble et al., 1997). The underfunding of rehabilitation services for disabled persons who want to work, in the wealthiest country in the world, whose government purports to value economic self-reliance, is a conundrum. Political leadership and advocacy are obviously needed. The movement to adopt evidence-based practices within state and local vocational rehabilitation and mental health agencies may help to overcome the political inertia (Ganju, 2004). There is also hope that private foundations and industries will add resources to enhance access to evidence-based services (Drake et al., 2006a).

IMPROVING OUTCOMES FOR THOSE WITH LIMITED SUCCESS

Short-term (1–2 years) and long-term (3–12 years) studies, reviewed above, show that about 60–70% of clients who receive supported employment attain at least one competitive job, but that only about half of them become steady workers over the years. In other words, some portion of clients, perhaps a third, do not attain competitive employment; another portion, perhaps another third, have limited success and do not become steady workers; and the last third become steady workers. The barriers that limit success for the middle third are multiple and complex. Factors such as socialization into disability, medication nonresponsiveness, inability to use medications effectively, co-occurring medical illnesses, and lack of psychosocial supports are probably involved. Current research, however, focuses on two substantial barriers: economic disincentives and cognitive deficits.

Disincentives within the benefits system are often seen as a barrier to employment by beneficiaries (General Accounting Office, 1996). Many people who are exposed to supported employment decide that work is not their goal once they receive benefits counseling, grasp how little they will actually gain economically, and understand what they may risk by going to work (e.g., removal from Social Security rolls and loss of health insurance). Some of these clients decide to work as volunteers, even though they have good employment skills, and others decide to declare themselves retired or to work under the table. Currently, efforts are under way at the Social Security Administration and the Centers for Medicare and Medicaid Services to reconsider benefit regulations in order to offer more encouragement to people who want to work. These efforts include the Medicaid Buy-In program, the Ticket-to-Work program, extended waivers of Social Security review, research programs, and so forth. Whether these efforts will increase vocational outcomes remains to be seen, but the willingness to experiment with changing regulations is encouraging and likely to be at least partially successful.

Another strategy to avoid the disincentives of benefits is to engage clients in supported employment very early in the course of their illness, before they acquire disability benefits and before they are socialized within the mental health system. Nuechterlein et al. (2005) have been studying this strategy in a clinic for people experiencing a "first episode" of schizophrenia with truly remarkable results: More than 90% of the participants were working and/or attending school at 6 and 18 months follow-up. If these results are replicated, the findings could fundamentally alter basic assumptions regarding disability, treatment, and rehabilitation.

Another promising area of current research focuses on cognitive deficits. Research shows that persistent cognitive deficits, such as problems of attention and problem solving, rather than lack of work skills, symptoms of illness, substance abuse, or other problems, constitute the most significant client-level barrier to employment success for people with psychiatric disabilities (Green, 1996b; McGurk & Mueser, 2004). In theory, functioning on the job might be improved by several new interventions that address cognitive deficits: (1) better job matches to avoid specific cognitive limitations; (2) compensatory strategies, such as posted reminders, to help clients overcome specific cognitive problems; (3) errorless learning training to address job-specific problems; (4) cognitive enhancement training to improve cognitive functioning through the use of computerized practice sessions that aim to stimulate the development of neurological connections; or (5) medications to enhance cognitive performance, such as those under development for dementia. All of these approaches are under active investigation, with some early studies showing positive results (McGurk, Mueser, & Pascaris, 2005).

ENHANCING SUCCESS FOR STEADY WORKERS

Long-term follow-up studies show that the majority of clients who become steady workers nevertheless decide to limit their work to part-time employment and do not give up benefits completely (Salyers, Becker, Drake, Torrey, & Wyzik, 2004a; Becker et al., 2007; Drake et al., 2006b). Anecdotally, many of these people indicate that they and their employers would prefer full-time employment, but clients are hesitant to give up benefits, especially health insurance, completely, and employers are often unable to offer adequate or any health insurance. Whether the Medicaid Buy-In legislation, other changes in disability benefits, or other improvements in alleviating symptoms or cognitive deficits will enable people to work full-time is unclear at this point.

SUPPORTED EDUCATION

Thus far our discussion has focused on employment; we now turn to analogous supported education services that have been developed to help people with psychiatric disabilities whose goal is to pursue education rather than work. *Supported education* refers to assisted postsecondary education in integrated educational settings for people with disabilities (Unger, 1990). Education is often the primary goal of younger clients, who have peers still in school and whose educations may have recently been disrupted.

PERSONAL EXAMPLE

Carolyn Mellon Gets an Academic Job

Carolyn was a 55-year-old woman with eccentric ideas, a flamboyant appearance, and a history of schizoaffective disorder. She had delusional ideas about a past job as a secretary in a university and thought of herself as a professional academic, though she had no college degree and had not worked in many years. Her mental health team noted that Carolyn's psychotic thinking had decreased with age, but she remained socially isolated and without a meaningful work role in her life. When a supported employment specialist joined the team, she automatically met with Carolyn to discuss employment. Because initial applications to the local university did not result in interviews, the employment specialist helped Carolyn to identify the local library as an appropriate work setting for an intellectual person. The mental health team agreed that library work without much contact with the public would be a good job match. Subsequently, the employment specialist helped Carolyn to secure a library job restacking books, initially on a trial basis and then as a permanent job. Carolyn took great pride in working with books and intellectuals, and the employment specialist helped Carolyn and her supervisors to resolve occasional interpersonal problems. Carolyn stayed in the job for more than 10 years and was highly celebrated when she retired at age 67.

Approaches to supported education are less standardized than approaches to supported employment because there has been relatively little research on supported education (Carlson et al., 2003). It makes sense that supported education should incorporate principles that parallel those of supported employment, with an emphasis on functioning in routine educational settings, attention to client choice, highly individualized services, integration with mental health services, and follow-up supports as needed. In practice, however, supported education programs have used a range of approaches that include self-contained classrooms, on-site supports, and mobile supports, with varying degrees of integration with mental health services (Carlson et al., 2003). The self-contained classroom approach, which is more analogous to preemployment vocational training programs, is the only one to be studied with experimental designs (Mowbray, Brown, Furlong-Norman, & Sullivan Soydan, 2000).

Although supported education has not been standardized and studied rigorously, a common approach is to combine supported education with supported employment. In routine practice settings, many young clients with psychiatric disabilities express educational goals or combined educational and employment goals, rather than exclusively employment goals. Many older individuals also desire to get more education to improve their job possibilities. Therefore, many employment specialists and multidisciplinary teams help these clients to pursue education, using the same approach that they use for employment. In fact, in the Nuechterlein et al. study (2005), described above, combined supported education and supported employment showed great success in achieving educational outcomes as well as employment outcomes among young people with a first episode of schizophrenia. The majority of clients pursued a combination of school and work. As a corollary, secondary prevention argues for early intervention with young people, helping them to pursue both educational and vocational goals, before they become disabled and obtain disability payments.

SUMMARY AND CONCLUSIONS

The field of vocational rehabilitation for people with psychiatric disabilities has moved rapidly over the last 15 years toward an evidence-based approach to supported employment, because supported employment has by far the strongest research support among vocational interventions. The success of supported employment has, in fact, raised expectations for treatment and rehabilitation in general, changed the way most mental health practitioners think about rehabilitation, and supported the ideologies of recovery, inclusion, and community integration with strong data. We now know that most people with mental illness want to work competitively and can do so (see previous example). Moreover, employment seems to help them in other areas of their lives, and long-term benefits appear to be even better than short-term benefits.

The success of supported employment has inspired and invigorated movements to reconsider financing of mental health and vocational services, to change benefit and insurance plans, to develop innovations that would improve vocational outcomes further, and to develop supported education services. Despite some challenges, supported employment continues to expand in the United States and internationally because it addresses a basic need expressed by most people with mental illness to work and contribute to society.

Chapter 10

Social Functioning

Impaired social functioning is the hallmark of psychiatric disabilities. Even more than difficulties in working and supporting themselves, problems with communication and close relationships often make people with psychiatric disabilities appear different to others and may partly account for the social stigma they so often experience. In this chapter we consider the common challenges in social functioning experienced by people with psychiatric disabilities, and the rehabilitation approaches for addressing these problems.

We begin by defining social functioning and considering the specific life domains typically included in it. We next consider the importance of social functioning in relation to psychiatric disability (including how disabilities are defined), its impact on the course of psychiatric illness, and its relationship to quality of life. Next, we discuss the determinants of social functioning, including symptoms, cognitive functioning and social cognition, and social skills. We then describe social skills training, and review its effects on social functioning. Next, we discuss the effects of social skills training in other rehabilitation approaches in regard to social functioning, including family psychoeducation, assertive community treatment, supported employment, and peer support/psychosocial clubhouses. We conclude by summarizing what is known about psychiatric rehabilitation for social functioning and suggest future directions for research in this area.

WHAT IS SOCIAL FUNCTIONING?

Social functioning can be defined as the quality and depth of an individual's interpersonal relationships, and the person's ability to meet socially defined roles and expectations.

PERSONAL EXAMPLE

Mary Hoffman Is Socially Anxious

Mary Hoffman, a 53-year-old woman with a 25-year history of schizophrenia, had few friends and experienced debilitating anxiety during brief conversations with acquaintances and strangers. Mary worked part-time at a grocery store, but she was in a constant state of fear about interacting with her coworkers and customers. When faced with these interactions, Mary would often clam up and appear expressionless, barely nodding at the other person. On the mornings Mary was scheduled to work she always experienced a struggle, and she contemplated leaving her job on many occasions to avoid these interactions. She recognized that her most difficult challenges were meeting new people and opening up to existing friends and family members. Mary said she had the most trouble starting and maintaining conversations and going along with the flow of "small talk." She explained, "I never know what to say after a 'Good morning!' or 'Hello.' " She also said she found it very difficult to talk about her feelings and to tell people about herself. Mary expressed that she felt comfortable talking only with her mother and father, and she even avoided confiding in a friend whom she had known for more than 10 years. She wanted to have closer relationships and to feel more comfortable conversing with her coworkers.

Social functioning is a multifaceted concept whose nature can be best understood by considering several different life domains, including *role functioning*, *social relationships*, *self-care and independent living skills*, and *leisure and recreational activities*. A fifth domain of social functioning that is widely accepted as important, but is difficult to systematically measure, is *community reintegration*. We describe these domains below.

Role Functioning

Role functioning concerns an individual's ability to meet socially and culturally defined roles such as worker, student, parent, homemaker, or other caregiver (e.g., for an aging parent). Some of roles are defined more or less straightforwardly by society. For example, the role of a worker includes working on a sufficiently regular basis, meeting one's own basic living needs and possibly (if the individual is the designated wage earner for a family) the needs of others as well. The role of a student involves attending class and completing assignments with sufficient regularity to pass courses toward earning a degree or certificate. The role of parent involves feeding, clothing, sheltering, protecting, showing love and affection, and ensuring that a child's educational, medical, and social needs are met. The role of homemaker may be less fully defined socially, but typically includes activities such as preparing meals, housecleaning, and doing laundry.

The specific nature of role functioning is defined by a combination of societal, cultural, family, and individual factors. What defines a role is a patterned set of social behaviors that produce specific and desirable products or outcomes that are expected by others (e.g., money, a degree or certificate useful in getting a good-paying job, happy and healthy children). As the failure of an individual to meet his or her social roles often shifts the burden of responsibility to others, problems in role functioning can have profound effects on people's social environment, including their relationships with others.

Social Relationships

Social relationships involve the ability to have sustained connections with other people that are meaningful, enjoyable, and mutually rewarding. Examples of common important relationships of this type include those with family members, friends, and intimate partners. Social relationships of a different sort are also involved in other aspects of daily living, such as relationships with people at work, treatment providers (e.g., doctor, nurse, rehabilitation specialist), landlords, or salesclerks. These types of relationships are primarily functional in nature (i.e., aimed at getting instrumental needs met), whereas those with friends and partners are primarily affiliative relationships (i.e., aimed at having interpersonal needs met, such as acceptance and affection). Family relationships often serve a combination of instrumental and affiliative functions.

The quality of social relationships with friends and intimate partners is generally determined by a combination of subjective perspectives (e.g., each individual's satisfaction with the relationship) and objective aspects (e.g., how often do the two people see each other? Is there reciprocity between them in terms of giving and receiving?). Similarly, the quality of relationships with family members is often evaluated in terms of both subjective satisfaction with those relationships, and objective indicators of the person's contributions to the household and the extent of the relatives' caregiving activities (Schooler et al., 1979; Tessler & Gamache, 1996).

Self-Care and Independent Living Skills

A wide range of skills are needed to care for oneself, to present oneself to others in a socially appropriate way, and to live independently and safely without supervision. Self-care skills typically include the ability to attend to hygiene and grooming, dress appropriately for the weather and social situations, and respond to medical needs, such as seeing the doctor, taking medication, and adhering to special dietary restrictions. Independent living skills encompass a broader-range of abilities, such as cleaning and maintaining one's apartment, appropriate interactions with one's landlord and neighbors, cooking, doing laundry, money management, shopping, and using public transportation.

Self-care and independent living skills are similar to role functioning in that they both involve the ability to meet socially defined expectations. They differ only in the nature of those expectations. For role functioning, the expectations are social in nature and other people typically depend on individuals to meet those expectations. For self-care and independent living skills, the societal expectation is for relative self-sufficiency, with the recognition that some interdependency and social exchange will occur cooperatively in some of these areas, such as cooking and cleaning. These skills have their greatest social impact when they are lacking, when an adult is unable to meet them on his or her own and requires help from others.

Leisure and Recreational Activities

In addition to work and relationships, how people spend their free time is an important determinant of their perceived quality of life. Leisure and recreational activities include fun and entertaining pursuits, such as hobbies, sports, watching TV or going to the movies, hiking, communing with nature, and reading. Other activities may also be included that involve personal meaning, growth, fulfillment, or health maintenance or improvement, such as keeping a journal, artistic expression, exercise, or spiritual enrichment.

Although some leisure activities can be done alone, many others are social in nature, and participating in them with others can help form or strengthen bonds with others.

Community Integration

Community integration is a natural by-product of successful adjustment in the previously reviewed domains of role functioning, quality of relationships, self-care and independent living skills, and use of leisure time. Community integration can be conceptualized as the extent to which individuals with a disability live side by side others without such disabilities and participate regularly in social activities in their communities (Wong & Solomon, 2002). The social rejection due to psychiatric disabilities deals a heavy blow to many consumers, who yearn not only to have rewarding relationships with others, but to be members of the broader communities in which they live (Carling, 1995). Social integration can encompass a wide range of activities and behaviors, such as attending public meetings (e.g., municipal or school board meetings), having regular interactions with nondisabled persons, volunteering, and participating in shared activities such as attending a place of worship or joining a local organization).

WHY IS SOCIAL FUNCTIONING IMPORTANT?

Social functioning is a major concern for persons with psychiatric disabilities for four reasons. First, problems in social functioning, including role functioning, close relationships, and self-care/independent living are explicitly included in the diagnostic criteria of some psychiatric disorders. For example, impaired social/occupational functioning is included in the diagnosis of schizophrenia according to both DSM-IV (American Psychiatric Association, 1994) and ICD-10 diagnostic criteria (World Health Organization, 1992). Furthermore, the determination of psychiatric disability benefits, such as Supplemental Security Income (SSI) and Social Security Disability Insurance (SSDI), usually hinges on a combination of having an established psychiatric disorder and its impact on functioning. Thus, impaired social functioning is central to the definition of psychiatric disability, and efforts to reduce those impairments can be construed as treatment for the disability.

Second, although for some individuals social difficulties emerge in the wake of a psychiatric disorder, for many others these impairments preceded the onset of their disorder for many years (Robins, 1966; Zigler & Glick, 1986). Poor premorbid social functioning is especially common in schizophrenia (Addington & Addington, 1993; Cannon-Spoor, Potkin, & Wyatt, 1982), but is also present in other disorders (Zigler & Glick, 1986). Thus, before developing a psychiatric disorder, many individuals lacked close friends, had never had an intimate relationship, had few leisure and recreational activities, dropped out of school, and worked little or not at all. Marginal social functioning can increase vulnerability to developing a psychiatric disorder, but it can also be a subtle sign of the gradual development of schizophrenia that presages the onset of more florid psychotic symptoms (Häfner, 2000; Häfner & an der Heiden, 2003). Because of the long-standing nature of social difficulties in many consumers, these problems are usually affected only minimally by pharmacological treatments, thus necessitating direct and concerted psychiatric rehabilitation efforts to improve them.

Third, quality of social relationships and frequency of social contacts are predictive of the course of psychiatric disabilities, including symptom relapses and rehospitalizations (Erickson et al., 1989; Rajkumar & Thara, 1989; Strauss & Carpenter, 1977). The prevailing hypothesis that accounts for this association is the *stress-buffering theory of social support* (Bebbington & Kuipers, 1992; Callaghan & Morrissey, 1993; Mor-Barak, Miller, & Syme, 1991). According to this theory, which is incorporated into the broader *stress-vulnerability model* of psychiatric illness (Liberman et al., 1986; Zubin & Spring, 1977), social support buffers the negative effects of stress on the biological vulnerability, which is root cause of the psychiatric disorder. For example, socially supportive people can help to minimize the effects of stress on someone by anticipating potential problems and taking steps to prevent them, problem solving with or on behalf of the person, and helping the person cope more effectively with stress. Thus, improving the ability of people with a psychiatric disability to participate in meaningful and rewarding relationships may enhance the social support they receive, which in turn may contribute to a better course of illness.

Fourth, social functioning is a highly valued dimension of life experience, and for this reason alone it is important to improve it. Social acceptance and connection is widely accepted as a fundamental human need, yet for all the reasons described above it is often not met in individuals with psychiatric disabilities. These consumers often have few friends (Breier, Schreiber, Dyer, & Pickar, 1991; Randolph, 1998) and identify improved social relationships as an important treatment priority (Bengtsson-Tops & Hansson, 1999; Wiersma, Nienhuis, Giel, & Sloof, 1998), but also report that such needs are not sufficiently addressed by mental health services (Middelboe, Mackeprang, Hansson, Werdelin, Karlsson, et al., 2001). In addition to the importance of close relationships, having a sense of purpose, which is often involved in fulfilling roles such as worker, student, or parent, lends meaning to life and is a common theme in consumers' writings about recovery (Mead & Copeland, 2000; Ralph, 2000). Finally, the desire to live independently is common among consumers, as described in greater detail in Chapter 8. Thus, efforts to improve social functioning may help people with psychiatric disabilities lead more meaningful and rewarding lives and may improve the course of their mental illness.

DETERMINANTS OF SOCIAL FUNCTIONING

Understanding the factors that are related to social functioning in persons with psychiatric disabilities may be helpful in targeting specific areas for improvement and developing rehabilitation strategies designed to address them. Four different factors related to psychiatric disabilities can have an impact on social functioning, including *symptoms*, *cognitive functioning*, *social skills*, and *environmental and resource factors*.

Symptoms

Specific psychiatric disorders are defined mainly by the presence of symptoms, such as psychotic symptoms, negative symptoms, depression, anxiety, and manic or hypomanic symptoms. All of these symptoms can interfere with social functioning. *Negative symptoms* are defined in terms of the absence of emotions, motivation, and behaviors that are ordinarily present in individuals. Common negative symptoms include apathy, anhedonia (loss of pleasure), alogia (poverty of speech or content of speech), and blunted affect (flattened facial expression and voice tone). Negative symptoms are most prominent in persons with schizophrenia but are also frequently present in depression. Negative symptoms can have a major impact on social functioning (Mueser, Douglas, Bellack, & Morrison, 1991; Pogue-Geile, 1989; Sayers, Curran, & Mueser, 1996). The lack of social drive characteristic of negative symptoms as well as difficulties initiating and following through on actions can have obvious effects on social relationships as individuals may invest little energy into developing and nurturing relationships, and they may be undependable in meeting expectations and obligations in relationships, including role responsibilities. Anhedonia and the expectation that normally pleasurable events will not be enjoyable results in apathy and an unwillingness to pursue potentially rewarding activities, which can be detrimental to establishing and maintaining close relationships. Blunted affect and alogia may make people less rewarding to interact with. Finally, a low energy level and lack of drive can lead to inattention to hygiene and living needs and consequent dependence on others for getting those basic needs met.

Psychotic symptoms, such as delusions and hallucinations, can influence social functioning in many different ways. Delusions are often social in nature, and acting upon them may be detrimental to existing relationships. For example, an individual may falsely accuse family members of trying to poison him or her, or avoid family friends because of a belief that they are working together to control his mind. Delusional beliefs can be particularly problematic in establishing intimate relationships, where they can serve as a barrier to developing a shared reality or perspective on the world with another person. Delusions can make people unable to fulfill the roles of worker, parent, or student, which typically require some ability to negotiate social relationships. Delusions can also lead to severe neglect or harm to oneself and for this reason are sometimes grounds for involuntary hospitalization. Hallucinations can be distracting and interfere with close communication with others. Command hallucinations (auditory hallucinations that command the individual to do things) sometimes lead people to hurt themselves or others.

Cognitive functioning can also have a significant impact on the broad range of social functioning (Green, 1996b; Green, Kern, Braff, & Mintz, 2000; McGurk, Mueser, Harvey, Marder, & LaPuglia, 2003). Difficulties with attention can make it hard for people to track conversations with others and to remain focused on relevant stimuli in their environment. Problems with psychomotor speed can make interactions with others feel awkward when the natural "give and take" of conversation is disturbed by the longer period of time the person needs to process the social information (Mueser, Bellack, Douglas, & Morrison, 1991a). Problems with psychomotor speed can also increase the time required to do a wide range of different tasks, such as working, cooking, dressing oneself, or participating in recreational and leisurely activities. Difficulties with memory can contribute to socially awkward situations when an individual forgets someone's name or the topic of conversation. Memory problems can also interfere with daily living activities (such as remembering what to buy at a store), as well as learning new tasks at home, work, or elsewhere. Problems in executive functions such as the ability to grasp abstract concepts, to plan, and to solve problems can contribute to a host of difficulties, including task performance (e.g., work, cooking) and resolving interpersonal conflict (i.e., problem solving).

In addition to the effects of impaired cognitive functioning in the areas of attention, psychomotor speed, learning and memory, and executive functions, problems in *social cognition* may also have a significant bearing on social adjustment. Social cognition involves the ability to accurately perceive and process social information (Corrigan & Penn, 2001; Penn, Corrigan, Bentall, Racenstein, & Newman, 1997). Examples of social cognitive skills include recognizing emotions in others, understanding important contextual factors in socially appropriate behavior (such as understanding whether one's relationship with another person is personal or professional), and the ability to perceive nuances during social interaction with others (such as understanding when someone is hinting at something). Problems in social cognition are common in people with psychiatric disabilities, especially in schizophrenia (Penn, Addington, & Pinkham, 2006). For example, people with schizophrenia have greater difficulties perceiving emotional expressions in others (Kohler et al., 2003; Mueser, Penn, Blanchard, & Bellack, 1997), as well as performing *theory of mind* tasks that require a person to temporarily adopt another person's perspective in order to solve a problem. Since understanding communication from others is the vital part of effective social functioning, especially in close relationships, problems in social cognition can be a significant obstacle to rewarding social relationships.

Social Skills

Social skills can be broadly defined as interpersonal behaviors or abilities that are critical for helping people to get their instrumental or affiliative needs met. Social skills can be divided into four broad categories, including nonverbal skills, paralinguistic skills, interactive balance, and verbal content (Bellack et al., 2004; McFall, 1982; Trower, Bryant, & Argyle, 1978; Wallace, Nelson, Liberman, Aitchison, Lukoff, et al., 1980). *Nonverbal social skills* include behaviors such as eye contact, interpersonal proximity, body orientation and gestures, and facial expression. *Paralinguistic features* include vocal characteristics of speech, such as voice tone, volume, inflection, and fluency. The nonverbal and paralinguistic features of social skills together are often more important to conveying the overall meaning and feeling of what is said than the actual verbal content.

Interactive balance refers to the flow of conversation between two people, including the latency of response and the relative amount of time each person talks. Adequate response latencies are critical to maintaining a natural and comfortable flow of conversation, and talking for relatively similar amounts of time can be important for ensuring that one person is not monopolizing or carrying most of the conversation. *Verbal content* is the actual choice of words and use of language, rather than the way in which it is spoken. Problems related to vocal content often occur when an individual is not aware of contextual factors that may govern the appropriateness of what is said in certain social situations (i.e., problems in social cognition). For example, appropriate disclosure of personal information depends on a variety of factors, such as familiarity with the other person and whether that person is a friend or coworker. Disclosing too much personal information too early can make other people feel uncomfortable.

Ample research shows that people with psychiatric disabilities, especially those with schizophrenia, often have impairments in social skills (Mueser & Bellack, 1998). The question of why these impairments are so common is a complex one, because social skills are multidetermined. Three factors related to psychiatric illness have been linked to poorer social skills: premorbid social functioning, negative symptoms, and cognitive impairment (Mueser et al., 1991b; Mueser, Bellack, Morrison, & Wixted, 1990a; Mueser, Blanchard, & Bellack, 1995b; Penn, Mueser, & Spaulding, 1996). Social skills are generally learned through natural interactions with family, with friends, at school, and on the job. The poor premorbid social functioning of some people with psychiatric disabilities (Zigler & Glick, 1986) may be partly due to the fact that they never learned effective social skills during their formative years, either because of a lack of opportunity or because of other problems (e.g., cognitive impairments). Some individuals who develop a psychiatric disorder had good social skills and functioned well socially before the onset of their psychiatric illness, but may have experienced a deterioration in their social skills because of illness-related factors such as negative symptoms, cognitive impairments, or disuse owing to lack of opportunity to use the skills in appropriate situations (e.g., during long-term hospitalization or protracted homelessness). Depression may also contribute to poorer social skills, although studies on this effect are inconsistent (Tse & Bond, 2004). It is also possible that demoralization related to developing a psychiatric disability, and the experience of social stigma, discourages some consumers from becoming socially involved with others, leading to a loss of their social skills.

Environmental and Resource Factors

The environment in which people live, and the resources to which they have access, have a bearing on their social, leisure, occupational, and independent functioning, whether or not they have a psychiatric disability. For example, living in an impoverished area with a high crime rate, few jobs, rampant substance abuse, and a lack of shared community resources (e.g., parks, YMCA, etc.) can pose a challenge to self-sufficiency, to establishing leisure activities, and to making enduring and meaningful social connections. The downward socioeconomic drift associated with developing a psychiatric disability, coupled with the impact of poverty on increasing vulnerability to serious psychiatric disorders (Dohrenwend, Levav, Shrout, Schwartz, Naveh, et al., 1992, 1998; Fox, 1990), leaves many individuals with limited resources and access to normative social roles.

Two additional environmental factors specific to mental illness may also influence social functioning. First, for individuals living in the community, the stigma of mental illness can lead to reduced social, vocational, and other opportunities (see Chapter 2). Past experiences with discrimination may lead some people to stop trying to improve their lot in life and to passively accept the status quo (Wahl, 1999b). Second, institutional settings, such as state hospitals or group homes, can limit opportunities for consumers to improve their social, occupational, and independent functioning because they are insulated from the community and a different norm of appropriate social behavior prevails. In these settings, the protection of the person and others, "compliance" with treatment and the regulations of daily living, and meeting basic living needs are of greatest importance, and minimal effort may be directed toward rehabilitation and improved psychosocial functioning. Indeed, in some settings efforts by consumers to assert more control over their lives may be met with either resistance or outright hostility by staff members. The net result of such environments is that people often do not have an opportunity to function more effectively, and a deterioration in functioning over years of institutionalization may occur (Wing & Brown, 1970).

SOCIAL SKILLS TRAINING

Because problems in social functioning can be a product of so many different factors in people with psychiatric disabilities, including both illness-related and other factors, a wide range of treatment and rehabilitation approaches may be helpful. For example, because severe symptoms can interfere with social adjustment, pharmacological treatment, teaching relapse prevention skills, and helping people develop effective strategies for coping with persistent symptoms can all improve social functioning. Although a wide range of rehabilitation methods may indirectly influence the quality of social adjustment in people with psychiatric disabilities, only one approach has been developed that specifically targets social functioning and has been repeatedly evaluated in controlled research designs: social skills training. In this section, we describe social skills training procedures, including techniques, logistics, generalization, training curriculum, and the incorporation of skills training into other rehabilitation methods. We then summarize the results of research on skills training.

Social Skills Training Procedures

Social skills training is a systematic approach to teaching interpersonal skills based on social learning theory. Social skills training evolved gradually as a rehabilitation approach over several decades (Liberman, DeRisi, & Mueser, 1989b), with refinements continuing up to the present day. In the 1940s, Salter (1949) first engaged people in role plays in an approach called *conditioned reflex therapy*, which was followed in the 1950s by Wolpe's use of instructions and role plays to teach assertiveness skills in order to inhibit feelings of anxiety (Wolpe, 1958). In the 1960s, Bandura's (1969) work on social learning theory demonstrated the power of modeling as a teaching device, and social skills training procedures began to incorporate role modeling as an integral part of the training process.

By the mid-to-late 1960s, social skills training had been packaged as an approach to teaching more effective interpersonal behaviors. Whereas early applications of social skills training focused on assertiveness or "standing up for one's rights" in nonclinical populations, success in this area soon led to using the methods to address other areas of social functioning, and in clinical populations as well. Since the development of its procedures, social skills training has become one of the most widely studied and implemented tools for changing social behavior across a wide range of individuals and situations, including persons with psychiatric disorders, substance use disorders, and developmental disabilities, as well as in numerous other applications in the general population, such as in schools, industry (e.g., teaching customer relations or supervisory skills), prisons, and for couples and families (Mueser, 1998).

Although the application of social skills training techniques varies, depending on the content, population, and setting where it is provided, the core ingredients are the same: complex social behaviors are broken down into component steps, which are then taught, using a combination of modeling (demonstrating) the skill, engaging the individual in role play to practice the steps of the skill, providing positive and corrective feedback about the person's role-play performance, conducting additional role plays to improve performance, and making a plan for the individual to practice the skill on his or her own. The steps of group-based social skills training are summarized in more detail in Table 10.1.

Before engaging consumers in social skills training, the trainer's efforts must first address the consumer's motivation to participate in such training. People are most interested in changing their behavior when they perceive that such changes will help them achieve personally meaningful goals. Therefore, prior to skills training, mental health practitioners meet with consumers individually to explore and identify their personal goals and to consider how skills training may help them achieve these goals. Examples of personal goals that consumers can set and pursue in skills training groups include having rewarding conversations with people, making friends, developing more leisure activities, getting closer to someone, resolving conflicts with people, getting one's needs met from health and mental health providers, being more assertive, avoiding drug and alcohol use, and being more effective or comfortable with social interactions on the job (e.g., with one's boss, coworkers, or customers). Once personal goals are established, the format and procedures of skills training are described in order to set accurate and positive expectations for consumers' participation in training sessions (Bellack et al., 2004; Liberman et al., 1989b).

Logistics

Social skills training is most often conducted in a group format, although individual applications are also feasible. There are several advantages of group, as opposed to indi-

TABLE 10.1. Steps of Group-Based Social Skills Training

1. Establish a rationale for the learning the skill.
   - Elicit, from group participants, reasons for learning the skill.
   - Acknowledge all contributions.
   - Provide additional reasons not mentioned by group members.

2. Discuss the steps of the skill.
   - Break down the skill into three or four steps.
   - Write the steps on a board or poster.
   - Discuss the reason for each step.
   - Check for understanding of each step.

3. Model the skill in a role play.
   - Plan the role play in advance.
   - Explain that you will demonstrate the skill in a role play.
   - Use two leaders to model the skill.
   - Keep the role play simple.

4. Review the role play with the participants.
   - Discuss whether each step of the skill was used in the role play.
   - Ask group members to evaluate the effectiveness of the role model.
   - Keep the review brief and to the point.

5. Engage a consumer in a role play of the same situation.
   - Start with a consumer who is more skilled or is likely to be compliant.
   - Request the consumer to try the skill in a role play with one of the leaders.
   - Ask the consumer questions to make sure he or she understands the goal.
   - Instruct group members to observe the consumer.

6. Provide positive feedback.
   - Elicit positive feedback from group members about the consumer's skills.
   - Encourage feedback that is specific.
   - Cut off any negative feedback.
   - Praise effort and provide hints to group members about good performance.

7. Provide corrective feedback.
   - Elicit suggestions for how the consumer could use the skill better next time.
   - Limit the feedback to one or two suggestions.
   - Strive to communicate the suggestions in a positive, upbeat manner.

8. Engage the consumer in another role play of the same situation.
   - Request that the consumer change one behavior in the role play.
   - Ask the consumer questions to check on his or her understanding of the suggestion.
   - Try to work on behaviors that are most critical and changeable.

9. Provide additional feedback.
   - Be generous but specific when providing positive feedback.
   - Focus first on the behavior that the consumer was requested to change.
   - Engage consumer in two to four role plays giving feedback after each one.
   - Use other behavior-shaping strategies to improve skills, such as coaching, prompting, and supplemental modeling.

10. Assign homework.
   - When possible, tailor the assignment to each consumer's level of skill.
   - Give an assignment to practice the skill.
   - Ask group members to identify situations in which they could use the skill.

Note. Adapted from Bellack, Mueser, Gingench, and Agresta (2004). Copyright 2004 by The Guilford Press. Adapted by permission.

vidual, skills training. First, group-based skills training may be more economical because training is provided to multiple consumers at the same time. Second, training in groups provides consumers with more role-modeling opportunities because they are able to observe each other performing the skill. Third, teaching social skills in a group can create a positive milieu in which consumers support each other and provide helpful feedback as they work toward improving skills and achieving personal goals. Giving feedback and support to other people may bolster consumers' feelings about themselves as they are able to help other people, which is akin to the concept of the "helper principle" in self-help groups (Campbell, 1997; Gartner & Riessman, 1977; Madara, 1988). Receiving feedback from one's peers can be helpful because of the very high credibility associated with such feedback.

Skills training in groups is usually done with four to eight consumers. Conducting groups is easier with two coleaders, as one can take primary responsibility for teaching the core curriculum and the other can attend to group process issues, such as making sure that all consumers are paying attention, understanding the material, and actively participating. When working with very impaired consumers, such as persons with significant cognitive impairment or very severe psychotic symptoms, a smaller group size is preferable, such as three to five consumers.

Skills training sessions usually last between an hour and an hour and a half, but, as with the size of the group, the duration of sessions can be reduced when working with individuals with limited attention spans. The frequency of sessions depends mainly on the setting where the training takes place. In general, more frequent skills training sessions over shorter periods of time leads to better skills acquisition. Thus, when feasible, conducting multiple training sessions per week (such as twice a week) is preferable to less frequent sessions, with a minimum of at least weekly sessions.

The duration of a skills training program depends on the specific areas of functioning targeted by the program, the setting where skills training is provided, and the level of cognitive functioning of the participants. When skills training is conducted on an outpatient basis, sessions are usually provided for at least 3 months, and often 6 months to a year or longer. Some skills training programs fade the intensity of sessions over time in order to promote maintenance of the skills when training has ended. Skills training can be provided for briefer periods of time in places where consumers live temporarily, such as acute care inpatient settings or homeless shelters. For example, in an inpatient setting in which consumers were hospitalized for an average of 2–4 weeks, a 2-week conflict resolution skills group was developed in which two skills ("expressing negative feelings" and "compromise and negotiation") were taught on an alternating weekly basis (Mueser, Levine, Bellack, Douglas, & Brady, 1990b). Group sessions were conducted three times per week (Monday, Wednesday, Friday), and consumers could begin participating within a few days following their admission to the hospital and remain in the group until their discharge.

Skills training can also be conducted individually, either to provide makeup sessions to consumers who have missed group sessions or just as an individual-based intervention. When such a format is utilized, the same training steps are used as described in Table 10.1, with the clinician often taking the roles of other people in role plays. When possible, other individuals can be selectively included in sessions to conduct role plays with the consumer. Individual-based skills training provides more time and flexibility for tailoring the training to meet the specific needs of the consumer. In addition, with individual-based skills training it is often easy and convenient for training to take place out of the office and in community settings, such as in the consumer's apartment or in a store (see the following section).

Programming Generalization

Although skills training conducted in settings such as community mental health centers, supervised residences, or hospitals provides consumers with an opportunity to learn the rationale for specific social skills and to practice and hone their skills in role plays, the generalization of skills from those settings to more naturalistic ones does not spontaneously occur for most individuals. To address this contingency, social skills training programs must also "program generalization" of newly acquired skills to consumers' natural environments where the skills are needed. There are three approaches to helping consumers apply skills taught in training sessions to their day-to-day lives.

First, homework assignments are routinely given at the end of each skills training session, aimed at helping consumers try the skill on their own. These assignments are then reviewed at the beginning of the next skills training session, with an emphasis on practicing the skill and receiving feedback from other group members and the leaders on how to further improve their skills. A homework assignment is most likely to be followed through and successful if the assignment is individually tailored to the client's personal goals and circumstances and the consumer is actively involved in getting the assignment and when and where it will be completed.

Second, *in vivo* trips to the actual settings where targeted social skills will be used can promote generalization of social skills. These trips can be conducted either individually or in a group to a wide range of settings such stores, restaurants, parks, or museums, to a medical clinic, or to various types of entertainment such as a play, movie, or carnival. Participating in community trips can be reinforcing in its own right and can provide opportunities for consumers to practice skills in "real-world" settings, with the help and support of other group participants (when applicable) and the leader(s). When *in vivo* trips are integrated into a skills training program, they are typically conducted once every week or two, and at a minimum monthly. Naturally, there are some social skills that cannot be readily practiced during *in vivo* trips, such as skills for resolving interpersonal conflicts, expressing intimate feelings, or refusing invitations to use substances.

Third, the generalization of skills can be enhanced by involving significant others as natural supports to consumers learning how to apply new skills (Tauber et al., 2000). Examples of significant others who can be involved in helping consumers practice their skills in naturally occurring social situations are family members, friends, residential counselors, or hospital staff members. Collaboration with significant others typically involves meeting with and informing them about the consumer's goals for participating in skills training, explaining the nature of social skills training (i.e., its emphasis on helping people gradually develop more effective skills through practice and positive reinforcement) and the targeted skills (i.e., specific steps of the skills), addressing and resolving concerns about the consumer's goal or the targeted skills, and identifying real-life situations where consumers can practice specific skills with the support or prompting of the significant others.

Involving and collaborating with natural supports can be critical to the success of skills training interventions for two reasons. First, working with significant others, and giving them a role in helping consumers learn specific social skills, maximizes the chances that they will support consumers in pursuing their goals and minimizes the possibility of their undermining those goals either deliberately (e.g., because they do not approve of them) or inadvertently (e.g., because they do not understand how specific social skills will help consumers to achieve their goals). Second, when natural supports are involved in skills training, consumers can be reminded to use their skills in situations where they may otherwise forget to use them and can experience the naturally rewarding consequences of more effective social skills.

For example, in one community residence where skills training was provided, a staff member observed two consumers loudly arguing, with one consumer upset by the other's frequent requests for cigarettes. Both consumers were participants in the skills training group, and so the staff member interceded and prompted them to use steps of the skill "compromise and negotiation" to resolve their disagreement. The consumers responded by using the skill and arriving at a compromise that was satisfactory to both of them. The staff member indicated that before being involved in the skills training group, he would have intervened and either split up the two consumers or mediated a resolution. Instead, the experience of successfully resolving the disagreement through the use of a social skill helped the consumers to feel good about their own skills and led to a mutually agreed-upon resolution.

Curriculum

Social skills training can be used to help consumers address a wide range of social, leisure, vocational, independent living, and health-related needs, and such a program requires a curriculum. Developing a skills training curriculum involves identifying the critical skills for functioning in specific areas, breaking down those skills into smaller steps, identifying role-play situations that can be used to help people learn the steps of the skill, and trying out the skills with consumers. Thus, developing a social skills curriculum is a time-consuming process. Fortunately, extensive curricula have already been developed. Two widely used approaches to social skills training curricula have been developed by Robert P. Liberman, Charles Wallace, and their colleagues at the University of California, Los Angeles (UCLA), and by Alan Bellack and his colleagues.

The UCLA skills training curriculum includes a series of social skills training *modules*, each focused on a different content area, that together are referred to as the Social and Independent Living Skills (SILS) program (Kopelowicz & Liberman, 1994; Liberman, Wallace, Blackwell, Eckman, Vaccaro, et al., 1993). Each module includes the same core set of resources, including a leader's manual, participants' workbooks, standardized *in vivo* and homework assignments to practice skills, questionnaires to assess learning of information taught in the modules, and a videotape of role-play demonstrations of the skills. Social skills are taught using the steps of skills training listed in Table 10.1. In addition to teaching the core steps of each social skill, using a combination of videotaped role plays and in-session practice, problem solving is also taught to help participants solve potential resource problems related to using particular skills (e.g., money, time, expertise needed to use the skill) and potential outcome problems related to using the skill (e.g., what could the person do if using the skill does not achieve its intended objective?). Social skills training topic areas that have been developed as part of the SILS program include basic conversational skills, friendship and intimacy, medication self-management, leisure for recreation, workplace fundamentals, substance abuse management, symptom self-management, and community reentry (for long-stay inpatient settings in which consumers are being prepared for discharge into the community).

An alternative approach to skills training curricula is taken by Bellack et al. (2004). These authors developed curricula to address a broad range of interpersonal situations. For each specific social skill, the following components were developed: a brief rationale for learning the skill, the specific steps of the skill, examples of role-play situations in which the skill could be practiced, and tips for leaders teaching the skill.

A total of 66 different skills were developed, organized into the following categories: basic social skills, conversational skills, assertiveness, conflict management, communal living, friendship and dating, health maintenance, vocational skills, and substance use. Using these curricula, skills training can be provided focusing on any one or a combination of topic areas.

These two approaches to packaging social skills curricula each have their own unique advantages and disadvantages. The primary advantage of the UCLA SILS program is that the curriculum and training methods are so rigorously specified that relatively little training of practitioners is required to implement the program successfully and achieve the desired outcomes (Corrigan, MacKain, & Liberman, 1994; Wallace et al., 1992). The primary disadvantages of this approach are that it requires access to audiovisual equipment, that some clinicians and some consumers do not like its highly structured format, and that skills training is limited to the specific topic areas for which modules have been developed. The primary advantage of the approach developed by Bellack and colleagues is that the skills training curricula are highly flexible and can be organized in a variety of ways (and supplemented with additional curricula if desired) to address a wide range of different needs. The primary disadvantage of this flexible approach is that skills training leaders require more training and supervision to conduct social skills groups.

In addition to the broad curricula focusing on social and independent living skills previously described, additional skills training curricula have been developed to address other specific areas of need. For example, several skills training programs have been designed to address the problem of substance abuse in people with psychiatric disabilities (Bellack, Bennet, & Gearon, 2006a; Mueser et al., 2003b; Roberts, Shaner, & Eckman, 1999). These programs typically provide skills training aimed at addressing a variety of problem areas related to substance abuse, such as skills for establishing relationships with people who do not abuse substances and skills for resisting invitations to use substances. This use of skills training is often integrated with motivational interviewing designed to help consumers identify personal goals they can achieve, in part, by developing a sober lifestyle (Bellack, Bennet, Gearon, Brown, & Yang, 2006b).

A specific application of social skills training has been in reducing the risk of being infected with or spreading infectious diseases such as sexually transmitted diseases, HIV/AIDS, and hepatitis C. People with psychiatric disabilities are at increased risk for contracting such infectious diseases (Rosenberg, Goodman, Osher, Swartz, Essock, et al., 2001a), and reducing the risk of infection is a high priority. For example, AIDS risk reduction programs involve teaching people about risk factors for acquiring or spreading the AIDS virus (e.g., unprotected sex with an infected partner) and training in steps to protect themselves and others (e.g., use of condoms, avoidance of sharing drug paraphernalia used to inject or snort substances) (Kalichman, Sikkema, Kelly, & Bulto, 1996; Susser, Valencia, Berkman, Sohler, Conover, et al., 1998).

Another example of a social skills training program designed to address health issues in people with psychiatric disabilities is the Helping Older People Experience Success (HOPES) program (Pratt, Bartels, Mueser, & Forester, in press). Older individuals with psychiatric disabilities have increased vulnerability to a wide range of medical disorders because of a combination of factors such as living a sedentary lifestyle, high rates of smoking, poor nutritional diet, and the metabolic effects of some psychotropic medications (e.g., antipsychotic medications) (Daumit, Pratt, Crum, Powe, & Ford, 2002; Felker, Yazel, & Short, 1996; Lambert, Velakoulis, & Pantelis, 2003). These problems are compounded by inadequate health care, including failure to detect diseases and inappropriate treatment (Druss et al., 2000a; Jeste, Gladsjo, Lindamer, & Lacro, 1996). As a result of medical comorbidity and poor independent living skills, older individuals with psychiatric disabilities are at high risk for institutionalization and premature mortality (Felker et al., 1996; Meeks & Murrell, 1997; Semke, Fisher, Goldman, & Hirad, 1996). To address the needs of the consumers, the HOPES program was developed, which combines training in basic interpersonal skills (e.g., conversational skills, friendship-making skills) with training in skills for medication self-management, interactions with healthcare professionals, and independent living. Training in basic interpersonal skills and independent living skills is designed to help older individuals strengthen their social supports and independence, with training in specific health-related concerns aimed at addressing health and mental health needs.

A further example of the various problem areas that social skills training can address is Corrigan and Holmes's (1994) program focusing on the problem of crime victimization in people with psychiatric disabilities. People with mental illness are more likely than those in the general population to be victims of crime such as rape and robbery (Gearon & Bellack, 1999; Goodman et al., 2001; Hiday, Swartz, Swanson, Borum, & Wagner, 1999). To address this problem, a "street smarts" skills training program was developed to educate consumers about how to avoid high-risk situations, to prevent victimization, and on social skills for extricating themselves from potentially harmful interpersonal situations.

PERSONAL EXAMPLE

Mary Hoffman Conquers Her Social Problems

Mary joined the Helping Older People Experience Success (HOPES) program (Pratt et al., in press) with the goal of making more connections with people at her job and getting closer to friends. From the start of Mary's participation, she was enthusiastic about the curriculum related to communication, leisure time, and friendships. She was able to share with group members the importance of learning and practicing these skills, and how using the skills could help her reach her goal. Mary often updated the group on ways she used the skills in her own life, and this motivated other group members to try to implement skills in their everyday lives. Despite her initial anxiety and concerns about participating in role plays, Mary valued them and with practice was able to perform many components of the skills. In role plays Mary proved to be particularly skilled at initiating conversations, but had difficulty in maintaining conversations, particularly when it came to asking people questions about themselves. She also found it hard to choose good and interesting conversation topics and spent a great deal of time practicing appropriate self-disclosure at work and at a chess club that she joined while participating in the program.

As Mary's participation in HOPES progressed, she became more comfortable sharing personal information with her friend of 10 years. She believed that their friendship had developed and that she no longer felt anxious about asking her friend to join her in a leisure activity or for support and help if she needed it. When Mary finished the HOPES program, she was meeting her friend three times a week for a morning walk followed by breakfast at their favorite restaurant. Mary also initiated activities with some of the HOPES group members, organizing a weekly visit to the community senior center for lunch and a bingo game. She was the leader in this venture, planning the time and day and helping other group members identify methods of transportation to and from the center.

Role of Skills Training in Other Rehabilitation Approaches

In addition to the many applications of social skills training described in the preceding section, skills training procedures are often incorporated into broad-based programs that include a variety of rehabilitation methods. A number of examples are briefly described here.

Social skills training has been integrated into several different models of family psychoeducation. In the behavioral family therapy model (Falloon et al., 1984; Mueser & Glynn, 1999), family members (including the consumer) are provided basic information about the consumer's psychiatric illness and the relevant treatment principles, and are then taught a core set of skills for expressing feelings and making requests. Training in problem solving follows. All the skills are taught with the use of social skills training procedures. A slightly different family program was developed by Barrowclough and Tarrier (1992), in which education is combined with teaching family members skills for managing stress and working on goals together. Yet another variation is McFarlane's (2002) multifamily group program, in which family members learn problem solving and work together to address common problems or goals.

The Illness Management and Recovery (IMR) program is a comprehensive program designed to help people learn how to manage their psychiatric illness in the context of pursuing personally meaningful "recovery" goals (Gingerich & Mueser, 2005). This program (see Chapter 5) is aimed at improving illness self-management based on the stress-vulnerability model of psychiatric illness (Liberman et al., 1986; Zubin & Spring, 1977). Thus, the primary focus is on improving medication adherence, decreasing substance abuse, improving stress management and skills for coping with persistent symptoms, and increasing social support. Social skills training is used to help people strengthen their social supports and is integrated with a other techniques (e.g., motivational interviewing, training in relaxation skills, teaching skills for coping with symptoms) to improve the individual's overall capacity for illness self-management.

Aside from the integration of social skills training with other rehabilitation methods in some programs, skills training can also be provided as an adjunctive rehabilitation approach. For example, social skills training has been provided as an adjunct to supported employment (Wallace, Tauber, & Wilde, 1999) or other vocational rehabilitation approaches (Mueser, Foy, & Carter, 1986; Tsang & Pearson, 2001) for people with psychiatric disabilities. The programs described here are only examples of how social skills training procedures are have been integrated or otherwise combined with other rehabilitation methods. There are many other examples and potential combinations.

Research on Social Skills Training

Since the development of social skills training methods and their application to people with psychiatric disabilities, skills training has been one of the most extensively studied approaches to psychiatric rehabilitation. The specific focus of research on social skills training has varied from study to study, with some investigators examining the effects of skills training on social skills, and others evaluating its broader impact on social functioning and the course of psychiatric illness. Similarly, a wide range of experimental designs have been used to study social skills training, including rigorous single-case research designs and randomized controlled trials (RCT). Consistent with the extensive research literature on social skills training, and the ever growing number of studies on it, the topic has been frequently reviewed in the scientific literature. The methods and conclusions of research reviews of social skills training are summarized in Table 10.2.

TABLE 10.2. Reviews of Research on Social Skills Training (SST) for Schizophrenia

Reviewer	Method of review	Number of studies	Focus of review	Conclusions
Donahoe & Driesenga (1988)	Narrative	39	Severe mental illness	• Consumers learn new social skills, retain them over time, and generalize them to other situations • Unclear effects on stress reduction, quality of life, symptoms, hospitalization
Benton & Schroeder (1990)	Meta-analysis	27	Schizophrenia 1972–1988	• Consumers learn, maintain, and generalize new skills • SST improves assertiveness, hospital discharge, relapse rate • Marginal benefits of SST for symptoms and functioning
Halford & Hayes (1991)	Narrative	5	RCTs of schizophrenia 1983–1986	• Consumers can learn and maintain skills • Unclear generalization of skills and impact on community functioning
Corrigan (1990)	Meta-analysis	73	Adults with psychiatric disorders 1970–1988	• Consumers can learn and maintain skills • SST reduces symptoms • SST effects stronger in outpatient than inpatient settings
Bellack & Mueser (1993)	Narrative	6	RCTs of schizophrenia 1983–1992	• SST improves skills and social functioning • SST has no impact on symptoms or relapses
Dilk & Bond (1996)	Meta-analysis	68	Severe mental illness 1970–1992	• SST has moderate effects on skill acquisition, reduced symptoms, improved personal adjustment • Limited research on effects of SST on role functioning
Penn & Mueser (1996)	Narrative	6	RCTs of schizophrenia 1984–1995	• Consumers can learn and maintain new skills • SST has less prominent effects on social functioning and symptoms • Longer duration of SST more effective

Study	Type	N	Focus	Findings
Smith, Bellack, & Liberman (1996)	Narrative	9	RCTs of schizophrenia 1983–1995	• Consumers learn and retain new social skills • Some evidence that skills generalize to improved social functioning
Wallace (1998)	Narrative	6	Recent RCTs of schizophrenia	• Specific and highly structured SST improves social functioning and quality of life
Heinssen, Liberman, & Kopelowicz (2000)	Narrative	27	Schizophrenia 1994–1999	• Consumers learn, retain, and generalize new social skills
Huxley, Rendall, & Sederer (2000)	Narrative	13	Schizophrenia 1994–1999	• Traditional SST improves social skills but has limited effects on functioning • SST based on UCLA SILS program leads to generalization of skills and improved social functioning
Bustillo, Lauriello, Horan, & Keith (2001)	Narrative	6	RCTs of schizophrenia 1983–1998	• SST improves social competence, which may translate into more adaptive functioning
Pilling et al. (2002a)	Meta-analysis	9	RCTs of schizophrenia 1980–1999	• No effects of SST on relapse, treatment adherence, global adjustment (two studies), social functioning (one study), quality of life (one study)
Bellack (2004)	Narrative	5	RCTs of schizophrenia 1986–2001	• SST improves social skills and social role functioning • SST appears to improve satisfaction and self-efficacy • No effects of SST on symptoms or relapses

Note. RCT, randomized controlled trial; SILS, Social and Independent Living Skills; SST, social skills training.

An inspection of the summary of research reviews discovers generally favorable findings supporting social skills training for 13 of the 14 reviews. The most negative review was a meta-analysis (Pilling, Bebbington, Kuipers, Garrety, Geddes, et al., 2002a), which has been criticized on several methodological grounds, such as overrestrictive inclusion criteria and not controlling for quality of study (Bellack, 2004; Mueser & Penn, 2004).

The research on social skills training can be summarized with three general findings. First, people with psychiatric disabilities are capable of learning new social skills and maintaining them over time. Second, social skills that are learned in one setting show some, but limited generalization to other settings. Third, skills training tends to improve the quality of social and leisure functioning, but does not have a consistent impact on symptom severity, relapses, or rehospitalizations.

The actual magnitude of the effect of skills training on social functioning is a topic of much debate, with most reviews concluding there is some impact but not a large one. The relatively modest effect of skills training on social functioning has led some critics to dismiss the approach (Pilling et al., 2002a). Alternatively, it has been argued that the effect of skills training on social functioning is greater than the effect of any other rehabilitation approach, and its modest effect may be partly due to the inherent challenges of improving functioning in the complex and multidetermined domain of social relationships and community adaptation (Mueser & Penn, 2004). Clearly, there is a need for more research on social skills training aimed at both understanding and improving its impact on social functioning.

Research has also evaluated predictors of response to social skills training. The most important finding has been that the degree of cognitive impairment predicts improvement from skills training. Specifically, poor memory has been found to consistently predict slower acquisition (Bowen, Wallace, Glynn, Nuechterlein, Lutzker, et al., 1994; Kern, Green, & Satz, 1992; Mueser et al., 1991b; Silverstein, Schenkel, Valone, & Nuernberger, 1998; Smith, Hull, Romanelli, Fertuck, & Weiss, 1999). Additional efforts may be needed to improve the ability of people with cognitive impairment to benefit from skills training, such as more intensive or longer training, or combining skills training with cognitive rehabilitation (Brenner, Roder, Hodel, Kienzle, Reed, et al., 1994).

In addition to studying the effects of social skills training on social functioning, research has also evaluated its effects on other areas of functioning. For example, two studies have shown that social skills training is more effective than other interventions for treating substance abuse in people with psychiatric disabilities (Bellack et al., 2006b; Jerrell & Ridgely, 1995). Two other studies have also evaluated the providing of supplementary skills training as to whether it improves the outcome of consumers in supported employment programs (Mueser, Aalto, Becker, Ogden, Wolfe, et al., 2005a; Wallace & Tauber, 2004), with mixed results.

OTHER REHABILITATION APPROACHES

Because of the centrality of impaired social functioning to psychiatric disabilities, quality of social functioning is often evaluated in studies of different psychiatric rehabilitation programs. In this section, we provide a brief summary of what is known about the impact of rehabilitation approaches (other than social skills training) on social functioning, including family psychoeducation, assertive community treatment, supported employment, and psychosocial clubhouses/peer support programs.

Family Psychoeducation

Family psychoeducation programs are broadly aimed at educating families about the nature of psychiatric disabilities and the principles of their treatment. As a result of improved understanding about psychiatric illness and closer collaboration with the treatment team, these programs have repeatedly been shown to reduce relapses and rehospitalizations (Pitschel-Walz, Leucht, Bäuml, Kissling, & Engel, 2001). Relapses and rehospitalizations can have a demoralizing effect on people with psychiatric disabilities and interfere with the quality of their social relationships (Glynn, 1998). Therefore, it might be expected that family psychoeducation programs improve consumers' social functioning if for no other reason than through reducing relapses and rehospitalizations. Furthermore, many family psychoeducation programs also work toward helping consumers improve their social functioning (Anderson, Reiss, & Hogarty, 1986; Mueser & Glynn, 1999).

Research on family psychoeducation provides some support for its effects on social functioning. Several studies have shown that compared to usual services, consumers who participate in family psychoeducation programs show significant improvements in social functioning (Barrowclough & Tarrier, 1990; Brooker et al., 1994; Clarkin, Carpenter, Hull, Wilner, & Glick, 1998; Falloon, McGill, Boyd, & Pederson, 1987; Zhang, He, Gittelman, Wong, & Yan, 1998) and negative symptoms (Dyck et al., 2000). However, these improvements tend to be small (Barrowclough & Tarrier, 1998). One study that compared more intensive family intervention (including monthly multiple family support groups and home-based behavioral family therapy) with less intensive intervention (family support groups alone) found consumers in both groups improved in social functioning, but there was no difference between the groups (Mueser et al., 2001). Overall, the findings suggest that family psychoeducation may improve social functioning, chiefly by reducing risk of relapse and rehospitalization.

Assertive Community Treatment

Assertive community treatment (ACT) programs are designed to deliver rehabilitation and treatment in people's natural living environment to consumers who tend not to access clinic-based community mental health services, and consequently are prone to frequent hospitalizations and severe psychosocial impairment (Stein & Santos, 1998). As described in Chapter 7, ACT programs themselves are not a form of rehabilitation, but rather a different organizational structure for delivering services in the community that does not rely on consumer motivation. From its inception in the 1970s, ACT was aimed at helping consumers get the broad range of their needs met, including both psychiatric treatment (e.g., medication), housing and daily living needs, and social needs. For these reasons, and because of early positive reports on the effects of ACT on social functioning (Stein & Test, 1980a), there has traditionally been an expectation among treatment providers that ACT improves social functioning.

With over 30 controlled studies evaluating the effects of ACT, there is now ample data on its effects on a number of major domains, including hospitalizations, symptom severity, housing stability, and social functioning. Overall, the results indicate that ACT does not have a consistent effect on social functioning, with only three of 13 studies that examined social functioning reporting significant effects (Bond, Drake, Mueser, & Latimer, 2001a). The primary effect of ACT is on reducing rehospitalizations and improving stable housing in the community. It should be noted that research on ACT has typically studied ACT teams that were not systematically providing consumers with social skills training, and concerted training may be required and have a significant impact on social functioning (Mueser, Bond, Drake, & Resnick, 1998).

Supported Employment

For many people, the workplace environment provides natural opportunities for meeting, socializing, and making friends. Furthermore, the fact that people with psychiatric disabilities often are capable of working in competitive jobs and enjoying the benefits of working, such as a sense of purpose, more economic resources, and improved self-esteem, have lead some to assert the old adage that "work is therapy" (Harding, Strauss, Hafez, & Liberman, 1987). Furthermore, most cross-sectional studies report a modest relationship between social and vocational functioning (Bond, Drake, & Becker, 1998). For these reasons, one might expect that supported employment programs, which are effective at helping consumers get competitive jobs (Bond, 2004), would also have an impact on social functioning.

Only limited research on supported employment has addressed this question. Bond and colleagues (2001b) found that obtaining a competitive job was associated with increased satisfaction with leisure time, but satisfaction with social relationships was not reported. Evaluation studies of supported employment have generally failed to detect any positive effects on either social functioning or satisfaction with social relationships (Drake et al., 1999; Drake, McHugo, Becker, Anthony, & Clark, 1996; Fabian, 1992; Mueser et al., 2004a). These findings are consistent with the general observation that the impact of psychiatric rehabilitation programs tends to be on the specific domains that are the focus of intervention, with relatively little crossover effects to other domains of functioning (Bustillo, Lauriello, Horan, & Keith, 2001; Mueser et al., 1997c).

Psychosocial Clubhouses/Peer Support Programs

Psychosocial clubhouses and peer support programs offer a different approach to helping consumers get their social needs met. Rather than focusing on teaching specific social skills thought to be critical for effective social interactions, these programs offer consumers an accepting social milieu based on the shared understanding that all members have a psychiatric disability, which can reduce anxiety and enable consumers to feel more comfortable simply by being who they are.

There is great intuitive appeal for the notion that psychosocial clubhouses or peer support programs improve the quality of consumers' social functioning. However, only limited research has addressed this question, in part because of the difficulties inherent to evaluating the effects of these types of programs. Peer support programs are especially difficult to study experimentally because participation in peer support is usually due to personal choice, so it is difficult to randomly assign an individual to these programs. Surveys of clubhouses indicate that consumers value group membership and recreational activities (Bond et al., 1995), although participation in a clubhouse does not appear to improve social functioning (Dincin & Witheridge, 1982). One large retrospective study reported that participation in a peer support program over the previous four months was related to four out of five indices on the Recovery Assessment Scale (RAS) (Corrigan, Salzer, Ralph, Sangster, & Kech, 2004), including willingness to ask for help and reliance on others. The relationship between these dimensions of the RAS and social functioning are not clear, but they suggest that participation in peer support is associated with a stronger social orientation. These associations could reflect the characteristics of consumers who are most likely to participate in peer support, rather than the effects of such participation.

One controlled study of a psychosocial rehabilitation program found that consumers assigned to that program, compared to two other vocational rehabilitation programs, reported significantly greater increases in satisfaction with their social relationships (Mueser et al., 2004a). However, other differences in social functioning were not evident, such as number of friends and depth of interpersonal relationships. Further research is needed to evaluate the impact of peer support and psychosocial clubhouses on the quality of social relationships.

SUMMARY AND CONCLUSIONS

Problems in social functioning are a fundamental part of psychiatric disabilities; they span a broad range of domains of interpersonal adjustment, including the quality of personal relationships, use of leisure time, role functioning, and self-care and independent living skills. Although common psychiatric symptoms such as depression, anxiety, anger, and mania interfere with social adjustment across a great number of psychiatric disorders, the quality of social functioning tends to be most impaired in individuals with schizophrenia spectrum disorders, for whom a "disorder in relating" has long been viewed as a core aspect of such illness (Strauss, Carpenter, & Bartko, 1974). Common difficulties in the interpersonal domain include having few friends, lack of reciprocity and intimacy in close relationships, dependence on others for meeting one's basic living needs, conflict with others, and problems in meeting social role expectations, such as being a parent, homemaker, student, or worker.

Social impairments in people with psychiatric disabilities are determined by a host of different factors, including decreased social drive, cognitive impairment, poor social skills, and symptoms. For people with schizophrenia spectrum disorders, problems in social functioning often precede the onset of the disorder by many years and are a long-standing life challenge. Difficulties in social relationships are only made worse by the social stigma associated with mental illness, leading to fear and avoidance of people with psychiatric disabilities and self-stigma for those with such disabilities. As a result of the pervasiveness of social impairments in people with psychiatric disabilities, and their multidetermined nature, these problems are among the most challenging of all aspects of mental illness, and in the absence of rehabilitation are relatively stable over the long term.

Efforts to improve social functioning have been at the forefront of the psychiatric rehabilitation field since its inception. Broadly speaking, three different approaches are frequently used to help individuals improve their social functioning. First, based on the assumption that symptoms and relapses can interfere with social functioning, improved management of the psychiatric illness is often employed as an indirect means of improving social functioning. Second, social skills training is often employed to teach more effective social behaviors by breaking down complex skills into their component steps and using the principles of social learning theory to teach these steps. Third, environmental approaches may be used that focus on either creating a more accepting and rewarding social milieu for the consumer (such as family psychoeducation) or involving consumers in a social milieu specifically intended to provide interpersonal contact in a rewarding and accepting environment, such as a psychosocial clubhouse.

Among these three approaches, research evidence indicates that improved illness management (i.e., reduced relapses and rehospitalizations) has a small benefit in improving social functioning. However, considering that many social difficulties predate the onset of the psychiatric illness, and many other social problems are not related to symptoms, simply providing effective treatment for psychiatric disorders is usually insufficient to have a major impact on social functioning. Research on social skills training indicates that it improves social functioning, including quality of social relationships and use of leisure time, although the research is not entirely consistent and gains are often quite modest. Finally, research on psychosocial clubhouses and peer support programs indicate that although consumers who participate in these programs enjoy their relationships in those settings, there is no evidence that participation in such programs actually improves social functioning. This limitation may be due to the fact that those individuals who experience the greatest difficulties in their social functioning are also least likely to participate in such programs.

Despite many years of research in psychiatric rehabilitation, problems in social functioning remain among the most stubborn challenges of mental illness. Although improving social functioning in consumers with psychiatric disabilities may seem a daunting challenge, substantial progress has been made in developing and validating social skills training methods to help them improve the quality of their social relationships. Social skills training is hard work, and it requires extensive practice combined with ample encouragement and support from both the mental health practitioner and other social supports. However, the payoffs for this hard work can be immense and provide a major boost to an individual's quality of life. Considering the evidence supporting the effects of skills training on social functioning, and the relative lack of evidence supporting other approaches, access to social skills training, including rigorously standardized programs, should be a priority for all people with psychiatric disabilities.

Although the research supporting social skills training for improving social functioning is stronger than for any other rehabilitation approach, much work remains to be done to improve its effectiveness. For example, skills training is usually offered in groups, but many consumers have difficulty in accessing such groups (e.g., in rural areas), or refuse to attend clinic-based groups. Guidelines for individualizing skills training procedures and providing training in consumers' natural environments are needed. There is also a need for more research on strategies for compensating or overcoming the rate-limiting effects of cognitive impairment on learning these skills (Smith et al., 1999b). Potential strategies include more intensive skills training, increased involvement of natural supports to help consumers use skills in their daily social interactions, and the incorporation of cognitive rehabilitation methods into skills training.

Because social functioning can be conceptualized as the "fit" between an individual and his or her social environment, efforts to improve that fit can either focus on the person, the environment, or both. Skills training primarily focuses on improving the social competence of the individual, while recognizing that some modicum of support is also necessary in the environment. A different approach that holds promise for the future is to address the environment to improve the fit with the consumer. Family psychoeducation is one approach to developing a more supportive social milieu in the family for the person with a psychiatric disability, and research indicates that certain programs are effective at achieving this (see Chapter 11). However, systematic efforts to create more supportive social milieus outside the family, such as in residential settings or long-stay hospitals, are lacking. Although such approaches may be worth pursuing for some settings, they do not appear to be feasible for consumers who are socially isolated, but are living in the community.

An alternative to modifying the environment is to help consumers find natural social opportunities in which they can have their needs met with a minimum of interference from their psychiatric disability. Research on supported employment has shown that with help, people with psychiatric disabilities can find competitive jobs in the community without requiring major efforts to train either their vocational or social skills (see Chapter 9). Just as there may be specific jobs in the community that are employment "niches" providing a good fit between an individual's vocational interests and skills and the requirements of a job, there may also be similar social niches (Rapp, 1998b). For example, at Thresholds in Chicago, a large innovative psychiatric rehabilitation program, some individuals with psychiatric disabilities have been helped to find such niches in local theater groups that provide opportunities for social contact with others in a social group that is more accepting of personal idiosyncrasies, including those related to having a mental illness, than other social groups. Social niches may be challenging to find for some individuals with psychiatric disabilities, but an advantage to locating such a niche could be the greater speed at which a person is able to have his or her social needs met.

Social functioning is a complex and critical aspect of the quality of a person's life. As each person's specific needs and desires differ, and the specific factors that contribute to impaired social functioning vary, rehabilitation of social functioning must be individually tailored. Fortunately, rehabilitation tools continue to be developed and refined. This rich technology for psychiatric rehabilitation that is currently available provides a solid basis for skilled and knowledgeable practitioners to help consumers achieve their social goals and improve their social functioning.

Chapter 11

Family Interventions

Societal beliefs about psychiatric illnesses are a determining factor in how families of persons with these disorders are treated. These cultural beliefs affect families in regard to whether they are provided with a diagnosis, informed of the course and treatment of a disorder; whether they are included in the treatment process, or whether they are offered assistance in coping with the disorder (Solomon, 1998b). At the height of the era of asylum treatment, families were considered passive contributors to the cause of such disorders by not having protected their relatives from the stresses of societal changes that were happening at the time, which were then believed to be the principal causal agent of mental illness (Terkelsen, 1990). Separation from the family was therefore considered to be a means of protecting the patient from the stress resulting from community pressures (Terkelsen, 1990).

Subsequently, families, most specifically parents, were viewed by mental health practitioners as the primary causal agents of their relatives' mental illness. Based on psychodynamic and family interactional theories of etiology, separation of the relative with a psychiatric disability from the family continued, as separation was thought to be the essential means to resolve parental pathogenesis (Lefley, 1996). Consequently, family members were not only ignored and uninformed regarding their relative's illness and treatment, but also blamed for having caused the disorder. Despite the popularity of these psychodynamic causal explanations of mental illness, these theories lost credibility owing to a lack of supporting evidence. Family therapies based on systemic dysfunction did not demonstrate the clinical efficacy that was hypothesized (Hatfield, 1997; Mueser & Glynn, 1999).

With accumulating scientific evidence of the neurobiological basis of psychiatric disorders, a combination of biological and environmental factors has emerged as an explanation for the onset and course of the illness (Mueser & Glynn, 1999). Family dysfunction is now seen as a possible consequence, rather than a cause, of the illness (Lefley, 1996). These new theories resulted in a paradigmatic shift by psychiatric practitioners away from blaming and pathologizing the family to an increasing recognition and acceptance that a family is an invaluable resource to both the relative with a psychiatric disability and the professional (Hatfield, 1994a). This new attitude precipitated a need to understand the family's experience of coping with a relative with a severe psychiatric disability. Eventually, research findings of the family environment prompted the development of interventions to assist the family in managing the ill relative's behavioral manifestations of the illness and to improve outcomes for the person with the psychiatric disability.

This chapter presents information on the family's experience of having a relative with a psychiatric disability and how this led to the development of a diversity of interventions to address the family's needs. The provision of services to families within routine care is assessed, along with the barriers to offering such services. Subsequently, each of the family interventions is described, as well as the research evidence related to their effectiveness. The final section presents issues and interventions related to persons with psychiatric disabilities as parents.

THE FAMILY EXPERIENCE OF MENTAL ILLNESS

Having a relative with a psychiatric disability affects all members of the person's immediate family, whether the family member is the primary caregiver or not. Although reactions differ by individuals, as well as by their role relationships to their relative with a psychiatric disability, the effects of the illness are felt by parents, spouses, siblings, and children—all experience the illness as life changing (Tessler & Gamache, 2000).

As the primary locus of care has shifted from hospitals to community, there has been increasing awareness of the importance of families in assuming the responsibility of caring for persons with psychiatric disabilities. At least three-quarters of persons with psychiatric disabilities have some type of ongoing contact with their families (Lehman et al., 1998b; Mandersheid & Sonnenschein, 1997). Thirty to 65% of persons with a psychiatric disability are estimated to live with their families (Beeler, Rosenthal, & Cohler, 1999; Goldman, 1982; Guarnaccia, 1998). Regardless of whether families reside with a relative with a psychiatric disability, they often provide support and assistance to this relative (Baronet, 1999; Carpentier, Lesage, Goulet, Lalonde, & Renaird, 1992). Families are often put in the position of assuming the role of caregiver, for which they are neither trained nor psychologically prepared (Doornbos, 2001; Lefley, 1996; Hatfield, 1987b). Families need not only to learn to cope with the vicissitudes of the illness, but also need to deal with the vagaries of the various service delivery systems, from the mental health, social welfare, social security, to, in some instances, the criminal justice system.

For the most part, parents and spouses rather than other family members, such as siblings or children, provide care for a relative with a psychiatric disability. Therefore, most of the research related to the experience of caregiving has focused on parents and spouses. Nevertheless, a few studies have assessed the role of siblings in the provision of care, coping with, and the reactions of siblings toward, their ill brother or sister (Gerace, Camilleri, & Ayres, 1993; Horwitz, Tessler, Fisher, & Gamache, 1992; Horwitz, 1993; Johnson, 2000; Kinsella, Anderson, & Anderson, 1996). Because care is usually provided on the basis of a hierarchy of family obligations, siblings may assume care for an ill sibling as parents age and become too frail or die (Lefley, 1987). Because persons with psychiatric disabilities are an aging cohort, siblings are likely to be put in the position of taking on more responsibility for the care of their ill sibling. Horwitz and colleagues (1992) found that the quality of the relationship between the siblings was a predictor of whether a well sibling would assist an ill one. Three distinct patterns of care by siblings have been determined: collaborative with the primary care providers; assistance in crisis situations, and detachment; and constructive or unhealthy escape from the brother or sister with a psychiatric disability in order to protect their own psychological stability (Gerace et al., 1993; Kinsella et al., 1996). A recent focus group study assessed the complex feelings of siblings of a brother or sister with a psychiatric disability and how the illness impacted their own sense of self and their relationship to their family of origin, partners, and friends. These siblings described "a sense of chaos and personal vulnerability that they associated with the constant presence of mental illness in the family" and their feelings about their families' increasing exhaustion and isolation as the illness progressed (Lukens, Thorning, & Lohrer, 2004, p. 497).

Family Burden

Because coping with a relative with a psychiatric disability impacts the full range of family life—home environment, work, leisure, income, and relationships with those inside and outside the nuclear family—the illness places an enormous burden on a family. There has been extensive research on family burden, dating back to 1950s with the classic study of spouses by Clausen and Yarrow (1955). In the 1960s the term *burden* was first used in this context by Hoenig and Hamilton (1966), who conceptualized it as having two components, objective burden and subjective burden. Objective burden is defined as the directly observable concrete costs that result from having a member with a psychiatric illness, including the financial costs of care as well as the daily disruptions imposed on the family due to the psychiatric illness. Subjective burden is a family member's personal discomfort or emotional strain that is experienced as a direct consequence of the illness. Although, conceptually, a number of researchers note the distinction between objective and subjective burden, their scales usually measure only burden, which mostly relates to subjective burden. The distinction of these concepts from general distress is that burdens are associated with problems specifically emanating from the psychiatric illness, whereas distress relates to poor mental health, psychological morbidity, or life strain not attributed to the relative's illness. Research has found that having a high degree of burden leads to high stress and poor physical and mental health (Maurin & Boyd, 1990; Rose, 1996).

Baronet (1999) conducted a review of 28 studies on caregiver burden in regard to mental illness. Respondents for most of the studies were female, of middle age, white, high school educated, and of lower middle income. More than half were parents, about a quarter were spouses, and a few were siblings and other relatives. The relative with the psychiatric disability typically had a schizophrenia spectrum disorder or an affective disorder. Not surprising, more objective burden was related to tasks of caregiving, whereas subjective burden was associated with disruptive behavior on the part of the person with mental illness. The objective burdensome activities included the provision of transportation, assistance with money management, housework and cooking, continuous supervision, limitations of caregivers' personal activities, and provision of financial assistance. The primary subjective burden concerns were related to safety and potential violence of the relative toward him- or herself or others, "excessive demands and high dependency toward the caregiver, night disturbances, embarrassing behaviors, symptomatic behaviors, worries about the future, and uncooperative attitude leading to conflicts and family hardships" (Baronet, 1999, p. 822).

Fifteen of the 28 studies assessed a diversity of variables related to burden. With regard to sociodemographic characteristics, the caregiver's being younger, being white (Horowitz & Reinhard, 1995; Pickett, Vraniak, Cook, & Cohler, 1993; Stueve, Vine, & Struening, 1997), and living with the ill relative (Jones, Roth, & Jones, 1995; Pickett, Greenley, & Greenberg, 1995) were related to higher burden. Younger age of the caregiver was specifically associated with stigma, fears regarding safety, and higher levels of overall burden (Greenberg, Kim, & Greenley, 1997; Pickett et al., 1995; Horwitz & Reinhard, 1995; Stueve et al., 1997). Burden was not associated with the gender, education, or family income of either the caregiver or the relative with a psychiatric disability, nor with the caregiver's relationship to the relative with mental illness (Baronet, 1999), although the issues of burden differed by the relationship (Jungbauer, Wittmund, Dietrich, & Angermeyer, 2004; Lukens et al., 2004).

The presence of symptomatic behavior had the strongest and most consistent relationship with high level of burden, but diagnosis was not related to burden (Baronet, 1999). However, when coping self-efficacy was assessed as a mediator, symptomatic behavior had less explanatory power (Solomon & Draine, 1995f) (see Figure 11.1). Webb and colleagues (Webb, Pfeiffer, Mueser, Gladis, Mensch, et al., 1998) found that coping styles for dealing with different symptom problems were correlated with perceptions of caregiver burden. Similarly, accommodating coping, or adjusting to realistic goals when faced with uncontrollable events, is associated with positive well-being among midlife parents of children with psychiatric disabilities (Seltzer, Greenberg, Floyd, & Hong, 2004). These findings demonstrate that the strength of their internal psychological resources helps families with managing the situation of having an ill relative (Solomon & Draine, 1995f).

Negative symptoms are more problematic for families than positive ones (Fadden, Bebbington, & Kuipers, 1987; Hooley, Richters, Weintraub, & Neal, 1987; Oldridge & Hughes, 1992), owing to their stable, ongoing nature and to misinterpretation as signs of character flaws of the relative with a psychiatric disability, as opposed to symptoms of the disorder (Mueser & Glynn, 1999). This explanation is consistent with research by Greenberg and colleagues (1997) who found that control attribution, or the belief that the behavior of the relative with a psychiatric disability was within that person's own control, was associated with greater family burden.

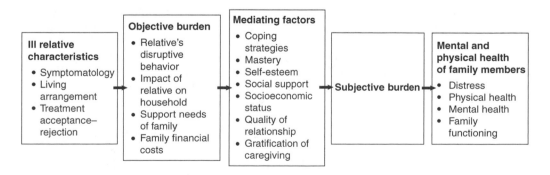

FIGURE 11.1. Family consequences of subjective and objective family burden.

Baronet's review concluded that external resources like social support produced mixed results, but there were varying means to operationalize the concept of social support for the family. It may also be that social support has an indirect relationship to burden affecting the well-being of family members (Webb et al., 1998). A recent study by Magliano, Fiorillo, Malangone, Marasco, Guarneri, et al. (2003) did find that a more supportive social network was associated with lower burden. Further, it is important to note that the perception of the sufficiency of professional support and the receipt of practical advice from providers were related to decreased objective burden (Biegel, Milligan, Putnam, & Song, 1994; Reinhard, 1994). Similarly, recent research on outpatient commitment found that those families whose relative was receiving sustained mandatory treatment had decreased subjective burden, as compared with those whose relative had either brief or no mandatory treatment (Groff, Burns, Swanson, Swartz, Wagner, et al., 2004). Again, this indicates the importance of formal support to reducing the stress of families.

Recent research by Jungbauer and Angermeyer (2002) found that burden varied by the phases of the disorder, specifically assessing individuals with schizophrenia. The onset of schizophrenia is a time of high stress, owing to the shock and feeling of helplessness. At this point families frequently do not connect the psychotic experiences to mental illness and attempt to put forth other explanations. As new episodes occur, the burden again intensifies, but is usually not as great as in the initial episode. At other times, family members experience chronic everyday burdens of coping with their relative.

Given the nature of schizophrenia, families also experience a sense of loss or "chronic sorrow" for who and what the relative was before the illness and for the loss of potential of what the relative could have been (Atkinson, 1994; Davis & Schultz, 1998; MacGregor, 1994; Miller, Dworkin, Ward, & Barone, 1990). Unlike the grief at the death of a relative, this can be an ongoing grieving process, as family members are continually confronted with their loss. The degree of burden has been found to be correlated with such grief (Solomon & Draine, 1996).

PERSONAL EXAMPLE

A Family Consultant Helps the Madison Family

Mary Jane Madison, a widowed mother in her late 60s, was very concerned about her son, Bill, who had paranoid schizophrenia and abused alcohol but refused treatment. He was hospitalized on a number of occasions and was in prison as a result of an assault against his mother. The mother was afraid to have him live with her. For a time he was receiving Supplemental Security Income and living in an apartment, where he worked for the landlord. The mother sought family consultation to get help with her son. She was worried that the landlord was taking advantage of her son and that Bill's abuse of alcohol and noncompliance with treatment would result in his getting into further trouble.

The family consultant worked with the mother to educate her about schizophrenia and about available treatment resources. Armed with this information, the mother realized that her son was entitled to have a case manager. Therefore, she pushed to get a case manager for Bill. Subsequently, the case manager arranged for a more structured living arrangement, medication, and a representative payee, so Bill wouldn't spend his money on alcohol. He successfully remained out of the hospital for the next 4 years.

For the most part, family burden has been assessed for family caregivers, usually mothers and spouses, whereas burden can be independent of caregiving. However, most of the research on the burden of spouses has been focused on individuals with depression and dementia, rather than schizophrenia, with the exception of a recent study (Jungbauer et al., 2004). Family members who are not involved in the care of the relative still experience burden, and there is some evidence that their burden does not significantly vary from that of the primary caregiver (Baronet, 1999; Magliano et al., 1999). For siblings, there is also the anticipated burden of their responsibility when their parents are gone (Lukens et al., 2004).

Positive Aspects of Caregiving

Some families find the term *family burden* offensive, for it portrays caregiving as a totally negative experience, rather than reflecting the positive aspects of the family and of caregiving. Therefore, a more neutral term has been proposed, caregiving consequences (Van Wijngaarden, Schene, Koeter, Becker, Knapp, et al., 2003). Szmukler and his colleagues (Szmukler, 1996; Szmukler, Burgess, Herman, Benson, Colusa, et al., 1996) have suggested assessing the experience of caregiving more globally, including positive and negative experiences, and have developed the Experience of Caregiving Inventory to do just this. There has been limited research on what is called the gratification of caregiving, or the positive aspects or consequences of caregiving. Bulger, Wanderman, and Goldman (1993) found that of the 60 parents of adults with schizophrenia whom they interviewed, all had a relatively high score on gratification, and no interviewee reported a total absence of gratification. These participants experienced gratification more frequently than burden. The quality of the relationship was likely the reason for the low level of burden. Similarly, Pickett, Cook, Cohler, and Solomon (1997) found that family caregivers with lower levels of burden rated their relationship with the child with a psychiatric disability more positively. Greenberg (1995) determined that the ill person's contributions to household tasks and companionship resulted in lower levels of caregiving burden and greater caregiver gains, such as personal strengths, new insights, and greater intimacy with others.

Even with the adversity of the experience of having a relative with mental illness, families are quite resilient. Mental illness may result in increased family bonds and commitment of family members to each other, and, over time, growth and development of the family as a unit and of its members as individuals. They learn coping skills and ways to adapt to the illness. Through education about the illness and learning about the available community resources, a family can come to terms with the illness and adapt to the stressors (Marsh, Lefley, Evans-Rhodes, Ansell, Doerzbacher, et al., 1996; Mannion, 1996).

Expressed Emotion

Although families are no longer considered the causal agents of psychiatric illness, there is concern that certain family environmental factors exacerbate a psychiatric illness and hasten the return of the ill person to the hospital. This relationship was serendipitously discovered in Britain when researchers assessed the impact of community care of discharged psychiatric patients. In a retrospective study, Brown, Carstairs, and Topping (1958) found that patients who were released to live with siblings or in community lodges fared better in terms of avoiding rehospitalization than those released to the homes of parents or spouses. Subsequently, a prospective study was undertaken to assess the impact of the family environment on patient relapse (Brown, Monck, Carstairs & Wing, 1962). Whether these researchers employed psychiatric deterioration or hospitalization as an outcome indicator, they found that those who returned to close family relationships that were high in negative family affect were more likely to deteriorate and return to the hospital. Subsequently, a number of studies have replicated this empirical relationship (Butzlaff & Hooley, 1998; Kreisman & Blumenthal, 1995)

This family affect was termed *expressed emotion* (EE), which is operationally defined as criticism, hostility, and emotional overinvolvement of families, according to their expressed responses to a semistructured interview about the events and activities in the home and their attitudes and feelings toward their ill relative (Brown & Rutter, 1966). The Camberwell Family Interview (CFI) was developed to assess family EE. The responses are taperecorded and then analyzed by a highly trained rater for both voice intonations and content to determine whether families are high or low in EE. The assumption of the CFI is that the responses to this measure are indicative of the negative or intrusive interactional behaviors of family members that occur on a daily basis in the home environment, and therefore the CFI is a means to measure the family environmental climate. Furthermore, research has shown that negatively charged statements tend to produce negative responses by the relative with a psychiatric disability, resulting in negative interactions (Hahlweg, Goldstein, Nuechterlein, Magna, Mintz, et al., 1989). However, the direction of the causal relationship of EE to relapse is unknown. It is unclear whether EE is a response of families to their relative's behavior or whether it is the negative affect of family members that produces environmental stress, precipitating relapse. Although the evidence seems to support the latter, but not the former explanation, there is yet a third possibility. This possibility combines the two explanations by characterizing the family member(s) and relative with a psychiatric disability as parts of an interactive process, with both parties being integral to generating EE (Strachan, Leff, Goldstein, & Doane, 1986). This hypothesis requires empirical examination.

Estroff and her colleagues (Estroff, Zimmer, Lachecotte, & Benoit, 1994), on the basis of their research, hypothesized that there may be a relationship between high EE and patient violence within these families, as violence is frequently a factor in the decision to admit a person to a psychiatric hospital. Many families of persons with psychiatric disabilities are confronted with threats, intimidation, and physical assaults and fear for their own safety. Estimates are that 10–40% of families experience some violence from an ill relative (Solomon, Cavanaugh, & Gelles, 2005). Some families find that they are put in the position of taking out a restraining order against a relative with a psychiatric disability in order to protect themselves (Solomon, Draine, & Delaney, 1995a).

A few studies have found a relationship between EE and family members' beliefs about mental illness, and these beliefs may play a role in the relapse of their relative (Barrowclough & Hooley, 2003; Wearden, Tarrier, Barrowclough, Zastowny, & Rahill, 2000). Families who are hostile and critical or have high EE are more likely to attribute the symptoms of the illness as residing within the personal control of the relative with a psychiatric disability, than those with low EE (Brewin, MacCarthy, Duda, & Vaugh, 1991; Barrowclough, Johnston, & Tarrier, 1994; Weisman, Lopez, Karno, & Jenkins, 1993; Weisman, Nuechterlein, Goldstein, & Snyder, 1998). Overinvolved families, however, hold beliefs similar to those of low EE families and attribute behaviors of the ill relative to symptoms of the disorder (Brewin et al., 1991).

Recently, Buzlaff and Hooley (1998) conducted a meta-analysis of the relationship of EE and psychiatric relapse. These reviewers confirmed that EE is "a significant and robust predictor of relapse in schizophrenia" (p. 547), but found that the relationship was strongest for those with the most long-standing illnesses. They further concluded that

EE is a stronger predictor of relapse for affective and eating disorders than for schizophrenia spectrum disorders. Similarly, a narrative review of a diversity of psychiatric disorders, including depression, posttraumatic stress, personality disorders, and alcoholism, confirmed the robustness of the empirical relationship of EE and outcomes of these disorders (Wearden et al., 2000). There is evidence that EE, or aspects of it, is a state rather than a trait and can change over time (Boye, Bentsen, Notland Munkvold, Lersbruggen, et al., 1999; Schreiber, Breier, & Pickar, 1995). Unstable EE patterns have been found to be associated with higher levels of perceived burden (Boye et al., 1999).

Although these EE studies have been the precipitant for the development of family interventions, the EE construct has engendered criticism by families and professionals alike (Solomon, 1996). High and low EE has come to connote good and bad families, respectively, which may be directly or indirectly communicated to families by practitioners. This then leads to once again blaming families and causing them to feel guilty, now for affecting the course of the illness rather than causing the onset of the disorder (Bernheim & Lehman, 1985; Platman, 1983). In the past some psychiatric rehabilitation programs discouraged contact with families on the assumption that overinvolved family members can undermine rehabilitation of their relative with a psychiatric disability (Beard et al., 1982; Dincin, Selleck, & Streicker, 1978). Similarly, in the early years of the Program for Assertive Community Treatment (PACT), persons with psychiatric disabilities were thought to need "constructive separation" from their families in order not to create pathological dependence (Stein & Test, 1980b). Furthermore, EE has been criticized for blinding practitioners to the potential support and assistance that families provide to a relative with a psychiatric disability. In addition, when families believe that the negative attributes of EE apply to them, they become more alienated from the mental health treatment system, which can have negative consequences for the relative with a psychiatric disability (Hatfield, Spaniol, & Zipple, 1987).

FAMILIES' NEEDS AND VIEWS OF PROVIDERS

Family members desire information about the disorder in terms of diagnosis, prognosis, and treatments, as well as assistance from mental health professionals, as they come to realize that they lack the expertise to undertake the responsibilities of their caregiving roles for their relative with a psychiatric disability. Noncaregiving relatives, including siblings and children, also want information about the illness to enhance their coping with the disorder (Biegel et al., 1994; Doornbos, 2001; Greenberg, Greenley, & Kim, 1995; Hatfield, 1987a; Kinsella et al., 1996). Needs of families differ by diagnosis and according to whether they participate in self-help groups (Mueser, Bellack, Wade, Sayers, & Rosenthal, 1992a). Hatfield (1983) studied what families considered as essential information for them to assist in helping an ill relative, and the highest priorities included knowing the appropriate expectations, learning how to motivate the ill relative, and understanding the disorder. She found that there was a good deal of discrepancy between what families want and what they receive from family therapists. Families also wish to learn skills to cope with the illness and its effects on family members, and to receive support for themselves in dealing with the stresses and strains (Lefley, 1996; Marsh, 1998; Hatfield, 1994a).

Despite these needs, families report a lack of understanding of the caregiving experience on the part of mental health practitioners (Doornbos, 2001; Solomon, Beck, & Gordon, 1988a, 1988b), as many practitioners often seem to have no awareness of the burdens faced by families (Kaas, Lee, & Peitzman, 2003). For example, Mueser and colleagues (Mueser, Webb, Pfeiffer, Gladis, & Levinson, 1996) found that professionals, in comparison to families themselves, underestimated the degree of burden associated with negative and positive symptoms in people with bipolar disorders, as compared with those with schizophrenia. Further, families often feel rejected, ignored, and blamed for their relatives' illness by mental health practitioners (Fisher, Benson, & Tessler, 1990; Kaas et al., 2003). Lefley (1996) described the stress that families experience because of the system's indifference to them as "iatrogenic burden." A number of researchers found that families were generally dissatisfied with the services they receive from mental health practitioners (Grella & Grusky, 1989; Hanson & Rapp, 1992; Solomon, 1994; Spaniol & Zipple, 1988), although some of these researchers did find that families had a relatively good amount of contact with case management services. In the latter case, families were more satisfied with this type of service, often more satisfied for their relatives with psychiatric disabilities than for themselves (Grella & Grusky, 1989; Solomon, 1994; Solomon & Draine, 1994b). Although some families feel that practitioners offer them little support, they frequently place unrealistic demands on them to control their relatives' behavior. Hanson and Rapp (1992) noted that families often feel as though practitioners want family members to function like ward attendants in a hospital.

Families want to be and believe they should be involved in the treatment planning process for an ill relative. They feel that they have much to offer practitioners by being included in the treatment process (Doornbos, 2001). For example, family caregivers are in a position to monitor compliance with medication, as well as the side effects of medications. Family members are frequently the first to notice prodromal symptoms of the disorder and signs of substance abuse in a relative (Herz, 1985). Families are, therefore, able to provide information to practitioners that would not otherwise be available to them (Doornbos, 2001). Without ongoing contact with practitioners, families often give up trying to communicate information to practitioners who can intercede to prevent a crisis (Leazenby, 1997). Although collaborative relationships between practitioners and families are promoted, a recent survey of families found that they received little information regarding their relatives' treatment plan (Marshall & Solomon, 2000).

BEST-PRACTICE GUIDELINES FOR FAMILIES

Recognizing the stress of a psychiatric disability on a family, recent best-practice guidelines issued by the American Psychiatric Association (1997), expert consensus panel guidelines (McEvoy et al., 1999), and rigorous reviews of the Schizophrenia Patient Outcomes Research Team (PORT) (Dixon, Goldman, & Hirad, 1999a; Dixon & Lehman, 1995; Lehman et al., 2004), and the World Schizophrenia Fellowship (1997) have all recommended that family members in contact with their relatives with psychiatric disabilities should be offered some type of psychosocial family intervention. Similarly, the Joint Commission on Accreditation of Healthcare Organizations (JCAHO), a private not-for-profit agency that establishes standards and conducts reviews, set family education as a priority for those with psychiatric diagnoses (JCAHO, 1997). Further, the President's New Freedom Commission on Mental Health (2003) has recommended the implementation of evidence-based practice, and included in this list of evidence-based practices is family psychoeducation.

The recent PORT recommendations specified that family interventions should have the key elements of being at least 9 months in duration and including "illness education, crisis intervention, emotional support, and training in how to cope with illness symptoms and related problems" (Lehman et al., 2004, p. 202). The rationale provided was that randomized trials showed that family interventions combined with adequate pharmacotherapy reduce 1-year relapse rates. Other benefits resulting from the provision of such interventions were reduced hospital admissions, reduced family burden, and improved relationships between family members and their relative with a psychiatric disability. Evidence indicates that interventions lasting less than 6 months are not as effective in reducing relapse (Lehman et al., 2004).

An expert panel that included practitioners from a variety of disciplines, as well as family members, persons with psychiatric disabilities, and researchers, has recently issued recommendations for competencies for psychiatric rehabilitation practitioners in working with persons with psychiatric disabilities. Within this listing of competencies, there is a specific set of recommendations for working with families (see Table 11.1). These include understanding the family experience, engaging the family in treatment and rehabilitation,

---

TABLE 11.1. Rehabilitation Practitioners' Competencies for Working with Families of Persons with Psychiatric Disabilities

1. Understand unique issues of family members, including parents, spouses, siblings, offspring, and caring others.
   - Identify impact of mental illness on family relationships and dynamics that may put members at psychological and physical risk.

2. Engage families in the treatment and rehabilitation process.
   - Approach families with tolerance, respect, and compassion.
   - Acknowledge their strengths, expertise, and contributions.
   - Communicate effectively with families.
   - Invite and facilitate family expression of concerns, questions, and needs.
   - Value family involvement in the treatment and rehabilitation process.
   - Educate and prepare families to effectively participate in the treatment and rehabilitation process.
   - Seek family input and collaboration in service planning and support activities.
   - Provide needed supports and resources for family involvement (e.g., transportation, child care).
   - Develop strategies to resolve issues related to confidentiality.

3. Become knowledgeable about family interventions and supports.
   - Identify local, regional, and national family support services.
   - Make appropriate referrals to support resources (e.g., respite care).
   - Obtain information about effective family interventions.
   - Provide family interventions and/or make referrals.

4. Address expressed needs of families.
   - Conduct family assessment.
   - Develop a service plan for the family.
   - Provide information about diagnosis and treatment.
   - Promote development of effective coping skills.
   - Address needs of persons with psychiatric disabilities who are parents, including provision of interventions to them and their children, appropriate referrals, and assistance with linking to needed services.
   - Address specific needs of young siblings and aging parental caregivers.

Note. Data from Coursey, Curtis, Marsh, Campbell, Harding, et al. (2000a, 2000b).

addressing the needs of families, and being knowledgeable about appropriate community resources for meeting family needs (Coursey et al., 2000a, 2000b).

FAMILY SERVICES IN ROUTINE CARE

There has been limited research on the extent to which families receive services as a part of routine care provided to a relative with a psychiatric disability. A few studies have examined the provision of support to families in focused, small samples in various types of settings (Bernheim & Switalski, 1988; Greenberg et al., 1995; Marshall & Solomon, 2000, 2003, 2004b; Solomon, 1994; Solomon & Marcenko, 1992; Solomon, Beck, & Gordon, 1988a, 1988b; Young, Sullivan, Burnam, & Brook, 1998). There was a great deal of diversity in terms of the degree of services received by families reported in these studies. This variance was due to the operationalization of "provision of services." For example, in their study of rural and small urban centers in Wisconsin, Greenberg et al. (1995) found that as many as 80% of family respondents reported receiving information about mental illness at some time from mental health professionals or other sources. However, this is a broad time span and there is a lack of clarity as to what "other sources" means. When responses were limited to "mental health professionals only," just over half of the respondents received information from this source. Marshall and Solomon (2000) found that almost three-quarters of a sample of National Alliance for the Mentally Ill (NAMI) members received information on diagnosis and medication, but little other information. This is a sample that one would expect to receive information from mental health practitioners, given its members' knowledge and their advocacy position. Similarly, Young and his associates (1998) found that about half of families caring for a relative with schizophrenia treated in two public mental health clinics, one a Veterans Administration (VA) facility, had had no communication with the clinic in the past year.

As a part of the PORT project, a larger-scale study than previous ones examined the services received by families of adults with schizophrenia. This study employed a representative sample of national Medicare data and one state's Medicaid data (Dixon, Lyles, Scott, Lehman, & McGlynn, 1999b). Dixon and her colleagues (1999b) found that less than 1% had a claim for family therapy in the Medicare outpatient data and less than 10% in the Medicaid data. In another aspect of the study, a random sample of persons diagnosed with schizophrenia who were receiving community care from public and private facilities in two states, one Southern and one Midwestern, were interviewed. These individuals with psychiatric disabilities reported that of those who had contact with families, 30% of their families had received advice and support about their illnesses. However, given the general nature of the question asked, it is unclear as to whether the families' information came from practitioners employed in the mental health system, as many families currently receive information from informal supports, reading material distributed by federal agencies and national mental health organizations, or from various websites.

BARRIERS TO SERVICES AND SUPPORTS TO FAMILIES

Although many professional and governmental guidelines recognize the need to provide services and supports to families, such services are being offered on a limited basis. Service provision to families may be hindered by a diversity of factors, which include practitioner, family, and organizational factors. (See Table 11.2). Irrespective of the fact that

TABLE 11.2. Barriers to Services and Supports to Families of Persons with Psychiatric Disabilities

Organizational factors

- Lack of financial support (i.e., uncovered health benefit)
- Lack of support by administrators
- Agency confidentiality policies that prevent release of information to families

Practitioner factors

- Attitude of blaming families for relative's illness
- Belief that family involvement is harmful to the ill relative
- Conflict in working with both the client and his or her family
- Lack of time
- Lack of expertise
- Views of families as having lost hope or given up on the ill relative
- Belief that families lack time and transportation to service
- Interpretation of confidentiality policies as preventing release of information to families

Family factors

- Avoidance of mental health service for fear of blame
- Negative experiences with mental health providers
- Family members' concerns that their involvement is not wanted by their relative

theories of family causality have been discredited, some practitioners still retain attitudes of blaming a family for its relative's disorder. A recent study of experienced social work practitioners and students found that although most agreed with the biological basis of severe psychiatric disorders, they still held to beliefs of the culpability of families for their relatives' mental illness. Moreover, experienced practitioners tended to hold these beliefs to an even greater extent than students (Rubin, Cardenas, Warren, Pike, & Wambach, 1998). This simultaneous retaining of both biological and family causality among both family members and practitioners was also found in a study by Marshall, Solomon, Steber, and Mannion (2003). Other researchers have found that practitioners believe that family involvement is frequently harmful or unnecessary to clients and that many practitioners are in conflict about treating both the client and the family. In addition, practitioners do not think that they have the necessary time or expertise to include families in the treatment process (Kaas et al., 2003). Other family factors that prevent practitioners from serving families include practitioners' perceptions that families have lost hope or have given up on being able to make changes, avoid services from mental health practitioners for fear of the stigma of mental illness, or lack time or transportation to the services. Some families avoid mental health services because they are concerned that they will be blamed for their relative's disorder, as they remember past negative experiences with mental health practitioners. Other family members are concerned that their relative with a psychiatric disability does not want them involved or communicating with the practitioner (Fisher et al., 1990; Kaas et al., 2003; Solomon, 1996).

In a study of psychiatric staff members at two large hospitals, Wright (1997) found that practitioners' work schedules and caseload size determined whether they became involved with families, rather than their attitudes about families. Organizational support in terms of leadership and financial support are important factors in whether these services are provided. Frequently, reimbursement for family sessions that do not include the relative with psychiatric disability is not available (Dixon et al., 2001a). Issues related to confidentiality of treatment information are also a major impediment to practitioners' even communicating with families regarding their clients, as they feel that this violates their clients' trust. Some interpret confidentiality policies very rigidly, such that it prohibits them from having any contact with families, even when families initiate contact to give rather than request information about an ill relative (Bogart & Solomon, 1999; Marshall & Solomon, 2003). However, confidentiality policies do not preclude practitioners from having contact with families. Bogart and Solomon (1999) proposed a model for practitioners to share information with family members. This model includes a release form for the relative with a psychiatric disability to sign, which specifies to whom and what information can be provided. For the most part, clients are quite willing to sign such a release form (Marshall & Solomon, 2004a, 2004b).

FAMILY INTERVENTIONS

In response to the family experience of coping with, and in some cases caring for, a relative with a psychiatric disability, researchers partnering with providers have developed a variety of interventions to address the needs of families. These interventions enhance a family's capability to improve the outcomes for a relative with a psychiatric disability. Hatfield (1994a) has categorized these interventions as clinical and nonclinical. As the categorization implies, clinical interventions were developed by mental health professionals, and nonclinical ones were mostly developed by family members. The clinical category consists of psychoeducational and other family-focused interventions that are incorporated into interventions for purposes other than working with families of persons with psychiatric disabilities, whereas the nonclinical domain includes family support and advocacy groups, family education, family consultation, planned lifetime assistance programs, and other family support services. Table 11.3 compares two major interventions: family psychoeducation and family education.

Clinical Interventions

Psychoeducational Interventions

Psychoeducation has not been consistently defined, but as the name implies, psychoeducational interventions have both an educational and psychotherapeutic component. Originally, these interventions were created by mental health professionals in response to the EE research, with the intention of enhancing the family members' ability to cope with their relative's illness and thereby lowering their expressed emotion behavior. This change in behavior was expected to reduce the likelihood of the ill relative's relapsing. Rather quickly, these interventions were offered to both high- and low-EE families. These psychoeducational programs are offered as part of an overall clinical treatment package for persons with psychiatric disabilities. Consequently, in most models, the relative with a psychiatric disability is required to be in treatment. They have two primary objectives: providing information regarding the disorder and its treatment, and teaching strategies to cope with the illness, which include problem-solving skills, coping and communication skills development, and crisis management. Ultimately, these objectives lead to the goals of improving the quality of life for both the family and the relative with a psychiatric dis-

TABLE 11.3. Comparison of Psychoeducation and Family Education

Psychoeducation	Family education
• Adjunctive to relatives' treatment	• Freestanding, independent of relatives' treatment
• Duration—9 months to 2 years	• Duration—a few hours to 12 weeks
• Precipitant: EE research	• Precipitant: Family experience, burden, and coping with illness
• Theoretical framework: behavioral management, cognitive-behavioral approach, family systems, social support	• Theoretical framework: coping and adaptation, social support
• Primary objective: reduce relapse for relative and increase functioning	• Primary objective: reduce family burden, increase coping skills
• Relative included in part or all of intervention	• Relative excluded, at least initially
• Developed and provided by mental health professionals	• Developed and provided by family members or family–professional teams
• Extensive randomized controlled trials (RCTs) attesting to effectiveness in reducing relapse—considered evidence-based practice	• Limited controlled research—a few controlled trials; emerging evidence base

ability, improving the functioning of the family as a unit, and reducing family environmental stress (Mueser & Glynn, 1999). Typically, these interventions last at least 9 months, but may continue for as long as 5 years, are often diagnosis specific, and are primarily focused on outcomes for the relative with a psychiatric disability, and secondarily on the well-being of family members (Solomon, 1996, 2000; Dixon et al., 2001a). Psychoeducational programs are provided by a mental health professional or a team of professionals, from a diversity of disciplines, including psychology, social work, family therapy, and psychiatry.

Over the past 25 years a variety of psychoeducational interventions have been developed and implemented in a number of countries, including European countries, China, India, Australia, and Japan. None of these interventions employ traditional family therapies (Dixon, Adams, & Lucksted, 2000a). They differ not only in their theoretical orientation but also in their format, duration, and locus of service delivery. For example, these interventions may be delivered to an individual family member, to a family unit, or to multiple families. In many of these interventions the relative with a psychiatric disability is included in all or part of the intervention. The locus of delivery may be the family's own home, a clinic setting, or some other location. The points at which these interventions are initiated also vary, such as at hospital discharge or at any time during the individuals' treatment. For the most part, these interventions have focused on families with a relative with schizophrenia, but they have also been designed for those with relatives with bipolar, major depression, schizophrenia and substance abuse, alcohol abuse, and posttraumatic stress disorder (PTSD) (McFarlane, Dixon, Lukens, & Lucksted, 2003). These psychoeducational interventions have a strengths-based perspective and view family members as competent therapeutic agents. They also promote a collaborative relationship between the family and the practitioner (Lam, 1991).

Three prominent examples of these interventions are Behavioral Family Management, by Falloon and colleagues (1984), Family Psychoeducation, by Anderson and her associates (1986), and McFarlane's (2002) Multifamily Groups. All of these interventions have been determined to be effective in at least two randomized studies.

- Falloon's intervention is a sequential approach that starts with assessment, then moves to intervention strategies including communication and problem solving training, and ends with ongoing review. This intervention encompasses the teaching of illness management strategies, employing behavior modification techniques. A behavioral analysis of the strengths and needs of the family unit and each family member is conducted. The focus is to help each family member to function at his or her best within the given situation of coping with a relative with schizophrenia. This intervention was originally delivered in the families' homes, although it has been delivered in clinics as well.

- Anderson's intervention, based on a family system's framework, starts establishing an alliance with a family at the point of the relative's admission to the hospital. Once a relationship is formed, the practitioner serves as a representative for the family with the hospital system. The second phase is a day-long survival skills workshop, which provides information about the disorder to a group of families. This format helps to reduce isolation and stigmatization of the family. Upon the relative's discharge from the hospital, individual family sessions begin and contacts are made with the family and the relative with a psychiatric disability during regularly scheduled sessions, phone consultations, and times of crisis. The duration is open-ended and contingent on the needs and negotiations with family members and the relative with a psychiatric disability. The ongoing sessions are used to apply information from the workshop and to deal with the process of social adjustment, and eventually employment, for the relative with a psychiatric disability (Anderson et al., 1986).

- McFarlane's intervention is a second-generation treatment model, as it combines aspects of two family psychoeducational interventions, family behavioral management, and multiple-family approaches. The first stage is for the practitioner to meet individually with each family to build an alliance and join with that family. The next stage is a workshop, as in Anderson's model. Unlike Anderson's intervention, however, this model employs problem-solving groups attended by both families and their ill relatives. This is a long-term intervention with a closed membership. Thus, the families receive support and problem-solving suggestions from one another. Consequently, this intervention has the advantage of being social support group as well. For the first year the multifamily group focuses on social stabilization of the relatives with psychiatric disabilities, and in the second year the group moves to emphasize social and vocational rehabilitation for their ill relatives. This intervention has been combined with assertive community treatment (ACT) to create Family-Aided Assertive Community Treatment (FACT; see Chapter 6 for a discussion of this model) (McFarlane, 2002).

As is apparent from these brief descriptions of the psychoeducational interventions each provides more than mere information about the disorder, but works with the family therapeutically. Mueser and Glynn (1999) have put forth a model that closely resembles that of Falloon and associates (1984), but is called behavioral family therapy (BFT), in order to reflect this therapeutic element. Behavioral family therapy is the most widely used of the family interventions and has the broadest applicability to a diversity of disorders. This approach includes an educational component and a skills training component addressing communication and problem solving. The extent to which these skill training aspects are employed is contingent on an assessment of the family needs (Mueser, 2005).

RESEARCH ON PSYCHOEDUCATIONAL INTERVENTIONS

Numerous reviews of controlled studies of family psychoeducation have consistently concluded that these interventions are more effective in reducing relapse, by delaying, if not preventing it, as compared with standard treatment without family psychoeducation. Consequently, the interventions are cost-effective owing to reduced days of hospitalization (e.g., Lam, 1991; Strachan, 1986; Mari & Streiner, 1994). Psychoeducation is currently considered evidence-based practice (EBP) (Dixon et al., 2001), and McFarlane's multifamily intervention is a part of the Robert Wood Johnson Implementing EBPs Project (Mueser, Torrey, Lynde, et al., 2003) and one of the Substance Abuse and Mental Health Services Administration implementation resource kits (U.S. Department of Health and Human Services, 2003b).

Since 1995 there have been at least 14 narrative and meta-analytic reviews of these interventions. Table 11.4 describes the outcomes of these reviews. The reviews have consistently concluded that these interventions produce lower rates of relapse. One review by Pharoah, Rathbone, Mari, and Streiner (2004) was a bit more equivocal, but this review included briefer family interventions, with a criterion of five or more sessions. There is some indication that such gains are maintained for at least 2 years. Most of these reviews were conducted on studies that focused on relatives with schizophrenia or schizophrenia spectrum disorders; only one focused specifically on depression (Baucom, Mueser, Shoham, Dauito, & Stickle, 1998). Baucom and colleagues (1998) included only two studies on depression and compared behavioral marital therapy with cognitive therapy. They concluded that behavioral treatment is more effective in reducing marital distress, whereas cognitive therapy is more effective in alleviating depression. In the majority of the studies included in the reviews, the family psychoeducational intervention was combined with psychopharmacological treatment, and frequently, case management. This factor has resulted in some reviewers concluding that these family interventions have increased medication compliance, which has likely contributed to the observed reductions in relapse.

Although some reviews were limited to interventions of at least 3 months, beneficial effects seem to depend on the duration of an intervention's being at least 9 months (Dixon & Lehman, 1995; Penn & Mueser, 1996), a conclusion reached by earlier reviews as well (Lam, 1991). Some noted that employing an insight oriented perspective in family interventions may actually result in negative outcomes (Penn & Mueser, 1996; Mueser & Glynn, 1999; Baucom et al., 1998). Most reviews concluded that there was no particular advantage of one family intervention over another. The fact that most psychoeducational interventions have a number of common elements may be why there is no advantage in using one model over another (Baucom et al., 1998). A report by the World Schizophrenia Fellowship (1997) noted that lack of clarity about the efficacy of a particular model in comparison with others may deter service systems and practitioners from implementing family psychoeducation. The critical elements of the interventions are not clear, but education alone does not seem to be effective. There is some evidence that the minimal intervention needs to include education, family support, psychopharmacology and case management for the relative with a psychiatric disability. A few studies assessed whether a multifamily or single-family format is more effective, but there was no clear conclusion

TABLE 11.4. Review Studies of Family Psychoeducation, 1995–2004

Reviewers	Type of review	Criteria	No. of studies	Findings
Baucom et al. (1998)	Narrative	Manual-based intervention, RCT, depression diagnosis	2	Behavioral marital therapy more effective than cognitive therapy in reducing marital distress; cognitive therapy may be more effective for alleviating depression
Baucom et al. (1998)	Narrative	Manual-based, RCT, schizophrenia diagnosis	11	Behavioral family intervention and supportive family therapy effective in reducing relapse; family system possibly effective in reducing relapse; intervention needs to be at least 9 months; insight-oriented approaches have negative outcomes
Dixon & Lehman (1995)	Narrative	RCT, patients diagnosed with schizophrenia; outcomes systematically described	15, and 1 review by Mari and Steiner	Reduces rates of relapse; suggestive improvement in patient functioning and family well-being; multifamily group may be superior for some subgroups
Dixon, Adams, & Lucksted (2000a)	Narrative	Studies between 1994 and 1998	15	Cultural factors influence effectiveness; families with relatives with recent onset disorders not included in same intervention with long-term families; interventions need to be professionally led and to include support, information, and crisis intervention
Falloon, Held, Coverdale, Roncone, & Laidlaw (1999)	Narrative	High-quality methods, > 6 months, compared to pharmacology plus CM	21	Significant advantage in clinical outcomes; reduces major exacerbation of illness, reducing residual symptoms, stress; help with stress management, economic benefits; enduring benefits of clinical and social recovery for up to 5 years; intervention using only education has limited effects; improved adherence and relationship with professionals; less clinical and social benefit; small advantage of multiformat over single format; social skills component has advantages

Goldstein (1995)	Narrative	Unclear	8 first-generation, 4 second-generation	Systematic psychoeducational family intervention reduced relapse beyond routine care, drug treatment, and ancillary crisis services
McFarlane et al. (2003)	Narrative	RCT, quasi-experimental required to measure outcome regarding relapse	11	Culturally and contextually specific adaptation; longer participation required for positive outcomes; > 6 months; with problem solving, coping skills training, social support and communications skills training needed for positive outcome; multiformat more effective for first episode than single format; some studies show improvement in family and relative psychosocial outcomes
Mueser & Glynn (1999)	Narrative	Follow-up > 18 months; RCT compared to routine care or another family intervention	11	Reduced relapse and hospitalization, suggestive of improved social functioning of the family and relative; all models equally effective; most interventions are behavioral; insight-oriented therapy has poor outcome
Pharoah et al. (2004)	Meta-analysis	RCT and quasi-experimental; schizophrenia spectrum disorders: > 5 sessions; compared to standard care	28	Reduced relapse at 1 year; may decrease relapse up to 2 years; no difference in dropouts from treatment; improved medication compliance; reduced cost—only few assessed cost—Behavioral Family Treatment compared to family support—equal results; group vs. single intervention—equivocal; better outcome for interventions by developers than for others
Pilling et al. (2002b)	Meta-analysis	Schizophrenia diagnosis; family sessions specific to provision of support and treatment; minimum—one of following: psychoeducational, problem solving, crisis management, or intervention with relative	18	Reduced relapse in first 12 months, single family intervention reduced rehospitalization; in first year: no difference in suicide rates; lower rates of treatment; noncompliance; increased compliance with medication; some evidence of reduced family burden; single family intervention more effective than group

(continued)

TABLE 11.4. *(continued)*

Reviewers	Type of review	Criteria	No. of studies	Findings
Pitschel-Walz et al. (2001)	Meta-analysis	Schizophrenia diagnosis	25	Relapse rates reduced by 20%; intervention > 3 months more effective than standard care; longer-term intervention more effective than shorter; combined family intervention and patient intervention more effective than drug treatment; family intervention and patient intervention = family intervention and patient drug treatment; all family interventions have similar positive outcomes, but those that are more intensive and of longer duration have better outcomes; multifamily groups more effective than single family unit; outcomes did not differ for up to 24 months; some studies showed reduced burden, lowered EE, increased knowledge of schizophrenia, better compliance, better social adjustment and quality of life, and lower cost to society
Penn & Mueser (1996)	Narrative	RCT compared with standard care on relapse	16	Lower rates of relapse over 1–2 years; interventions of longer duration, more beneficial outcomes, > 9 months; psychodynamic interventions not effective (only 1 study); improved social function of patient and reduced family burden (only 1 study); all family interventions equally effective
Cuijpers (1999)	Meta-analysis	At least pre–post design, outcome measure classified as burden	16	Family interventions had considerable effects on burden; > 12 sessions, larger effects; effects found for components of burden, psychological distress, family functioning, relationship with relative; most studies had moderate effects, few studies had large effects

on this issue. Dixon (1999) indicated that maximum benefit may be for first-break patients. In addition, practitioners were cautioned about paying attention to cultural issues; at least one study had no effect for a Hispanic sample, whereas studies in China that were mindful of the cultural context reported positive outcomes (Dixon et al., 2000a; Penn & Mueser, 1996).

Few studies evaluating psychoeducation have assessed family outcomes, such as family functioning and family burden. There were mixed findings among those studies that did assess these outcomes, but generally there seemed to be a tendency for improvement in psychosocial outcomes for families and their ill relatives, such as in family burden, family functioning, family stress, and social role functioning of the relative (see Table 11.2). One reason for the lack of strong conclusions regarding outcomes for families may be the inconsistency in the use of outcome measures. That is, with few studies in a given review assessing the same outcomes, it was difficult to come to strong conclusions. However, Cuijpers (1999) conducted a review of just the effects of burden and its component parts as an outcome of family interventions and concluded that family interventions do have an effect on burden and its components. Stronger effects on burden, however, required at least 12 sessions.

The compelling positive results for psychoeducation are somewhat tempered, in that most studies were not conducted under usual practice conditions. There is only limited evidence of the effectiveness of these interventions within the usual practice arena (Dixon et al., 2000a). Pharoah and associates (2004) indicated that research carried out by the developers of an intervention has stronger results than research conducted by others. When cost was assessed, these psychoeducational interventions were found to be cost-effective. A limitation of these interventions is that they are designed for persons with psychiatric disabilities who are engaged in treatment and have regular contact with their families, and that their families are willing to be involved in these lengthy and time consuming interventions (Pitschel-Walz et al., 2001). The lengthy time commitment required of participants has been a major criticism of these interventions.

Nonclinical Interventions

Several nonclinical interventions have also been shown to have positive impacts on family members. These include family education, consultation and mutual support groups.

Family Education

Family education programs were generally developed by families themselves to respond to their needs for practical advice and information, which they felt were not being met by mental health practitioners. Families generally feel that they do not need treatment themselves, but rather a more hands-on type of assistance in meeting a myriad of problems that they encounter (Hatfield, 1994a). Treatment in the present context refers to family therapy provided from a perspective of family pathology or deficit, as opposed to providing cognitive-behavioral interventions that teach basic skills in managing psychiatric illness. Many family education programs were "grassroots" efforts, created by families associated with NAMI (Lefley, 1996). The goals of these family educational interventions are to reduce families' stress and burden, to increase families' coping skills, and to improve families' quality of life. These educational interventions emphasize the competencies of families, rather than their deficits (Solomon, 1996). Families are taught the skills needed to cope with the existential problems resulting from the illness of an ill relative and how to manage relapse, should it occur (Lefley, 1996). These interventions are not based on a presumption of family pathology.

The major stimulus for family education programs has come from health education, parent education for those with disabled children, and adult education (Hatfield, 1994b). The underlying conceptual basis for family education interventions emerged from findings regarding stress, coping, and adaptation and the need for social support (Hatfield, 1987a, 1990; Marsh, 1992). The coping and adaptation framework focuses on the strengths, resources, and adaptive capacities of families. Families learn to cope with the behaviors of a disorder by modifying their own behaviors, cognitively neutralizing the meaning of the experience, and/or managing the emotional consequences of the problems that arise from their relative's disorder (Pearlin & Schooler, 1978). Adaptive coping is the family members' use of behavioral and cognitive strategies to reduce their stress and burden resulting from their relative's illness. In addition, these interventions employ aspects of social support, which help to buffer stress through emotional support, practical advice, and information sharing. Particular programs may have a different conceptualization. For example, NAMI's Family-to-Family education program (FFEP) employs a trauma model of recovery, viewing mental illness in the family as a traumatic event from which family members need to recover and learn to care for themselves (Burland, 1998).

Family education programs are generally freestanding rather than part of a comprehensive service package for the relative with a psychiatric disability (Solomon, 1996). These are usually group approaches, but these programs are often paired with support groups, so participants can continue to benefit from the support aspect when the educational program is completed. Generally, these programs are delivered in community settings, such as churches, schools, or other locations that are convenient and accessible to family members (Solomon, 2000). Because they are independent of the mental health system, the stigma of attending a mental health agency is avoided. Moreover, family members who have had negative experiences with mental health practitioners are more likely to attend these interventions when they are independent of the mental health system. These programs are frequently led by family members, although they sometimes have professionals speak on a specific topic, such as new medications (Battaglino, 1987). Programs of this kind may also be facilitated by an individual who has the dual role of professional and family member or cofacilitated by a professional and a trained family member. Most educational groups have an open admission policy for anyone with a relative with a psychiatric disorder, regardless of whether the relative is receiving treatment or not. This is in contrast to psychoeducation interventions that require the relative with a psychiatric disability to be in treatment. Families whose ill relatives deny the illness and/ or are resistant to treatment (estimates are as high as 50%; Kessler et al., 2001) are in great need of assistance. Usually the ill relative does not participate in these education programs, at least not initially, so that family members can be comfortable in speaking honestly about their own concerns without feeling hampered by the presence of their relative with a psychiatric disability (Solomon, 2000).

Family education programs are usually group interventions that commonly have a didactic component that provides information on a diversity of disorders, usually schizophrenia and major affective disorders; course of the disorders; treatment modalities; means to creating a supportive environment, including information on environmental theories and family blaming; coping with a disorder on a daily basis as well as in crises; available community resources; and planning for the future. Many of these programs also have an experiential component whereby participants engage in practicing skills in order to handle situations likely to arise during the course of an illness. Much of the educational content of these programs is very similar to that of psychoeducational programs. Frequently, these programs have a highly specified curriculum manual, such as the Journey of Hope Program in Louisiana, the family education program of the Training, Education, Consultation (TEC) Family Center of the Mental Health Association of Southeastern Pennsylvania, and FFEP. Some assign homework to participants between sessions. There may be supplemental material employed, such as videos or informational material that is distributed. Generally, these programs are brief interventions that range from a couple of hours on a given day to 10 or 12 weekly sessions, each lasting 1–2 hours (Solomon, 2000).

FFEP, sponsored by NAMI, is widely offered throughout the United States, Puerto Rico, and Canada. This program is continuing to expand internationally. This is a train-the-trainer model in which family members are trained and then, in turn, train others. In this way the program becomes self-sustaining (Dixon, 1999). There is no cost to participants for this particular program, the cost is assumed by organizational donations (e.g., local NAMI chapters) and local governments (Dixon, Lucksted, Stewart, Burland, Brown, et al., 2004). For other programs there may be a nominal fee, and others may be totally supported by contributions from local governmental entities. However, a recent study of state support of family interventions found that three-quarters of the states had no policy on this issue, and that the states' allocated financial support was minimal, ranging from $11,500 to $150,000 (Dixon et al., 1999a).

Because many of these programs were designed with parents in mind, particularly those who have an adult child with schizophrenia, other family members do not always feel these interventions to be relevant to their needs. A number of programs have been developed specifically for spouses, children, and siblings, as well as for those with specific disorders such as bipolar and borderline personality disorder. The spouse groups, for example, focus specifically on their own concerns rather than those of parents, such as dealing with intimacy issues and marital role responsibilities (e.g., Mannion, Mueser, & Solomon, 1994).

RESEARCH ON FAMILY EDUCATION

Although these interventions have proliferated to a great extent, the evaluation of their effectiveness is limited in both amount and degree of rigor. Most of the evaluation studies conducted on family education have been naturalistic studies rather than randomized designs and have indicated positive outcomes (Dixon, Stewart, Burland, Delahanty, Lucksted, et al., 2001b; Pickett-Schenk, Cook, & Laris, 2000). To date, there have been at least six randomized trials and one quasi-experimental design of family education (Abramowitz & Coursey, 1989; Dixon et al., 2004; Pickett-Schenk, Steigman, Bennett, & Lippincott, 2005; Posner, Wilson, Kral, Lander, & McIlwraith, 1992; Reilly, Rohrbaugh, & Lackner, 1988; Smith & Birchwood, 1987; Solomon, Draine, Mannion, & Meisel, 1996a, 1996b, 1997).

In contrast to the findings on psychoeducation, there is no evidence that these interventions affect relapse or rehospitalization rates. However, these interventions are not primarily designed to affect the outcomes for the relative with a psychiatric disability (Solomon, 1996). All have found positive outcomes for family members, but most of them have employed different outcome measures, resulting in little consistency of findings. Families that participated in these trials have been found to gain knowledge about the disorder and a greater understanding of and satisfaction with mental health services, to be quite satisfied with these interventions, and to be more satisfied with the mental health treatment system. These studies have reported reductions in burden; improved self-care; less distress, fewer depression symptoms, and less anxiety; improved relationships with their relative with psychiatric disability, improved coping behaviors, and an increased sense of self-efficacy in dealing with their relative's illness (Abramowitz & Coursey, 1989; Dixon et al., 2004; Posner et al., 1992; Reilly et al., 1988; Smith & Birchwood, 1987; Solomon, Draine, Mannion, & Meisel, 1996a, 1996b, 1997).

There is some evidence that these gains are maintained for as long as 6 months, but no studies have assessed outcomes beyond this period of time (Dixon et al., 2004; Solomon, 1996). Solomon and colleagues (1996a) did find a secondary benefit for the relative with a psychiatric disability, in that this person's attitude toward medication compliance, even without his or her being involved in the intervention, was improved. Dixon and her colleagues (2004), who conducted one of the most rigorous studies, including a fidelity assessment, with positive outcomes, indicated that these findings provide support for family education to achieve the status of evidence-based practice.

Family Consultation

Family consultation, sometimes called supportive family counseling or family systems consultation, is a process in which an individual family member or an entire family unit (the consultee) turns to a mental health practitioner "for the purpose of clarifying a situation, reaching a decision, solving a problem, or accomplishing an objective" regarding a relative with a psychiatric disability (Mannion, 2000, p. 6; Bernheim & Lehman, 1985; Bernheim, 1982). The consultant may be either a professionally trained practitioner or a trained family member. This is an individual approach to providing advice, support, and/or information that is determined to be needed by the family or a family member in collaboration with the consultant. However, based on research, this approach has been adapted for a group process, whereby a group of family members is facilitated by a professional and a family member, and families share their problems and strategies for solving them (Mannion, Draine, Solomon, & Meisel, 1997). This approach is truly a process of collaboration between the practitioner and the family member. The consultant collaborates with the family unit or individual family member to determine the objectives that will be worked on and then to develop a plan for accomplishing these objectives. This is a very flexible approach, in which the direction is jointly decided. The practitioner works as a consultant (Solomon, Marshall, Mannion, & Farmer, 2002). As in family education, the theoretical basis for this intervention is relieving stress, coping, and adaptation. Mannion (2000) has developed a manual for the implementation of this intervention in routine care at community mental health agencies.

Frequently, the relative with a psychiatric disability is not included in the meetings with the consultant. The exclusion of the relative from some parts of this intervention enables family members to be free to express negative emotions and concerns that may upset their relative if present. This intervention is especially attractive to families whose relatives with psychiatric disabilities refuse or resist mental health services (Solomon, Marshall, et al., 2002; Solomon, 2000).

Besides helping the family to learn new skills to cope with the relative's disorder, the consultant evaluates the use of the skills by the family member(s), provides information about available resources in the community, and in a few cases, may accompany the family to a mental health agency. The consultant generally provides educational materials that are relevant to meet the needs of the family. The consultant may refer families to support groups, and families may simultaneously attend support groups and other family education programs. Frequently, this intervention can be provided over the phone, especially once a relationship has been established. This makes it easy for family members to contact the consultant as questions arise. Having the consultant available long range so they can obtain advice as situations with their ill relative change is an aspect that families particularly like (Budd & Hughes, 1997). Ascher-Svanum, LaFuze, Barrickman, Van Dusen, and Fompa-Loy (1997) conducted a survey of families of persons with psychiatric disabilities and found the preferred family intervention was advice by a professional over the phone. Usually, this intervention is highly focused on one or two particular objectives and is of very short duration, but also available over time when needed.

RESEARCH ON FAMILY CONSULTATION

The research on the family consultation intervention is very limited. In a few studies that researched a comprehensive intervention for persons with psychiatric disabilities, consultation was a component of the package (Mingyuan, Hegin, Chengde, Jianlin, Qingfeng, et al., 1993; Xiang, Ran, & Li, 1994; Zhang, Wang, & Li, 1994). But these investigations do not enable one to disentangle the assessment of family consultation. One arm of a randomized study of family education assessed family consultation (Solomon et al., 1996a, 1996b, 1997). This study determined that participants in family consultation improved their sense of self-efficacy in coping with a relative's disorder and that these gains were maintained for a period of 6 months.

Family Support and Advocacy Groups

Family support groups provide emotional support, empathy, information, and opportunities to share feelings with others who have a common experience of having a relative with a psychiatric disability. These groups are usually peer led, open-ended in terms of both duration and new entrants, and offered in an environment that is nonjudgmental and free of stigma. These groups also afford opportunities for engaging in advocacy efforts. Support is provided through group meetings in which participants can network with other family members who have common concerns (Solomon, 1998b). Participants are in a position to learn from others about practical means of coping with their relatives' illness and to gain in self-esteem through the process of assisting others (Marsh, 1998). Members share solutions to common problems, engage in role modeling, and provide positive reinforcement to others (Lefley, 2003). Participants exchange information about the illness, available resources, and strategies for coping and managing the illness and their own reactions. The aims of these groups are to increase knowledge, decrease burden, and increase skills and means of coping with their relatives' illness. These support groups have some of the elements of family education, but they are not quite as structured or formalized in regard to the provision of information.

Like family education programs, these groups generally meet in accessible community locations. The groups are facilitated by family members and usually meet for an hour or two every couple of weeks. Often these groups sponsor guest speakers on topics of concern to the membership (Ballaglino, 1987). Most of these support groups today are sponsored by NAMI, although there have been support groups for families since the 1960s, prior to the formation of NAMI in 1979. Generally, such groups also engage in public education about mental illness, antistigma campaigns, resource development, and legislative advocacy and provide representation on local boards and committees (Lefley, 2003). In some cases, these groups have developed service programs for persons with psychiatric disabilities to fill the gaps in the community service system (Lelfley, 2003). Lefley (1996) has noted that engagement in these advocacy activities can be very therapeutic for family members. However, families' needs for support, assistance, and information must be met before they are interested in engaging in advocacy work. Therefore, support groups that have been meeting for a long period of time have often moved into focusing more on advocacy than providing support and information. This is problematic for new members wishing to join established groups. As a consequence, some groups are developing strategies to meet the needs of new entrants by having them individually meet with members who are willing to serve the function of supporting the basic needs of new members. New membership is essential for the continuing existences of these groups, and if the groups do not provide for the needs of new entrants, these potential members will find that there is little purpose for them to return to the group (Solomon, 2000). As noted in discussing family education programs, some of these are paired with support groups. These education programs provide an opportunity for the development of new support groups from an established educational group.

RESEARCH ON SUPPORT AND ADVOCACY GROUPS

Research on support groups for families has examined the differences between members and nonmembers and the benefits gained by those who participate in these groups. There has been only one randomized study of family support groups. The reason for the limited use of these studies is that the randomized design is antithetical to the nature of self-help groups generally. The randomized study compared mutual support groups, psychoeducation based on McFarlane's model, and standard care outpatient services. Each intervention lasted 6 months, 12 biweekly sessions with each session being for a period of 2 hours. The peer leader of the support group was elected by the group members and trained by the researchers. A researcher helped to facilitate the group, encouraging its members to develop and go through the various stages, from engagement to termination. Although this differs from the format of a natural support group, the investigators found that the results of this support group included improvements in the functioning of the relative with psychiatric disability and fewer hospitalizations, as compared with the other two conditions (Chien & Chan, 2004).

Less rigorous research has indicated that support group participation results in a number of positive outcomes. These include improved coping skills, increased knowledge, increased perceptions of social supports, less subjective burden and lower psychological distress (Biegel & Yamatani, 1986; Citron, Solomon, & Draine, 1999; Heller, Roccoforte, Hsieh, Cook, & Pickett, 1997; Norton, Wandersman, & Goldman, 1993; Mannion, Meisel, Solomon, & Draine, 1996). Heller and colleagues (1997) found that longer participation resulted in greater benefits. Those who typically participate in these groups tend to be white, female, highly educated, and middle class (Mannion et al., 1996). Therefore, the results are biased by the nature of those who join and by those who stay in these groups.

Although the data on support groups are essentially derived from participants attesting to their satisfaction with these groups, Glick and Dixon (2002) recommend that family support groups should be included in treatment plans and that practitioners make referrals to these groups. They noted that this does not occur very often. For example in a study in Canada, Looper and his colleagues (Looper, Fielding, Latimer, & Amir, 1998) found that psychiatrists referred only 10% of their patients and families to the local Alliance for the Mentally Ill. Glick and Dixon (2002) hypothesized that practitioners do not include these referrals in treatment plans because of a lack of awareness of such services, a belief that they are not useful, and a mutual distrust between families and practitioners.

It is also important to note that a plethora of self-help books for families about mental illness have been published over the past two decades. One of the earliest was *Surviving Schizophrenia: A Family Manual* by E. Fuller Torrey (1983). In addition, the Expert Consensus Treatment Guidelines for Schizophrenia (McEvoy et al., 1999) included "A Guide for Patients and Families," which was distributed to families. This contained information on symptoms, course, medications and side effects, psychosocial treatment and rehabilitation, services and living arrangements, and what families can do to help, as well as a list of support groups and other readings.

Planned Lifetime Assistance Programs and Other Support Services

Given the number of aging parents who care for their ill relatives, many families are concerned about what will happen to a relative with a psychiatric disability when older parents become disabled or are gone. Small nonprofit agencies have been developed by families to handle special needs trusts (SNTs). Community mental health agencies could also serve this function, but are not likely to do so. These programs offer estate plans or living trusts for persons with disabilities that provide funds for goods and services that are not otherwise covered in programs like Medicaid or Supplemental Security Income (SSI), such as dental care and education. They also prevent persons with psychiatric disabilities from putting their benefits in jeopardy, as these benefits, such as SSI, are needs-based programs that do not allow individuals to have more than a specified amount of money. Should their funds exceed an allocated amount in any given month, they loose their benefits until they spend down the money (Tarutis & Boyd, 2001). These trusts can be established with a relatively limited amount of money. For example, PLAN (Planned Lifetime Assistance Network) of PA (Pennsylvania) requires $5,000 to establish a trust. There is a national organization of PLANs. PLAN of PA also serves as a representative payee for persons with psychiatric disabilities (independent of whether they have a trust or not), as well as other disabilities, and provides case management services. It will assist in paying bills for persons with disabilities, should this be desired or needed.

Research on Planned Lifetime Assistance Programs

There has been no evaluation of the effectiveness of planned lifetime assistance interventions. But there has been research on when and why families engage in future planning, including planning for residential placement (Hatfield & Lefley, 2000; Kaufman, 1998; Smith, 2004). Hatfield and Lefley (2000) found that personal issues of the caregiver, such as lack of knowledge regarding planning, the characteristics of the relative, and unfamiliarity with the service system, including housing options, are obstacles to future planning. Subjective burden and perceptions of aging prompt planning for placement, but being overwhelmed with daily hassles can prevent families from taking steps toward residential placement (Rimmerman & Keren, 1995; Smith, 2004).

Respite Care

Respite care is another type of assistance for families. Respite care offers concrete temporary relief to family caregivers (U.S. Department of Health and Human Services, 1999). This service may be provided by an individual coming into the home to assist temporarily

PERSONAL EXAMPLE

The Madison Family Revisited: Consultant Assists Bill's Sister

Bill's mother died. Prior to her death she had Bill's older sister promise to take care of him. Subsequently, Bill would call his sister and make demands of her. Being the well sibling, she felt very guilty about her brother's illness. More over, she was afraid of him and felt compelled to meet his demands. She too sought out the family consultant, who helped her with understanding the illness and how to set limits with Bill. The consultant also referred her to a psychoeducation program at a local community mental health center. This program provided support to her, helped with her feelings of isolation, and assisted her in problem solving around the issues of dealing with her brother.

with the ill relative while the caretaker family member goes shopping or visiting. Other programs may take the ill relative on an outing to relieve the caretaker for a short period of time or may stay with the ill relative while the family goes on vacation. These types of services offer benefits to both the family members and the relative with a psychiatric disability.

PARENTING ROLE OF PERSONS WITH PSYCHIATRIC DISABILITIES

For years, persons with psychiatric disabilities were seen as asexual beings and not likely to achieve the role of parenthood (Nicholson & Blanch, 1994). Currently, more than half of those with psychiatric disabilities become parents (Nicholson, Biebel, Katz-Leavy, & Williams, 2002). Yet even today, little is done in terms of family planning for those with psychiatric disabilities. A lack of education about birth control may be the reason for the high number of unplanned pregnancies among women with psychiatric disabilities (Mowbray, Oyserman, Zemencuk, Ross, & Scott, 1995b). Given the view of this population by many providers, there has been little consideration or provision for them as parents. Currently, persons with psychiatric disabilities are rarely asked by practitioners whether they have any children (Nicholson, Geller, Fisher, & Dion, 1993; DiChillo, Matorin, & Hallahan, 1987). However, the fertility rates of women with psychiatric disabilities are comparable to those of women in the general population (Nimgaonkar, Ward, Agarde, Weston, & Ganguli, 1997), and their number of children is consistent with or slightly higher than that of the general population (Caton, Cournos, & Dominique, 1999; Mowbray, Oyserman, Bybee, McFarlane, & Rueda-Riedle, 2001; White, Nicholson, Fisher & Geller, 1995). Parenthood is a central source of meaning to mothers with psychiatric disabilities (Mowbray, Oyserman, & Ross, 1995a; Sands, 1995). Estimates are that two-thirds of women with psychiatric disabilities are mothers (Nicholson & Henry, 2003). In a study of parents of adults with psychiatric disorders, parents reported that 57% of their children had biological offspring (Gamache, Tessler, & Nicholson, 1995).

Most research on parenthood of persons with psychiatric disabilities has focused on the impact on their children, with little examination of their parenting experiences per se (Mowbray et al., 1995a). Few studies have examined the role of the father with a psychiatric disability (Nicholson & Henry, 2003), but then most such fathers are not married to the mothers and even fewer have responsibilities for child care (Oyserman, Mowbray, & Zemencuk, 1994). The research that assessed the experience of mothers with a psychiatric disabilities has found that many of the pertinent issues are common to all parents, particularly low-income single mothers. However, some issues are specific to mothers with psychiatric disabilities. Some mothers struggle with the combined stressors of raising their children and coping with their psychiatric illness, frequently with minimal supports (Nicholson, Sweeney, & Geller, 1998a; Oyserman et al., 1994; Mowbray, Schwartz, Bybee, Spong, Rueda-Riedle, et al., 2000). A particular stressor for mothers with psychiatric disabilities is the possible loss of custody of their children, as they are at high risk for this (Nicholson et al., 1998; Park, Solomon, & Mandel, 2006; Sands, Koppelman, & Solomon, 2004). Estimates are that 28–65% lose custody of their children (Mowbray et al., 2001). Routinely, or periodically when the person with a psychiatric disability decompensates, family members may assume part or all of the responsibility of child rearing (Nicholson, Sweeney, & Geller, 1998b). Consequently, parenthood has produced a new burden for families of persons with psychiatric disability. However, little attention has been paid to this issue in either research or service provision (Gamache et al., 1995).

Mothers feel that because they have a psychiatric disability they are put in the position of having to prove themselves, as mental health practitioners frequently hold the mother responsible for a child's problems. They often have difficulty knowing whether the stresses of caring for a child are "normal" or a result of the illness. Some report having difficulty in managing a child's behavior. The needs of child rearing sometimes conflict with managing the illness. For example, a mother may stop taking her medication, so that she is not slowed down, in order to keep up with her young child. Like other mothers, mothers with psychiatric disabilities make sacrifices for their children (Nicholson et al., 1998a, 1998b). Moreover, mothers do not know how to tell their children about their illness and the reason for their taking medication (Nicholson & Henry, 2003).

However, there is limited service provision targeted to parents with psychiatric disabilities. A national survey of state mental health authorities regarding women with psychiatric disabilities who have children was conducted to determine the nature of their policies and programs. The investigators found that the majority of the states have parent training programs, but most are not designed to meet the needs of persons with psychiatric disabilities (Nicholson et al., 1993; Nicholson & Blanch, 1994). These researchers concluded that persons with psychiatric disabilities are not identified as parents; pregnancy is addressed policywise as a medical condition; the mother–child relationship is not a primary focus of the public mental health sector, but seen as the responsibility of social or child welfare services; and the clinical and programmatic needs of mothers are not a priority. These researchers, as well as Oyserman and colleagues (1994), note that there are some specialized programs for this population, including programs for pregnant women. For example, Thresholds, a psychiatric rehabilitation agency in Chicago, has a comprehensive program that mothers attend 3–5 days a week, followed by monthly home visits. This program includes clinical and rehabilitation services along with education and support, such as training in stress and household management, and education in child development. A nursery and a child care setting are also part of this program, with child care workers modeling caregiving activities and conducting periodic assessments of a child's development (Oyserman et al., 1994).

Nicholson and Blanch (1994) noted that effective rehabilitation for parents with psychiatric disabilities requires a comprehensive approach, whether it is offered within a given program or by assessing the mother's needs, strengths, and capabilities and then making arrangements for appropriate services. This rehabilitation approach can certainly enhance the capabilities of mothers with psychiatric disabilities and contribute to positive outcomes for them and their children. A recent pilot study of an integrated treatment approach to parent training showed promise. The Integrated Family Treatment offered home-based services including parent skill training, modeling, and coaching, as well as linkage to various environmental supports (Brunette, Richardson, White, Bemis & Eelkema, 2004b).

The National Mental Health Association has been sponsoring a program called the Invisible Children's Project, a planning program for local communities to engage in a consensus process in providing services and developing policies that support families in which there is parental mental illness. Communities apply for grants, and awards are about $10,000, to implement a consensus process to design a responsive service system to address the needs of these families. The funds are used for coalition building to help facilitate the establishment of coordinated and comprehensive services for meeting the needs of the entire family.

SUMMARY AND CONCLUSIONS

Cultural beliefs regarding families of persons with psychiatric disabilities have clearly changed over the last 30 years. Families are now viewed less as toxic agents and more as competent integral members of the rehabilitation team and as ongoing support systems for their relatives with psychiatric disabilities. The welfare of family members is increasingly seen as essential to the recovery process of their relative with a psychiatric disability. By meeting the needs of family members for information, education, support, and coping skills, benefits accrue to the entire family, including the relative with mental illness. Families whose needs are met through one or more family interventions attain a better quality of life for themselves and their relatives with psychiatric disabilities. Over the years there has been increasing recognition of the need to develop more specialized interventions for specific family members, for designated diagnoses, and for identified characteristics of relatives with psychiatric disabilities and their families. Most recently, a family role for persons with psychiatric disabilities has been recognized—that of parent. This role requires new interventions to ease the burdens of parenthood for such families.

Although some of these interventions clearly incur additional costs for the mental health system, they also have the potential for financial savings through cost offsets resulting from possible reductions in costly mental health service utilization, particularly reductions in hospitalizations and emergency room visits. With the range of family interventions, rehabilitation practitioners do not necessarily have to provide these interventions themselves; rather, they need to be competent and comfortable in working with families and knowledgeable about available community resources to facilitate family access to the appropriate interventions. They need to have an understanding and an appreciation of the family experience and to realize that caregiving can be a 24-hours, 7-days-a-week, 52-weeks-a-year job.

Chapter 12

Psychosis and Cognitive Impairment

Ever since researchers and clinicians first described serious mental illnesses such as schizophrenia, deficits in cognitive processes have been considered central to these illnesses. Kraepelin (1919/1971) believed that cognitive deficits led to "annihilation of intrapsychic coordination." Bleuler (1911/1950) described the nature of deficient processes, attributing poor cognitive functioning to the loss of associations between thoughts. Since these original formulations, research and development of cognitive interventions for people with schizophrenia and other disabling psychiatric disorders have largely represented two independent traditions. First, an extensive literature on *cognitive rehabilitation* has developed over the past four decades, seeking to improve information processes so that people with psychiatric disabilities are better able to perceive and comprehend their world (Storzbach & Corrigan, 1996). This body of work has reflected laboratory-based approaches to cognition, focusing on the improvement of discrete information processes like attention, memory, and decision making. The first half of this chapter reviews processing deficits and intervention strategies that remediate these deficits.

Second, researchers, largely from Britain, have extrapolated the principles and practices of *cognitive therapy* to some of the symptoms and dysfunctions of schizophrenia and other disabling psychiatric disorders. Consistent with the *zeitgeist* in cognitive therapy, researchers in this arena have crafted interventions that help people to think about and act upon their belief systems. The second half of this chapter explains these kinds of deficits and the approaches that help people with psychiatric disabilities to address them.

Cognitive rehabilitation and cognitive therapy are fundamentally adjunctive services. Rather than being stand-alone rehabilitation strategies, they are best suited to be appended to other rehabilitation programs. Hence, job coaches might use these approaches for employees with cognitive deficits that are interfering with work. Case managers might adopt cognitive therapy for a person whose delusions are interfering with successful living in his or her home.

COGNITIVE REHABILITATION OF PROCESSING DEFICITS

Information or cognitive processing refers to the interconnectedness of the components of thought (e.g., attention, memory, and executive functioning), which are necessary for people to perceive, understand, and act upon their world. There was a time when cognitive processing deficits manifested by people with psychotic disorders were thought to be *derivative* (i.e., they emerged from the more apparent symptoms of the disorder or from medication effects), but now researchers have convincingly shown that many of the processing deficits are present before the onset of the disorder and remain after most symptoms have remitted (Bellack, Gold, & Buchanan, 1999; Green, 1999; Twamley, Jeste, & Bellack, 2003). Hence, cognitive processes are important treatment targets in their own right. Given this assertion, the question then is, what is the relevance of processing deficits to psychiatric disability and rehabilitation? Several issues are addressed here to answer this question. First, a profile of deficit areas relevant to cognition is provided. Then we review evidence indicating that impairments in specific cognitive processes interfere with social functions, which, in turn, undermines the achievement of goals in the major life domains. This section then provides a summary of research on the impact of treatment strategies on cognitive impairments and psychiatric disabilities. This summary includes a brief review of medication effects (Chapter 7 reviews medication issues more thoroughly) and a more comprehensive discussion of rehabilitation approaches. Much of the research reviewed in this chapter was completed in studies of people with schizophrenia. Hence, research on this illness is used as the framework for understanding general principles and practices related to cognitive rehabilitation. The nature of cognitive deficits and the corresponding rehabilitation strategies should parallel those related to principles used in other diagnoses.

What Are Relevant Processing Deficits?

Many of the goals of pharmacological and psychotherapeutic interventions seek to diminish the impact of the symptoms of serious mental illness. Symptom remediation, however, does not guarantee positive outcomes in all functioning domains. For example, many people experience fewer psychotic symptoms and diminished depression but still are unable to fully enjoy relationships or to meet work goals. In like manner, cognitive processing impairments are an independent barrier to achieving life goals. Literature reviews suggest that about three-quarters of people with serious mental illness like schizophrenia show abnormal functioning on process measures (Palmer, Heaton, Paulsen, Kuck, Braff, et al., 1997). Findings from a meta-analysis of more than 200 studies comparing cognitive processes between people with schizophrenia and normal controls showed moderate to large effect sizes, with the largest deficits being in memory and attention (Heinrichs & Zakzanis, 1998). Although research clearly shows that people with serious mental illness have significant deficits in cognitive processes, the way in which processes were defined and cognition was measured differs significantly across studies. Information processing is a frequently used paradigm for understanding these diverse deficits (Corrigan, 1996).

Information-Processing Impairments

The fundamental assumption behind information-processing paradigms is that the macro aspect of sensory input is divided into discrete bits of information (e.g., visual stimuli can be described in terms of color, contrast, depth, location, and relative size) and that the macro experience of human cognition can be divided into composite functions (e.g., attention, memory, and executive) that interact in some meaningful order (e.g., serially, in parallel distribution) (Corrigan & Stephenson, 1994). Hence, the process of knowing can be understood by studying the various components of the information process individually and together. From a methodological standpoint, breaking down information processing and cognition into theoretical elements greatly enhances the study of these phenomena. The range of research questions increases geometrically with the number of defined elements. Similarly, methodological precision is enhanced as the questions of cognitive research narrow from "How does a person know?" to "How does a person attend, recall, recognize, or react?"

An information-processing paradigm also has several advantages for understanding cognitive functioning (Ingram & Kendall, 1986). The specificity and organization of this approach facilitates the identification of cognitive deficits. Findings about specific cognitive functions seem to coincide with biological research in neuroscience, which suggests putative associations between information processing and structures of the central nervous system. Moreover, measurement strategies used in defining information processes have been adapted for the assessment of cognitive deficits. In turn, variations of these assessment instruments have been used as rehabilitative tools.

STAGE THEORY

The first information-processing theories were bottom-up, serial search models of cognition (Sternberg, 1966, 1967) like the one illustrated in Figure 12.1. According to this perspective, information processing is serial, in that it manipulates information in a stepwise fashion one byte at a time; functions include information intake and encoding, storage and retrieval, transformation and conceptualization, and response selection and action.

PERSONAL EXAMPLE

Keiko Fukuoka Can't Remember What Was Said

Keiko was severely distressed by voices from the devil when she was first admitted for a medication evaluation. Her speech was also marked by loose associations, so people had difficulty understanding her. These symptoms remitted almost entirely after 6 weeks of atypical antipsychotic medication.

Even though she continued on the medication, her attention was poor. This did not seem to result from being sedated by her medication. When others talked with Keiko, she seemed wide awake. However, she had great difficulty in following the content of a medication management skills class. Even when the peer instructor repeated the information, she could not remember it. As a result, she was having difficulty taking her medication as prescribed in her new apartment. Keiko was also having trouble with her supervisor at work. She was forgetting phone messages and misplacing files.

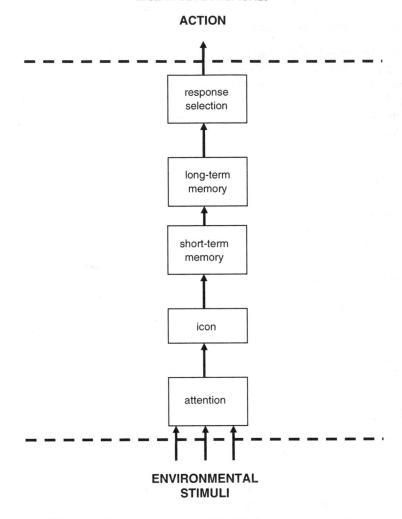

FIGURE 12.1. Bottom-up model of information processing.

These models are bottom-up models, because processing is *initiated* by attention to incoming information. We now take a closer look at these functions, beginning with attention.

As represented in Figure 12.1, the relative infinity of information in the research participant's environment is significantly reduced by an attentional filter. Broadbent (1958, 1977) believed that this filter was a selective process whereby individuals may focus attention on only a few of several channels of incoming information. For example, research participants in a study may attend to a complex auditory message while ignoring the written message on a computer screen. However, information from the visual channel typically dominates attentional processing (Posner, Nissen, & Klein, 1976). Attended information then becomes the figural "snapshot" that is available in iconic memory for a very short time (Averbach & Coriell, 1961; Sperling, 1960). Most of this information is lost as the icon decays or is replaced by subsequent incoming information, so that only a few bytes of original information remain. This information is encoded vis-à-vis extant memory traces so that the information has meaning beyond its stimulus qualities—for example, that a conglomeration of lines and curves, shades, and hues is perceived to be the image of a human being.

The amount of information that can be held in short term-memory is relatively limited and decays quickly (Miller, 1956). Short-term memory, often called working memory, refers to an individual's ability to report what is currently on his or her mind. Depending on the individual's previous experience with incoming information, his or her mental set, and environmental conditions, some information in short-term memory is consolidated into long-term memory (Atkinson & Shiffrin, 1968). Investigators believe that information in long-term memory is sorted into categories, memory structures that are defined by a set of unique and descriptive attributes. Information in long-term memory may be retrieved in the future; two forms of retrieval have been described: recognition and recall (Mandler, 1972; Rabinowitz, Mandler, & Patterson, 1977). In terms of recognition, individuals may *compare* incoming information to categories in the memory store, thereby recognizing the data: "Oh, I know you, you're Mr. Jones." Alternatively, the executive mechanism of an individual may initiate a more active and cognitively demanding memory search to recall a perceptual instance. "Let's see. In the past, I've seen Mr. Jones and Ms. Smith at the street corner."

The recall process also suggests the manner in which motoric responses are generated. A response may be elicited in reaction to an external stimulus (comparison function) or to an internal decision (executive function). The generated response may come from several motoric actions arranged hierarchically in the long-term store (Broen & Storms, 1966; Hull, 1952). Positions in the response hierarchy vary in arousal level and are determined on the basis of past learning history and present situational demands. In highly familiar situations, the arousal of certain reactions exceeds that of most others and individuals tend to respond automatically—that is, with little conscious consideration of response alternatives and with little cognitive effort (Hasher & Zacks, 1979, 1984; Schneider & Shiffrin, 1977). In less familiar situations, the arousal of a range of responses that exceeds a response–strength ceiling becomes conscious. Individuals select a response from these alternatives or, if unsatisfied with the options, search their memories again for alternatives.

The cognitive processes in bottom-up models, and their juxtaposition to neighboring processes, readily suggest clinical problems. For example, according to Figure 12.1, cognitive deficits may result from (1) an overrestrictive attentional filter that results in a person's missing key information, (2) sensory icons that are quickly disrupted by subsequent information, (3) inaccurate encoding of incoming information, (4) rapid decay of information from short-term memory, (5) diminished consolidation to long-term memory, (6) inability to retrieve information in the long-term store, (7) an impoverished set of responses available for selection, and (8) random selection of responses from the response hierarchy. Similarly, these problem foci suggest specific rehabilitation strategies. For example, remediation of attentional deficits may include self-instructional strategies in which people tell themselves to focus their attention on narrow stimulus bands, repeated practice on attentional tasks, and differential reinforcement for attention to targeted stimuli.

The Link between Processing Deficits and Social Disabilities

Although some rehabilitation providers may argue that improving a person's memory or attentional abilities is an important goal in its own right, most agree that cognitive remediation is best understood as an important step in helping people better perceive and understand social situations, which, in turn, is an essential step in achieving most life goals. Hence, the development of cognitive rehabilitation strategies rests on identifying specific cognitive impairments that interfere with social functioning and/or the pursuit of life goals (Bellack et al., 1999). Research suggests that 20–60% of social functioning variance is due to cognitive processes (Green, Kern, Braff, & Mintz, 2000). Summaries by Green (1996b, 1998) have found three sets of correlations, as outlined in Figure 12.2; he divided the social functioning sphere into three progressively more complex domains for these summaries. *Psychosocial skill training* represents the discrete behaviors that provide the necessary foundation for interpersonal interaction. *Social problem solving* is the more dynamic and reactive strategy to resolve barriers to situational goals. *Community outcomes* is the most macrolevel construct, representing the attainment of social roles commensurate with most life goals, such as working, living independently, and establishing relationships.

Psychosocial skill acquisition was shown to be significantly associated with memory, especially with verbal recall, and with attention and vigilance (Bowen et al., 1994; Corrigan, Wallace Schade, & Green, 1994; Kern et al., 1992; Lysaker, Bell, Bioty, & Zito, 1995; Mueser et al., 1991b). Correlations between executive functioning and skill acquisition were found in some studies but need to be further replicated. Social problem solving was also associated with verbal recall and vigilance, but not with executive functioning (Bellack, Sayers, Mueser, & Bennett, 1994; Corrigan et al., 1994; Penn, Mueser, Spaulding, Hope, & Reed, 1995; Penn, Van Der Does, Spaulding, Garbin, Linszen, et al., 1993). Community outcome was associated with verbal recall and executive functioning (Buchanan, Holstein, & Breier, 1994; Goldman, Blake, Marks, Hedeker, & Luchins, 1993; Jaeger & Douglas, 1992; Johnstone, Macmillan, Frith, Benn, & Crow, 1990; Lysaker, Bell, & Beam-Goulet, 1995; Wykes, Sturt, & Katz, 1990). An interesting pattern emerges in considering the sum of these findings in Figure 12.2. That is, the more complex social functioning constructs seem to be associated with the more complex cognitive

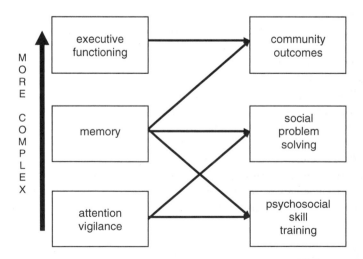

FIGURE 12.2. The associations between cognitive processing and social functioning. Cognitive processes represent the three core concerns: attention, memory, and executive functioning. Social functioning includes psychosocial skill acquisition, social problem solving, and community outcome.

processes. It is important to note that most of these findings represent cross-sectional correlations, so the direction of the association is not clear. Future research needs to discern whether cognitive processes, in fact, are causes of social functioning or whether this correlation represents some other kind of association.

The Impact of Interventions

Green and Nuechterlein (1999) have framed the connection between cognitive and social functioning impairments as the *delta question*; that is, what changes in cognitive processes correspond with changes in functional outcome? Three overall principles address the delta question by describing approaches that improve cognitive processes and, it is hoped, social dysfunctions: restoration, compensation, and reorganization (Bellack et al., 1999; Spaulding, Fleming, Reed, Sullivan, Storzbach, & Lam, 1999). *Restoration* represents the impact of "mental exercising," which leads to regaining part or all of the original cognitive process. *Compensation* provides an external cognitive prosthetic or crutch that improves cognitive functioning. *Reorganization* is a more elaborate form of compensation whereby people set up their environments so they are better able to understand task demands, given their limited cognitive abilities. Both pharmacological and rehabilitation interventions may achieve the goals implied by these principles.

Psychopharmacological Interventions

Psychotropic medications have complex effects on the cognitive deficits relevant to psychiatric disability. Conventional antipsychotic medication, for example, has shown a mixed pattern of impact (Blanchard & Neale, 1992; Medalia, Gold, & Merriam, 1988; Mishara & Goldberg, 2004; Spohn & Strauss, 1989). Low-to-moderate doses of conventional antipsychotic medications seem to improve impairments in attention and vigilance, but have no measurable effects on memory. High doses of conventional antipsychotics (defined as more than 700 chlorpromazine equivalents) may actually decrease vigilance and memory from the symptomatic baseline. Given the role of learning in the skill training component of rehabilitation, deficits in vigilance and memory may undermine a person's participation in his or her rehabilitation program (Corrigan & Penn, 1995).

More widely used atypical antipsychotic medications seem to have a better profile in terms of ameliorating cognitive impairments. Summaries of more than 20 studies have shown that people with psychoses who are treated with atypical medications are likely to experience better attentional abilities and response speed (Keefe, Silva, Perkins, & Lieberman, 1999; Meltzer & McGurk, 1999); memory and executive processes seemed less responsive to these medications and may actually show a mildly averse effect. Antidepressant medications largely have positive effects on cognitive processes (Curran, 1995). Mood-stabilizing drugs like lithium may have negative consequences, however, by slowing cognitive speed (Pachet & Wisniewski, 2003).

All benefits that occur because of psychotropic medications seem to be restorative in character; that is, there is direct improvement in basic functions rather than compensation or reorganization by some external prosthesis. Despite this positive profile, research has failed to show that the cognitive abilities of people with serious mental illness returned to "normal" levels after medication use alone (Keefe et al., 1999; Rund & Borg, 1999). Plenty of room remains for improvement in cognitive functioning, which may be facilitated by rehabilitation approaches. Chapter 7 more completely summarizes the role of medication in psychiatric rehabilitation.

Rehabilitation Interventions

Two types of cognitive rehabilitation currently exist: *targeted programs* that seek to remediate individual processing deficits, with social impairments improving as a secondary result, and *integrated programs* that combine cognitive and social interventions to directly address the interpersonal deficits that arise from interpersonal dysfunctions.

TARGETED PROGRAMS

Three types of targeted rehabilitation programs have emerged in the literature that correspond with the three principles of cognitive rehabilitation (Kurtz, Moberg, Gur, & Gur, 2001; Twamley et al., 2003); these are summarized in Figure 12.3. Interventions promoting restoration are largely repetitive exercises that require specific attention, memory, or executive functioning activity. Repeated practice is assumed to restore the corresponding deficit. Compensatory approaches teach the person some sort of cognitive skill that is meant to augment the impaired cognitive function. Reorganizational approaches help people to offset cognitive limitations by environmental cues. Each of these approaches is discussed more thoroughly below. These three types of targeted approaches may conceivably be used to remediate deficits in the three core impairment areas: attention, memory, and executive functioning. The interaction of approaches with deficit areas yields a matrix of possible interventions, as outlined in Figure 12.3

Restoring Cognition through Repeated Practice. Repeated practice has a more than 40-year history of development and evaluation (Bell, Bryson, Greig, & Wexler, 2001; Bell, Bryson, & Wexler, 2003; Green, Ganzell, Satz, & Vaclav, 1990; Karras, 1962, 1968; Medalia, Aluma, Tryon, & Merriam, 1998; Meiselman, 1973; Van der Does & Van den Bosch, 1992; Wagner, 1968). In short, the intervention instructs participants through multiple trials of an attentional, memory, or executive functioning task, with the hypothesis that repeated practice will strengthen performance on the specific skill as well as generalize to related cognitive functions. Two examples from Bell et al. (2001, 2003) illustrate this approach. In a visual tracking task meant to improve sustained attention, participants see a black line moving across a red background on a computer screen. Yellow cubes appear along the line as it moves. Participants are instructed to focus on the

	Attention	Memory	Executive Functioning
Restorative: through repeated practice			
Compensatory: through learning strategic cognitive shortcuts			
Reorganizational: through environmental cues and other manipulations			

FIGURE 12.3. Examples of the three types of targeted cognitive rehabilitation for the three core cognitive concerns.

end of the line and click the mouse whenever a yellow cube appears. A "ta-da!" sound is heard when a response is correct and a discordant sound when it is wrong. The speed and duration of the black line and yellow cubes are changed to increase task difficulty.

In a sequence recall task meant to enhance memory, participants are instructed to remember 2–10 words displayed on a computer screen. After a delay, one of the words is displayed and the participant must click on a numbered line to indicate its position on the original list. As in the visual tracking task, correct responses are acknowledged with a "ta-da!" and errors with a discordant sound. Task difficulty is adjusted by changing the length of the list, the number of times a list is presented, the amount of time to study a list, and the delay between presentation of the list and subsequent target words.

Errorless learning approaches have been used to augment repeated practice (Kern, Liberman, Kopelowicz, Mintz, & Green, 2002). In using errorless learning, tasks begin with simple components and progress to more complex ones only after the person has met a 100% criterion. This approach assumes that learning is more durable if mistakes are minimized or totally eliminated during training. In addition, performance on repeated practice has been enhanced with monetary reinforcers. For example, participants may be paid a nickel each time they correctly identify a yellow cube in the visual tracking task. The combination of repeated exercise and monetary reinforcement has been directly used to improve social perception by having participants practice on videotaped vignettes of social interactions (Corrigan, Nugent-Hirschbeck, & Wolfe, 1995b).

Compensating for Deficits via Cognitive Prosthetics. Compensatory strategies have been most commonly used to improve memory (Koh, 1978; Koh, Grinker, Marusarz, & Forman, 1981; Larsen & Fromholt, 1976; Van der Gaag, Kern, Van den Bosch, & Liberman, 2002). Four have been shown to be particularly powerful, with the first three helpful for enhancing the recall of verbal information.

1. *Encoding.* People are instructed to put a new concept into their own words. One way to do this is to associate a personally meaningful word or phrase with the concept to be learned. For example, Harry was to learn that his friend Mark lived on Monroe Street, so he encoded it as "one of the M presidents, like the streets in downtown Chicago."

2. *Chunking.* Chunking is organizing information into meaningful bits. For example, the number 17086144770 can be more easily recalled as the phone number 1 (708) 614-4770.

3. *Categorization.* Categorization is organizing information into meaningful groups. Consider this list for example:

Red	Rose	Duck	Horse	Black
Dog	Apple	Blue	Lily	Orchid
Tulip	Pear	Crow	Brown	Mouse
Lime	Cat	Lemon	Grape	Yellow

A person may be better able to recall these items when reorganizing the list into colors (red, blue, brown, black, yellow), animals (dog, cat, duck, crow, horse, mouse), flowers (tulip, rose, lily, orchid), and fruit (lime, apple, pear, lemon, grape).

4. *Self-instruction* (Meichenbaum & Cameron, 1973; Van der Gaag et al., 2002). This task is especially useful for helping a person to recall the steps in a personally rele-

vant behavior like those related to brushing one's teeth, taking medicine, or lighting a charcoal grill. When doing self-instruction, first, a model demonstrates the steps of a multicomponent behavior and says these steps aloud. Consider the steps to paying the phone bill:

> First, I get out my phone bill.
> Then I get out my checkbook.
> I separate the stub that needs to be returned to the phone company from the statement.
> I then write down the amount on the stub in the ledger of my checkbook and subtract it from my balance. Then, I turn to the corresponding blank check and fill in the date, amount, and payee. I then sign it.
> I put the check and stub in the return envelope. I put my return address on the envelope and then a postage stamp.
> I then put the envelope in the mailbox in my apartment building.

After reviewing the steps aloud, the participant is asked to repeat the steps while also demonstrating them. Sometimes the steps are written on a piece of paper to remind the person.

Reorganizing One's Environment to Offset Deficits. Two major reorganizing approaches have been developed and evaluated: shaping and environmental adaptation. *Shaping* is a strategy that developed out of operant behavior therapy and primarily involves differential reinforcement of successive approximations to a goal behavior. In this sense, it reorganizes complex behaviors into steps, with the first being relatively easy and the rest progressively becoming more difficult. For example, the complex task of introducing oneself—with the goal being smiling, shaking hands, and saying, "Hi, my name is X. Nice day, isn't it?"—would include six steps:

> Step 1: Walk up to another person.
> Step 2: Look the person in the eye.
> Step 3: Smile.
> Step 4: Say, "Hello."
> Step 5: Say, "My name is X."
> Step 6: Say, "Nice day, isn't it."

Using shaping, the person would first be reinforced for doing step 1 alone. Once this step is mastered, the next goal for which reinforcement is given is step 2 *and* step 1. Steps continue to be added until the person is able to master all six steps at once, which is the goal behavior. What has been a complex and cognitively overwhelming task for the person has been broken down and reorganized into doable steps.

Shaping has been applied to the cognitive deficits that result from psychiatric disability (Silverstein, Menditto, & Stuve, 1999, 2001; Menditto, Baldwin, O'Neal, & Beck, 1991). Typical applications use time as the unit to shape. Participants are begun on a cognitive task (such as a practical language or math task or office work such as folding, cutting, and stapling) for a short period of time (e.g., 5 minutes) and "shaped" up to 30 minutes or more (Bellus, Kost, Vergo, Gramse, & Weiss, 1999; Menditto, Baldwin, O'Neal, & Beck, 1991; Silverstein, Hitzel, & Schenkel, 1998; Spaulding, Storms, Goodrich, &

Sullivan, 1986). Reinforcers used in these programs were typically points or tokens that were part of a token economy (see Chapter 18 for more information on setting up token economies).

Environmental adaptation is the second reorganizational approach to cognitive rehabilitation; that is, otherwise complex environments are simplified so that people with cognitive impairments can accurately perceive and understand the reorganized setting (Heinssen, 1996). Research by Velligan and colleagues (2000; Velligan, Lam, Ereshefsky, & Miller, 2003) has identified two types of cognitive deficit that govern environmental alterations: apathetic and distracted. The "apathetic" individual tends to miss relevant environmental cues or is unable to organize multitask processes into meaningful steps. Relevant alterations may include using checklists for complex tasks, placing signs and equipment for daily activities in obvious places, and using labels or electronic devices (like computer-driven medication dispensers) to cue behavior.

Those with distracted patterns tend to be overwhelmed by attending to too much information in a situation, including cues that are irrelevant to the goals of the situation (Velligan et al., 2003). For example, a "distracted" person may not be able to clearly understand a message from her employer because she is also listening to a radio talk show in the background instead of tuning it out. Environmental alterations for such individuals may include organizing supplies to minimize incorrect use (placing complete outfits—shirt, pants, and underwear—in separate boxes in a closet) or minimizing background noise by turning off radios and television.

The Use of Computers in Targeted Cognitive Rehabilitation. As evident in the preceding discussion, cognitive rehabilitation frequently includes the use of computers. In fact, a variety of software packages have been developed to advance the cognitive rehabilitation agenda, though not necessarily for psychiatric disabilities. They have such names as *Jigsaw* (produced by Encyclopedia Britannica), *Captain's Log*, and *Foundation*. Packages specific to cognitive rehabilitation have been used along with other programs that, although developed for general education or entertainment purposes, may have properties relevant to rehabilitation goals. These include *Where in the World Is Carmen San Diego*, *Thinking Things 3*, and *Spell It Deluxe*. See Medalia and Revheim (1999) for a discussion of these software packages. The important issue for the rehabilitation provider is to discern which of these and other computer programs, if any, will benefit program participants.

Computers and sophisticated graphics have a natural allure for both rehabilitation providers and consumers. They offer the promise of cutting-edge technology that conceivably may remediate fundamental deficits. However, the promise of computer technology may have gotten ahead of the evidence that actually supports it. Certain criteria have been developed to help providers discern whether any particular computer package will be useful for the cognitive needs of participants:

- There is evidence that the computer package improves functioning in people with cognitive processing deficits.
- There is some evidence that the computer package improves cognitive deficits related specifically to the psychiatric disabilities of program participants.
- Improvement in these cognitive deficits yields some meaningful change in a person's life. It does not just teach participants to press the computer keys faster.

- The amount of time needed to gain benefits by participating in the program is not excessive. For example, daily, hour-long participation in a cognitive rehabilitation to improve attentional participation from the 50th to the 60th percentile would likely not be cost-effective.
- The requirement for associated computer hardware does not mean additional excessive costs. For example, a provider needs to consider whether buying virtual reality goggles that cost $10,000 is worth the expenditure.

INTEGRATED SOCIAL AND COGNITIVE REHABILITATION PROGRAMS

In order to improve social functioning by enhancing cognitive processes, innovators have developed several programs that purposefully integrate cognitive and social rehabilitation approaches. Two integrated programs have been well developed and studied: integrated psychological therapy and cognitive enhancement therapy.

Integrated Psychological Therapy. Integrated psychological therapy (IPT) combines cognitive retraining with social skills training to help people overcome processing deficits so they can better understand and interact with the social world (Brenner, Hodel, Roder, & Corrigan, 1992; Brenner, Roder, Hodel, Kienzle, Reed, et al., 1994; Roder, Mueller, Mueser, & Brenner, 2006; Spaulding et al., 1999). IPT is a highly structured approach that is conducted in hour-long group meetings, three to five times a week for several months to a year or more. Participants pass through five subprograms that begin by targeting basic cognitive processes and progress to social cognitive processes and social skills.

    1. *Cognitive differentiation.* Participants in this subprogram use repeated practice to improve stimulus discrimination during a card sorting task. When they show mastery of this task, they move to concept formation, which includes word problems involving antonym and synonym recognition. Finally, systematic search strategies are learned through a variation of "Twenty Questions."

    2. *Social perception.* One goal of this subprogram is to help participants discriminate between important social information and environmental noise. To accomplish this, program participants view a series of slides in which actors interact in different social situations and display emotions of varying intensity. As the program progresses, emotions and interactions increase in complexity and distress. Participants are instructed to report observable characteristics of the actors. They are asked to interpret the intent of actions and the emotion displayed by the actors.

    3. *Verbal communication.* This subprogram extrapolates skills learned in subprograms 1 and 2 to improve participants' ability to pay attention to the statements of others and to improve their ability to accurately understand what is being said. During initial exercises, participants are rewarded for repeating verbatim the comments of partners. Literal repetition is quickly replaced with paraphrasing partners' statements. Reciprocal communication is improved with questions that foster the mutuality of listening and talking. Participants are taught the utility of basic question words (*who, what, when, where*) and prompted to use them in conversation. Participants are instructed to continue free communication without immediate prompts.

    4. *Social skills* and 5. *Interpersonal problem solving.* The last two subprograms, which closely parallel more traditional behavior skills training, are reviewed in Chapter

10 (Liberman, 1988). Briefly, individual social skills are modeled by group leaders, participants rehearse the skills in role plays, and feedback is provided by peers. The IPT social skills subprogram is facilitated by focusing on cognitive components of the task. Similarly, acquisition of traditional problem-solving steps is enhanced by accentuating cognitive aspects. For example, selecting a solution to a problem involves cognitive analysis of the success and failure of similar solutions in other situations.

Cognitive Enhancement Therapy. Cognitive enhancement therapy (CET) seeks to remediate social impairments caused by deficits in cognitive processes by focusing on social cognition (Hogarty & Flesher, 1999; Hogarty, Flesher, Ulrich, Carter, Greenwald, et al., 2004). Social cognition, defined as the collection of mental operations fundamental to social interactions, which include the human ability to perceive the intentions of others (Brothers, 1990), has been shown to be a qualitatively distinct paradigm from information processing (Corrigan & Penn, 2001; Penn et al., 1997a). Note the bidirectional nature of social cognition: that is, a person acts on social information that reciprocally acts on that person.

CET is a complex program, both in theory and in practice, that seeks to meet the complex needs of social cognition. Like IPT, CET prescribes a series of exercises to be performed daily over several months or more of treatment. CET begins with exercises that address deficits in basic, nonsocial cognitive processes: attention, memory, and executive functioning. An example of an attention-enhancing task is *time estimates*, adapted from Ben-Yishay (1996). For this task, a 12-second clock is presented on a computer screen with four equidistant dots between each second. The instruction for participants is to press a lever when the second hand reaches a predetermined criterion time, such as 5, 10, or 20 seconds. A beep accompanies each movement of the second hand. Early or late responses to the targeted time will remove one of the interval dots, thus providing participants with visual feedback for having under- or overestimated the time. Rehabilitation providers can provide motivational cues as well: "Nice job on that one!" Providers can fade any of the three cues: auditory beeps, visual dots, or motivational feedback.

Basic cognitive activities are slowly augmented by strategies that are meant to enhance social cognition. These activities are largely conducted in small groups that focus on socialization, graduated in difficulty, and manipulated by coaching and cueing. Specific examples of small-group activities include the elaboration of motivational accounts, the formation of "condensed messages" (typically eight- to ten-word "telegrams" that reflect an interpersonal crisis in need of resolution), and the solving of real-life social dilemmas, in which the pros and cons of specific decisions are reviewed.

McGurk and colleagues (McGurk & Mueser, 2004; McGurk, Mueser, & Pascaris, 2005; McGurk, Mueser, Feldman, Wolfe, & Pascans, 2007) sought to enhance the outcomes of supported employment by integrating it with cognitive retraining. Immediate effects showed improvement in cognitive processes and, of perhaps even greater significance, employment goals. These effects were seen remarkably at 1 year and 2 to 3 year follow-ups.

THE EVIDENCE REVISITED

Cognitive rehabilitation seems to hold significant promise, which has not yet been realized in the evidence. Its principles and practices are both theoretically elegant and methodologically precise, leading to hypotheses that identify the cognitive roots of disabilities.

In addition, cognitive rehabilitation is linked to exciting computer-based technologies. Despite these assets, there is a lack of research showing that interventions of this kind lead to meaningful change. As reviewed above, there is research suggesting that some cognitive interventions yield improvements in measures of attention, memory, or executive functioning. What research has failed to find is that improvement in these measures is related to change in real-world phenomena linked to a person's life goals. We believe that the future promise of cognitive rehabilitation rests with this latter issue. As rehabilitation researchers and providers use the methods outlined here, they need to evaluate their impact on a person's ability to work, live independently, develop relationships, and perform other activities basic to key life goals.

COGNITIVE THERAPY FOR DEFICITS IN THOUGHT CONTENT

The major form of content deficit found in people with psychiatric disabilities encompasses the delusions found in many people with psychoses. Delusions are false beliefs that often impede people in achieving life goals because they impair complete understanding of social situations. This section reviews the form and impact of delusions, as well as cognitive therapy principles that help people overcome the disabilities that result from delusions.

Specific Deficits Related to Delusions and Other Thought Content

Delusions have traditionally been regarded as fixed, false beliefs, held with absolute conviction, and not amenable to reason (DSM-III-R; American Psychiatric Association, 1987). Widely acknowledged problems with the standard psychiatric definition, however, has led to phenomenological studies in which the experience of delusions are better described and understood. The DSM-IV (American Psychiatric Association, 1994) reflects this recent work; rather than "held with absolute conviction," the standard definition of delusions includes fluctuating rates of *conviction, preoccupation*, and *distress* caused by the false belief, as well as *action* taken in accordance with the belief (Garety & Freeman, 1999; Garety & Hemsley, 1994; Strauss, 1969). Examples of these factors or dimensions are summarized in Figure 12.4. The four dimensions are relatively independent of one another (Garety & Hemsley, 1994; Strauss, 1969) and have helped shift the conceptualization of delusions from categorical entities to those that are multidimensional (Appelbaum, Grisso, Frank, O'Donnell, & Kupfer, 1999; Blackwood, Fordyce, Walker, St. Clair, Porteous, et al., 2001; Garety & Freeman, 1999).

Accounts of delusional experiences have noted certain themes particular to people with schizophrenia. Persecutory, or paranoid, delusions (in which a person believes that others have malevolent intentions toward him or her) are most commonly observed (Bentall, 2001); grandiose delusions (in which a person has an exaggerated sense of his or her importance, power, knowledge, or identity), ideas of reference (in which apparently innocuous events are believed to have some special significance for the person), and delusions of control (a so-called passivity symptom whereby a person believes his or her actions are controlled by external forces) are also commonly reported (Frith, 1999). Delusions are evident not only in the most serious forms of mental illness in the schizophrenia spectrum, but also in association with other psychiatric illnesses, including affective psychosis (Goodwin, Alderson, & Rosenthal, 1971), mania (Taylor & Abrams, 1975), depression (Maher & Spitzer, 1993), and paranoia (Kendler, Gruenberg, &

Dimensions	Definition and Scale	Examples
Conviction	The degree to which the person believes the delusion is true. *On a 7-point scale, where 1 = not at all certain and 7 = absolutely certain, how certain are you that this belief is true?*	Jack is absolutely sure that the CIA is following him because he joined a radical student group in college. Shirley is not at all certain that the voices she hears in her head are from the devil.
Preoccupation	The amount of time the person spends thinking about the delusion. *On a 7-point scale, where 1 = never and 7 = all of the time, how much time do you spend thinking about the belief?*	Jack rarely thinks about the CIA following him; "After 8 years, I have learned how to live with it." Shirley cannot get the thoughts about devil voices out of her head no matter how she tries to block them.
Distress	The degree to which thinking about the belief upsets the person. *On a 7-point scale, where 1= not at all distressed and 7 = absolutely upset, how upset does thinking about this belief make you?*	Jack is not really distressed about the thought of being followed by the CIA. Shirley is highly anxious when she thinks about the devil voices.
Action	The motivation to act to control the delusion. *On a 7-point scale, where 1 = no desire to 7 = active effort, how much do you want to change or otherwise control these beliefs?*	Jack has learned how to live with "the CIA following me." He is not motivated to act further on these beliefs. Because Shirley is so tormented by the thought that the devil is speaking to her, she is trying to actively control her thoughts.

FIGURE 12.4. The four dimensions of delusions. Each might be assessed using a multipoint scale. Shirley's example shows how delusions (believing the devil may be talking to her) often arise from hallucinations (hearing voices).

PERSONAL EXAMPLE

Elaine Otumwe Says, "Do You Know Me? I'm Famous."

Elaine Otumwe was plagued by many psychotic symptoms, including delusions of reference. She reports that the news media seems to have some unexplainable fascination with her, because the local *News Gazette* runs a headline story about her almost every day. She admits that the story is not always in her name: "Sometimes they mix up the stories and get the specific incident wrong." Elaine believes that people on the street are beginning to take note of her fame. Last week she noticed several small groups at the local coffee shop talking about her. She does not know what to make of this; she does not feel particularly famous or great. Nor, for that matter, does she feel as though she is being hounded by the news. The frequent stories are just the everyday burden of living in a large metropolitan area.

Elaine's delusions are beginning to interfere with her life goals. She recently decided not to move out of a halfway house into her own apartment even though she can afford it, given the income from her job as a taxi dispatcher. When looking at a one-bedroom walk-up just a mile from her job, she was certain that the landlady recognized her and was going to increase her monthly rent because of her notoriety.

Tsuang, 1985). Evidence in support of a continuum of delusional beliefs also comes from studies conducted on nonclinical groups. Failures in *reality discrimination* (i.e., the inability to distinguish between real and imaginary events) can be experimentally demonstrated in individuals without apparent disorders (Perky, 1910; Bentall & Slade, 1985; McKellar, 1968; Posey & Losch, 1983; West, 1948; Young, Schnefter, Klerman, & Andreasen, 1986). Verdoux and colleagues (Verdoux, Maurice-Tison, Gay, van Os, Salamon, et al., 1998) found that research participants with no psychiatric history demonstrated some semblance of delusional ideation, which may include attenuated versions of beliefs regarding persecutory, mystic, and guilt experiences. Such findings suggest that delusions represent a dimensional phenomenon lying on a continuum with normality. Two models have been developed to explain the creation and maintenance of delusions as clinical phenomena: attributional bias and metarepresentation.

Attributional Bias

People without psychiatric disabilities typically demonstrate an attributional bias that is self-serving when explaining the causes of events. Positive outcomes in social situations are attributed to characteristics of the *individual*, such as a proactive orientation or an intrinsic quality. Nondelusional research participants often attribute negative outcomes to something *outside* themselves. Such biases are exaggerated among people with persecutory delusions. Specifically, as compared with nonclinical and depressed controls, people with paranoid ideation take too much credit for success (internal attribution of positive events), whereas responsibility for failure is excessively denied (external attribution of negative events) (Candido & Romney, 1990; Bentall, Kinderman, & Kaney, 1994; Kinderman & Bentall, 1997; Lyon, Kaney, & Bentall, 1994). People with paranoid ideation tend to personalize their attributions; in order to protect their self-esteem, those with persecutory delusions are more likely to blame other people rather than situational factors when things go wrong (Bentall et al., 1994; Kinderman & Bentall, 1997). Blaming others leads to false beliefs of the type that are observed in paranoid delusions.

Deficits in Metarepresentation

Metarepresentation, which sometimes is also studied as theory of mind (ToM; Frith, 1994), is the normative psychological ability to understand the intentions and behaviors of other people. ToM influences the way in which one attributes the causes of events in the social world to oneself and to others. The generation of causal attributions that are external and personal, as compared with those that are external and situational (i.e., delusional beliefs that are explained by another person's behavior rather than by circumstances) may be influenced by poor ToM abilities because they are constituents of a social-cognitive domain that involves anticipating and interpreting the behavior of others (Bentall, 1994; Kinderman & Bentall, 1997; Kinderman, Dunbar, & Bentall, 1998). Conversely, in order to appropriately generate external *situational* attributions, rather than blame other people (i.e., a personalizing bias) for negative events, one must have an appreciation of the mental states and intentions of others. A person must be able to imagine the world from the other's perspective and the way in which his or her own experiences affect reactions toward others. Deficits in metarepresentation such as disordered ToM abilities cause a person to misinterpret the intentions of others, which, in turn, may contribute to delusional ideation (Frith, 1994; Frith & Corcoran, 1996; Corcoran, 2001).

Interventions to Remediate These Deficits

Aaron Beck (1976), Albert Ellis (1977), and others (Freeman & Davis, 1990; Kendall, 1982) have developed cognitive therapy as a means for addressing the depression and anxiety that results from the content of certain thoughts. As outlined in Figure 12.5, Ellis described the problems caused by thoughts in terms of ABC: antecedents, beliefs, and consequences. The presumed relationship between antecedent and consequence is illustrated at the top of the figure (i.e., a student worries about failing a class test). This minor worry can become significant depression or anxiety when mediated by a belief such as "I must be a stupid student. I am worthless because I have no discipline to study for tests." The central goal of cognitive therapy is to teach people to identify these hurtful, usually irrational thoughts and obtain evidence that counters or reframes them. "Everyone fails a test once in a while. It does not mean I am a bad person." In this way, the person can control the psychological distress that results from these thoughts. Specific methods to facilitate the identification of and to counter irrational thoughts are summarized later in this section.

In the past decade or so, researchers have applied this model to delusional thoughts. Figure 12.6 provides several examples in which B is the delusional belief. Not only can delusional beliefs cause extreme psychological distress, but their consequences may undermine life goals. Hence, cognitive therapy may help people cope with delusions so that they do not undermine a person's work and independent living goals. Three review articles have summarized more than 20 outcome trials examining the impact of cognitive therapy on delusions (Dickerson, 2000; Gould et al., 2001; Rector & Beck, 2001). The results of studies on cognitive therapy for delusions have largely been positive, with investigations showing participants to have less conviction of and preoccupation with delusions after weekly trials of cognitive therapy. Follow-up analyses suggest that these effects are maintained over time when continued cognitive therapy is provided.

Less common have been studies that examined the effects of diminished conviction and preoccupation on corresponding symptoms or psychosocial domains. One study showed diminished delusions correlated with improved self-esteem (Haddock, Bentall, & Slade, 1996). A second study showed improved quality of life scores for individuals who

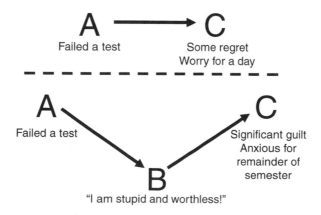

FIGURE 12.5. The ABCs that describe how irrational thoughts cause symptomatic reactions. A is the antecedent, the situation that leads up to a possible symptom. C is the consequence, the result of the antecedent. B is the intervening belief that can evolve an otherwise mild or benign consequence into depression or anxiety.

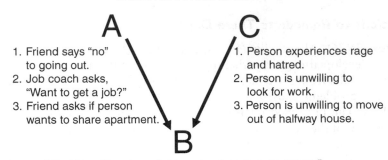

A
1. Friend says "no" to going out.
2. Job coach asks, "Want to get a job?"
3. Friend asks if person wants to share apartment.

C
1. Person experiences rage and hatred.
2. Person is unwilling to look for work.
3. Person is unwilling to move out of halfway house.

B

"That friend has been talking about me in a mean way."
"I don't need a job. I am a rich and famous rock star."
"The CIA will get me if I move out of the halfway house where the nurse protects me."

FIGURE 12.6. Using the ABCs to illustrate how delusions may cause psychological distress or undermine life goals.

participated in cognitive therapy, as compared with those who did not (Jackson, McGarry, Edwards, Hulbert, Henry, et al., 1998). Additional work in this area is especially important. What secondary gains do people realize when learning how to control their delusions? Given that delusions in cognitive therapy are described to the person as barriers to attaining personal goals (e.g., Harry is unable to get a good job because he believes he is George Washington), how does diminished conviction and preoccupation improve goal attainment?

The three reviews have also summarized the limitations of research on cognitive therapy for schizophrenia and other disabling psychiatric disorders, suggesting future directions for investigation in this area. One recurring concern about past research involves an inclusion criterion for research participation—namely, the research participant must be distressed by his or her delusions. As a result, many people with delusions are being excluded from research participation. Many people with delusions that inhibit their life goals are either not distressed by the delusions or do not realize that the associated distress is due to such a belief system. A related problem is the high rate of attrition of research participants; large numbers of people drop out of cognitive therapy because of dissatisfaction (Drury, Birchwood, Cochrane, & MacMillan, 1996b; Jackson et al., 1998; Haddock, Tarrier, Morrison, Hopkins, Drake, et al., 1999). If the effects of cognitive therapy are going to expand beyond the group of people who admit distress with their beliefs, then researchers need to think further about how engagement and other aspects of cognitive therapy should be framed for this group.

Another important problem with past research has been the lack of control for concurrent treatments. Researchers need to determine how cognitive therapy augments other psychosocial treatments. For example, what are the relative contributions of cognitive therapy to a treatment regimen that includes skills training and vocational rehabilitation? This limitation may be addressed using various research methods including multifactorial and dismantling designs. This kind of research can help to identify the specific active ingredients that lead to thought mastery as well as other psychosocial benefits.

Applying Cognitive Therapy to Delusions

Four steps are important in applying cognitive therapy to the needs of people with delusions.

1. Engage with the person to develop a collaborative therapeutic relationship.
2. Identify, assess, define, and otherwise make sense of the delusional beliefs that are causing problems for the person.
3. Strategically challenge these beliefs.
4. Once the person has become somewhat uncertain about the beliefs, help the person to develop counter beliefs.

ENGAGEMENT

Engagement is central to successful cognitive therapy for delusions. People with schizophrenia or other psychiatric disabilities have repeatedly been told that they should stop these crazy thoughts. As a result, people with delusions may be unwilling to talk with rehabilitation providers about their "odd" beliefs. In addition to the range of fundamental skills that foster any kind of therapeutic relationships, two tasks help counselors to break down this wall. First, providers challenge the stigmatizing idea that delusions are qualitative marks that distinguish the psychotic person from the "sane" population. Instead, as outlined earlier in this chapter, participants are educated to realize that delusions are just one of many examples of *problematic beliefs*. All people, whether challenged by psychiatric disability or not, have extreme beliefs that guide their lives, beliefs that cannot be shown to be true. Consider as an example some of our private thoughts regarding religion; empirical proof for such private phenomena as a god and miracles is impossible.

Framing delusions as being on the same continuum as normal experiences leads to the second task of engagement: identifying the *person's* goals of cognitive therapy. Rather than having the rehabilitation provider set the goal—"get rid of those crazy delusions"— the person decides the direction. The purpose of cognitive therapy, called collaborative empiricism by Beck (1976), is to determine how certain beliefs hurt the person and how these beliefs can be reframed or in some other way controlled so that the negative impact is diminished.

> Harry Summerfield believed he was George Washington, the first president of the United States, and that he did not work because "the president does not need a salary!" Hence, a therapeutic goal was to determine how to reconsider his being George Washington so that Harry did not have to give up on work and a social life. In this instance, neither the provider nor the client needed to argue about whether Harry's being Washington was true, only what to do about that belief so that the delusion did not narrow his life goals severely.

ASSESSING DELUSIONS

Consistent with basic psychopathological research reviewed above, delusions have been described by three dimensions, which are useful in defining the experience for individuals and in evaluating the impact of cognitive therapy (Chadwick, Birchwood, & Trower, 1996).

1. *Conviction.* How certain is a person about his or her delusional belief? Likert scale items can reliably represent this dimension, ranging from high (consistently certain the belief is true) to low (frequently uncertain about the truth of the belief).
2. *Preoccupation.* How much time does the person spend thinking about delusions? This can be directly assessed by asking the person how often he or she spends time think-

ing about the belief. Note that both conviction and preoccupation can change significantly over the normal course of a delusion, even without cognitive therapy. Hence, repeated measures are needed to obtain a relatively reliable picture of the current status of delusions.

3. *Accommodation.* Can the person conceive of beliefs or experiences that disconfirm the delusions? Individuals who can generate more examples of accommodation are likely to receive greater benefit from cognitive therapy (Brett-Jones, Garety, & Hemsley, 1987). Hence, accommodation in some ways represents readiness to change. Brett-Jones and colleagues (1987) have developed a method for more directly assessing readiness to change in a person with delusions, called Reaction to Hypothetical Contradiction. A plausible hypothetical event that challenges a delusion is proffered, and the individual is asked how such an event might alter the belief, if at all. People who are more open to hypothetical contradictions are more likely to benefit from cognitive therapy.

> Let us contrast an assessment of Harry's delusion about being George Washington with one concerning Joan Arnowicz, who believed she was getting communications from outer space. Prior to cognitive therapy, Harry was highly convinced that he was George Washington: "No doubt about it; I'm the first president!" Joan was less certain about outer space communications. "Sometimes it seems like aliens are sending me messages through my teeth; other times, I'm not so sure. I wonder if my mind is playing tricks on me again." Preoccupation also differed. Harry did not spend a lot of time thinking about being George Washington. "It's just who I am. Why should I need to think about it?" Joan, however, was significantly stressed by her delusions. She rarely had them out of her mind.
>
> Both Harry and Joan seemed willing to accommodate alternative explanations. When Harry read a history book that said Washington died more than 200 years ago, he wondered how this fit with his delusion. After Joan met a physicist from the local university who said direct communication with aliens was not physically possible, she felt a brief period of relief.

CHALLENGING BELIEFS

Rehabilitation providers who have engaged with participants, and have helped them to conceive of delusions from a cognitive perspective, use the same menu of belief challenging strategies as those adopted by cognitive therapists in addressing other psychiatric disorders. The place to begin is to obtain evidence that challenges a belief. The providers and the person jointly look for evidence that diminishes the person's conviction about a belief. As this evidence amasses, the individual is more easily able to generate counters to the delusion.

A second way to challenge delusions is through empirical testing. Consistent with the typical approach of cognitive therapy, the rehabilitation provider and the person jointly set up a test to see if reality corresponds with the assumptions outlined by the delusion. The steps in this kind of test include defining evidence that would challenge a delusion, identifying ways to search for this evidence, actually engaging in a study to look for such evidence, and examining the impact of the search on the ongoing beliefs (Chadwick et al., 1996; Fennell, 1989). Rehabilitation providers need to make sure that all phases of evidence gathering are part of a collaborative process. Some frustrated providers may assume the role of debater and try to unilaterally disprove a delusion. In this case, the provider has abandoned the basic principle of collaborative empiricism and has likely diminished engagement with the person. This pitfall can be avoided by remembering the primary assumption of the collaborative approach—namely, that all aspects of cognitive therapy are controlled jointly by the provider and the person. In fact, the provider may want to highlight the individual's control and power in the therapy situation when the person seems to be responding poorly to a specific component of the intervention.

When trying to find evidence that challenged Harry's belief about his being George Washington, the provider asked Harry to check out with respected others whether he could possibly be Washington. They first developed a survey about Washington, which Harry then administered to his minister and to the instructor in his composition class at night school. Results from both people added to Harry's uncertainty about being Washington. An equally important task was to challenge Harry's belief that work was not necessary because he had the president's salary. In particular, Harry asked these respected others whether they thought pursuit of a regular job was possible even if he was, in fact, George Washington. Affirmative responses from both endorsed his burgeoning desire to get work.

DEVELOPING COUNTERS

Once the person seems less certain about a problem belief, the rehabilitation provider helps the person to develop counters that may be used in the future when he or she is hampered by the delusional belief. For example, a counter to Harry's belief that he was George Washington might be, "No, that's impossible. I can't be the first president cause he's been dead for 200 years!" Like most other elements of cognitive therapy, central to developing counters is to ensure that the participant has an active role in generating counters and in trying them out to make sure that they are relevant and potent. Once again, frustrated providers may err by constructing counters on their own and imposing them on the person.

Role reversal is an excellent way to identify meaningful counters. In this approach, the provider assumes the voice of the delusion, stating different versions of it. The participant, in turn, argues against the delusion, providing counters that challenge it. Role reversal is particularly powerful because the provider can invoke statements that the participant has actually used to defend his or her belief. Consider this example with Harry and his rehabilitation provider:

REHABILITATION PROVIDER (RP): Harry, for this exercise, I'm going to argue that I am George Washington. And you are going to come up with reasons why that can't be so. Ready?

HARRY (H): Yep, let's do it.

RP: You know, Harry, it might seem strange, but sometimes I think I am George Washington.

H: You mean, like the first president of the United States, the Father of Our Country?

RP: That's me.

H: But that's impossible. he died more than 200 years ago.

RP: Yeah, but I am from Virginia and Washington was from Virginia.

H: Sure, but you know not everyone from Virginia could be George Washington.

RP: Maybe . . . , but when I walk down the street, it seems that everyone is staring at me. It must be because I am famous and the first president.

H: You know, sometimes I walk down the street and people stare at me too. I'm wondering if people are just being friendly and making eye contact. Or perhaps they are nosy. It doesn't have to mean they think you are the president.

RP: But sometimes I just feel special.

H: Me too. I think we are all special.

From this kind of interaction, Harry might identify counters that are poignant for him. These may include, "I am still special even if I am not George Washington, which is, of course, impossible because he died 200 years ago."

Role reversal is essentially a controlled argument in which the person struggles with and overcomes the problematic belief. Rehabilitation providers must keep in mind two caveats as they engage a person in this exercise. First, providers should not give up on the reversal too easily, as in the following exchange:

RP: You know, Harry, it might seem strange, but sometimes I think I am George Washington.

H. But that's impossible. He died more than 200 years ago.

RP: Wow, you are right. I never thought of it that way. I will stop thinking I am Washington.

In this case, the rehabilitation provider does not mirror the true tension that the person feels when holding to a problematic belief. The exchange between provider and person needs to progress through several give-and-takes to make sure that multiple facets of the delusion are challenged. Alternatively, the provider should not try to *win* the role reversal. In such a case, all the provider has done is to prove to the person that he or she is right for having a delusional belief. The provider should be attentive to how the participant is responding to the exercise and back off a bit when the person is unable to counter any part of the role reversal.

SUMMARY AND CONCLUSIONS

Many people with psychiatric disabilities are not able to achieve life goals because of cognitive deficits. Typically, these deficits are discussed in terms of process (how they think) and content (what they think). Process approaches frequently rely on information processes that represent the combination of individual processes (e.g., attention, memory, and executive functioning) to yield an integrated thinking person. Cognitive rehabilitation may facilitate improvement in these deficits in terms of three principles: restoration ("mental exercising" returns normal functioning), compensation (prostheses assists people with cognitive tasks), or reorganization (environmental manipulation help the person with cognitive tasks). Two types of interventions incorporate these three principles: (1) Targeted approaches seek to improve individual processes through repeated practice, mnemonic strategies, or lists and prompts. (2) Integrated programs attempt to ensure that improvements in cognitive functioning lead to better social functioning and achievement of life goals.

Delusions are common disabilities related to thought content. According to cognitive therapy, delusions are represented as extremes on a continuum. Steps to challenge delusional thoughts include engagement, belief definition, challenging the belief, and developing counters. Preliminary research on both cognitive rehabilitation and cognitive therapy for people with psychiatric disabilities has been encouraging. Outcome studies have shown the discrete cognitive processes and content areas that have improved after participating in these services. Future research in this area, however, must show how improvement in specific cognitive deficits leads to meaningful change for the person. Namely, how does being better able to attend to an information task translate into achieving work goals? Framing cognitive interventions in terms of real world goals can significantly benefit the ongoing development of treatment in this arena.

Chapter 13

Managing Criminal Justice Involvement

In recent years mental health professionals as well as criminal justice personnel have had growing concerns regarding the increasing numbers of individuals with severe mental illness involved with the criminal justice system. Current estimates are that 25–50% of persons with severe mental illness come in contact with the criminal justice system at some point during their illness (Silberberg, Vital, & Brakel, 2001; Solomon, 2003). However, adults suffering from mental illness have long been placed in jails and prisons (Quanbeck, Frye, & Altshuler, 2003). The large number of persons with mental illness housed in jails in the early 19th century is what prompted Dorothea Dix to begin her crusade to lobby state legislatures to develop state psychiatric facilities in order to improve the care of those with psychiatric disorders (Grob, 1966; Torrey, Stieber, Ezekiel, Wolfe, Sharfstein, et al., 1992). But the depopulation of these facilities in the mid-20th century, more stringent criteria for civil commitment, and the inadequacy of the community mental health system developed to replace these facilities have all been factors implicated in the recent influx of individuals with psychiatric disorders into the criminal justice system (Engel & Silver, 2001; Fisher, Wolff, & Roy-Bujnowski, 2003; Lamb & Weinberger, 1998).

Currently, there are more individuals incarcerated in this country than ever before. Between the mid-1970s and today, the rate of incarceration increased dramatically after a period of almost 50 years of stability, as displayed in Figure 13.1 (Visher & Travis, 2003). Consequently, there is an incentive on the part of criminal justice sector to reduce the numbers of individuals incarcerated, particularly those who could more appropriately be served elsewhere. Recently, criminal justice and mental health officials, along with researchers, policy makers, advocates, consumers, and family members have collaborated to develop innovative programs and policies to reduce the criminalization of these individuals (Crisanti & Love, 2002). This chapter first addresses whether severe mental ill-

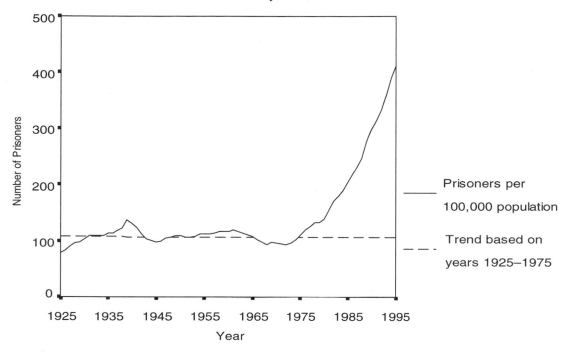

FIGURE 13.1. Prisoners per 100,000 population sentenced to state or federal prison on December 31 of the year. Data from Maguire and Pastore (1997). Figure reprinted from Draine (2003, p. 12). Copyright 2003 by Elsevier. Reprinted by permission.

ness contributes to engagement in criminal behavior, then presents the extent of criminal justice involvement by persons with mental illness, causative factors and theoretical explanations for these high rates of involvement, and the existing legal–mental health intervention strategies that have emerged to prevent and remedy the current situation.

DOES MENTAL ILLNESS LEAD TO CRIMINAL BEHAVIOR?

In the last decade there have been a few studies, all conducted in Nordic countries, that employed birth cohort designs to address this question. These studies have consistently found that those with severe psychiatric disorders, particularly schizophrenia, are at increased risk of committing nonviolent offenses, and at higher risk for violent offending (Arseneault et al., 2000; Brennan et al., 2000; Rasanen, Tiihonen, Isohanni, Rantakallio, Lehtonen, et al., 1998). Tengstrom and his colleagues (Tengstrom, Hodgins, Grann, Langstrom, & Kullgren, 2004) point out that community studies as well as diagnostic studies of convicted offenders have documented consistent findings with birth cohort studies. These investigations found that individuals with mental illness have higher rates of convictions for crimes, mainly violent crimes, than those without mental illness. Tengstorm and associates (2004), as well as others (Monahan, 1997; Wessely, Castle, Douglas, & Taylor, 1994), further acknowledge that regardless of the fact that the rates of these crimes are elevated among persons with mental illness, the percentage of those with mental illness who offend is very low, often in the single digits. Furthermore, because the rate of mental illness in general is low and the risk of violence among this population is moderate, the contribution of violence to society by individuals with mental illness is slight (Swanson, 1994).

Although the results from these birth cohort studies seem particularly convincing in regard to a causal link between mental illness and criminal behavior, they are correlational designs that have not always taken into account the primary potential statistical confounds (Hiday, 2006). Possible biases need to be considered when the evidenced is used to support a causal relationship between mental illness and violent behavior, which has generally been operationalized as criminal behavior (Arboleda-Florez, Holley, & Crisanti, 1998). Major causal variables that need to be controlled for are substance misuse, psychopathy/antisocial personality disorder, history of victimization, community disorganization, and socioeconomic status (Hiday, 2006; Arboleda-Florez et al., 1998).

In regard to substance abuse, there are few persons diagnosed with schizophrenia without substance abuse included in investigations correlating mental disorders with violent behavior (Hiday, 2006). The risk of violence is markedly higher among persons with substance abuse disorders than among those with schizophrenia or other psychotic disorders (Eronen, Angermeyer, & Schulze, 1998). Further, much of the relationship between mental illness and criminal behavior is explained by psychopathy, more than by substance abuse (Tengstrom et al., 2004; Hiday, 2006). Among offenders with schizophrenia, two groups have been identified: early-onset offenders, who have a consistent pattern of antisocial behavior from childhood; and late starters, who have no history of antisocial behavior or criminality prior to onset of the mental disorder. Those in the early-onset group, in whom psychopathy is very high, are very similar to criminal offenders without mental illness (Tengstrom et al., 2004). In addition, a history of child abuse has been found to be associated with violent reactive behavior and criminal offending in general population studies, but has not been addressed in studies of persons with mental illness, even though, as a group, persons with severe mental illness have extremely high rates of child abuse and victimization. Another often neglected variable is the community from which persons with mental illness come. Such communities are characteristically of low socioeconomic status and high unemployment rates, are resource deprived, and tend to have prevalent violent behaviors both inside and outside the residents' home environments, which results in violent behaviors being a learned response pattern (Hiday, 2006). Consequently, Hiday (2006) states that "each of these factors . . . has a high prevalence among persons with severe mental illness who are violent, which makes each a potential confounder in the association between severe mental illness and violence. Not only may each of them alone be a partial cause of violence of persons with major mental disorders, but also when they occur at the same time, which they commonly do, they may explain much of the association between severe mental illness and violence" (p. 321). Given that arrest for major criminal offenses often used as a proxy for violence, this statement could use the term *violent criminal offending* or *criminal offending*, rather than *violence*.

PREVALENCE OF PERSONS WITH MENTAL ILLNESS IN THE CRIMINAL JUSTICE SYSTEM

The Bureau of Justice Statistics estimated that 283,800 mentally ill offenders were incarcerated in state and federal prisons and local jails in the United States at midyear 1998 (Ditton, 1999). This figure is based on surveys conducted by the Bureau, which found that 16% of state prison inmates, 7% of federal inmates, and 16% of those in local jails reported either a current mental or emotional condition or an overnight stay in a mental hospital. In addition, approximately 16% of 547,800 probationers responded positively to the same two criteria for mental illness (Ditton, 1999, p.1). Prior studies estimating the rates of mental illness among those incarcerated have ranged from 8 to 16%, contingent on the methodology, the institutional setting, and the operational definition of mental illness employed (Ditton, 1999). These figures are comparable to estimates based on clinical studies suggesting that 6–15% of individuals in local jails and 10–20% in state prisons have severe mental illness (Lamb & Weinberger, 1998; Lovell & Jemelka, 1998).

Epidemiological studies conducted by Teplin and her colleagues (Teplin, 1990, 1994; Teplin et al., 1996) have found rates of severe psychiatric illnesses, including depression, mania, and schizophrenia, to be higher among jail detainees than in the general population. These investigators interviewed 728 randomly selected male detainees entering Chicago's Cook County jail. Using the National Institute of Mental Health Diagnostic Interview Schedule (DIS), they found that 6.4% of jail detainees met the current diagnostic criteria for these severe psychiatric diagnoses and 9.48% met lifetime criteria, as compared with 1.8% current and 4.4% lifetime rates for the Epidemiologic Catchment Area (ECA) sample. Two-thirds of this jail detainee sample had a disorder other than antisocial personality disorder in their lifetimes, and half of them had an episode within the 2-week period prior to the interview (Teplin, 1994). These investigators concluded that the prevalence rates in the jail sample were significantly higher than in the five-city sample of the ECA and these results were not due to an artifact of race or age (Teplin, 1990).

During the past 30 years, a number of small-scale studies have been conducted that attempted to estimate the prevalence of incarcerated individuals with mental illness; these estimates varied from as low as 5% for those with psychosis to more than 90% with a psychiatric disorder of those who were referred for mental health evaluations (e.g., Fisher, Packer, Simon, & Smith, 2000; Lamb & Grant, 1982, 1983; Whitmer, 1980; Teplin, 1990; Schuckit, Herman, & Schuckit, 1977). A recent study by Fisher, Packer, Banks, Smith, Simon, et al. (2002), employing the DIS with a sample of male detainees in two jails in Massachusetts, found that 10% met the lifetime criteria for schizophrenia, major depression, and bipolar disorder, with more than half of those meeting the criteria reporting at least one psychiatric hospitalization.

There is some evidence to indicate that a large portion of individuals with mental illness among jail inmates were previously homeless. Although homeless persons generally tend to have a higher rate of criminal activity than the general population, those with psychiatric illnesses among the homeless population have an even higher rate of criminal activity (Fischer, 1988; Lamb & Grant, 1982, 1983; Martell, Rosner, & Harmon, 1995; McNeil, Binder, & Robinson, 2005; Michaels, Zoloth, Alcabes, Braslow, & Safyer, 1992; Snow, Baker, & Anderson, 1989; Solomon & Draine, 1999). Belcher (1988) observed that persons who were mentally ill and homeless were particularly vulnerable to engaging in criminal behavior as a result of a lack of structure and resistance to engagement with psychiatric treatment services. Some studies have found that individuals in this population tend to be charged with minor offenses, whereas others determined that a number were charged with serious crimes, but even these serious charges seem to be survival strategies (Solomon & Draine, 1995c, 1995d). However, only a few of these investigators asserting that individuals with mental illness are generally arrested for minor offenses made comparisons to the nature of charges among those charged who did not have mental illness, and the fact is that most individuals from the general population are charged with minor offenses.

Given the large numbers of individuals incarcerated, even a small proportion who have mental illness is a large number of individuals. This situation presents difficulties for law enforcement and correctional staff members. Borum, Deane, Steadman, and Morrissey (1998) surveyed officers in three jurisdictions and determined that encounters with individuals with mental disorders were frequent and were seen as a significant problem for their police departments. Similarly, other research has found that correctional staff members perceive the presence of psychological problems among inmates as second only to overcrowding as their most significant concern (Gibbs, 1983).

It is therefore not surprising that criminal justice officials whose institutions are overcrowded and underresourced feel that they are burdened with being the primary institutional provider of mental health care. Jails and prisons in the United States today house more individuals with mental illness than do all of the state hospitals (Sigurdson, 2000), and their numbers have exponentially increased from 1955 to 1985, rising from 185,780 to 481,393 (Palermo, Gumz, & Liska, 1992). As based on a national survey of jails regarding the treatment of persons with mental illness, psychiatrist E. Fuller Torrey has claimed that jails have become the largest de facto mental institutions in the country; the Los Angeles County jail provides mental health treatment to 3,300 of the 21,000 inmates housed per day in this facility (Torrey et al., 1992; Torrey, 1995).

POLICE DECISIONS:
INCARCERATION VERSUS PSYCHIATRIC TREATMENT

The current incarceration of large numbers of persons with severe psychiatric disabilities in prisons or jails is due in part to the behaviors of police officers. The police have a duty to intervene in the lives of persons with mental illness on the basis of two common-law principles: "The power and authority of the police to protect the safety and welfare of the community, and the state's paternalistic or parens patriae authority, which dictates protection for citizens with disabilities who cannot care for themselves, such as those who are acutely mentally ill" (Lamb, Weinberger, & DeCuir, 2002, p. 1266). When police are dealing with individuals who are mentally ill and pose a threat of danger to themselves or the community, both principles are operating.

The police have a great deal of discretion in how a disturbing incident or minor crime is handled. The police are generally the first to respond to a mental health crisis situation. They are then put in the position of identifying an individual as one in need of psychiatric treatment and then transporting the individual to a treatment facility, or making the determination that the illegal activity takes precedent and arresting the individual. Consequently, police officers assume the role of primary gatekeepers in determining whether the mental health or criminal justice system is the most appropriate means to meet the needs of the individual and to protect community safety (Lamb et al., 2002). They also have the option of dealing with an occurrence informally, attempting to calm the situation. On the basis of an observational study, Teplin and Pruett (1992) categorized the individuals with mental illness who were dealt with in informal dispositions by police as neighborhood characters, troublemakers, or quiet "crazies." These investigators found that more than 70% of persons with mental illness were handled with these informal dispositions, but mentally ill suspects were still arrested twice as often as suspects who were not mentally ill (46.7 vs. 27.8%) and hospitalizations were initiated for only 13.3% of the mentally ill suspects. These findings were quite consistent with Bittner's (1967) study that was conducted more than two decades earlier. Thus, Teplin and Pruett (1992) concluded that police function as "streetcorner psychiatrists," and Bittner (1967) referred to these practices as "psychiatric first aid." However, a more recent study that employed two large-scale, multisite field research data sets examining police behavior found that police were not more likely to arrest mentally disordered suspects, when controlling for factors that are known to influence police discretion (Engel & Silver, 2001). In fact, in these analyses mental illness was found to serve as a protective factor against arrest.

There are a variety of structural factors that keep police from transporting to treatment facilities individuals who have committed a minor crime (an alleged major crime leaves little discretion—the person is arrested) and appear to be mentally ill. Taking individuals to a psychiatric emergency service can take a great deal of police officers' time, thus keeping them from performing their other duties. Furthermore, police officers frequently wait at these facilities only to find that individuals are not admitted, owing to stringent commitment requirements, or, if admitted, are quickly released. In addition, officers are sometimes treated with hostility by staff members of these mental health facilities and with a lack of respect for their judgment regarding an individual's need for treatment. Knowing these response patterns may prevent officers from even attempting these options, as arrest may be a more efficient disposition from their perspective (Lamb et al., 2002; Teplin & Pruett, 1992). Teplin and Pruett (1992) found that "it is common practice for police to obtain a signed complaint from a third party (thus facilitating arrest) even in situations where psychiatric hospitalization was thought to be the more appropriate disposition" (p. 147). This procedure gives them the option of arresting the individual in the event that hospitalization is not forthcoming. Thus, police may resort to "mercy bookings" even though these bookings may be unconstitutional, but detaining individuals with mental illness who are not suspected of a crime is not prohibited in most states (Lamb et al., 2002). Taking into custody an individual who appears to be in need of mental health care may be perceived as a better alternative to doing nothing, as the police believe that the individual is more likely to receive the needed care if arrested (Laberge & Morin, 1995; Lurigio, 2000). They are of the opinion that the person will, in all probability, be evaluated and treated by a mental health professional. Families and others, such as landlords, have been found to call the police to handle unmanageable individuals and to provide transportation to mental health emergency facilities (Bonovitz & Bonovitz, 1981; Bonovitz & Guy, 1979; Hiday, 1999). Families have also reported the use of restraining orders, with the expectation that the ill relative will violate the order and be arrested and thus receive needed treatment (Solomon et al., 1995a).

Although police are the first to respond to psychiatric crises, they frequently feel ill equipped to identify and intervene in cases involving mental illness (Borum et al., 1998). In other situations, persons who have been evaluated as mentally ill by a mental health professional may not be deemed so by law enforcement personnel, and therefore transport to a treatment facility is not seen as an option. In other cases, mental illness may be assessed as drug or alcohol intoxication, especially if at the time of the incident the person was using such a substance. It is also possible that in the confusion or chaos of the situation, signs of mental illness may not be observed (Lamb & Grant, 1982; Lamb et al., 2002). Moreover, if the individual engages in violence, the likelihood of arrest increases (Robertson, Pearson, & Gibb, 1996).

CAUSAL FACTORS AND THEORETICAL EXPLANATIONS FOR CRIMINAL INVOLVEMENT

The criminalization hypothesis has been put forth as one of the explanations for persons with mental illness being placed in the criminal justice system. This hypothesis has come to mean that persons with mental illness, who prior to deinstitutionalization would have been in mental hospitals, are now entering the criminal justice system. Researchers have operationalized criminalization in terms of arrests, prosecution, and incarceration in prisons and jails (Lamb & Weinberger, 1998). Thus, *criminalization* has taken on a diversity of meanings since the term was first coined by Abramson (1972), who observed increasing numbers of persons with severe mental illness being arrested for minor offenses instead of being treated in the mental health system. The research to test this hypothesis has included examining police encounters with persons with mental illness, arrest rates, prevalence of mental disorders among jail and prison populations, and referrals of mentally ill offenders to forensic units (Hiday, 1999). The results of these studies have been mixed, showing some support for this hypothesis (e.g., Engel & Silver, 2001; Hiday, 1999; Teplin, 1985). But because of the lack of longitudinal data, the direct connection between deinstitutionalization and criminal justice involvement cannot be tested (Teplin, 1993).

The "psychiatricization" of criminal behavior has been put forth as another explanation as to why there are high rates of persons with mental illness found in the criminal justice system (Hiday, 1999; Melick, Steadman, & Cocozza, 1979; Monahan, 1973). This theory assumes a shift in responsibility from the criminal justice system to the mental health system, suggesting that deviant behavior is being interpreted as a psychiatric problem. In support of this, Melick and her colleagues (Melick, Steadman, & Coccozza, 1979) showed that over a 30-year period, starting in the mid 1940s, the number of males being admitted to psychiatric hospitals in New York with histories of arrest steadily and consistently increased. In addition, the trend to hospitalize individuals with substance abuse and antisocial personalities has contributed support for this hypothesis (Hiday, 1999).

The hydraulic or balloon theory of social control proposes that when there is a change in the population of one institution that serves the societal function of social control or keeping from view those whom society sees as deviant, there will be an inverse change of equal magnitude in another social control institution. Therefore, when there is a reduction in state psychiatric hospitals, there is an increase in jails and prisons. This hypothesis was tested by Penrose (1939) for 18 European countries, where he consistently found an inverse relationship between the populations of prisons and psychiatric hospitals. More recently, Teplin (1991) reviewed the research in relation to this hypothesis and concluded that the results were mixed, contingent on the types of studies assessed.

A theory related to the hydraulic perspective is the criminological concept of incapacitation, which is based on the assumption that if individuals who have a propensity to commit crimes are incarcerated, their ability to engage in criminal behavior will be eliminated and, consequently, crime rates will be reduced (Fisher et al., 2003). Confinement, regardless of type of institution, reduces criminal activity. Data in support of this theory have resulted from comparisons of arrests prior to 1960, which typically showed arrest rates for psychiatric patients to be lower than those for the general population, whereas arrest rates after the 1960s were equal to or higher than those for the general population (Harry & Steadman, 1988; Rabkin, 1979). There is little question that deinstitutionalization has increased the capacity of persons with severe mental illness to engage in criminal activity. This population now spends more time in the community, where there is greater opportunity to engage in criminal behavior. Similarly, this is the situation for the use of drugs and alcohol by this population.

Another explanation is that persons who are mentally ill are dangerous, and dangerous people are likely to engage in criminal activity, particularly violent crimes (Hiday, 1999; Lamb & Weinberger, 1998). For years it was thought that persons who were mentally ill were no more likely to be violent than the general public. However, recent research has shown that individuals who are mentally ill are moderately more violent, especially when abusing substances and when experiencing certain active psychotic symptoms. The relationship between mental disorders and violence/illegal behavior is further compounded when individuals are nonadherent to prescribed medications (Lamb & Weinberger, 1998; Link, Andrews, & Cullen, 1992; Mulvey, 1994; Monahan, 1992; Swartz, Swanson, Hiday, Borum, Wagner, et al., 1998). Psychopathy, usually measured by the Hare Psychopathy Checklist, composed of factor 1—selfish, callous, and remorseless use of others, and factor 2—chronically unstable and antisocial lifestyle, has been determined to be a significant predictor of violent criminal recidivism (Hare, Clark, Grann, & Thorton, 2000; Harris, Rice, & Quinsey, 1993; Monahan, Steadman, Silver, Appelbaum, Robbins, et al., 2001). Swanson, Swartz, Estroff, Borum, Wagner, et al. (1998) also noted that the high crime areas in which many persons with severe mental illness live may be seen as dangerous and threatening to them and thus produce a violent response. However, most studies do not find persons with mental illness being arrested for the more serious offenses (Hiday, 1999).

CONSENSUS FOR IMPROVING RESPONSE REGARDING CRIMINAL JUSTICE INVOLVEMENT

Recently, the Council on State Governments (CSG) established the Criminal Justice/Mental Health Consensus Project to respond to the critical needs of persons with mental illness involved in or at risk of being involved in the criminal justice system. The objective of this 2-year effort was to develop policy recommendations to improve the response to this population (Thompson, Reuland, & Souweine, 2003). CSG partnered with a number of national criminal justice and mental health organizations. The report (available at *www.consensusproject.org*) resulted in 50 policy statements and hundreds of recommendations that reflect the numerous points within the criminal justice system at which changes can be made to improve the response of the system to persons with mental illness—from "initial contact with law enforcement, to pretrial issues, adjudication, and sentencing, to incarceration and reentry" (Thompson et al., 2003, p. 35). A series of policy statements, along with approaches to implementing the policies, are presented. The themes included the need to (1) improve collaboration between the mental health and criminal justice systems, (2) have training and cross-training of criminal justice and mental health practitioners, and (3) have accessible and effective mental health services that are responsive to individuals who are difficult and not successfully engaged with community-based mental health services.

STRATEGIES AND INTERVENTIONS FOR MANAGING CRIMINAL INVOLVEMENT

To address the issues of criminal justice involvement of persons with mental illness, there needs to be a collaborative effort that includes representatives of the criminal justice and mental health systems, as well as families and consumers. An interagency task force for planning and continuing oversight should consist of representatives from mental health governmental entities and agencies, the local jail and prison, police and/or sheriff's department, the probation and parole departments, district attorney's office, pretrial services, and district courts (Schnapp & Cannedy, 1998). In some locations these task forces have also included members of the National Alliance for the Mentally Ill (Finn & Sullivan, 1988). In some cases, these task forces have been established in response to horrific incidents between law enforcement and persons with mental illness. For example, the Crisis Intervention Team (CIT) model was initiated in Memphis, Tennessee, as a result of a person with mental illness being killed in a situation that could have been avoided (Perez, Leifman, & Estrada, 2003). "Suicide by cop" is the most difficult situation for officers to cope with. This is an incident in which an individual engages in life-threatening behavior with the intent to provoke the police "to fire at the suicidal individual in self-defense or to protect civilians" (Lamb et al., 2002, p. 1269).

A number of specialized strategies and interventions have emerged from such planning groups to respond to the needs of persons with severe mental illness involved in the criminal justice system. These have been developed to intersect at various points in the criminal justice system, ranging from initial police contact, court hearings, incarceration in prisons and jails, to community reentry upon release from incarceration. A Sequential Intercept Model has been developed that proposes "points of interception," or opportunities for interventions to keep people with mental illness from entering or getting more deeply involved in the criminal justice system (*darla.neoucom.edu/CJCCOE/about.html*). The points are outlined in Table 13.1. The following section describes the various prominent current interventions and an assessment of their effectiveness, which is relatively limited.

The development and establishment of mental health–legal interventions to address the issue of persons with mental illness being in contact with the criminal justice system have been proliferating at an expanded rate. A precipitant of this situation has been the willingness of the government to expand resources for their development and implementation. In 2000 the federal government passed the America's Law Enforcement and Mental Health Project Act, which instructed the attorney general of the United States to fund demonstration projects. This resulted in the Mental Health Court Grant Program's funding a number of courts, and reauthorization of this legislation has occurred (*www.mentalhealthcourtssurvey.com*). Legislation entitled the "Mentally Ill Offender Treatment and Crime Reduction Act" recently passed both houses, authorizing $5 million for states and communities to use for such purposes as jail diversion, treatment of individuals with serious mental illness while incarcerated, and community reentry programs (*Consensus Project Newsletter*, 2005).

These interventions are designed to bring mental health treatment and the criminal justice system together in ways that will promote the mental health of persons with psychiatric disorders who come into contact with the criminal justice system, at the same time enabling them to meet their responsibilities for their criminal actions. A legal

---

TABLE 13.1. Sequential Intercept Model

- The ultimate intercept: best clinical practices in an accessible mental health system
- Prearrest diversion: law enforcement/ emergency services (e.g., CIT)
- Postarrest: initial detention/initial hearings
- Postinitial hearings: jail, courts, forensic evaluations, and forensic commitments
- Reentry from jails, state prisons, and forensic hospitalization
- Community corrections and community support

Note. Data from Ohio Criminal Justice Coordinating Center of Excellence (*darla.neoucom.edu/CJCCOE/about.html*).

approach entitled *therapeutic jurisprudence* offers a helpful way to think about and understand the design of these interventions and their effectiveness. Therapeutic jurisprudence proposes to examine how knowledge, theories, and insights from mental health and related disciplines can help shape "legal rules, legal procedures, and the roles of legal actors (such as lawyers and judges)" that are "consistent with the principles of justice and other constitutional values" (Winick, 1997, p. 185). Within this framework, these legal mechanisms are assessed in terms of whether and how they produce therapeutic or antitherapeutic outcomes. Therapeutic jurisprudence elicits the examination of these consequences with the use of social science "to identify them and to ascertain whether the law's antitherapeutic effects can be reduced, and its therapeutic effects enhanced, without subordinating due process and other justice values" (Winick, 1997, p. 185). This approach views the law and its procedures as having the potential to be a therapeutic agent, and therapeutic jurisprudence has grown considerably since its inception by Wexler and Winick in the early 1990s. Therapeutic jurisprudence has been applied in a diversity of areas, including psychiatric rehabilitation (Spaulding, Poland, Elbogen, & Ritchie, 2000; Wexler & Winick, 1991b).

Using this framework does not presume that any combination of mental health considerations with the legal process is inherently therapeutic and legally responsible. For example, Wolff's (2003) assessment of specialized mental health courts found them inconsistent with the legal principle of equal treatment under the law and proffers an alternative model of having a mental health professional participate in the courtroom proceedings. Consequently, therapeutic jurisprudence requires consideration of the law

---

PERSONAL EXAMPLE

Ken Monroe's Pathway into the Criminal Justice System

Ken Monroe, a 35-year-old African American man with a diagnosis of paranoid schizophrenia, had never been engaged in any long-term treatment and had had no contact with any mental health professional in more than 2 years. Just prior to his entanglement with the criminal justice system, he had an exacerbation of his symptoms of paranoia. His paranoia was focused on his family and neighbors, whom he thought were out to get him. To protect himself, he checked into a motel. While he was residing in the motel, his paranoia persisted and he soon became concerned that other motel guests were also out to get him. This paranoia reached a state in which he felt that these individuals were going to do him physical harm, so he wanted the police to protect him from them. He then devised a plan that involved throwing objects out the windows of his second-story motel room onto the cars in the parking lot. These objects ranged from books to the room's TV set. He felt that this was the only avenue available to him, as he was too paranoid to use the telephone or leave his room.

Ken was extremely pleased when the police responded to his actions, having been called by the motel manager. However, his elation was quickly diminished when he found that he was the one being arrested, not the other motel guests. He was initially charged with violating an obscure section of the criminal code related to projecting missiles, but was later pleaded down to simple assault. Ken subsequently spent almost a year in jail, as he was denied bail. For 6 months he was pretrial status and was then sentenced to 11½ to 23 months, of which he served another 5½ months, and the rest of his time on parole in the community.

and its procedures, as well as mental health outcomes, and calls for social scientists to evaluate these interventions in light of social science research methods (Wexler & Winick, 1991a). To date, none of these interventions have been evaluated in this context. Wolff's (2003) proposal, based on an analytic assessment, requires hard scientific evidence generated by employing a solid research investigation of the two alternative approaches, as well as the usual legal processing of individuals with psychiatric disorders to determine which enhances the therapeutic outcomes while maintaining legal considerations.

Intervention with Persons with Mental Illness at Police Contact

Police encounters constitute 7–10% of all law enforcement contacts (Deane, Steadman, Borum, Veysey, & Morrissey, 1999). Although, for the most part, these contacts occur without incident, a number of police perceive such encounters with mentally ill persons as operationally problematic and they feel ill equipped to handle these situations (Borum et al., 1998; Hails & Borum, 2003). The first-generation efforts to respond to the needs of police included the training of law enforcement personnel regarding recognition of and managing mental illness, as well as the availability of and access to mental health resources (Hails & Borum, 2003; Lamb et al., 2002). Although these trainings have not been systematically evaluated, they are thought to be helpful and not likely to be harmful. However, they are thought not to be sufficient to change the behaviors of police in their encounters with individuals with mental illness. There is a need for the establishment of specialized programs (Borum, 2000). Currently, cross training between law enforcement and mental health personnel is considered to be most effective (Schnapp & Cannedy, 1998). Mental health personnel need to have more knowledge about the criminal justice system and its mechanics, just as officers need to be knowledgeable about mental health resources.

Because of the perceived deficiencies of the first-generation responses, a second generation of specialized responses has been established. These are collaborative efforts between mental health and criminal justice personnel and are highly focused, very sophisticated, and quite promising (Hails & Borum, 2003). These programs are referred to as prebooking, pre-arrest, or police-based diversion programs, as the diversion occurs prior to arrest or charges being filed by the police (Steadman, Deane, Borum, & Morrissey, 2000). Arrests are avoided by having the police make direct referrals to mental health treatment, thereby, keeping persons with severe mental illness from entering the criminal justice system (Hails & Borum, 2003). On the basis of the results of surveys of police departments in U.S. cities with populations of more than 100,000, Deane and her colleagues (1999) categorized the specialized police programs into three groups:

1. Police-based specialized response—Use sworn officers who have special mental health training to provide crisis intervention services and to act as liaisons to the formal mental health system (some have additional services as a secondary response).
2. Police-based specialized mental health response—Police departments hire mental health consultants who provide on-location and telephone consultation to officers in the field.
3. Mental health-based specialized response—Mobile crisis teams are developed, which are part of community mental health service delivery systems, but have established specific arrangements with police departments to respond to special needs at the location of an incident.

These investigators also found that two-thirds of all departments that responded, including those without specialized response programs, rated themselves as being at least moderately or very effective in managing persons with mental illness in crisis. There has been virtually no systematic research on these programs, but the limited research seems to indicate that they have promise in regard to reducing arrests and the use of force by police officers (Hails & Borum, 2003; Lamb, Weinberg, & Gross, 1999; Lamb, Shaner, Elliot, DeCuir, & Foltz, 1995; 2004; Steadman, Deane, Morrissey, Westcott, Salasin, et al., 1999b; Scott, 2000). In the evaluation of these programs, it is difficult to be sure that diverted individuals are truly those who would likely have been arrested, if not for the existence of these diversion programs, and not merely psychiatric crisis clients. This sampling problem complicates evaluation of these interventions (Draine & Solomon, 1999).

The Memphis CIT model has become the model of choice nationally and has been replicated in a number of cities. As of 2003, this model had been implemented in 18 jurisdictions (Hails & Borum, 2003). This program has been designated a model by the National Alliance for Mental Illness and the American Association of Suicidology. As opposed to training all officers to handle mental health crises, the CIT model selects to train and deploy officers who have the greatest interest, the most amenable attitudes, and the most appropriate interpersonal skills to function as the first-line response to specialized mental health calls (Hails & Borum, 2003). The two main features of this program are a crisis intervention team staffed by specifically trained police officers and a crisis triage center, based in an emergency department at a regional medical center. The service program has a no-refusal policy and a quick police turnaround time of less than 30 minutes (Steadman, Stainbrook, Griffin, Draine, Dupont, et al., 2001b). A recent evaluation of this program found that diverted individuals had improvements in symptoms 3 months after being diverted (Cowell, Broner, & Dupont, 2004). This program also resulted in reduced criminal justice costs, but treatment costs were higher for diverted individuals. Consequently, the program was associated with higher costs (Cowell et al., 2004). Another study found that this program had a low arrest rate as compared with diversion programs in other locations (Steadman et al., 2000).

Another prebooking program that is considered a model program by the National Institute of Law Enforcement and Criminal Justice and by Torrey and colleagues (1992) is Montgomery County Emergency Services (MCES) in Pennsylvania. This is both a pre- and postbooking service (postbooking is discussed below). MCES is situated in a freestanding psychiatric hospital, which in a crisis can dispatch an ambulance and staff members who are trained as both emergency medical technicians and psychiatric crisis specialists; police can also transport an individual to the facility. MCES has a no-refusal policy for police, and police spend an average of 20 minutes in the drop-off process. If an ambulance is sent, police just need to provide a statement at the scene of the incident (Draine & Solomon, 1999; Steadman et al., 2001b). A recent evaluation found that diversion did not significantly impact future arrests at 3 or 12 months a compared with an in-jail mental health program (Blank, Draine, & Solomon, 2003). On the basis of an assessment of the aforementioned two programs, as well as one other, Steadman and associates (2001b) determined the essential elements of prebooking diversion programs, as shown in Table 13.2.

Postbooking Diversion

Postbooking programs are more common than prebooking ones (Desai, 2003) and are designed to reduce the length of incarceration (Draine & Solomon, 1999). Among the

**TABLE 13.2. Essential Elements
of Prebooking Diversion Programs**

- High visibility
- Single point of entry
- No-refusal policy
- Streamlined intake procedure
- Legal foundation for police referrals
- Cross training of staff

postbooking programs, there are three types: prearraignment, postarraignment, and mixed, which includes both pre- and postarraignment (Steadman, Morris, & Dennis, 1995). Jail diversion programs have been developed to move individuals with mental illness who are charged with misdemeanors, and in some cases nonviolent felonies, from the criminal justice system to the mental health system for treatment (Desai, 2003; Shafer, Arthur, & Franczak, 2004). These postbooking diversion programs have three main objectives: (1) to screen and identify individuals with severe mental illness; (2) to have mental health professionals negotiate a treatment plan for detainees between the mental health and criminal justice personnel, and (3) after the plan is negotiated, to have designated staff associated with the criminal justice system serve as a liaison between the detainee and community mental health services. This negotiated disposition can be an alternative to prosecution, a condition of reduced charges, or a condition of probation (Desai, 2003). Some postbooking programs are court based and some are jail based. These programs have three tiers of jail diversion: release from jail with the condition of participating in psychiatric treatment, deferred prosecution—that is, postponing legal proceedings for a period of time during which the individual participates in treatment— summary probation, which is in lieu of jail time, whereby the individual is placed under probation for a period of time and is to attend treatment (Shafer, Arthur, & Franczak, 2004; Steadman, Cocozza, & Veysey, 1999a).

Steadman and associates' (Steadman et al., 1995) examination of national post-booking diversion programs found six key features among the most effective programs, which are indicated in Table 13.3. Definitions of jail diversion vary by program. One program defined jail diversion as "anything that's done to reduce potential time in jail and replace it with involvement in the mental health system" (Steadman et al., 1995, p. 1634). Another program indicated that the only goal is "keeping mentally disordered persons out of jail to prevent jail overcrowding and disruption" (Steadman et al., 1995, p. 1634). Overall, these researchers concluded that the most effective programs were those that were a "part of a comprehensive array of other jail services, including screening, evaluation, short-term treatment, and discharge planning (i.e., linkage), that are integrated with community-based mental health, substance abuse, and housing services" (Steadman et al., 1995, p. 1634).

Desai (2003) conducted a research review of the benefits of jail diversion, including both pre- and postbooking evaluations. She noted that as a concept, diversion has been enthusiastically received, but there is very little evidence of the benefits and costs. On the basis of her assessment, she concluded that diversion programs are likely to be effective in reducing incarceration for a 1-year period of time, but was unable to determine if these programs reduce future arrests.

TABLE 13.3. Key Features of Effective Jail Diversion Programs

- Integration of community-level services—mental health, judiciary, and social services
- Regular meetings among key players
- A designated liaison or boundary spanner who manages interactions between correctional, mental health, and judicial staff
- A strong leader who has good communication skills and understands all components of all systems as well as informal networks
- Early identification of detainees who have mental health treatment needs and meet the diversion criteria
- Diversion case managers who have experience in both mental health and criminal justice systems

Note. Data from Steadman, Morris, and Dennis (1995).

Three studies have evaluated postbooking diversion programs. Lamb and colleagues (Lamb, Weinberger, & Reston-Parham, 1996) followed persons charged with misdemeanors from a court-based program and compared those who were diverted with mandated treatment to those diverted without mandated treatment. Individuals who received judicial monitoring of their mandated treatment had better outcomes than those who were referred for treatment but did not have court monitoring. Steadman and his colleagues (1999a) also evaluated a court-based diversion program and compared diverted and nondiverted individuals. These investigators determined that the groups did very similarly at the 2-month follow-up interview, but those who were nondiverted did not get released during the follow-up period. These researchers did find that two factors were important in diversion decisions, community risk and availability of specialized diversion programs. Shafer and his associates (2004) compared the outcomes of individuals who were diverted with those not diverted, as based on a process of collaborative decision making between criminal justice and mental health personnel. This evaluation employed a quasi-experimental design; consequently, the groups were not initially equal. All participants showed improvements over time, irrespective of their diversion status. Both groups had reductions in a number of criminal and violence indicators, but there were no significant differences between the groups. A recent investigation assessed rediversion into postbooking jail diversion programs and found that about 20% of individuals were rediverted, usually shortly after diversion, and some were diverted more than once (Boccaccini, Christy, Poythress, & Kershaw, 2005). Other studies described diversion programs, and one such study found that 80% of individuals remained engaged in the services (Broner, Nguyen, Swern, & Goldfinger, 2003). Thus, there are limited data indicating the effectiveness of these diversion programs. To conduct sound methodological studies is extremely challenging, both in terms of the feasibility of implementing rigorous research and in establishing these diversion programs, as they require overcoming numerous barriers to the cooperation of the mental health and criminal justice systems (Desai, 2003; Draine & Solomon, 1999).

Mental Health Courts

Although diversion programs are the most well known of the efforts to stop the flow of persons with severe mental illness into the criminal justice system, the newest postarrest initiative is the establishment of mental health courts (Wolff, 2002, 2003). These courts are based on a rehabilitative philosophy (Petrila, 2003). Currently, there are few mental health courts, but with the Federal Mental Health Courts program, as previously mentioned, they are already expanding in number and are expected to increase even further with reauthorization legislation. As of 2004, there were 110 mental health courts (*www.mntalhealthcoutsurvey.com/*, November 29, 2004). These courts evolved from the perceived success of drug courts and are consistent with other specialty courts, such as family and juvenile courts (Steadman, Davidson, & Brown, 2001a; Watson, Hanrahan, Luchins, & Lurigio, 2001). Therapeutic jurisprudence has been philosophically influential in the development of these courts (Boothroyd, Poythress, McGaha, & Petrila, 2003). As drug courts proliferated, the number of individuals with mental health problems on their dockets increased, resulting in some courts developing special mental health tracks within the drug treatment courts (Watson et al., 2001).

The concept of mental health courts has become extremely broad—"almost any special effort by the courts to better address the needs of persons with serious mental illness who engage with the criminal justice system can qualify as a mental health court" (Steadman et al., 2001a, p. 458). The function of mental health courts seems similar, in some cases, to postarrest diversion. Consequently, Steadman and his associates (2001a) have suggested employing the following criteria for identifying a mental health court: (1) handles all individuals identified for referral to community mental health services on initial booking on a single court docket, (2) employs a court team approach to arrive at treatment and supervision plans, with a person designated as the court liaison to ensure linkage, and (3) establishes designated appropriated treatment slots prior to the judges' making rulings, which includes continued monitoring under the aegis of the court, with possible criminal sanctions, including reinstituting charges or sentences. The primary goal is to divert these individuals away from the criminal justice system to a treatment program (Boothroyd et al., 2003). Court staff members collaborate with mental health providers to implement a therapeutic intervention. These courts vary in terms of eligibility criteria, such as charges, usually misdemeanors or nonviolent felonies, specific diagnosis, and prior and/or current involvement with the mental health system, but all require that eligible individuals voluntarily agree to participate before they are placed in the court program. Defendants must be willing to accept treatment. If defendants agree to participate, they may then have their charges or jail sentences deferred (Goldkamp & Irons-Guynn, 2000; Watson et al., 2001; Wolf, 2003). Initially, these courts focused on defendants shortly after their arrest, but some courts have expanded their scope to accept referrals from other courts, as well as from attorneys, police, friends, relatives, or others aware of individuals who are mentally ill and in the criminal justice system (Goldkamp & Irons-Guynn, 2000).

Some critics have concerns that mental health courts may be coercive and/or may be vehicles for coerced treatment. However, these courts may contribute to keeping participants in treatment, therefore increasing the likelihood of successful outcomes. The issue of voluntariness in mental health courts is complicated by the question of an individual's competency to comprehend and make a decision to participate, which needs to be determined before an individual can be a mental health court candidate (Goldkamp & Irons-Guynn, 2000). Similarly, questions are raised about the court's use of sanctions for noncompliance with treatment, such as using more restrictive treatment alternatives or even incarceration, and whether these mechanisms are appropriate for producing desired outcomes (Goldkamp & Irons-Guynn, 2000). One of the greatest concerns is the extent to which the procedures used in these courts differ from those of conventional courts, leaving open the question of whether there is insufficient protection of due process.

Goldkamp and Irons-Guynn's (2000) process assessment of four mental health courts determined that each found the community mental health treatment and funding resources insufficient to meet the needs of the population they served. The insufficiency of the treatment system may well be the reason that these individuals are involved in the criminal justice system. Therefore, there is some irony in designing a program that places these offenders in the very systems that previously failed them (this is also true for diversion programs). A primary policy question is whether these courts have increased the available services for individuals with severe mental illness and/or co-occurring substance abuse, or simply made them a priority group of people who are displacing others in need of treatment. This priority status may result in an incentive to become involved with the criminal justice system in order to receive needed treatment (Petrila, Pothress, McGaha, & Boothroyd, 2001; Steadman et al., 2001a). Petrila and his associates (2001) have noted that in some instances the task forces developed to create these courts have gained additional funding for mental health services.

Evaluations of these courts have been very limited. Four outcome evaluations have been undertaken. One, of Broward County, Florida, considered by some to be the first mental health court, employed a quasi-experimental design. This evaluation found that defendants in a regular court were more likely not to have been receiving services before or after their court appearances, in comparison to those in the Broward County Mental Health Court. In addition, comparison court defendants who had been receiving treatment were more likely to discontinue treatment than defendants in the mental health court. Mental health court defendants also received a greater volume of services than those in the comparison court, but comparison defendants tended to use more costly services than mental health court defendants, such as crisis or emergency services or intensive residential treatment (Boothroyd et al., 2003). However, the intensive services received by the treatment court clients did not result in improved clinical outcomes, which was explained by a lack of control over the type and quality of services received (Boothroyd, Mercado, Poythress, Christy, & Petrila, 2005). Seattle's two mental health courts were assessed with basically pre- posttest designs, and both had decreased booking rates and decreased annualized jail lengths of stay; increased linkage, increased treatment hours, improved functioning, and prevention of deterioration (Trupin & Richards, 2003). The Clark County, Washington, mental health court was assessed with a pre-posttest design and was found to have reduced arrest rate for both new crimes and probation violations, and clients received more supportive services and fewer emergency services (Herinckx, Swart, Ama, Dolezal, & King, 2005). Cosden, Ellens, Schnell, Yasmeen, and Wolfe (2003) conducted a randomized study of a mental health treatment court with an assertive community treatment model (see Chapter 6, "Case Management") as compared with usual court processing. Defendants in both conditions improved over the course of a year in terms of life satisfaction, alleviation of distress, and independent living, and those involved in mental health court had reductions in substance abuse and in new criminal activity. Defendants in both conditions were equally likely to spend time in jail, but those from the mental health court tended to spend time for probation violations as opposed to new criminal charges, which was the case for those in the control condition. This was explained by the fact that those in the mental health court condition were under greater scrutiny than those in the other condition and were therefore more likely to be caught on violations of the stipulations of their probation. This situation was also found for those on probation and parole in other studies (Solomon & Draine, 1995e; Solomon, Draine, & Marcus, 2002). Thus, these evaluations indicate that mental health courts show promise, but there are certainly issues to be mindful of. Anecdotal reports by judges, public defenders, prosecutors, and staff members of the sheriff's department in the Cosden and colleagues (2003) study indicated that more thought was given to their clinical needs and the available mental health resources for offenders with mental illness who were not involved in the experimental program, because of the collaborative nature of the project.

Jail and Prison Mental Health Programs

The jail has become the institution of last resort, the one place that is unable to refuse admittance to persons with severe mental illness (Belcher, 1988; Lamb & Weinberger, 1998). Jails hold presentence individuals and those serving short-term sentences, usually less than 1 year, or those awaiting adjudication, whereas prisons are for those with longer sentences. Persons with severe mental illness, on average, stay in jails and prisons two to three times longer than others without mental illness and therefore cost more to incarcerate (Axelson & Wahl, 1992). Persons with mental illness are more likely to be denied early release and to serve out their sentences, because the community mental health services they need do not exist, or there is no housing for them or they have no one to put up bail (Haimowitz, 2004; Hartwell, 2003). For example, a 1997 study of the Riker's Island facility found that inmates with mental illness spent 215 days, on average, in jail, whereas the general inmate population was incarcerated for an average of 42 days (Butterfield, 1998). Ditton (1999) found that inmates with mental illness were sentenced to prison for terms that averaged 12 months longer than the terms for other inmates. Pennsylvania's Department of Corrections estimates that incarceration costs $140 per day, or $51,000 per year, for an inmate with mental illness, as compared with $77 per day for the average inmate (Lamberg, 2004).

Jails are generally ill equipped to provide appropriate treatment for inmates with mental illness, yet they are required by law to protect and provide at least minimal care for these inmates. Treatment is also needed for troublesome behaviors in order to achieve effective management of these facilities (Osher, Steadman, & Barr, 2003; Steadman & Veysey, 1997). Yet Steadman, Holohean, and Dvoskin (1991) found that 45% of persons with severe mental illness and functional disabilities did not receive any treatment in New York state prisons. Generally, jails do not have any policies or procedures for managing inmates with psychiatric disorders. Small jails provide very little in terms of services, other than screening for mental illness and suicide prevention, and larger jails, those with more than 1,000 inmates, tend to provide a greater array of services (Steadman & Veysey, 1997). A jail's mental health services may include intake screening and psychiatric evaluation, crisis services, and short-term treatment, which can include suicide prevention, case management, counseling, psychiatric medication, and discharge planning (Watson et al., 2001). The American Psychiatric Association (1989) recommends that these services, as well as access to inpatient care, be provided by all jails. However, there are no clear criteria for what constitutes adequate care in jails and prisons (Osher et al., 2003). Some large city jails have inpatient psychiatric units. For example, the Philadelphia local jail system has a 60-bed inpatient acute care unit and arrangements for long-term psychiatric care by transferring patients to the local state hospital forensic unit or, in some cases, to a specialized locked general hospital psychiatric unit. Veysey, Steadman, Morrissey, and Johnson (1997) determined that jails relied heavily on prescribed medication and that most detainees with mental illness were prescribed medication. In addition, persons were sometimes housed in specialized mental health units (segregated from the general population) and some received other mental health services, including individual and group therapy and case management (Veysey et al., 1997). The weakest of the services provided is also the most important: discharge planning and follow-up (Steadman et al., 1995; Morris, Steadman, & Veysey, 1997). Some jails do have external case managers who visit inmates, which is an important link to continued care for these inmates upon release from jail (Veysey et al., 1997). Frequently, with mental illness inmates are put in isolation owing to the poor quality of mental health services in the facility and the lack of proper staffing to manage this population (Schaefer & Stefancic, 2003). However, there are standards for treatment of offenders with mental illness within jails and prisons issued by the National Commission on Correctional Health Care (Maier & Fulton, 1998).

PERSONAL EXAMPLE

Doris Cummings's Community Reentry from Jail and Her Later Return to Jail

Doris Cummings, a white female in her early 40s, was released from incarceration after serving more than a year and a half in jail for two separate charges of fire setting. One offense related to a dispute with a neighbor, when Doris set off firecrackers over her neighbor's patio, which resulted in a fire. The other charge stemmed from an incident while she was incarcerated, when she set her mattress on fire in her jail cell.

Doris had a diagnosis of schizophrenia for more than 15 years, with only an intermittent treatment history. Doris was frequently requested to leave treatment programs because of her disruptive behavior, which the providers attributed to her co-occurring borderline personality disorder. While incarcerated, Doris refused all medication, regardless of the presence of active symptoms. She received minimal treatment while incarcerated (consisting of seeing a psychiatrist who prescribed medication, which she did not take), as the jail had no provision for specialized housing for female inmates with mental illness.

Upon discharge, she returned to her previous living arrangement (next to the same neighbor who was the complainant in her initial charge). The household consisted of her mother, who had a 30-year history of untreated schizophrenia, and a father who was a practicing Jehovah's Witness. Her father's religious beliefs resulted in his being opposed to her taking her prescribed medication. He believed that prayer was the answer to her mental health problems. She was placed under administrative supervision because she was charged in a county that was unfamiliar with her record (her neighbor literately lived in a different county). The parole department at her release was unaware of her psychiatric history, and therefore no provision was made for intensive supervision. The only discharge plan that was made for her upon release was a requirement to make financial restitution to the victim, in this case her neighbor, and she was requested to go to her local mental health agency. But she was merely given a card with the name and phone number for a local mental health agency and was told to call for an appointment. With no supervision and her father's opposition, Doris did not go for treatment.

Subsequently, Doris was rearrested twice on technical violations of her parole: failure to pay her restitution and failure to comply with mental health treatment. She was later arrested on new charges that stemmed from a traffic violation, which escalated into an assault charge because of her erratic and bizarre behavior at her preliminary arraignment. During this hearing she was found sitting in the judge's office, which she had trashed and from which she had to be forcibly removed. Consequently, Doris was sent to jail, where she stayed until she completed her sentence. She was again released to the community with no provision for criminal justice supervision or treatment, because she had served her full sentence.

Some jails and prisons have developed or made arrangements for specialized programs for persons with mental illness. For example, Bucks County, Pennsylvania, contracts with a private mental health center to provide on-site psychiatric services in the local jail. The staff includes psychologists, a psychiatrist, and a case manager. Services include 24-hour crisis coverage, psychiatric evaluations, medication management, individual and group psychotherapy, case management, community placement, and coordination of aftercare services (Torrey et al., 1992; Draine, Blank, Kottsieper, & Solomon, 2005). Edens, Peters, and Hills (1997) reviewed seven treatment programs for treating prison inmates with co-occurring disorders. Primary program components included "an extended assessment period, orientation/motivational activities, psychoeducational groups, cognitive-behavioral interventions such as restructuring of 'criminal thinking errors,' self-help groups, medication monitoring, relapse prevention, and transition into institution or community-based aftercare facilities" (Edens et al., 1997, p. 439). A number of the programs reviewed were modified therapeutic community approaches to being responsive to individuals with mental illness by employing less confrontation. Some prison mental health programs even provide social skill training, employing several modules from the University of California, Los Angeles (UCLA) Social and Independent Living Skills Program (Welsh & Ogloff, 2003). Most of these programs have not been evaluated. Lovell and colleagues (Lovell, Allen, Johnson, & Jemelka, 2001; Lovell & Jemelka, 1998), however, evaluated an intermediate-care residential program for male prisoners with mental illness. This program provides medication monitoring, skills training, and a supportive milieu to assist participants in coping with life in prison. The program was found to be clinically successful and cost-effective. At exit, participants were less symptomatic, had significant reductions in assaults and infractions, and had higher rates of work and school involvement (Lovell et al., 2001). Another research study of a residential treatment unit found that the program was effective in reducing risk and improving management of inmates with psychiatric disorders (Condelli, Bradigan, & Holanchock, 1997; Condelli, Dvoskin, & Holanchock, 1994).

Forensic Hospitalization

There are also forensic hospitals and forensic units within larger state hospitals that are designed with maximum security in order to serve persons with mental illness involved in the criminal justice system. These facilities are administered by either the state departments of corrections or state departments of mental health. Individuals who are "incompetent to stand trial" (IST), "not guilty by reason of insanity" (NGRI), and "guilty but mentally ill" (GBMI), as well as other detainees/offenders who are not able to be managed in a jail or prison, spend time in these facilities. A detainee who is determined by a psychiatric evaluation to be IST is one who is not capable of understanding the nature and purpose of the criminal proceedings and, consequently, cannot assist counsel with his or her own defense. These individuals who are IST may be treated within the jail (such facilities are usually large urban jails with available mental health services) or, frequently, are sent to a psychiatric facility to be treated in order to be restored to competency. Once so restored, a defendant returns to prison or jail and continues with the criminal proceedings. When an offender receives an NGRI verdict, the individual remains in a psychiatric hospital as long as he or she is believed to be suffering from a psychiatric disorder. Generally, defendants judged NGRI remain hospitalized for periods of time far longer than they would have spent in prison and can be released to the community only by court approval. In both Oregon and Connecticut there is a Psychiatric Security Review Board that oversees these NGRI acquitees and can revoke their conditional releases and return acquitees to hospitals. These boards are composed of mental health and criminal justice experts (Bigelow, Bloom, Williams, & McFarland, 1999; Bloom, Williams, & Bigelow, 2000). Those adjudicated GBMI are sent to and treated in a psychiatric hospital until they are declared to be sane. It is important to note that neither legal incompetence nor legal insanity is equivalent to mental illness. A person with severe mental illness can still meet the legal definitions of competence and/or sanity (Hiday, 1999; Lovell & Jemelka, 1998; Schaeffer & Stefancic, 2003). It is also important to note that these specific groups constitute a relatively small portion of persons with mental illness involved in the criminal justice system.

Community Corrections Supervision and Reentry

Although discharge planning for incarcerated individuals with mental illness has long been viewed as essential, inmates rarely receive it. Recently, New York City was required by court decree to provide discharge planning services to inmates with mental illness (*Brad H v. City of New York*, 2000; Barr, 2003; Osher et al., 2003). Community-based supervision of persons with mental illness must ensure access to treatment, as well as the safety of the individual and the community (Sommers & Baskin, 1995). However, when offenders serve their full sentences incarcerated, then no provision is made for community treatment, even if they were receiving treatment while incarcerated (Barr, 2003). There are no outcome studies to guide evidence-based transitional planning practice, but there is guidance from a multisite research study of jail mental health programs and from guidelines issued by such organizations as the American Psychiatric Association and the American Association of Community Psychiatrists to develop a best practices model (Osher et al., 2003). Based on these sources, the APIC (Access, Plan, Identify, and Coordinate) model was created for inmates with co-occurring disorders, which are quite prevalent among those involved with the criminal justice system. This model is composed of four components designed to "assess the inmate's clinical and social needs, and public safety risks; plan for the treatment and services required to address the inmate's needs; identify required community and correctional programs responsible for postrelease services; and coordinate the transition plan to ensure implementation and avoid gaps in care with community-based services" (Osher et al., 2003, p. 83). This model requires a great deal of collaboration between the various systems—mental health, substance abuse, and criminal justice—and is designed to be flexible enough to be used by small jails as well as very large ones. The phrase *transition planning* is employed in this model rather than *discharge planning*, because transition "implies bidirectional responsibilities and requires collaboration among providers" (Osher et al., 2003, p. 82).

Similar psychosocial interventions are employed for both offenders being released or diverted from jails or prisons and for those under community supervision in lieu of being incarcerated. Probation is for those offenders who do not serve any of their sentences incarcerated, and parole is for those who are released from jail or prison to serve the rest of their sentences in the community. However, offenders can find themselves incarcerated should they violate the stipulations of their probation or parole. The mandatory conditions of serving time in the community usually include no commission of another crime, regular reporting, no possession of a firearm or other dangerous weapon or of illegal substances; special conditions can be designed for a designated offender by the releasing authority (e.g., the judge) to achieve specific goals (Carroll & Lurigio, 1984). Special conditions or stipulations for persons with severe psychiatric disorders generally require access to appropriate treatment and supervision by probation/parole officers to ensure participation in treatment. In some cases, there are specialized caseloads, including exclusively mental health caseloads that are meaningfully reduced in size, and officers have specific training in skills and knowledge regarding the specialized population. These officers also engage in specific supervision practices, such as the use of integrated mental health and criminal justice resources and of problem-solving strategies for addressing probationer noncompliance (in contrast to threats of incarceration), as persons with mental illness have high rates of technical violations (Skeem, Encandela, & Louden, 2003; Skeem & Emke-Francis, 2004; Skeem & Petrila, 2004). The practices of specialized officers include continuous monitoring, more communication with treatment agencies, and greater flexibility to allow for mistakes without immediate incarceration (Veysey, 1994). Currently, supervised release is generally oriented toward surveillance and punishment, rather than its traditional orientation of offender rehabilitation and community reintegration (Lurigio, 2001). Psychiatric illness among parole/probation populations is often ignored unless psychiatric symptoms were an explicit part of the individuals' offenses, specified in their release plans, or florid at discharge (Carroll & Lurigio, 1984). The use of stipulations with the potential to violate the parolee or probationer is similar to outpatient commitment orders, whereby the court retains jurisdiction to modify or revoke the conditional release (Silberg et al., 2001).

The use of specialized forensic case management is one of the prominent innovative community-based approaches to serving persons with mental illness. This strategy provides linkages between the mental health, substance abuse, and criminal justice systems. The case managers are cross trained in all of these systems. There must be clear lines of communication between case managers and the probation/parole authorities, as case managers may use sanctions for leverage (Healey, 1999). TASC (originally Treatment Alternatives for Street Crime, now Treatment Alternatives for Safe Communities) agencies designed a case management model that evaluations found to be effective in linking criminal justice to treatment systems, particularly substance abuse treatment. This model has been extended to include individuals with co-occurring substance abuse disorders who are involved in the criminal justice system (Godley, Finch, Dougan, McDonnell, McDermit, et al., 2000). Some case management programs have employed intensive case management and others have used Assertive Community Treatment (ACT; see Chapter 6, "Case Management") or what has been referred to as Forensic Assertive Community Treatment (Hartwell, Friedman, & Orr, 2001; Lamberti, Weisman, & Faden, 2004). A recent survey of members of the National Association of County Behavioral Health Directors to identify assertive community treatment programs serving persons with mental illness and criminal justice histories and collaborating with criminal justice agencies found that there were 16 programs that met these criteria (Lamberti et al., 2004). A limited fidelity assessment by the researchers found that a common deviation from the model was inadequate availability of a psychiatrist (Lamberti et al., 2004). The primary referral sources for most of these programs were local jails, more than two-thirds included probation officers as team members, and half of the programs had a supervised residential component (Lamberti et al., 2004). In some cases, the forensic case management program provides services while the offenders are in the jail, plans for community services prior to release, and then continues to provide services to offenders in the community.

One of the most highly recognized of these forensic assertive community treatment programs is Project Link in Rochester, New York, which incorporates assertive community treatment with intensive case management. This program also has a treatment residence for those with chemical dependence. The program is very well integrated with the criminal justice system, as staff members work with police, in the courtroom, and in the jail, where they arrange for services prior to release. This program received the Gold Award from the American Psychiatric Association (Wagner & Gartner, 1999; Weisman, Lamberti, & Price, 2004). Preliminary research has found this program to be effective in reducing number of days hospitalized and incarcerated, service use, and number of arrests, and to be cost-effective. It has also found improvement in community adjustment of offenders served (Lamberti, Weisman, Schwarzkopf, Price, Ashton, et al., 2001; Weisman et al., 2004). Thresholds Jail Project, a modified ACT, which also received the Gold Award, had a drop in jail days for those served (Guardiano & von Brook, 2001; Lurigio, Fallon, & Dincin, 2000). Wilson, Tien, & Eaves (1995), using a quasi-experimental design, found similar results for an ACT program with experimental participants spending less time incarcerated than comparison participants. Solomon and Draine (1995e) compared modified forensic ACT with forensic intensive case management (FICM) and with usual care, employing a randomized design. No differences in psychosocial and clinical outcomes were found, but a higher proportion of clients served by ACT (60%) were incarcerated than those served by FICM (40%) or those in usual care (36%). Although these differences were not statistically significant, they were in the opposite direction of expected effects.

Three studies evaluated case management services for forensic clients. Ventura, Cassel, Jacoby, and Huang (1998) assessed two case management models. One provided jail-based case management service, which planned for release. The other was a community-based case management service that was provided after release to some, but not all, of those who had received jail-based case management. Recipients of community-based case management who received up to an hour of service per month were less likely to be rearrested than those who did not receive the service. More than an hour of case management per month did not significantly relate to rearrest. Jail-based case management alone did not relate to rearrest. Frankel, White, Wilzor, Lamon, and McAuliffe (1998) examined Forensic Outreach Services, an 8-week intensive case management service. Using the offenders as their own controls, investigators found a 94% drop in reincarceration rates over a 30-month period. Given the reduction in incarceration, the investigators determined that this program was cost-effective. Draine and Solomon (1994) followed 65 homeless offenders leaving jail, for six months after they were assigned to intensive case management, to assess whether the nature and intensity of case management services predicted a return to jail. The investigators found that "less satisfaction with quality of life, fewer case management services provided in clients' homes, more service time face to face with case managers, and more services involving interaction with other providers were associated with return to jail" (p. 245).

Solomon et al. (2002) examined the extent to which the receipt of case management services explained incarceration for technical violations of probation and parole, versus incarceration for new offenses, by 250 offenders with severe mental illness who were receiving specialized psychiatric probation and/or parole services. Offenders who received intensive case management services from the community mental health system were six times more likely to be incarcerated for technical violations than those incarcerated for a new charge. These researchers concluded that a service that primarily engages in monitoring, which can be the situation with case management, has a tendency to observe violations of criminal sanctions, hence resulting in high rates of offenders returning to jail. This finding is very similar to that of other studies of probation and parole services for persons with mental illness that found that intensive supervision for offenders with mental illness frequently results in higher rates of reincarceration (Lovell, Gagliardi,

& Peterson, 2002; Petersillia & Turner, 1993). If case management essentially performs monitoring and brokering without providing rehabilitation to change offenders' behavior or seeking community accommodations for them, then consequences like reincarceration are likely to occur. Petersilia and Turner (1993) noted that intensive supervision was primarily oriented to surveillance and supervision, as opposed to service and treatment.

SUMMARY AND CONCLUSIONS

Currently, there is a high proportion of persons with severe mental illness involved in the criminal justice system. These individuals tend to have long histories of psychiatric illness, but tend not to be engaged in treatment at the time of arrest. This situation may be due to the fact that the treatment system has struggled with these clients, "but [has] acknowledged defeat" (Whitmer, 1980). Hence, these individuals have been labeled "forfeited clients." The mental health system is quite resistant to working with persons who are or who have been involved with the criminal justice system. As the media have focused more attention on such persons, public policy makers have put more resources into the development of new interventions to address the needs of this population. However, mental health providers have to change their attitudes and not throw up their hands in defeat. They need to work with the criminal justice system and to have an understanding and knowledge of the criminal justice system. These clients need to receive more than minimal treatment, with more than an additional pair of eyes monitoring them; they need meaningful rehabilitation, including cognitive rehabilitation, social skills training, and supported employment, so that they have the tools needed to be integrated into the community and engage in prosocial behaviors. Otherwise, the cycle of reincarceration will not be broken.

Part III

SPECIAL POPULATIONS AND PROBLEMS

The chapters in Part III summarize the basic tools that constitute a rehabilitation team's interventions that help people with mental illnesses to overcome their disabilities. Subgroups within this population have special problems that require adapting rehabilitation programs to meet their exigencies. These include people with a history of trauma, who also abuse alcohol and other substances, who are involved in the criminal justice system, who also manifest aggressive behaviors, and who have significant personal health problems. Research shows that people with these problems are not rare, but rather commonly encountered. Hence, the rehabilitation team needs to strategize in preparing to help individuals with such special needs.

Chapter 14

Trauma and Posttraumatic Stress Disorder

Over the past decade there has been a growing awareness of the widespread problem of trauma in the lives of people with psychiatric disabilities. Trauma may play a role in the development of some psychiatric disorders and has a major impact on the course of psychiatric illness and the quality of life for people who have such disabilities. Rehabilitation practitioners need to be aware of the nature of trauma, the effects of trauma on people with psychiatric disabilities, and the common consequences of trauma such as posttraumatic stress disorder (PTSD), in order to identify it, to take steps to prevent further traumatization, and to help people deal with its consequences.

We begin this chapter with a review of the prevalence of trauma exposure in people with psychiatric disabilities. We next consider why traumatic experiences are so common in these individuals' lives. We then discuss the consequences of trauma (including more severe symptoms and PTSD) and other problems such as health difficulties and the frequent use of acute care services. We note that despite the high prevalence of trauma and PTSD in persons with psychiatric disabilities, these problems are not routinely assessed in mental health practice, and we consider possible reasons for this failure, as well as solutions to the problem. We then review various treatment approaches for helping people with psychiatric disabilities to cope with and overcome the effects of trauma on their lives. Next, we consider broader interpretations of the concept of "trauma," which include the experiencing of psychotic symptoms, coerced treatment, and the psychological effects of developing a mental illness. We conclude by discussing the trend toward developing more trauma-informed services for people with psychiatric disabilities.

PERSONAL EXAMPLE

Susan Franklin's Struggle with Schizophrenia and PTSD

Susan was a 40-year-old divorced woman with a diagnosis of major depression, who had experienced her first episode and hospitalization at the age of 26. Since then, she had multiple relapses and hospitalizations and made several suicide attempts. Susan struggled with bouts of severe depression throughout her life, as well as intermittent hallucinations and paranoid delusions. She also experienced significant anxiety, especially around people, that interfered with maintaining close relationships with people, working with her treatment team, and seeking employment, despite a desire to work. Susan lived alone and received supported housing services. She regularly saw her daughter and grandchild, but otherwise her only social contacts were her trips to see her doctor at the community mental health center and late-night grocery shopping.

As part of a new screening and assessment program at her local mental health center, Susan's case manager met with her to conduct a lifetime history of her trauma exposure, and to determine whether she met the criteria for posttraumatic stress disorder (PTSD). Susan had been in treatment for more than 15 years, but this meeting with the case manager was the first time anyone had specifically asked her about her traumatic experiences and their psychological consequences. Although Susan found it difficult to talk about these experiences at first, she also reported feeling relieved that at last someone had asked about them. During the assessment, Susan revealed that she had suffered multiple traumas both in childhood and in adulthood, but the events that caused her the most distress were having been sexually abused at the age of 10 by her brother, and then sexually abusing her younger cousin. The assessment confirmed that she met the criteria for PTSD owing to her sexual abuse by her brother, and after her case manager explained what that meant, she agreed to meet with a clinician about a new treatment program for PTSD at that center.

TRAUMA IN PSYCHIATRIC DISABILITIES

Psychological *trauma* refers to the experiencing of an uncontrollable event perceived to threaten a person's sense of integrity or survival (Herman, 1992; Horowitz, 1986; van der Kolk, 1987). The *Diagnostic and Statistical Manual of Mental Disorders*, 4th edition (DSM-IV; American Psychiatric Association, 1994) adopts a narrower definition of *traumatic event* as an event involving direct threat of death, severe bodily harm, or psychological injury, which the person at the time finds intensely distressing. Sources of trauma include combat exposure, natural disasters, and violent victimization such as rape or assault. In this chapter we adopt the DSM-IV definition of trauma, although we also consider other types of trauma as well.

Prevalence of Trauma Exposure

By almost all accounts, trauma is ubiquitous in people with psychiatric disabilities. Over the past two decades, numerous surveys evaluated past, recent, and ongoing trauma in the general population as well as in people with mental illnesses. For example, in the National Comorbidity Study, 56% of respondents reported exposure to a traumatic event during their lives (Kessler, Sonnega, Bromet, Hughes, & Nelson, 1995). Men are more likely to experience or witness physical assault, whereas women are more likely to be sexually victimized (Breslau, Davis, & Andreski, 1995; Breslau, Davis, Andreski, Peterson, & Schultz, 1997; Kessler et al., 1995). Although trauma is common in the general population, among persons with psychiatric disabilities, trauma exposure is even higher. Between 34 and 53% of consumers report childhood sexual or physical abuse (Goodman et al., 2001; Greenfield, Strakowski, Tohen, Batson, & Kolbrener, 1994; Jacobson & Herald, 1990; Rose, Peabody, & Stratigeas, 1991; Ross, Anderson, & Clark, 1994), and 43–98% report some type of traumatic event during their lives (Carmen, Rieker, & Mills, 1984; Howgego et al., 2005; Hutchings & Dutton, 1993; Jacobson, 1989; Jacobson & Richardson, 1987; Lipschitz, Kaplan, Sorkenn, Faedda, Chorney, et al., 1996; Mueser, Goodman, Trumbetta, Rosenberg, Osher, et al., 1998b; Walsh, Moran, Scott, McKenzie, Burns, et al., 2003).

The specific rates of trauma exposure vary from one study to the next, depending on the setting and characteristics of the consumers surveyed and the specific methods used to ascertain trauma exposure. Nevertheless, multiple studies indicate that sexual and physical abuse or assault are especially common in persons with psychiatric disabilities. For example, Figure 14.1 summarizes the findings from a large study that evaluated trauma exposure in childhood, adulthood, and over the past year in a mixed sample of consumers with schizophrenia spectrum or major mood disorders receiving public mental health services (Goodman et al., 2001). It can be seen that more than half the women reported a history of childhood sexual abuse, as well as about one-quarter of the men. Sexual assault in adulthood was also a problem for women, whereas physical abuse and physical assault were common for both men and women.

Although trauma is a common problem for people with psychiatric disabilities, it is even more common in some subgroups. Women who are homeless are especially vulnerable to interpersonal victimization, with rates ranging as high as 77–97% (Davies-Netzley, Hurlburt, & Hough, 1996; Goodman, Dutton, & Harris, 1995). Likewise, persons with comorbid mental illness and substance use disorders are more prone to trauma, in both childhood and adolescence and in adulthood (Kessler et al., 1995; Ouimette & Brown, 2002). Indeed, trauma is so common in people with psychiatric disabilities that it can be considered a "normative" experience for this population (Goodman et al., 1997). For example, one comprehensive study of trauma exposure found that 98% of people with

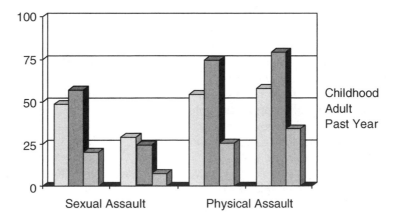

FIGURE 14.1. Rates of trauma in childhood, adulthood, and past month for men and women (*N* = 779) with psychiatric disabilities. Based on Goodman et al. (2001).

psychiatric disabilities had been exposed to at least one traumatic event involving the threat of death or injury to themselves or others (Mueser et al., 1998b).

Understanding the High Rate of Trauma in Psychiatric Disabilities

Why is trauma so common across the lifespans of people with psychiatric disabilities? This question is a complex one, because it seeks to address both the high rate of trauma in childhood and adolescence for people who later develop psychiatric disabilities, and the frequent victimization experienced by people after the onset of psychiatric illness. The answers to these questions likely involve multiple factors that differ in their importance between consumers. We first discuss how trauma in childhood and adolescence may contribute to the development of psychiatric disabilities, and then consider how having a psychiatric disability increases susceptibility to trauma.

Trauma in Childhood and Adolescence

Traumatic experiences in childhood are related to the subsequent development of psychiatric and substance use disorders in adulthood, as well as associated emotional problems such as anxiety, depression, and suicidal thinking (Browne & Finkelhor, 1986; Dube, Anda, Felitti, Chapman, Williamson, et al., 2001; Kendler, Bulik, Silberg, Hettema, Myers, et al., 2000; Kendler, Kuhn, & Prescott, 2004; Kessler, Davis, & Kendler, 1997b; Read, Perry, Moskowitz, & Connolly, 2001). Furthermore, adverse events in childhood contribute to the later development of medical problems such as chronic fatigue syndrome, lung disease, autoimmune disorders, diabetes, migraine, gastrointestinal disorders, and ulcers (Goodwin, Hoven, Murison, & Hotopf, 2003; Goodwin & Stein, 2004; Romans, Belaise, Martin, Morris, & Raffi, 2002; Talley, Fett, Zinsmeister, & Melton, 1994). Thus, exposure to trauma during the formative years of childhood and adolescence increases vulnerability to a range of problems in adulthood, which suggests that adverse events play a role in the etiology of mental illness.

One theory as to why early life trauma increases the risk of developing mental illness is illustrated by the stress–vulnerability model (Falconer, 1965; Zubin & Spring, 1977). This model proposes that psychiatric disorders are caused by a combination of *biological vulnerability* to a specific disorder (e.g., schizophrenia, major depression, bipolar disorder), determined by a combination of genetic and early environmental factors (e.g., obstetric complications), and exposure to *environmental stress* (e.g., emotional or physical abuse). Environmental stress can impinge on biological vulnerability to either precipitate the onset of a disorder or to worsen its course and outcome. However, the effect of stress on vulnerability can be mitigated by *coping skills* (e.g., social skills, problem-solving skills) and *social support*. Thus, according to this model, multiple traumatic events during childhood and adolescence could directly increase vulnerability to psychiatric illness by producing high exposure to stress, and indirectly increase vulnerability due to low social support and limited opportunities to develop healthy coping skills (e.g., owing to a lack of good role models).

Other theories have proposed a link between trauma exposure and the development of specific disorders. For example, Read and colleagues (Read, Perry, Moskowitz, & Connolly, 2001; Read, van Os, Morrison, & Ross, 2005) have proposed a neurodevelopmental model of schizophrenia that hypothesizes that exposure to early childhood abuse, especially sexual abuse, plays an etiological role in the development of schizophrenia through the alteration of basic brain functions responsible for the disorder. Another theory linking trauma exposure to psychiatric disability concerns the impact of the loss of a caregiver (Brown & Harris, 1978). Caregivers play enormously important roles in the lives of children, especially at an early age, and research has shown that the loss of a caregiver, especially a mother during the first years of life, is associated with a significant increase in the development of depression in adulthood. The specific mechanisms underlying this association are not known, but may include both biological and psychological factors.

Trauma after the Onset of Psychiatric Disability

A number of factors may account for the high rates of trauma in people after they have developed psychiatric disabilities. One factor is the circumstances in which many people with psychiatric disabilities live. Because psychiatric disorders often have a negative effect on the ability of people to work and support themselves, people with such disorders are often dependent on others and society for necessary living supports, which are often marginal at best. Furthermore, some psychiatric disorders, such as schizophrenia, occur more often in urban than rural areas (Torrey, Bowler, & Clark, 1997; Van Os, 2004). Consequently, many people with psychiatric disabilities have low incomes, reside in substandard housing, and live in impoverished neighborhoods (Eaton, 1994; Lögdberg, Nilsson, Levander, & Levander, 2004), which makes them vulnerable to crime (Carmen et al., 1984; Gearon & Bellack, 1999; Goodman et al., 2001; Hiday et al., 1999; Honkonen, Henriksson, Koivisto, Stengård, & Salokangas, 2004; Walsh et al., 2003).

Aside from the specific living circumstances of people with psychiatric disabilities, the disorders themselves and the effects of co-occurring substance use problems may also contribute to increased trauma exposure. People with psychiatric disorders, especially schizophrenia, often have cognitive impairments that interfere with their ability to plan ahead and to anticipate the thoughts and motives of others. Both of these problems can make it more difficult for people to protect themselves from others, and thus cognitive impairment is an established risk factor for interpersonal victimization (Mueser, Hiday, Goodman, & Valenti-Hein, 2003a; Sobsey, 1994).

Just as cognitive problems contribute to victimization, psychiatric symptoms can also play a role. Hypomanic or manic symptoms can include high levels of irritability and anger in a person who perceives another as interfering with his or her goals, leading to verbal and physical aggression and reciprocal aggression from the other person. Depression can contribute to victimization in a very different way. Low self-esteem is among the common symptoms of depression, along with reduced self-efficacy and lack of perceived control over one's life. These symptoms may cause people who are depressed to feel that they do not deserve to be treated better by others, or that they are powerless over their lives, and thus fail to escape from abusive situations. Depression is a very common symptom in victims of domestic violence (el-Bayoumi, Borum, & Haywood, 1998; Sisley, Jacobs, Poole, Campbell, & Esposito, 1999).

Psychotic symptoms can also contribute to victimization, especially when they involve paranoid delusions of command hallucinations (i.e., auditory hallucinations that instruct an individual to do something). Persistent psychotic symptoms are associated with increased anxiety and depression (Birchwood, Mason, MacMillian, & Healy, 1993; Garety, Kuipers, Fowler, Chamberlain, & Dunn, 1994; Mueser et al., 1991c). However, these symptoms can also lead to aggressive and violent behavior, aimed either at protecting oneself or appeasing the voices (Mackinnon, Copolov, & Trauer, 2004; McNeil, 1994; Trower, Birchwood, Meaden, Byrne, Nelson, et al., 2004). As violence is often reciprocal and people frequently respond to aggression by fighting back (Goodman et al., 2001), psychosis that leads to "defensive" aggression may have the paradoxical effect of resulting in violence and injury to them.

The common problem of substance abuse and dependence may also contribute to high levels of victimization (Hiday et al., 1999; Lam & Rosenheck, 1998). People with psychiatric disabilities and substance use problems are often at high risk for violence by virtue of using substances with others who see them as easy prey and may take advantage of them economically, sexually, and otherwise, using threats or actual violence to extract the desired resources from their victims. In addition, people who develop substance dependence problems may further increase their vulnerability through their efforts to obtain substances (such as by stealing or trading sex for money or drugs). Finally, substance use may contribute to victimization because the substances themselves can reduce inhibitions, which can lead to risky behaviors (e.g., spontaneous sexual encounters or starting fights) or reduce individuals' awareness of their surroundings, making them less able to protect themselves.

A final reason trauma that may be so common in adulthood is that early victimization may increase vulnerability to subsequent victimization, independent of psychiatric disability. Research indicates that people who are abused in childhood are more prone to revictimization over their lifetimes (Arata, 2002; Burnam, Stein, Golding, Siegel, Sorenson, et al., 1988; Nishith, Mechanic, & Resick, 2000; Wilson, Calhoun, & Bernat, 1999). The reasons for this revictimization are unclear. A possible explanation is that individuals who are abused as children may lack appropriate role models to learn how to protect themselves. Another possibility is that the exaggerated perceptions of threat that many abuse survivors experience, as reflected by PTSD symptoms such as hypervigilance and high autonomic arousal, may make them unable to distinguish between realistic and unrealistic threats.

Consequences of Trauma

Trauma exposure has been linked to a wide range of negative consequences in people with psychiatric disabilities. The majority of studies have focused on symptoms and have reported that higher levels of trauma exposure are related to more severe depression, anxiety, and psychotic symptoms (Beck & van der Kolk, 1987; Briere, Woo, McRae, Foltz, & Sitzman, 1997; Carmen et al., 1984; Figueroa, Silk, Huth, & Lohr, 1997; Goff, Brotman, Kindlon, Waites, & Amico, 1991; Muenzenmaier, Meyer, Struening, & Ferber, 1993; Schenkel, Spaulding, DiLillo, & Silverstein, 2005). Less research has evaluated other consequences of trauma, although some evidence points to more severe substance use problems and higher utilization of emergency and inpatient psychiatric services (Briere et al., 1997; Carmen et al., 1984; Switzer, Dew, Thompson, Goycoolea, Derricott, et al., 1999).

One consequence of trauma that has become a major focus of attention in recent years is PTSD in persons with a psychiatric disability. PTSD is a psychiatric disorder defined in terms of physiological and behavioral reactions following exposure to a traumatic event (American Psychiatric Association, 1994). According to DSM-IV, the major criteria for the diagnosis of PTSD include exposure to a traumatic event involving a threat to life or injury to self or others, accompanied by a strong negative emotional reaction at the time, and the persistence or emergence of the following symptom clusters 1 month or more after the traumatic event: reexperiencing the trauma (e.g., intrusive memories of the event, nightmares), avoidance of trauma-related stimuli (e.g., avoiding situations, thoughts, or feelings related to the traumatic experience), and overarousal (e.g., hypervigilance, exaggerated startle response). In addition, some degree of functional impairment due to the PTSD symptoms is required for the diagnosis.

Since the 1990s a number of studies have examined the prevalence of PTSD in persons with psychiatric disabilities (Cascardi, Mueser, DeGiralomo, & Murrin, 1996; Craine, Henson, Colliver, & MacLean, 1988; Howgego et al., 2005; McFarlane, Bookless, & Air, 2001; Mueser et al., 1998b; Mueser et al., 2001b; Mueser, Rosenberg, Jankowski, Hamblen, & Descamps, 2004b; Neria, Bromet, Sievers, Lavelle, & Fochtmann, 2002; Resnick, Bond, & Mueser, 2003; Switzer et al., 1999). As summarized in Figure 14.2, most studies have reported rates of current PTSD ranging between 28 and 43%. These high rates are in sharp contrast to the lifetime rate of PTSD in the general population, between 8 and 12% (Breslau, Davis, Andreski, & Peterson, 1991; Kessler et al., 1995; Resnick, Kilpatrick, Dansky, Saunders, & Best, 1993). Two studies have reported somewhat lower rates of PTSD among persons with psychiatric disabilities (14 and 13%). One of these studies differed from the others in that it focused on first admissions of those experiencing a psychotic episode (Neria et al., 2002), rather than individuals with a previously established psychiatric disability, suggesting that vulnerability to developing PTSD exists both before and following the onset of a psychiatric disability. The study by Resnick et al. (2003) found lower rates of PTSD than the other studies; however, the sample size was relatively small.

Research focusing on which individuals are most likely to have PTSD has revealed some interesting trends. Although, in the general population, women are more vulnerable to PTSD than men, among persons with psychiatric disabilities most studies have not found such a difference. However, rates of PTSD do differ across different diagnostic groups, with consumers who have major depression or borderline personality disorder most likely to have PTSD, followed by persons with bipolar disorder, and then people with schizophrenia or schizoaffective disorder (Bolton, Mueser, & Rosenberg, 2006; Mueser et al., 1998b; Mueser et al., 2001b; Mueser, Salyers, Rosenberg, Goodman, Essock, et al., 2004c). As in the general population, persons who have experienced the

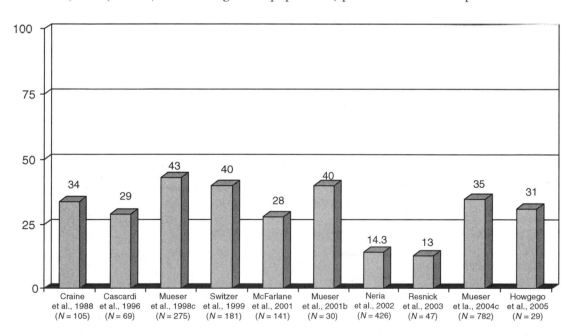

FIGURE 14.2. Rates of PTSD in samples of persons with psychiatric disabilities.

most extensive trauma history are most likely to have PTSD, especially individuals with a history of childhood sexual abuse.

The assessment and treatment of PTSD as an important consequence of trauma in persons with psychiatric disabilities have grown rapidly in recent years for two related reasons. First, PTSD is a well-defined syndrome and there are firmly established instruments for assessing its prevalence and severity. The clinical status of PTSD as a diagnostic entity makes it easier to measure and track over time, which also makes it a suitable target for intervention. In contrast, aside from PTSD there is no single, well-defined, cohesive syndrome that occurs in the wake of trauma that can be readily measured and made the focus of treatment. In addition, although there are many clinical correlates of trauma exposure (e.g., depression, substance abuse), their actual relationship to traumatic experiences is unclear. Second, there is extensive research literature on the treatment of PTSD in the general population, with a variety of different psychotherapeutic and pharmacological interventions shown to be effective (Bradley, Greene, Russ, Dutra, & Westen, 2005; Foa, Keane, & Friedman, 2000). In contrast, there are no empirically supported interventions for treating the broad range of other correlates of trauma exposure in the general population. The fact that much is known about the treatment of PTSD in the general population has given hope and provided an impetus for adapting those interventions to meet the unique needs of individuals with psychiatric disabilities and PTSD.

PTSD and the Course of Psychiatric Disabilities

In addition to the importance of PTSD as a syndrome associated with high levels of anxiety and depression, PTSD has also been hypothesized to interact with the course of mental illness. Mueser and colleagues (2002b) proposed a model, based on the stress-vulnerability model described earlier in this chapter (Liberman et al., 1986; Zubin & Spring, 1977), in which PTSD is hypothesized to mediate the associations between trauma exposure over a person's lifetime and the severity and course of mental illness. This model is summarized in Figure 14.3.

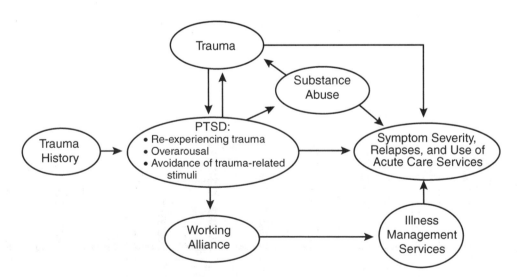

FIGURE 14.3. Interactive model positing relationships between trauma history, PTSD, and the course of psychiatric disabilities. Based on Mueser et al. (2002b).

According to the model, the symptoms of PTSD and associated problems can both directly and indirectly worsen the course of severe mental illness. The symptoms of PTSD can directly worsen the course of a mental illness in several ways. Chronic unwanted memories and other reexperiencing symptoms may be experienced as daily stresses that contribute to worsening symptoms and a higher vulnerability to relapses, like other forms of chronic stress. In addition, avoidance of trauma-related stimuli, which are often social in nature owing to the high rates of interpersonal victimization, can lead to avoidance of close personal relationships, and therefore less access to social support, which may also contribute to a worse course of mental illness. Social difficulties, such as in making friends and maintaining intimate relationships, are very common in persons with PTSD and are a major source of distress (Calhoun, Beckham, & Bosworth, 2002; Kuhn, Blanchard, & Hickling, 2003; Monson, 2005). Finally, the overarousal symptoms of PTSD can also contribute to worsening symptoms, as high levels of arousal can increase vulnerability to symptom relapses (Straube & Öhman, 1990; Zahn, 1986).

Several associated features of PTSD may also indirectly worsen the course of a psychiatric disability. Attempts to self-medicate the symptoms of PTSD through alcohol and drug abuse can precipitate relapses and impair functioning (Drake & Brunette, 1998; Linszen, Dingemans, & Lenior, 1994). Substance abuse may also have the indirect effect of increasing vulnerability to subsequent retraumatization, as previously discussed in this chapter. Finally, as discussed earlier, having PTSD may also increase susceptibility to retraumatization.

ASSESSMENT OF TRAUMA AND PTSD IN PERSONS WITH PSYCHIATRIC DISABILITIES

Despite the high rates of trauma exposure and PTSD reported in numerous studies, they are not routinely assessed in typical mental health practice. For example, among five studies of persons with psychiatric disabilities reviewed by Mueser and colleagues (2002b) that reported rates of PTSD between 29% and 43% following a standard assessment, PTSD was noted in 0–3% of their charts. Similarly, trauma history is rarely noted in the charts of people with psychiatric disabilities (Frueh, Cousins, Hiers, Cavanaugh, Cusak, et al., 2002; Read, 1997), which raises the question of why trauma and PTSD are not evaluated more systematically.

One reason for not assessing trauma and its consequences is the widespread belief that discussing such experiences can be upsetting to consumers and lead to the exacerbation of symptoms. Furthermore, clinicians may be concerned that reports of traumatic events by persons with psychiatric disabilities are not reliable or are delusional, despite the evidence that such assessments can be reliably conducted (Rosenberg et al., 2001b). The net result of the reluctance of consumers to talk about traumatic experiences, and of clinicians to ask, is that trauma-related problems often go undetected and untreated.

Another reason for the lack of assessment is the nature of PTSD itself. One of the major symptom clusters of PTSD is avoidance of trauma-related stimuli, such as situations, thoughts, or feelings that remind people of their traumatic experiences. A by-product of this avoidance is that traumatized individuals avoid talking about their experiences to anyone, including mental health practitioners.

Related to avoidance is the tendency of some people to minimize their traumatic experiences, even when directly asked about them. Minimization is most likely to occur when vague language is used to inquire about a person's trauma history, because such imprecision leaves much open to individual interpretation. For example, many individuals, especially men, who experienced sex as a child with an adult do not label these experiences as "sexual abuse" (Baker & Duncan, 1985; Lab & Moore, 2005). Similarly, individuals who report recent events of forced sexual behavior or significant physical aggression against them by partners or family members frequently do not label these experiences as sexual or physical "abuse" (Cascardi et al., 1996).

Avoidance and minimization of discussion about traumatic experiences may be due to the anxiety associated with memories of those experiences, but other factors may play a role as well. Although there are benefits to talking about personal secrets (Pennebaker, Barger, & Tiebout, 1989; Pennebaker, Kiecolt-Glaser, & Glaser, 1988; Wastell, 2002), there are also potential costs, such as rejection (Kelly & McKillop, 1996). Furthermore, negative reactions to a person's divulging traumatic experiences may be greater when the individual has a psychiatric disability, which can be due to the stigma of mental illness and the belief that the reports of trauma may be delusional or that the trauma was the consumer's own fault (Marley & Buila, 1999). Furthermore, a survey of staff responses to mental health consumers who revealed traumatic experiences indicated a lack of support or a lack of referrals to counseling (Read & Fraser, 1998), suggesting that the concerns consumers may have about how practitioners will respond to such revelations are not ill founded.

A final reason why trauma history and PTSD are often undetected is that clinicians do not know what to do with this information in their work with consumers. Eilenberg, Fullilove, Goldman, and Mellman (1996) found that when clinicians were mandated to assess trauma history in psychiatric outpatients, there was a significant increase in documented traumatic experiences, but little effect on the recognition of PTSD or treatment planning. Similarly, Cusack, Frueh, and Brady (2004) found that when trauma and PTSD screenings were included in the standard intake assessment at a community mental health center, rates of detected trauma and PTSD both increased, but not PTSD treatment services.

One study of mental health practitioners indicated that fewer than half believed they could detect PTSD symptoms in the consumers with whom they worked, only 28.2% indicated that they were comfortable with their knowledge of effective treatments of PTSD, and only 18.1% reported that they felt confident in their ability to treat PTSD (Salyers, Evans, Bond, & Meyer, 2004b). However, most clinicians indicated that they believed consumers would benefit from treatment specifically for PTSD (67.3%) and other trauma-related problems (74.1%). Thus, most practitioners believe they are ill equipped to assess and treat PTSD, even though they believe consumers would benefit from it. This apparent lacuna in training and clinical skills likely accounts for the lack of attention to PTSD and other trauma-related difficulties in treatment planning, even when assessment of these problem areas is standardized and required.

TREATMENT APPROACHES

The increased recognition of the high prevalence of trauma exposure and PTSD in persons with psychiatric disabilities has led to treatment approaches aimed at reducing the effects of trauma on their lives. Many of these approaches have been informed by research on the treatment of PTSD in the general population. Therefore, in this section we first describe empirically supported interventions for PTSD in the general population. We do not address treatment strategies for other consequences of trauma in the general population because of the lack of consistent evidence supporting any specific approaches. We then describe treatment programs designed for people with psychiatric disabilities. Although not described here, we also note that one standardized, broad-based group intervention has been developed to address PTSD in persons with a substance use disorder, the Seeking Safety program (Najavits, 2002), with some research suggesting that it has beneficial effects (Hein, Cohen, Miele, Litt, & Capstick, 2004), and several controlled trials under way.

Treatment of PTSD in the General Population

Research on the treatment of PTSD in the general population has shown that two cognitive-behavioral techniques are especially effective: exposure therapy and cognitive restructuring. *Exposure therapy* (formerly called *flooding* or *implosion therapy*) is a widely used technique in the treatment of anxiety disorders. The application of exposure therapy to PTSD involves having people systematically confront, rather than avoid, feared but safe trauma-related stimuli, such as thoughts and images of traumatic experiences, and situations that remind them of those experiences (Foa & Rothbaum, 1998; Keane, Fairbank, Caddell, & Zimering, 1989). As individuals talk about their traumatic experiences and become able to deal with situations that remind them of those experiences, they learn that the memories and situations cannot hurt them, and their anxiety gradually decreases (or *habituates*). This habituation of anxiety is accompanied by a reduction in the symptoms of PTSD.

Cognitive restructuring is a widely used technique for many psychiatric disorders (Beck, 1995). The core assumption underlying the use of cognitive restructuring is that all negative emotional reactions people have to different situations, including internal stimuli such as thoughts or images, are determined by specific thoughts or beliefs that they have about themselves, other people, or the world in general. The thoughts underlying negative feelings in any particular situation may or may not be accurate, but are frequently inaccurate or unrealistic in people with anxiety and depression problems. Cognitive restructuring involves helping people to identify the underlying thoughts related to negative feelings such as anxiety, depression, anger, or shame, to carefully examine the evidence supporting (and not supporting) those thoughts, and to change them when they are not supported by the evidence. Experiencing traumatic events such as childhood sexual or physical abuse; a sexual or physical assault; being a victim of domestic violence; a bad accident; or the unexpected death of a loved one can naturally shape people's thoughts and beliefs about themselves and the world, leading to exaggerated perceptions of risk, avoidance, and PTSD (Ehlers & Clark, 2000). Cognitive restructuring for PTSD focuses on helping people to alter inaccurate trauma-related thoughts and beliefs and replace them with more accurate and adaptive ones.

Although cognitive-behavioral programs for PTSD tend to emphasize either exposure therapy, cognitive restructuring, or their combination (Cloitre, Koenen, Cohen, & Han, 2002; Foa & Rothbaum, 1998; Resick & Schnicke, 1993), these programs also incorporate other strategies as well, such as providing education about PTSD and teaching anxiety management techniques. As with all cognitive-behavior therapy, homework assignments are given for people to practice the skills taught in sessions. Most cognitive-behavioral therapy programs for PTSD are quite time limited, lasting between 9 and 30 sessions.

There is a wealth of evidence from controlled research showing that exposure therapy and cognitive restructuring are effective treatments for PTSD, with many studies demonstrating the superiority of these methods over nonspecific supportive therapy (Bisson, Ehlers, Matthews, Pilling, Richards, et al., 2007; Bradley et al., 2005; Foa et al., 2000). Remission rates of PTSD following cognitive-behavioral treatment are often more than 50%, even in people whose traumatic experiences occurred many decades earlier, such as women with PTSD due to childhood sexual abuse (McDonagh-Coyle, Friedman, McHugo, Ford, Sengupata, et al., 2005). Research evaluating whether the combination of exposure therapy and cognitive restructuring is more effective than either one alone has failed to find an added benefit (Marks, Lovell, Noshirvani, Livanou, & Thrasher, 1998).

Finally, much attention has been drawn to a treatment approach called eye movement desensitization and reprocessing (EMDR), which has been purported to be a more rapid, more effective treatment for PTSD than the cognitive-behavioral approaches described above (Shapiro, 1995). EMDR involves helping people talk about upsetting experiences and developing alternative and more adaptive ways of looking at them. This work is interspersed by the use of distraction techniques (such as the clinician waving a finger back and forth in front of the person or tapping the table) thought to facilitate the processing of traumatic memories. EMDR has generated significant controversy in the scientific community because of frequent exaggerated claims about its superiority to other approaches, aggressive marketing of the intervention, lack of scientific basis for the development of the approach, and questions about the importance of the distraction component of the treatment (Herbert, Lilienfeld, Lohr, Montgomery, O'Donohue, et al., 2000; Herbert & Mueser, 1992; McNally, 1999). Controlled research indicates that EMDR is effective for the treatment of PTSD (Bisson et al., 2007), but does not suggest that the distraction component contributes to better treatment outcomes. As EMDR incorporates elements of both exposure therapy and cognitive restructuring, but no uniquely efficacious components, it can be considered a type of a cognitive-behavioral therapy.

Programs Focused on PTSD in People with Psychiatric Disabilities

Unfortunately, research on cognitive-behavioral treatment of PTSD in the general population has routinely ruled out individuals with challenging comorbid disorders, such as bipolar disorder, schizophrenia, treatment refractory depression, depression, or substance abuse, as well as problems such as self-injurious behavior or cognitive impairment. Although there are case studies documenting the successful use of cognitive-behavioral therapy for PTSD in people with a psychiatric disability (Mueser & Taylor, 1997; Nishith, Hearst, Mueser, & Foa, 1995), controlled studies have not been conducted until recently, leaving open the question of how best to treat PTSD in these individuals. Two programs have recently been developed to address PTSD in such individuals, based on cognitive-behavioral treatment methods shown to be effective in the general population (Frueh, Buckley, Cusak, Kimble, Grubaugh, et al., 2004; Mueser et al., 2004b). A third psychoeducational program addressing PTSD has also been developed for psychiatric inpatients (Pratt, Rosenberg, Mueser, Brancato, Salyers, et al., 2005). We describe one of these programs below.

Mueser and colleagues (2004b; Mueser, Bolton, Carty, Bradley, Ahlgren, et al., 2007) developed individual and group versions of a cognitive-behavioral treatment program for PTSD in persons with psychiatric disabilities, with a primary focus on cognitive restructuring for changing PTSD symptoms. The individual approach is briefly described here and summarized in Table 14.1. The program is provided over 12–16 weekly 1-hour sessions and is integrated with other mental health services. The first session begins with

TABLE 14.1. Overview of Cognitive-Behavioral Therapy Program for PTSD in Consumers with Psychiatric Disabilities

Module	Topic	Goals	No. of treatment sessions
1	Introduction	• Engage consumer in treatment • Provide treatment overview	1
2	Crisis Plan Review	• Decide on a crisis plan with consumer • Clarify with consumer's treatment team the plan for managing any crises	1
3	Psychoeducation Part I: Core symptoms of PTSD	• Help consumer to understand nature of PTSD • Make education relevant to consumer's own experience of symptoms	1–2
4	Breathing Retraining	• Improve consumer's ability to manage tension and anxiety associated with PTSD	1+
5	Psychoeducation Part II: Associated Symptoms of PTSD	• Help consumer understand how other problems and symptoms are related to PTSD and trauma	1–2
6	Cognitive Restructuring Part I: Thoughts and Feelings	• Clarify relationship between thoughts and feelings	1–2
7	Cognitive Restructuring Part II: Challenging Your Thoughts and Feelings	• Help consumer understand how trauma influences thinking • Facilitate changing maladaptive thoughts through weighing evidence and challenging unsupported beliefs • Instruct consumer in how and when to take appropriate action when needed	7+
8	Generalization Training and Termination	• Bring treatment to closure • Ease transition from PTSD treatment to care as usual with treatment team	2

a brief *orientation* to the program, including a discussion of the various treatment components and the role of homework. This is followed by developing a personal *crisis plan* for responding to an increase in symptoms (PTSD or other) or other problems that could threaten participation in the program (e.g., self-injurious behavior, substance abuse). The clinician then teaches the consumer *breathing retraining*, a commonly used anxiety management strategy for slowing the rate of respiration in order to reduce the flow of oxygen to the brain and associated feelings of overarousal. The next two sessions focus on *education* about PTSD. These sessions let consumers know that their PTSD symptoms are common reactions to trauma and that they are not alone, which solidifies their motivation to work on their PTSD symptoms.

Following the completion of education about PTSD, usually in session 3, the rest of the sessions are devoted to teaching *cognitive restructuring*. Consumers are first informed about the role of thoughts and beliefs in determining emotional reactions to events and are then taught how to identify, challenge, and change inaccurate thoughts that lead to negative feelings. Cognitive restructuring is taught as a skill for dealing with negative feelings, with practice initially focusing on any thoughts associated with negative feelings and then gradually focusing more on trauma-related thoughts and beliefs. Toward the end of treatment, if PTSD symptoms persist, other support persons (e.g., case manager, significant other) are identified who can help the consumer continue to practice the cognitive restructuring skill, and who may participate in a joint session with the consumer and the clinician.

One pilot study on this intervention has been completed, showing high levels of treatment retention and significant reductions in PTSD symptoms and depression (Rosenberg, Mueser, Jankowski, Salyers, & Acker, 2004a). A randomized controlled trial of the intervention has recently been completed (Mueser, Rosenberg, Xie, Jankowski, Bolton, et al., 2007). This study compared the effectiveness of the cognitive-behavioral treatment program for PTSD with usual services in 108 persons with psychiatric disabilities (59% major mood disorder without borderline personality disorder, 25% major mood disorder and borderline personality disorder, 16% schizophrenia or schizoaffective disorder), treated at four community mental health centers in New Hampshire or Vermont. Minimal exclusion criteria were imposed (hospitalization or suicide attempt in past 3 months). Assessments were conducted at baseline (before treatment), after the 4–6 month treatment program, and at 3- and 6-month follow-ups. Treatment retention in the cognitive-behavioral therapy program was good (81%). Analyses indicated that the cognitive-behavioral treatment program was more effective than usual services at reducing the severity of PTSD symptoms, other symptoms, and negative trauma-related beliefs, and improving knowledge about PTSD, perceived health, and the therapeutic alliance with the case manager (a separate therapist provided the cognitive-behavioral treatment for PTSD, not the case manager). Subsequent analysis also indicated that the cognitive-behavioral treatment program was more effective at reducing PTSD symptoms and diagnosis in people who had severe PTSD at baseline. This study supports the feasibility of treating PTSD in persons with psychiatric disabilities, and suggests that cognitive-behavioral treatment can be effective for PTSD in people with challenging problems, such as psychotic symptoms, suicidal ideation, and cognitive impairment.

Broad-Based Programs for Trauma Survivors with Psychiatric Disabilities

Several programs have been developed that focus on the broader range of trauma consequences in persons with psychiatric disabilities. The Trauma Recovery and Empowerment (TREM) model was developed to address these difficulties in women with psychiatric disabilities who are survivors of sexual or physical abuse, using a group format to engender mutual support and validation for individuals' traumatic experiences (Harris, 1998). TREM is based on four core assumptions about the effects of interpersonal trauma on women (Fallot & Harris, 2002). First, some current dysfunctional behaviors may have originated as effective coping strategies in response to trauma. Second, people who have been exposed to trauma in childhood and adolescence may not have had an opportunity to develop effective coping skills for adulthood. Third, trauma exposure can sever connections with family, community, and oneself. Fourth, women who have been abused often feel disempowered and unable to advocate for themselves.

To address these problems, TREM focuses on the development of "trauma recovery skills" in 11 different areas: self-awareness, self-protection, self-soothing, emotion modulation, relational mutuality, accurate labeling of self and others, sense of agency, problem

PERSONAL EXAMPLE

Susan Gets Treatment for Her PTSD

Susan's case manager arranged for her to meet with a clinician, who reviewed the results of her assessment with her. Susan had endorsed a moderate number of PTSD symptoms related to her sexual abuse by her brother, such as intrusive memories of the events. Susan also reported feeling wracked with guilt over her own sexual abuse of her younger cousin. One of her most upsetting symptoms was her inability to spend time with her young grandson, because he served to trigger her memories of these abuse experiences. The clinician described the treatment program, and Susan agreed to participate in it.

Soon after the program began, Susan found some relief from her anxiety with the breathing retraining technique, which, with practice, she learned to use in stressful situations. She was able to grasp the information covered in the educational sessions and completed worksheets both in the sessions and at home, in which she described her PTSD symptoms. Although she experienced increased distress early in treatment in response to the focus on her early abuse experiences, she also expressed relief at learning that her symptoms could be understood as PTSD and did not mean that she was "crazy."

Cognitive restructuring was introduced over the course of three sessions. Susan began practicing the skill using the cognitive restructuring worksheets. She brought worksheets she had completed at home to the sessions, where she and her clinician reviewed them together. Examination of her cognitive restructuring worksheets across sessions revealed a gradual increase in her understanding of the skill and ability to apply it to upsetting situations. Susan's primary feelings and automatic thoughts focused on guilt and shame about her victimization and perpetration experiences as a child. As she was able to challenge her belief that she was a "bad" person because of her childhood experiences, as well as the belief that she would hurt her grandson, she became much more able to care for him. Susan's psychotic symptoms primarily involved delusions of reference, whereby she believed that others could read her mind and know that she was a "bad" person for having, as a child, abused her younger cousin. Through cognitive restructuring, Susan challenged this delusion in a similar way that she had with other, less psychotic, beliefs. Over time this delusion became much less prominent and distressing to her.

Upon completion of treatment, the severity of Susan's symptoms was greatly reduced and she was functioning much better. Although she experienced some PTSD symptoms, she was able to care for her grandson on a regular basis and engage in other activities that she had previously avoided, including going to public places such as stores and restaurants. At a 3-month follow-up, she had maintained her gains and reported that she was enjoying life much more than she had before.

solving, parenting, sense of purpose, and decision making. These skill areas are taught through a combination of techniques, including education, cognitive restructuring, skills training, peer support, and limited exposure. Weekly group sessions last 75 minutes, are co-led by women, and are provided over a 9-month period. Pilot studies indicate that TREM is associated with a range of improvements in women with psychiatric disabilities, including improvement in areas related to PTSD, depression, and substance abuse (Fallot, McHugo, & Harris, 2005). A randomized controlled trial of the TREM program is currently under way. In addition, a number of variants of TREM have been developed to address the effects of trauma in other people, such as men with psychiatric disabilities, women with substance use disorders (Toussaint, VanDeMark, Bornemann, & Graeber, 2006), and adolescents.

Although TREM was developed to focus primarily on outpatients, some programs have been designed to address trauma consequences in inpatients with psychiatric disabilities. Talbot and colleagues (Talbot, Houghtalen, Cyrulik, Betz, Barken, et al., 1998) developed a 3-week program called Women's Safety in Recovery for inpatients and consumers in day treatment programs who have experienced childhood sexual abuse. Hour-long group sessions are held three times per week for 3 weeks and are co-led. The program is not intended to be comprehensive treatment for the effects of sexual abuse, but rather a "first-stage" intervention intended to promote mastery over life stressors through awareness and development of skills. The curriculum is divided into three modules, each taught for a week, including "control of the body" (i.e., recognizing how sexual abuse effects health through the participants' perceptions about their bodies, medical care, and self-harm), "control of the environment" (i.e., addressing safety concerns), and "control of the emotions" (i.e., dealing with painful, trauma-related emotions). A variety of techniques are employed in the group, including didactic presentations, group discussion, art therapy, problem solving, and homework. Research has not evaluated this program.

TRAUMA RELATED TO THE EXPERIENCE OF MENTAL ILLNESS

So far this chapter, we have focused on the relatively narrow DSM-IV definition of a traumatic event, which includes the experiencing or witnessing of a significant threat of harm or death accompanied by severe negative emotions such as fear or horror. However, the word *trauma* often has much broader connotations in the English language and may refer to the experiencing of any extremely shocking or disruptive event and the aftermath of coping with such an event. In recent years there has been growing interest in conceptualizing a range of different experiences related to mental illness as traumatic, and evidence that posttraumatic reactions similar to those in PTSD are common (Frame & Morrison, 2001; Jackson, Knott, Skeate, & Birchwood, 2004; McGorry, Chanen, McCarthy, Van Riel, McKenzie, et al., 1991; Meyer, Taimenen, Vuori, Aijala, & Helenius, 1999; Morrison, Bowe, Larkin, & Nothard, 2001; Priebe, Broker, & Gunkel, 1998; Shaner & Eth, 1989). These traumatic experiences can be broadly grouped into three types, including symptoms (especially psychotic symptoms) and associated behaviors, coerced or involuntary treatment, and the social stigma and personal effects associated with developing and being labeled with a mental illness. We describe the nature of each of these three types of trauma, then follow with a discussion of research and treatment considerations.

Psychiatric Symptoms

Several aspects of having an acute episode of psychiatric symptoms, or receiving treatment for it, have been described as traumatic (Shaner & Eth, 1989). Psychotic symptoms may be experienced as traumatic in a number of ways. For example, hearing a television news broadcaster directly refer to you during the evening news (a delusion of reference), believing that there is a conspiracy of people who want to kill you (a paranoid delusion), believing others can hear your thoughts out loud ("thought broadcasting"), hearing voices when no one is around (auditory hallucinations)—all can be terrifying experiences as they are perceived as direct threats or dramatic invasions of your privacy (i.e., your own mind). Furthermore, the loss of contact with reality associated with these and other psychotic symptoms can make these experiences even more frightening when the symptoms have remitted and people look back on them and contemplate their lack of control over them.

In addition, during periods of acute symptoms people may act in self-destructive, violent, disorganized, or socially embarrassing ways. For example, people may attempt suicide, strike out at others in fits of anger or because of misperceived threat, walk carelessly into traffic, take off their clothes, engage in sexual indiscretions or farfetched financial schemes, or claim to have extraordinary abilities they do not have (such as being a great inventor or being able to read minds). When the symptoms that lead to these behaviors (e.g., severe depression, psychosis, mania) have been reduced or eliminated, people often look back on such behaviors with mortification and may be terrified of a recurrence.

Involuntary and Coerced Intervention

The history of modern mental health treatment is replete with a wide range of coerced interventions imposed on individuals, such as electroshock therapy, insulin shock therapy, and psychosurgery. Similarly, in the past it was common for people with mental illness to be involuntarily hospitalized "for their own good," even when they presented no clear danger to themselves or others. The laws governing involuntary hospitalization and coerced treatment have changed substantially over the past several decades to prevent these types of abuses (Applebaum, 1994). However, involuntary and coerced treatment continues to play a significant role in the treatment of mental illnesses and is often described as traumatic by consumers (Campbell, 1989; Chamberlin, 1978; Millet, 1991).

Involuntary treatment for mental illness is legally sanctioned in most modern societies when symptoms lead to behaviors that pose a threat to the self or others and the individual lacks the insight or willingness to obtain the necessary treatment. Involuntary or coerced treatment can take many forms, with involuntary hospitalization being one of the most common types. Such hospitalization can involve a variety of assaults on a person's autonomy, such as being confronted by the police, physically subdued, handcuffed or placed in a straitjacket, admitted to a locked hospital ward, and injected with psychotropic medications. Once he or she is in the hospital, coercion or force may be used to impose other treatments on the individual, such as requiring the person to take part in specific "therapeutic" activities or to take medication as a condition of increased freedom and privileges in the hospital or discharge from the hospital. Finally, disruptive or aggressive behavior in the hospital may lead to a person's being physically subdued and placed in a seclusion room or in restraints, which can be experienced as traumatic, especially by a person with a history of sexual abuse.

In addition, when an individual is in a hospital, he or she may be exposed to other types of trauma, such as bizarre, threatening, disorganized, or violent behavior by other inpatients. Furthermore, because of the natural power differential between consumers and staff members in an inpatient setting, there is the potential for being exposed to physically, verbally, and even sexually abusive behavior from members of the staff. Exposure to traumatic experiences in the psychiatric hospital setting, which is presumed to protect rather than threaten the physical and psychological integrity of individuals with psychiatric disabilities, has been described as "sanctuary trauma" (Robins, Sauvageot, Cusack, Suffoletta-Maierle, & Frueh, 2005).

Social Stigma and Effects on the Self

A final aspect of mental illness frequently viewed as traumatic is the social stigma associated with developing and being labeled with a mental illness, and its effects on the individual's perception of self (Beale & Lambric, 1995; Roe, 2001; Wahl, 1997; Williams-Keeler, Milliken, & Jones, 1994). The loss of social opportunities because of the stigma of mental illness, along with challenges such as dealing with cognitive impairment, managing persistent symptoms, and preventing relapses, can be demoralizing and lead to a loss of self-worth and sense of place in the world. These effects can be compounded by mental health professionals who, in their misguided attempts to help consumers adapt to having a mental illness, encourage them to lower their hopes and ambitions (Deegan, 1990). Recovery from the trauma of developing or being labeled mentally ill, as well as from the experience of involuntary treatment, and the developing a positive self-identity and sense of purpose are prominent goals championed in the consumer movement (see Chapter 17 on peer support).

Treatment Considerations

PTSD symptoms clearly occur as a result of a person's developing a psychiatric disability and receiving coerced treatment for it. Mueser and Rosenberg (2003) have suggested that PTSD symptoms related to these experiences may include avoidance of treatment for mental illness, leading to a vicious cycle of relapses and rehospitalizations. However, research has not yet evaluated treatments for PTSD symptoms due to the experience of mental illness and its treatment.

As awareness has grown regarding the high prevalence of trauma in people with psychiatric disabilities, and the potentially traumatizing effects of some treatments imposed on individuals, there has been a movement toward changing treatment practices to ensure that they are more informed by an understanding of the effects of trauma and retraumatization (Fallot & Harris, 2001; Freeman, 2001; Harris, 1994; Harris & Fallot, 2001a; Harris & Fallot, 2001b). The interest in developing more trauma-informed services has been spurred by two related problems associated with traditional mental health services. First, as previously described, trauma history and PTSD have been frequently neglected in assessing the needs of persons with psychiatric disabilities. There are numerous poignant accounts of consumers whose trauma histories were ignored or discounted by mental health professionals (Pritchard, 1995), often with tragic consequences (Jennings, 1994). Furthermore, the potential for underdiagnosis of PTSD, or its potential misdiagnosis as another disorder, is significant, considering the mounting evidence that psychotic symptoms (e.g., auditory hallucinations, persecutory delusions) can occur in PSTD in the absence of schizophrenia or major mood disorders (Butler, Mueser, Sprock, & Braff, 1996; Hamner, 1997; Mueser & Butler, 1987; Sautter, Brailey, Uddo, Hamilton, Beard, et al., 1999; Sautter, Cornwell, Johnson, Wiley, & Faraone, 2002).

Second, in addition to the failure to recognize and address trauma-related problems, consumers have also complained about the retraumatizing effects of psychiatric practices that can trigger PTSD and related symptoms, such as the use of physical restraints or seclusion. For some individuals, the concept of "recovery" resonates more strongly with recovery from perceived abuses of the mental health treatment system, and personal trauma history, than with recovery from a psychiatric disability (Pritchard, 1995). To address concerns about recognizing and addressing trauma-related problems and avoiding retraumatization by the mental health system, many states are changing policies and practices to make them more trauma informed in light of the needs of consumers with a history of victimization (Jennings, 2004). Examples of such changes in practices include the education of staff members about the nature of trauma and its effects (including PTSD), systematic evaluation of trauma and PTSD, involvement of consumers in all aspects of decision making about their care, positive efforts to avoid humiliating and shaming consumers, monitoring of staff behavior, openness of institutions to outside parties such as advocates, training staff members in strategies for minimizing or eliminating the need for physical restraints, and involving consumers in developing personal advance psychiatric directive care plans for the management of possible future crisis situations in which their decision-making capacity may be compromised.

SUMMARY AND CONCLUSIONS

Traumatic experiences, such as sexual and physical assault, are common in persons with psychiatric disabilities, both in childhood preceding the onset of psychiatric disorders and in adulthood after such disorders have developed. Trauma exposure in childhood increases a person's risk of developing a psychiatric disability, and exposure throughout a person's lifetime is linked to a wide range of negative outcomes, including more severe symptoms, impaired functioning and health, substance abuse, and higher service utilization. The most amply documented psychiatric consequence of trauma in persons with psychiatric disabilities is posttraumatic stress disorder (PTSD), a syndrome characterized by reexperiencing a trauma (e.g., intrusive memories of the event, nightmares), avoidance of stimuli that remind the person of the traumatic event (e.g., avoidance of physical intimacy in a person with a history of childhood sexual abuse), and overarousal (e.g., hypervigilance, difficulty with sleeping). Most surveys of persons with psychiatric disabilities indicate *current* rates of PTSD between 28 and 43%, as compared with *lifetime* rates of PTSD in the general population between 8 and 12%.

Despite the high prevalence of trauma in people with psychiatric disabilities, PTSD and other consequences of trauma are rarely assessed or treated, and consequently these problems continue to worsen during the course of a psychiatric illness and contribute to a worse quality of life. Evidence-based practices are not yet available for treating the consequences of trauma in persons with psychiatric disabilities, but progress is under way with several interventions already developed that are either in the pilot-testing phase or undergoing rigorous controlled evaluation. Two general approaches to treating the consequences of trauma have been developed. The first focuses on treating PTSD, based on cognitive-behavioral evidence-based practices in the general population (e.g., use of cognitive restructuring and/or exposure therapy), with adaptations to accommodate the special needs of the individual with a psychiatric disability. The second approach involves targeting a broader range of trauma sequelae, including poor self-image and self-esteem, interpersonal problems, substance abuse, and lack of attention to health and other self-care behaviors.

In psychiatric nomenclature, and in the DSM series in particular, the word *trauma* refers to experiencing or witnessing an event that poses grave danger to the physical integrity of the self or another, which is accompanied by a strong emotional reaction, such as fear or revulsion. Common types of trauma according to this definition include physical and sexual abuse and assault, accidents, disasters, being in combat, and the sudden unexpected death of a loved one. However, the word *trauma* can also refer to any extremely upsetting event or set of events. When the term is used this way, a broader range of experiences related to psychiatric disabilities are frequently described as traumatic, including psychotic symptoms, being involuntarily hospitalized, being placed in seclusion or restraints, being exposed to other severely disorganized individuals, and coming to grips with having a mental illness and the social stigma associated with it. Efforts are under way to make psychiatric services more sensitive and less retraumatizing by assessing consumers' traumatic experiences, changing coercive practices to minimize treatment-related trauma, and providing opportunities for individuals to process their traumatic experiences and move forward in their lives.

Great gains have been made over just the past decade in understanding the importance of trauma and its impact on people with psychiatric disabilities, and these gains have recently been translated into standardized interventions designed to address its consequences. Furthermore, mental health services themselves are in the process of changing from more coercive, hierarchical-based systems to systems focused on empowering consumers, implementing shared decision making, and avoiding the potential trauma inherent in coercive treatments. Considering the progress made in recognizing the problem of trauma in psychiatric disabilities, and the substantial knowledge base that already exists for treating PTSD in the general population, there are good reasons for being optimistic that evidence-based practices for treating the consequences of trauma in psychiatric disabilities will become available over the next decade.

Chapter 15

Dual Diagnosis

Dual diagnosis or *dual disorder* refers to co-occurring, or coexisting, severe mental illness and substance use disorder (abuse or dependence on alcohol or other drugs). Nicotine is usually left out of these discussions, although, as we discuss in Chapter 16, the prevalence of nicotine addiction in this population is enormous. The problem of dual disorders first became apparent among young adults with severe mental illnesses living outside of hospitals after deinstitutionalization (Caton, 1981; Pepper, Krishner, & Ryglewicz, 1981). Since that time, co-occurring disorders have continued to be a primary focus of treatment and rehabilitation. Although the population of people with co-occurring mental and substance disorders is now recognized to be extremely heterogeneous, two important findings have been clearly established.

The first consistent and robust research finding is that substance use disorder is a common comorbidity among people with severe mental illness. Along with many clinical studies, community surveys such as the Epidemiologic Catchment Area Study (Regier et al., 1990) and the National Comorbidity Study (Kessler, Nelson, McGonagle, Edlund, Frank, et al., 1996) have established that approximately 50% of persons with severe mental illnesses self-report sufficient symptoms for a diagnosis of substance use disorder. Because people tend to underreport substance abuse and because having co-occurring disorders rather than a single disorder increases the likelihood of treatment (Regier et al., 1990), we estimate that more than half of all treated clients with severe mental illnesses have a co-occurring substance use disorder. This is a critical finding because it implies that clinicians should assume that the modal, or typical, client has a dual diagnosis rather than a single diagnosis.

The second robust research finding regarding co-occurrence is that people with dual diagnoses have a much greater rate of adverse outcomes than individuals who have men-

---

PERSONAL EXAMPLE

Louisa Martinez Gets Ineffective Treatment

Louisa was a young Hispanic woman who developed difficulties with depression and suicidal behavior in adolescence. Over 10 years, while her diagnosis evolved from major depression to bipolar disorder because of the emergence of manic episodes, Louisa failed out of college, experienced two divorces, made several suicide attempts, was hospitalized nearly 20 times, and was seen by numerous psychiatrists and mental health practitioners. Yet her alcoholism went undetected and untreated during all of her contacts with the mental health system. She had a remarkably parallel experience in the substance abuse treatment system. Over 5 years she entered several substance abuse treatment facilities and attended numerous Alcoholics Anonymous meetings without anyone recognizing that she needed to take medications and manage her bipolar illness as well as her alcoholism. She had never received coordinated mental health and substance abuse treatment by the same practitioner, and she remained unstable and miserable.

---

tal illness alone (Drake & Brunette, 1998). Many of these adverse outcomes appear to be causally related to substance abuse, because they tend to improve rapidly (or the risk of their occurrence tends to decrease rapidly) when people attain abstinence. Typical adverse outcomes include higher rates of relapse (Swofford, Kasckow, Scheller-Gilkey, & Inderbitzin, 1996), hospitalization (Haywood, Kravitz, Grossman, Cavanaugh, Davis, et al., 1995), victimization (Goodman et al., 1997), violence (Steadman et al., 1998), incarceration (Abram & Teplin, 1991), homelessness (Caton, Shrout, Eagle, Opler, Felix, et al., 1994), and serious infections such as HIV and hepatitis (Rosenberg et al., 2001a). This finding is also critical, because it implies that helping people to attain abstinence may be the most efficient way to reduce risk for the kinds of serious outcomes that people with mental illnesses themselves most wish to avoid.

EARLY CLINICAL AND RESEARCH APPROACHES

Ever since the high rate and adverse consequences of co-occurring disorders became apparent during the early 1980s, numerous clinical interventions have been developed and tested. Initial studies documented that the poor treatment received by Louisa Martinez was the norm. The traditional system of treatment in the United States, consisting of parallel or sequential interventions in a variety of mental health treatment settings and separate substance abuse treatment settings, was ineffective. These programs were not set up for people with co-occurring disorders; coordination between programs was absent or inadequate; and those with dual diagnoses rarely received simultaneous treatments for both disorders (Ridgely, Osher, Goldman, & Talbott, 1987). The urgent need to combine mental health and substance abuse interventions in more integrated systems of care in the United States became widely recognized in the 1990s. Increasing momentum since that time has resulted in a national consensus regarding the goal of integrating mental health and substance abuse interventions, at least for people with co-occurring severe mental illnesses and substance use disorders (U. S. Department of Health and Human Services; DHHS, 1999, 2002, 2003).

Clinical innovations for people with co-occurring disorders, public policy related to integrated treatments, and treatment effectiveness studies developed rapidly. Early studies of integrated treatment in the 1980s demonstrated that adding substance abuse counseling to community mental health treatment for people with dual disorders was helpful for those who were motivated and stayed with treatments (Mercer-McFadden, Drake, Brown, & Fox, 1997). However, the majority of people with dual disorders were not easily engaged in treatment and were not motivated to pursue abstinence, and they fared poorly (Hellerstein, Rosenthal, & Miner, 1995; Lehman, Myers, Thompson, & Corty, 1993). Many clinicians noted that outreach and motivational interventions were helpful in engaging clients with dual diagnoses in abstinence-oriented treatments (Mercer-McFadden et al., 1997). Early studies also showed that these clients did not readily fit into residential substance abuse programs and that inpatient dual-diagnosis treatments did not confer benefits after hospital discharge (Drake, Mercer-McFadden, Mueser, McHugo, & Bond, 1998c). Pharmacological approaches to these clients were largely unstudied during this era.

During the 1990s, dual-diagnosis programs began to integrate mental health and substance abuse interventions and to individualize the interventions based on the person's stage of motivation. For example, individuals who were engaged in mental health treatment but not motivated to pursue abstinence were helped by a series of motivational approaches (see Mueser et al., 2003b, for details). Several open clinical trials demonstrated that integrated interventions were effective in engaging people in treatment, helping them to reduce and eliminate their substance abuse, and helping them to stabilize their mental illnesses (Detrick & Stiepock 1992; Drake, McHugo, & Noordsy, 1993; Durell, Lechtenberg, Corse, & Frances, 1993; Meisler, Blankertz, Santos, & McKay, 1997). Similarly, modifications of traditional residential treatment programs seemed to be more effective (Blankertz & Cnaan, 1994; Sacks, 1997). By the mid-1990s, however, the field was still limited by a lack of controlled research (Drake et al., 1998c).

RECENT CLINICAL APPROACHES

Since the mid-1990s, a rapidly developing clinical research effort in the United States and elsewhere (particularly in the United Kingdom and Australia) has addressed the clinical interventions for people with co-occurring severe mental illnesses and substance use disorders. More than 40 controlled studies of psychosocial interventions have been completed in the past 10 years, and new studies are published almost every month (see Table 15.1). Furthermore, pharmacological approaches to treatment with considerable promise have begun to appear. The recent clinical research emphasizes several principles of care (Drake, Mueser, Brunette, & McHugo, 2004), specific psychosocial interventions (Mueser, Drake, Sigmon, & Brunette, 2005b), residential interventions (Brunette et al., 2004a), and psychopharmacological interventions (Brunette, Noordsy, Buckley, & Green, 2005). We first summarize specific approaches to intervention and then emerging principles of care.

Individual Therapies

A variety of individual therapies are now used to help people with dual diagnoses. These interventions often address mental health, substance abuse, or posttraumatic symptoms.

TABLE 15.1. Summary of Recent Intervention Studies

Type of intervention	Summary of findings
Individual therapy	Eight studies show inconsistent results for motivational counseling and cognitive-behavioral counseling on reducing substance use and improving other outcomes.
Group therapies	Eight studies show fairly consistent results on reducing substance use and improving other outcomes.
Family interventions	One study shows mixed results.
Structural interventions	Ten studies of assertive community treatment and other forms of intensive case management show mixed results on reducing substance use, but fairly consistent results on reducing hospitalization and homelessness.
Contingency management	Six studies show fairly consistent results on reducing substance use and improving other outcomes.
Housing interventions	Twelve studies of integrated dual diagnosis residential treatment show fairly consistent results on reducing substance use and improving other outcomes.
Rehabilitation interventions	No studies focused specifically on dual diagnosis clients.
Pharmacological interventions	Few controlled studies.
Legal interventions	Few studies and minimal evidence for improvements.

The individual counseling intervention is usually combined with other interventions as part of a comprehensive program. The most common approach, motivational counseling, involves helping people to identify their own life goals, recognize the extent to which substance use interferes with reaching those goals, and discuss their ambivalence about continued substance use (Mueser et al., 2003b). Motivational counseling is often followed by cognitive-behavioral counseling, which entails helping people to recognize their motives and risk factors for substance use, to develop alternative strategies for dealing with motives and risk factors, and to practice and then use these new strategies (Mueser et al., 2003b).

Only motivational counseling has been tested as a stand-alone individual dual-diagnosis therapy in controlled studies, and the studies all involve brief interventions of one to three sessions. Nevertheless, the findings are promising. The single-session interventions appear to help people connect with outpatient treatment (Baker, Lewin, Reichler, Clancy, Carr, et al., 2002; Swanson, Pantalon, & Cohen, 1999), and the three-session interventions actually show improved substance abuse outcomes several months after treatment (Graeber, Moyers, Griffiths, Guajardo, & Tonigan, 2003; Kavanagh, Young, White, Saunders, Wallis, et al., 2004).

Motivational and cognitive-behavioral counseling for substance abuse and psychosis have been experimentally tested in combination with a family intervention (Barrowclough, Haddock, Tarrier, Lewis, Moring, et al., 2001; Haddock, Barrowclough, Tarrier, Moring, O'Brien, et al., 2003). Outcomes at 12 months favored the experimental intervention in terms of global functioning, substance abuse, symptoms, and hospitalizations. Most of these gains had been maintained at 18 months, although the groups were no longer significantly different in regard to substance abuse outcomes.

Group Therapies

Group interventions are part of most dual-disorders programs and nearly all self-help approaches. A rich variety of group approaches are employed in practice, but few have been studied in well-controlled experiments. All of these group interventions, whether directed by professionals or within the self-help tradition, attempt to take advantage of several consistent findings: Most people with dual disorders are social beings, express social motivations for using substances, become trapped in networks of substance abusers and purveyors, and express the need for new social connections in the process of recovery (Drake, Wallach, Alverson, & Mueser, 2002). Group interventions provide information, discussion, feedback, and support. In addition, the social relationships that develop within group interventions are presumed to provide support for recovery, new friendships, and connections with long-term peer supports.

Early studies of group interventions for persons with co-occurring disorders were methodologically flawed and produced mixed results (Bond, McDonel, Miller, & Pensec, 1991; Lehman et al., 1993; Hellerstein et al., 1995; Jerrell & Ridgely, 1995), but recent controlled studies indicate more positive findings.

Two recent studies of group interventions tailored the discussions to the individual's stage of change and motivations to use substances, and both documented improved outcomes in substance abuse and other behaviors (Aubrey, Cousins, LaFerriere, & Wexler, 2003; James, Presto, Koh, Spencer, Kisely, et al., 2004). Meanwhile, two studies of a relapse prevention group for clients with bipolar and substance use disorders showed that substance abuse and abstinence outcomes were significantly better for the relapse prevention group (Weiss, Griffin, Greenfield, Najavits, Wyner, et al., 2000; Weiss, Griffin, Kolodziej, Ray, & Hennen, 2004). In addition, two studies compared alternative forms of active dual-diagnosis group interventions using experimental designs, and each showed improvements in hospital and substance abuse outcomes, without favoring one approach over the other (Drake, Yovetich, Bebout, Harris, & McHugo, 1997; Penn & Brooks, 1999). The variety of group interventions suggests that the active ingredient is something other than content, perhaps social support, or that an optimally effective approach has not yet been identified.

Self-help groups, such as Alcoholics Anonymous, Dual Recovery Anonymous (Hamilton & Sample, 1994), or Double Trouble (Vogel, Knight, Laudet, & Magura, 1998), are frequently used to support recovery from dual disorders, but these interventions have not been studied in controlled research. One cross-sectional study showed that participation in Dual Recovery Anonymous, as compared with participation in Alcoholics Anonymous, was associated with lower symptoms of mental illness and substance abuse and higher levels of personal well-being (Laudet, Magura, Vogel, & Knight, 2000).

Family Interventions

Interventions for families, delivered by professionals or peers, are widely advocated, effective, and rarely used, both in the mental health field and in the substance abuse field

(Dixon et al., 2001a; Stanton & Shadish, 1997). Effective family interventions address education, support, and skills. That is, they help family members to understand the illnesses and treatments their relatives are experiencing, they acknowledge the pain of the family members themselves and provide opportunities for them to support one another, and they enable family members to improve their skills for helping their relatives. For example, family members can learn and practice how to respond when their relatives are intoxicated, suicidal, or psychotic, all of which are difficult situations that require the family members to have some knowledge and training. Families can also learn skills for solving new problems as they arise and how to access efficiently the human service resources in their local areas. Effective interventions involve a substantial amount of time for meetings, usually over several months.

Although the research on family interventions for severe mental illness or substance abuse alone is robust (Dixon et al., 2001a; Stanton & Shadish, 1997), little research has examined the effects of family interventions for persons with dual disorders. We do know that family support for persons with dual disorders is associated with better outcomes over time (Clark, 2001). The Barroclough et al. (2001) study cited above showed positive gains as a result of counseling plus family intervention. Pilot work on a model combining individual family work, based on behavioral family therapy, with multiple-family support groups has yielded promising results for clients with co-occurring disorders (Mueser & Fox, 2002), and controlled work is currently under way.

Structural Interventions

Structural interventions involve changes in the organization of the health care system in which mental health and substance abuse services are delivered. The most common approach to increasing the intensity and integration of community-based services is to initiate assertive or intensive case management (described in Chapter 6). Intensive day rehabilitation or outpatient programs are also used, but we are unaware of any controlled studies of such programs.

Several studies have examined assertive community treatment or similar intensive case management approaches for persons with dual disorders in a controlled fashion (Carmichael, Tackett-Gibson, & Dell, 1998; Chandler & Spicer, 2006; Drake et al., 1998b; Drake et al., 1997; Essock, Mueser, Drake, Covell, McHugo, et al., 2006; Godley, Hoewing-Roberson, & Godley, 1994; Ho, Tsuang, Liberman, Wang, Wilkins, et al., 1999; Jerrell & Ridgely, 1995; Morse, Calsyn, Klinkenberg, Helminiak, Wolff, et al., 2006). In all of these studies, the more intensive and integrated services had superior outcomes in some but not all areas. However, the studies differ from one another in design, clinical model, implementation, measures, and positive outcomes, making conclusions somewhat unclear. The most consistently positive outcomes in relation to assertive or intensive case management are increased residential stability, decreased hospitalization, and decreased homelessness. Substance abuse outcomes are sometimes, but not consistently, improved in the assertive or intensive treatment condition. Substance abuse is difficult to assess, but at least two recent and well-done studies show that substance abuse treatment can be successful with various case management approaches (Essock et al., 2006; Morse et al., 2006). Substance abuse outcomes are probably related to the quality rather than the structure of substance abuse services and can probably be integrated in different ways (McHugo et al., 1999; Jerrell & Jerrell, 1997). None of the aforementioned studies show positive effects on incarceration outcomes, similar to other studies of assertive community treatment for people in the criminal justice field (Drake, Morrissey, & Mueser, 2006c). Moreover, there is some evidence that people with dual diagnoses and heavy involvement in the criminal justice system have difficulty in forming effective treatment relationships and do not respond to assertive community treatment and dual-diagnosis counseling over many years (Xie, Drake, & McHugo, 2006).

In sum, these outcomes are similar to those found in many previous studies of assertive community treatment (Mueser et al., 1998a) and indicate that people with dual diagnoses also benefit from assertive community treatment in terms of improving their residential stability and avoiding crises that lead to hospitalization and homelessness. As Essock and colleagues (2006) point out, the evidence suggests that integration of mental health and substance abuse services can be delivered in various case management models and does not require assertive community treatment. Finally, people with dual diagnoses who are heavily involved in the criminal justice system do not appear to be good candidates for assertive or intensive approaches to case management. An exception may be those with antisocial behavior that is induced by (rather than preceding) their substance abuse (Mueser et al., 2006a).

Contingency Management

Contingency management involves the systematic provision of incentives and/or disincentives for specific behaviors, such as substance use, for the purposes of modifying those behaviors and improving functional adaptation. Giving vouchers as rewards for negative results of urine toxicology tests shows great promise as a substance abuse intervention (Higgins, Alessi, & Dantona, 2002). Contingent incentives have been shown to reduce cigarette smoking among people with schizophrenia (Tidey, O'Neill, & Higgins, 2002), and an early study also demonstrated the effectiveness of positive reinforcement and response cost contingencies in reducing alcohol use among hospitalized veterans with schizophrenia (Peniston, 1988).

Contingency management interventions have recently been used successfully to reduce illicit drug use among people with severe mental illness. Studies utilizing rigorous within-subject designs (e.g., no treatment–treatment–no treatment) have demonstrated that contingent monetary- and voucher-based incentives are effective in reducing marijuana use among clients with schizophrenia, even among individuals who are not seeking treatment for their marijuana use (Sigmon, Steingard, Badger, Anthony, & Higgins, 2000). Contingent management of Social Security disability benefits (vs. noncontingent management) was also shown to lead to decreased alcohol and drug use in a recent experimental pilot study of people with severe mental illness and substance dependence (Ries, Dyck, Short, Srebnik, Fisher, et al., 2004).

Housing Interventions

Because substance abuse adversely impacts stable housing for persons with dual disorders and is strongly associated with homelessness (Drake, Osher, & Wallach, 1991), integrated residential programs for people with dual disorders are increasingly common (McCoy, Devitt, Clay, Davis, Dincin, et al., 2003). Ten recent controlled studies have examined a variety of these residential programs (Aguilera, Anderson, Gabire, Merlo, Paredes, et al., 1999; Anderson, 1999; Blankertz & Cnaan, 1994; Brunette, Drake, Woods, & Hartnett, 2001; Burnam, Morton, McGlynn, Petersen, Stecher, et al., 1995; De Leon, Sacks,

Staines, & McKendrick, 2000; Kasprow, Rosenheck, Frisman, & DiLella, 1999; Moggi, Hirsbrunner, Brodbeck, & Bachmann, 1999; Nuttbrock, Rahav, Rivera, Ng-Mak, & Link, 1998; Sacks, Sacks, McKendrick, Banks, & Stommel, 2004). In nearly all of these studies, despite variations in the specific residential service models, successful programs were more integrated (blending mental health and substance abuse interventions), more flexible (regarding entrance procedures, behavioral rules, and automatic discharges), and longer in expected tenure (e.g., 1 year or more in residence). Because of the difficulty of randomly assigning people to housing, all of these studies were either quasi-experimental or experimental studies with serious methodological problems. Nevertheless, highly supportive housing appears to be an important consideration, not only in achieving remissions but also in maintaining them (Drake, Wallach, & McGovern, 2005b).

Rehabilitation Interventions

Many studies, as well as self-reports, suggest that people with dual diagnoses have difficulty in attaining and sustaining substance abuse remissions without changing their lives considerably in terms of developing new relationships and meaningful activities that do not involve substance use (Drake et al., 2002). Furthermore, studies of supported employment often indicate that people with dual diagnoses do as well as those with a single diagnosis (Sengupta, Drake, & McHugo, 1998) and that having a job helps to reduce substance abuse (Salyers et al., 2004a). Rehabilitation interventions that address social and vocational functioning are therefore often incorporated into dual-diagnosis programs, but there have been no controlled studies of stand-alone rehabilitation interventions.

Pharmacological Interventions

Experimental studies of medications for people with dual diagnoses have been rare, largely because these individuals have been systematically excluded from medication trials. However, several lines of research are in progress (Brunette et al., 2005). Chapter 7 more thoroughly examines psychopharmacological issues and rehabilitation. People with co-occurring schizophrenia and substance use disorders who are prescribed conventional antipsychotic medications tend to continue to use substances and to experience higher levels of uncomfortable side effects than do those with single diagnoses (Salyers & Mueser, 2001). However, five quasi-experimental or retrospective studies show that the atypical antipsychotic clozapine may be helpful in treating substance use disorders in people with schizophrenia (Buckley, McCarthy, Chapman, Richman, & Yamamoto, 1999; Drake, Xie, McHugo, & Green, 2000b; Green, Burgess, Dawson, Zimmet, & Strous, 2003; Lee, 1998; Zimmet, Strous, Burgess, Kohnstamm, & Green, 2000). Three additional studies suggest that clozapine helps people with schizophrenia to reduce cigarette smoking (McEvoy, Freudenreich, McGee, VanderZwaag, Levin, et al., 1995; George, Sernyak, Ziedonis, & woods, 1996; McEvoy & Freudenreich, 1999). Studies of other atypical antipsychotic medications are even more preliminary, and they do not show similar promise (Green et al., 2003; Noordsy, O'Keefe, Mueser, & Xie, 2001).

Several studies show that valproic acid in combination with lithium is associated with improvement of alcohol disorders in people with bipolar disorders (Brady, Sonnes, & Ballenger, 1995; Hertzman, 2002). Little is known about the impact of other anticonvulsant medications on people with dual diagnoses. The antidepressant bupropion has helped with smoking cessation in two small studies of people with schizophrenia (Evins & Mayes, 2001; Weiner & Ball, 2001). Thus far, however, there is no experimental evidence that antidepressants affect the use of alcohol or other drugs of abuse by people with dual diagnoses.

The use of benzodiazepines is controversial for persons with primary substance use disorders, but the practice appears to be common for people with dual disorders. One prospective naturalistic study of people with dual disorders showed that prescribed benzodiazepines do not appear to improve outcomes and are associated with the development of benzodiazepine abuse (Brunette, Noordsy, Xie, & Drake, 2003b).

Disulfiram has been safely used in open clinical trials to decrease alcohol use in people with dual disorders (Mueser, Noordsy, Fox, & Wolfe, 2003c). Preliminary studies show that naltrexone may be associated with decreased alcohol use in comorbid persons with schizophrenia (Dougherty, 1997; Maxwell & Shinderman, 1997, 2000). A recent randomized clinical trial demonstrated positive effects of disulfiram and/or naltrexone on alcohol abuse for people with dual diagnoses (Petrakis, Nich, & Ralevski, 2006). Finally, people with schizophrenia are often treated with methadone replacement therapy, concurrent with psychosocial and psychiatric treatments (Miotto, Preti, & Frezza, 2001), but opioid replacement therapies have not been experimentally studied in people with dual disorders.

Mandated Treatment

Mandated interventions are commonly used with people with have dual disorders, in part because many are involved with the criminal justice system and under some sort of legal control or supervision. These interventions are more completely discussed in Chapter 13. In regard to people with dual diagnoses, legal directives include incarcerations, conditions of probation, conditions of parole, involuntary hospitalization, outpatient commitments, coercive medication, and guardianships for finances or other functions. More subtle, but still coercive, techniques are also used to shunt people into hospitals, group homes, and other supervised situations. Given the frequency with which mandatory interventions are used for this population, remarkably few studies have addressed them. A small number of controlled studies of outpatient commitment, which include large proportions of people with dual diagnoses, do not show evidence of efficacy (Swanson, Swartz, Borum, Hiday, Wagner, et al., 2000).

PRINCIPLES OF DUAL-DIAGNOSIS TREATMENT

There are clear inconsistencies across the studies heretofore reviewed, in terms of the types of interventions, the quality of research designs, and the use of specific outcome measures. Therefore, the simplest (though clinically unhelpful) conclusion is that the research in this area does not yet yield consistent findings based on randomized controlled trials that can be easily summarized by systematic review or meta-analysis. This conclusion ignores the evidence-based medicine principle that we should use a hierarchy of evidence rather than merely the highest level of evidence (Guyatt & Rennie, 2002). Further, the recent proliferation of controlled studies (experimental and quasi-experimental) permits some limited clinical recommendations regarding principles of dual-diagnosis treatments (see Table 15.2).

TABLE 15.2. Principles of Dual-Diagnosis Care

1. *Integrated treatment*. Combine and individually tailor the mental health and substance abuse interventions.

2. *Stagewise treatments*. Match treatments to the client's level of motivation and stage of recovery.

3. *Long-term retention*. Keep treatment, rehabilitation, and support available and easily accessible for as long as needed.

4. *Comprehensive services*. Address all areas of the individual's personal recovery.

5. *Interventions for treatment nonresponders*. Provide different approaches to intervention for clients who are not making progress toward recovery.

Integrated Treatment

The most consistent principle of care across recent studies is that effective dual-disorder interventions clinically integrate (i.e., combine and individually tailor) mental health and substance abuse interventions at the clinical interface (Drake et al., 2004). This definition of integration differs slightly from others, such as administrative, financial, organizational, and physical integration, but it often includes these other concepts. Clinical integration means that the same clinician (or clinical team) provides appropriate mental health and substance abuse interventions in a coordinated fashion and helps the individual learn to manage intertwined illnesses (Bellack & DiClemente, 1999; Carey, 1996; Minkoff, 1989; Mueser, Drake, & Noordsy, 1998b). In all of these interventions, the clinician or clinical team takes responsibility for blending the interventions into one coherent package. For the individual with a dual diagnosis, the interventions appear holistic and unitary, with a consistent approach, philosophy, and set of recommendations.

   Clinical integration implies that the interventions for individual disorders are modified as well as combined. That is, each treatment component aims to help people to manage both disorders by recognizing their inseparability. For example, social skills training addresses not only developing relationships, but also finding friends who are not substance abusers and learning to avoid and resist peer pressure and social situations that are associated with substance use (Mueser et al., 2003b). Relapse prevention addresses risk situations and coping strategies related to preventing episodes of substance abuse and/or mental illness (Drake et al., 2005b). Vocational rehabilitation focuses on employment that helps people to manage both illnesses (Becker, Drake, & Naughton, 2005). Similarly, family psychoeducation emphasizes the need to understand and cope with two (or more) intertwined disorders (Mueser & Fox, 2002).

Stagewise Treatments

Another consistent principle is that effective programs tailor interventions to the person's stage of treatment or recovery. Stagewise treatment is based on the concept of stages of change (Osher & Kofoed, 1989; Prochaska & Diclemente, 1984). Although there are different ways of conceptualizing progress toward recovery, commonly recognized stages of treatment include (1) engaging the person in a collaborative, trusting relationship (*engagement stage*), (2) helping the engaged person to develop motivation for recovery-oriented interventions (*persuasion or motivation stage*), (3) helping the motivated person to acquire skills and supports for managing both illnesses and pursuing personal goals (*active treatment stage*), and (4) helping the person who is in stable remission to develop and use strategies for preventing relapses (*relapse prevention stage*). Separate studies show that specific interventions can be used to engage people with dual diagnoses in treatment, to help them increase their motivation for controlling or managing their disorders, and to help them gain remissions (Drake et al., 2004). However, although there are numerous studies of relapse prevention for severe mental illness (Herz et al., 2000) and for substance abuse (McGovern, Wrisley, & Drake, 2005), there are currently no controlled studies of substance abuse relapse prevention specifically for this population (Drake et al., 2005b).

Engagement Interventions

Because many people with dual disorders have difficulty accessing and making use of treatment (Owen et al., 1996), effective programs emphasize engagement by providing outreach, practical assistance, and flexible and culturally competent services, as well as by using a motivational counseling style (Mercer-McFadden et al., 1997; Mueser et al., 2003b). For example, inner-city homeless persons with dual diagnoses are often engaged in integrated treatment programs through outreach to shelters and the streets by workers who have same-language capacity and cultural sensitivity, who help with housing and other practical matters, and who take the time needed to develop a trusting relationship. These approaches enable people to access services and to establish relationships with providers. Without outreach and a trusting relationship, failure to engage and dropout rates are high. Studies of residential programs also indicate that engagement strategies are critical, with more flexible programs encouraging people who are not yet abstinent to enter gradually without requiring abstinence.

Motivational Interventions

Even when people are engaged in treatment, they are often unmotivated to manage their own illnesses (Ziedonis & Trudeau, 1997). Effective programs provide motivational counseling interventions that are designed to increase readiness for more definitive interventions (Mercer-McFadden, Drake, Brown, & Fox, 1997; Carey, 1996). Motivational counseling helps people to identify their own goals and then to recognize, through a systematic examination of the advantages and disadvantages of current patterns, that substance abuse and mental illness interfere with attaining those goals (Miller & Rollnick, 2002). Research demonstrates that people who lack motivation can be reliably identified and effectively helped by motivational interventions (Carey, Maisto, Carey, & Purnine 2001). There are, of course, methods other than counseling to help people increase their motivation to manage illnesses. Contingency management and supported employment, described above, are two approaches that appear to enhance motivation.

Active Treatment Interventions

When people are motivated, effective programs of many types can help them to acquire the skills and supports needed to manage their own illnesses. As reviewed above, a wide range of interventions and combinations of interventions has been studied: counseling to promote adherence, cognitive and behavioral skills training, family and social network interventions, self-help, and medication.

Several approaches, ranging from behavioral tailoring to promote medication adherence to early warning sign recognition to prevent relapse, can be effectively used to help people to manage their mental illnesses and substance use disorders (Mueser et al., 2002a). The evidence showing that people who participate fully in different types of dual-disorder treatment groups tend to do well supports this conclusion.

Relapse Prevention Interventions

When people with dual diagnoses achieve stability, remission, or symptom control, they remain vulnerable to relapse. Relapse prevention plans are therefore recommended in most programs, but there have as yet been no outpatient studies of relapse prevention in regard to substance abuse for individuals with dual diagnoses. Many residential treatment programs incorporate relapse prevention approaches. For example, people in residential dual-diagnosis programs are often encouraged to have a job in the community and a specific relapse prevention plan before leaving (Brunette et al., 2001).

Long-Term Retention

Notwithstanding a few studies of brief interventions, most of the current research shows that longer treatment intervals are associated with better outcomes. This finding could, of course, be explained by self-selection, inasmuch as people who are more motivated or less ill may elect to stay in treatment longer, or by circularity, because people who relapse are dismissed from treatment programs and therefore have shorter treatment intervals. No studies have systematically varied the length of participation.

Most dual-disorder programs accept that the majority of people attain recovery gradually over months or years with appropriate supports in the community, rather than quickly in an intensive treatment program (Drake et al., 1998c; Xie et al., 2006). Learning to lead a satisfying and sustainable life, apart from substances of abuse, typically requires changing many aspects of one's life, such as activities, habits, stress management, friends, and housing (Alverson, Alverson, & Drake, 2000). Our 10-year prospective study indicates that this process takes time and often involves relapses en route to recovery (Drake et al., 2006b; Xie, McHugo, Fox, & Drake, 2005).

Comprehensive Services

Most dual-diagnosis programs offer a variety of services and individualize them according to needs. Typical services include individual and group counseling, medication management, peer group supports, family interventions, vocational services, liaison with the criminal justice system, money management, trauma interventions, housing supports, and other supports (Mueser et al., 2003b). These programs address substances of abuse and mental illnesses broadly in all programs rather than narrowly as discrete treatment interventions (Torrey, Drake, Cohen, Fox, Lynde, et al., 2002). For example, hospitalization during acute episodes provides important opportunities for accurate diagnosis, stabilization, and linkage with outpatient dual-disorder interventions (Greenfield, Weiss, & Tohen, 1995). Similarly, housing, social, and vocational programs can support the dually diagnosed person in acquiring skills and supports needed for recovery. These comprehensive programs are, of course, difficult to evaluate because the interventions are not discrete.

The extensive research on homelessness, housing, incarceration, and residential treatment indicates that people with dual diagnoses are prone to lose housing and often require extensive supports to maintain housing (Drake et al., 1991). They can lose their housing because of financial problems, behavioral problems, social network problems, absences due to institutionalizations, and other stressors. Studies of residential treatment indicate that during the initial stages of recovery, people need safe, stable, and secure housing that helps to support the process of recovery. Mature dual-disorder programs in the United States inevitably have an integrated housing component that offers long-term residence or permanent housing (Osher & Dixon, 1996). Ethnographers point out that housing is a primary need that precedes treatment (Hopper & Barrow, 2003) and that people with dual diagnoses need not just treatment but also housing, social supports, and meaningful activities to attain and sustain recovery (Alverson et al., 2000). This was also the lesson learned from the recent Homelessness Prevention Program, in which it was found that programs with direct access to housing were more successful in helping people attain and maintain stable housing (Banks, McHugo, Williams, Drake, & Shinn, 2002).

The psychological process of recovery involves not only managing one's illnesses but also pursuing personally meaningful and satisfying life goals (Mead & Copeland, 2000; Ralph, 1998; Rapp, 1998b; Torrey & Wyzik 2000). The person recovering from dual disorders often participates in employment, new friendships, self-help programs, renewed family relationships, exercise, hobbies, and other recovery-oriented activities. The personal change process is complex and involves developing new attitudes, habits, behaviors, friendships, and coping strategies. Hence, recovery typically takes months or years rather than days or weeks, as the individual modifies many aspects of daily behavior and consolidates them incrementally. Throughout the transformation to recovery, it is helpful for the individual to have a continuous relationship with one clinician who serves as a guide and support in pursuing a variety of goals.

Interventions for Treatment Nonresponders

Not all people with dual diagnoses respond to the same interventions. Treatments need to be tailored to the individual, empirically tested, and modified over time to reflect an algorithmic approach to rehabilitation. A number of ancillary interventions may be helpful to individuals who do not respond well to basic approaches. Residential treatment has been studied extensively in controlled research, but several other interventions are common in clinical practice, including money management (Ries et al., 2004; Ries & Comtois, 1997), intensive family interventions (Mueser & Fox, 2002), trauma interventions (Harris, 1998; Rosenberg et al., 2001b), contingency management (Sigmon et al., 2000; Shaner, Roberts, Eckman, Tucker, Tsuang, et al., 1997), conditional discharges (O'Keefe, Potenza, & Mueser, 1997), and medication (Brunette et al., 2005). Some of these may be instituted at the beginning of treatment for appropriate individuals. For example, early inclusion of family psychoeducation that addresses mental illness and substance abuse, for those individuals who live with their families, seems warranted, as does consideration of a trauma intervention for those who have clinically significant symptoms of posttraumatic stress disorder (PTSD). Contingency management shows promise as a technique to enable people who lack motivation to attain abstinence. Other interventions can be considered when individuals do not respond well initially. For example, long-term residential treatment is expensive but may be an effective approach for people who have cognitive problems or impulsive behavior and who have failed to respond to outpatient treatment. Little research has been done on these ancillary approaches to treatment, other than the previously reviewed studies of residential treatment.

Limits of Current Research

Although research on dual-diagnosis treatment has expanded rapidly, this is still a new field and the research is limited in numerous ways. The participants in most of these studies are heterogeneous with respect to mental illness diagnoses, substance abuse diagnoses, treatment histories, and other important characteristics such as motivational level. There is little consensus on specific clinical approaches, which continue to evolve rapidly, and most programs offer an individually tailored package of interventions, with the result that studies are not strictly comparable. There are relatively few true experiments, and most of the existing experiments have limitations, such as small study group size, treatment drift, and highly selected participants with supportive families. Other research methods vary significantly from study to study in terms of measures, length of follow-up, and other important features. Because persons with dual diagnoses are difficult to engage and retain in treatment, attrition is high in many studies. Each of these difficulties affects validity, practicality, and generalizability. Nevertheless, the field is progressing rapidly, with greater specificity of approaches and more experimental studies appearing regularly.

Current Research Questions

Current research questions encompass both clinical interventions and service system issues. Refining and testing specific interventions with the full range of clients, rather than with highly compliant or otherwise nonrepresentative clients, is clearly a priority. Currently available individual, group, family, self-help, and pharmacological interventions will undoubtedly become more effective as they are standardized, tested, and improved. In addition, we need to study how to sequence and combine interventions in relation to stages of treatment and recovery. For example, one set of interventions, such as client and family psychoeducation combined with outreach and motivational counseling, may be optimal for people who are not yet engaged in treatment and not yet motivated to pursue abstinence, whereas an entirely different set of interventions, such as group behavioral substance abuse counseling and medication, may prove best for those who are engaged in treatment and actively trying to achieve long-term abstinence.

Current studies typically examine persons with dual diagnoses as a group, although they are clearly heterogeneous. Another priority may be to develop and test typologies for the sake of developing more specific clinical recommendations and research. Short-term as well as long-term studies indicate a diversity of responses to standard dual-diagnosis treatment (Drake et al., 2004; Drake, O'Neal, & Wallach, in press; Mueser et al., 2005b). Xie, Drake, and McHugo (2006) recently identified four distinct courses in a prospective 10-year study: One group responded quickly to treatment and developed relatively stable abstinence; a second group responded quickly but continued to have a fluctuating course over many years; a third group (the largest) improved slowly and steadily over time; and a fourth group appeared to be completely unresponsive to standard treatments for 10 years. Characterizing these groups carefully may allow service matching to be more effective and may facilitate the development of new interventions for subgroups.

The development of treatment algorithms is also critical. Applying an algorithmic approach to dual-diagnosis treatment implies that simple and inexpensive interventions should be tried first, with interventions of increasing intensity added as people demonstrate nonresponsiveness to the simpler interventions. Some data are already available for a number of secondary interventions, such as treatment with disulfiram or clozapine,

---

PERSONAL EXAMPLE

Bill Williams Learns to Manage Dual Diagnosis

Bill began to have mood swings as an adolescent. Although a bright and ambitious young man, Bill drank heavily both when he was in a high-energy state and when he was feeling depressed. The combination of unstable moods and alcohol abuse resulted in his flunking out of college and having trouble maintaining a job. He rejected counseling in high school and college. By age 24, he attempted suicide, was hospitalized, and was referred to the local community mental health center. The treatment team recognized immediately that Bill had a dual-diagnosis problem. After 6 months of outreach, building an alliance, and providing dual-diagnosis education, they engaged Bill in a process of selecting interventions of his preference. An effective treatment plan was soon in place. The team psychiatrist prescribed lithium for bipolar disorder and disulfiram for alcoholism; Bill first attended a dual-diagnosis group and then Alcoholics Anonymous meetings regularly with a team counselor who was in recovery; and the team employment specialist helped him to attend community college part-time and work part-time. Bill was confident that he was learning to manage his illnesses and that he was making progress toward his goals of finishing college and working in a bank.

---

intensive family treatments, trauma interventions, and long-term residential interventions, but there have been no comprehensive attempts to develop algorithms.

Beyond developing and testing interventions for routine clients in routine treatment systems, transforming the systems of care is a challenge for administrators and services researchers. Thus, for example, the field needs studies of financing and contracting mechanisms, of dissemination and implementation, of training procedures for all clinicians, of computerized decision support systems, and of shared decision making. Service system interventions, rather than small programs utilizing highly trained specialized clinicians, will be required to have an impact on a problem that affects the majority of persons.

SUMMARY AND CONCLUSIONS

This chapter addresses rehabilitation services for people with co-occurring severe mental illnesses, such as schizophrenia and bipolar disorder, and substance use disorders, defined as abuse or dependence on alcohol or other drugs. Recent controlled research studies indicate that individual and group counseling, contingency management, intensive case management, and residential interventions are effective; promising approaches to family intervention and psychopharmacology are currently being tested. Principles of care include integration of mental health and substance abuse interventions, stagewise interventions that correspond to the individual's level of motivation, long-term care, comprehensive care, and algorithmic care based on treatment response. Future research is expected to refine the existing interventions, clarify a typology of dual-diagnosis clients, and improve attempts to match people to individualized treatments.

Chapter 16

Physical Health and Medical Care

Individuals with severe mental illnesses have substantially increased rates of medical morbidity and early mortality. These negative health outcomes have been largely attributed to four factors: (1) poor health care habits, such as having a bad diet, inactivity, smoking, and substance use disorders; (2) adverse effects of psychiatric medications, such as increasing obesity and cardiovascular disease; (3) inadequate medical care, such as failure to receive immunizations and other preventive interventions; and (4) high rates of suicide.

Recommendations to improve these individuals' health and longevity include improving health care behaviors, careful screening for and management of medication side effects, enhancing general and specialty medical care, and preventing suicides. Although there are few controlled studies to guide practice, several approaches in each of these areas have been proposed. Psychiatric rehabilitation staff can be helpfully involved in several ways, which we discuss below.

INCREASED MEDICAL MORBIDITY AND EARLY MORTALITY

Individuals with severe mental illnesses have increased rates of medical problems (i.e., physical morbidity) involving a variety of illnesses (Breakey, Fischer, Kramer, Nestadt, Romanoski, et al., 1989; Daumit, Pratt, Crum, Powe, & Ford, 2002; Dickey & Azeni, 1996; Dickey, Norman, Weiss, Drake, & Azeni 2002; Felker et al., 1996; Goldman, 1999; Jeste et al., 1996; Jones, Macias, Barreira, Fisher, Hargreaves, et al., 2004; McCarrick, Bertolucci, Goldman, & Tessler, 1986; Rosenberg et al., 2001a; Sokal, Messias, Dickerson, Kreyenbuhl, Brown, et al., 2004; Tsuang, Perkins, & Simpson, 1983). The most common serious medical problems in this population include obesity,

---

PERSONAL EXAMPLE

Eleanor Moore Receives Poor Medical Care

Eleanor Moore, a 55-year-old divorced woman with diagnoses of schizoaffective disorder and alcoholism, had been in and out of homelessness and hospitals for 10 years. She became sober during a court-ordered 3-month hospitalization, and upon discharge entered a housing program for people with co-occurring disorders. For 9 months after discharge from the hospital, she attended Alcoholics Anonymous regularly, made friends with others who were pursuing recovery, and worked part-time at a restaurant. Mrs. Moore's life seemed to be on a very positive course until she developed a respiratory infection and was discovered to have widely disseminated lung cancer. She died within 5 weeks. Her history revealed 40 years of heavy smoking, little medical care for the last 10 years, and a complete absence of smoking cessation interventions. During her most recent visit to the state mental hospital, her cancer was undetected because she received a minimal physical examination and did not have a chest X-ray, owing to the hospital's budgetary problems.

---

hyperlipidemia, Type II diabetes, cardiovascular disease, and blood-borne viral infections (Cimpean, Torrey, & Green, 2005). Obesity, defined as body mass index of greater than 30 kg/m², is epidemic among people with severe mental illnesses—for example, affecting 40–60% of people with schizophrenia (Catapano & Castle, 2004). Obesity predisposes a person to several serious diseases, such as hypertension, Type II diabetes, heart disease, cancer, and others (Flegal, Carroll, Ogden, & Johnson, 2002). Type II diabetes, which involves tissue resistance to insulin (Type I diabetes entails failure to make insulin), is approximately twice as prevalent (15%) among people with schizophrenia as among the general population in the United States (Dixon, Weiden, Delahanty, Goldberg, Postrado, et al., 2000b). Cardiovascular disease, which leads to heart attacks and strokes, is the leading cause of death and disability in the United States, and people with mental illnesses have even higher rates than the general population (Enger, Weatherby, Reynolds, Glasser, & Walker, 2004). Lethal blood-borne viral infections, such as HIV, hepatitis B, and hepatitis C, affect 30% or more of persons with severe mental illnesses (Rosenberg et al., 2001a). Chronic obstructive pulmonary disease is also much more common among persons with severe mental illness than among those in the general population (23 vs. 6%) (Himmelhoch, Lehman, & Kreyenbuhl, 2004).

As one consequence of high rates of medical comorbidity, people with severe mental illnesses have greatly reduced physical functioning (defined as physical limitations on usual daily activities such as walking, climbing stairs, and carrying groceries; Chafetz, White, Collins-Bride, Nickens, & Cooper, 2006). Their physical functioning resembles that of those in the general population who are 10–20 years older.

Another consequence is that individuals with severe mental illnesses are extremely vulnerable to early institutionalization in nursing homes (Bartels, Forester, Mueser, Dums, Pratt, et al., 2004). They enter nursing homes several years earlier than their non-mentally ill counterparts in the population, and one of the primary reasons for early institutionalization is the increasing burden of medical illnesses.

A third consequence is that individuals with severe mental illnesses experience worse mental health outcomes because of their medical problems. Many studies have documented that high rates of medical problems (often undetected) exacerbate mental health conditions (Koranyi, 1979; Felker, Workman, Stanley-Tilt, Albansese, & Short, 1998). In the Schizophrenia Patient Outcomes Research Team study, a greater number of current medical problems independently contributed to more severe psychosis and depression, and to greater likelihood of a previous suicide attempt (Dixon, Postrado, Delahanty, Fischer, & Lehman, 1999c).

Finally, the most serious consequence of medical problems is that people with severe mental illness experience high levels of early mortality (Allebeck, 1989; Baxter, 1996; Brown, 1997; Felker et al., 1996; Newman & Bland, 1991; Simpson & Tsuang, 1996; Tsuang & Woolson, 1978; Tsuang, Woolson, & Fleming, 1980a). On average, people with severe mental illnesses have a 20% shorter lifespan than others in the general population (Newman & Bland, 1991). Although some of these early deaths are due to suicide, most are caused by general medical illnesses (Brown, 1997). Suicide accounts for approximately 5–10% of deaths in persons with schizophrenia (Caldwell & Gottesman, 1990) and 10–15% of deaths among those with bipolar disorder (Harris & Barraclough, 1997). Many other illnesses also influence early mortality (Brown, 1997; Tsuang & Woolson, 1978). For example, these individuals have higher than expected death rates due to cardiovascular, pulmonary, gastrointestinal, endocrine, and infectious diseases (Brown, Inskip, & Barraclough, 2000; Buda, Tsuang, & Fleming, 1988; Mortensen & Juel, 1990; Tsuang, Woolson, & Fleming, 1980b).

REASONS FOR MEDICAL MORBIDITY AND EARLY MORTALITY

Poor medical health and early mortality among individuals with severe mental illnesses are due to several factors, including poor health care behaviors, side effects of psychiatric medications, inadequate medical care, suicide, and other factors. These are summarized in Table 16.1 and described in detail below.

Health Care Behaviors

People with severe mental illnesses tend to have sedentary lifestyles and unhealthy diets (Brown, Birtwhistle, Roe, & Thompson, 1999; Strassnig, Brar, & Ganguli, 2005), both of which are risk factors for obesity, high cholesterol, Type II diabetes, and cardiovascular disease (Cimpean et al., 2005). Unemployment, poverty, and poor social skills undoubtedly contribute to inactivity and dietary problems, and there may also be features of mental illness, treatment, and stigma that contribute to unhealthy lifestyles.

Another critical behavioral risk involves elevated rates of addictions, including high rates of nicotine dependence (Dalack, Healy, & Meador-Woodruff, 1998; Ziedonis, Kosten, Glazer, & Frances, 1994) and abuse/dependence involving alcohol and other drugs (Regier et al., 1990; Kessler, Crum, Warner, Nelson, Schulenberg, et al., 1997a). In one primary care clinic for people with severe mental illnesses, 78% smoked, 44% abused alcohol, and 31% abused other substances (Crews, Batal, Elasy, Casper, & Mehler, 1998). Overall, about half of the people with severe mental illnesses have a substance use disorder other than nicotine dependence (Regier et al., 1990), and the rates of nicotine dependence are even higher (Dalack et al., 1998; Ziedonis et al., 1994). These addictive behaviors predispose a person to several medical problems, including cancer, chronic respiratory diseases, and serious infections. As a direct result of their substance use, people with severe mental illnesses are also prone to engage in dangerous behaviors,

TABLE 16.1. Causes of Medical Morbidity and Early Mortality

Poor health care behaviors

- Toxic effects of substances, including nicotine, alcohol, and other drugs
- Inactivity
- Poor diet

Medication side effects

- Neurological (tardive dyskinesia)
- Endocrine (Type II diabetes mellitus)
- Metabolic (lipid changes, obesity)
- Cardiovascular (arrhythmias, coronary artery disease)

Inadequate medical care

- Inattention to physical health
- Poor access to health care
- Poor quality of health care

Suicide

- Intentional suicide
- Accidents, violence, overdoses related to substance abuse

Other factors

- Genetic or illness-related vulnerabilities

such as using drugs intravenously, sharing needles with other drug users, and having unprotected sex with multiple partners, all of which increase the risk of HIV and other blood-borne viral infections (Carey, Carey, & Kalichman, 1997; Rosenberg et al., 2001a).

Medication Side Effects

Psychiatric medications contribute substantially to excess medical morbidity and mortality through a variety of neurological, metabolic, and other adverse side effects (Marder et al., 2004). Psychotropic medications can cause obesity, high levels of cholesterol, Type II diabetes, and heart arrhythmias. Recently, there has been considerable concern about the relationship between second-generation antipsychotic medications and changes in glucose and lipid metabolism, known as the metabolic syndrome (Sacks, 2004). Some medications are more strongly implicated than others for specific problems. For example, nearly all antipsychotic medications are associated with weight gain, but clozapine and olanzapine are associated with the greatest weight gain (greater than 4 kg at 10 weeks) (Allison, Mentore, & Heo, 1999) and with the greatest changes in glucose metabolism (Henderson, Cagliero, Copeland, Borba, Evins, et al., 2005). Similarly, most antipsychotic medications can cause serious neurological side effects, such as tardive dyskinesia (persistent involuntary movements), but high-potency medications, such as haloperidol and fluphenazine, are highly prone to produce these problems.

Inadequate Medical Care

Primary medical care interventions, such as vaccinations for influenza, screening for common diseases, and other preventive care measures, have been shown to improve medical health for vulnerable populations (Blumenthal, Mort, & Edwards, 1995). However, people with mental illnesses have a decreased likelihood of receiving preventive medical care (Druss, Rosenheck, & Desai, 2002), including recommendations to reduce sexual risks, to stop smoking, and to remove firearms from the house (Carney, Allen, & Doebbing, 2002).

Many studies document that people with severe mental illnesses do not usually receive high-quality medical care (Felker et al., 1996). For example, one study found that only 50% of clients in community mental health centers had a regular nonpsychiatrist doctor (Crews et al., 1998). An extensive review estimated that approximately 50% of psychiatric clients had known medical problems that needed further evaluation or treatment and another 35% suffered from previously unidentified medical problems that needed further evaluation or treatment (Felker et al., 1996). In a primary care clinic for people with severe mental illnesses, for example, 87% of new clients received a new medical diagnosis, and a majority needed immunizations and medical screening (Crews et al., 1998). Even among homeless people, those with severe mental illnesses tend to receive less medical care than others (Folsom, McCahill, Bartels, Lindamer, Ganiats, et al., 2002). People with severe mental illnesses are also less likely to receive needed specialized medical procedures, such as cardiac interventions following heart attacks (Druss et al., 2000a).

The findings on medical care are not entirely consistent. One study using national survey data found that persons reporting a mental disorder were as likely as others to have a primary medical care provider, but were more likely to report inability to obtain needed care or delaying care because of financial problems (Druss & Rosenheck, 1998). Another study of clients in psychiatric centers found that they were more likely to report receiving medical care in the past year than persons in national surveys, but were less likely to receive dental care and much more likely to report barriers to medical care, such as difficulty in getting appointments and paying for medications (Dickerson, McNary, Brown, Kreyenbuhl, Goldberg, et al., 2003). Access to care and quality of care vary widely, and individuals who are most disadvantaged are probably at greatest risk. For example, the fairly recent exposé of high mortality in New York City's board-and-care homes illustrates the real impact of marginal care for persons with severe mental illnesses ("For mentally ill," 2002).

Suicide

People with severe mental illnesses of all types, including schizophrenia, bipolar disorder, and depression, have greatly increased rates of suicide, several times greater than the general population (Caldwell & Gottesman, 1990; Harris & Barraclough, 1997). Suicide often affects young men, those in the early phases of experiencing mental disorder and those with higher education and higher expectations (Drake, Gates, Cotton, & Whitaker, 1984; Pompili, Girardi, Ruberto, & Tatarelli, 2004). Depression and hopelessness often presage completed suicides. Co-occurring substance abuse increases the risk of suicide (Bartels, Drake, & McHugo, 1992). Affected individuals often withdraw from social contacts and drop out of treatment relationships prior to suicide. Current research thus suggests that those who are at highest risk for suicide are young people who become overwhelmed by the losses related to mental illness and hopeless about the possibility of recovering, those whose predominant mood is depression, those who use alcohol and drugs, and those who use social withdrawal rather than more positive coping strategies. There is also a strong likelihood that genetic factors influence suicide risk.

Other Factors

Some evidence indicates that metabolic abnormalities, such as in glucose metabolism, are present in people with schizophrenia before they are exposed to medications (Thakore, 2004). Thus, metabolic abnormalities may be an inherent part of the illness that is exacerbated by certain medications. The same situation also describes neurological abnormalities. The syndrome of tardive dyskinesia was clearly documented before the use of antipsychotic medications but can be precipitated by specific medications.

REASONS FOR INADEQUATE MEDICAL CARE

Inadequate medical care is a common theme in this literature, and many studies have examined the reasons. Medical problems among people with severe mental illnesses frequently go undetected because practitioners in psychiatric settings assume limited responsibility for general medical care, people with severe mental illnesses have limited access to primary care, and primary care providers often have limited knowledge about the health risks associated with mental illness and psychiatric medications (Marder et al., 2004). Another reason is that people with mental disorders sometimes have limited ability to describe their symptoms (Goldman, 1999). Moreover, coordination between psychiatric staff and primary care staff is often difficult (Crews et al., 1998). People with severe mental illness commonly demonstrate impairments in basic self-care skills (Velligan, Mahurin, Hazleton, Eckert, & Miller, 1997), and poor adherence to medication for general medical problems and poor health care follow-up are common problems (Crews et al., 1998). For example, patients with HIV who have psychiatric problems have poorer adherence to antiretroviral medications (Sternhell & Corr, 2002). For practitioners, it can be difficult to differentiate between somatic manifestations of psychiatric illness and general medical problems (Crews et al., 1998). People with mental illness report fears of being treated rudely, lack of financial resources, and many other perceived barriers when they seek medical attention (Carney, Yates, Goerdt, & Doebbeling, 1998; Dickerson et al., 2003; O'Day, Killeen, Sutton, & Iezzoni, 2005). Poverty, unemployment, and underinsurance are undoubtedly factors (Druss & Rosenheck, 1998). Inadequate medical care may also be related to neglect of self-care owing to symptoms of mental illnesses such as social withdrawal, paranoia, and psychotic thinking (Goldman, 1999).

Sternberg (1986) divided problems in obtaining adequate medical care into three groups: disease-related problems (e.g., medical problems and psychiatric problems overlap and are difficult to differentiate, and medical problems are often caused by psychiatric medications); patient-related problems (e.g., patients are often reluctant to seek medical attention and are poor historians); and health care system problems (e.g., poor access to health care for persons who are underinsured or destitute, and poor coordination between mental health and general medicine). Another category may be practitioner-related problems, inasmuch as medical providers may have biased perceptions of people with mental illnesses and their ability to follow through with treatments (Brunette, Drake, Marsh, Torrey, Rosenberg, et al., 2003a).

INTERVENTION APPROACHES

In this section we review attempts to help people with mental illnesses to improve their physical health and decrease their risk of early mortality. We address four categories of interventions, which are summarized in Table 16.2: attempts to help people improve their health care behaviors, to limit the serious side effects of medications, to improve the access and quality of medical care, and to prevent suicide.

Improving Health Care Behaviors

Changing behaviors of any kind generally involves altering attitudes, skills, and supports. These approaches can be used in relation to reducing substance abuse, smoking cessation, improving diets, increasing exercise, enhancing medical self-care, and eliminating dangerous behaviors. Examples of outcomes of the three approaches may be that people with severe mental illnesses increase their motivation to seek influenza vaccinations, learn shopping skills to ensure a healthier diet, and join peer support groups that promote regular exercise.

Because inactivity, poor diet, and obesity are such common problems for persons with severe mental illnesses (Brown et al., 1999), many experts recommend exercise and dietary counseling (Green, Patel, Goisman, Allison, & Blackburn, 2000; Ryan and Thakore, 2002; Richardson, Faulkner, McDevitt, Skrinar, Hutchinson, et al., 2005). A systematic review of evidence indicates that all behavioral interventions (e.g., cognitive-behavioral counseling or rewards for diet and/or exercise) report small reductions in, or maintenance of, weight, whereas the evidence for pharmacological interventions is less consistent (Faulkner, Soundy, & Lloyd, 2003). The research on these interventions is,

---

TABLE 16.2. Recommendations to Improve Physical Health and Longevity

Improving health care behaviors

- Health improvement interventions to focus on diet and exercise
- Smoking cessation programs
- Integrated dual-diagnosis interventions

Minimizing medication side effects

- Routine medical screening for side effects
- Education regarding side effects and polypharmacy
- Shared decision making

Improving medical care

- Ensuring access to prevention, primary care, and specialty care
- Connecting medical care and mental health care

Preventing suicides

- Basic suicide prevention techniques
- Medications for suicidal clients
- Addressing risk factors assertively

---

however, largely based on nonexperimental studies (Chue, 2004; Werneke, Taylor, Sanders, & Wessely, 2003). Sustained adherence to exercise programs presents a problem for individuals with mental illnesses, just as it does for those in the general population (Richardson et al., 2005).

Helping people with mental illnesses to overcome alcohol and drug abuse is discussed in Chapter 15. In this section we address smoking cessation. Given that 60–80% of people with severe mental illnesses are addicted to nicotine, this is a seriously neglected area. Research generally shows that people with severe mental illnesses are less likely to try to quit smoking and that those who do try are only half as successful as other smokers (Ziedonis & George, 1997). Nevertheless, many do quit smoking. Controlled trials of smoking cessation interventions support the use of bupropion (Evins, Cather, Deckersbach, Freudenreich, Culhane, et al., 2005) and nicotine replacement therapy (Chou, Chen, Lee, Ku, & Lu, 2004). Less well-controlled studies support the use of clozapine (George, Sernyak, & Ziedonis, 1995) or nicotine nasal spray (Williams, Ziedonis, & Foulds, 2004).

Minimizing the Side Effects of Psychiatric Medications

Medical practitioners who are prescribing and managing psychotropic medications are legally and ethically responsible for monitoring health-related side effects. Guidelines are rapidly being developed for routine monitoring of metabolic, endocrinological, neurological, cardiac, ophthalmological, and other side effects (Marder et al., 2004). For example, a practitioner should routinely give attention to the client's weight, waist circumference, body mass index, plasma lipids, and plasma glucose.

Risks can often be alleviated by changing medications when warning signs appear, for example, when weight gain exceeds 5% during the first few months of starting a medication (American Diabetes Association, American Psychiatric Association, American Association of Clinical Endocrinologists, & North American Association for the Study of Obesity, 2004). Other helpful steps include avoiding polypharmacy and using less dangerous medications. Even with optimal medication management, however, all medications have risks of side effects, and therefore attention to lifestyle changes, such as changes in diet and exercise, is critical.

One goal that has received little attention in the professional literature is to help people become more knowledgeable about their own medications and more active in choosing and monitoring those medications (Deegan & Drake, 2006). For example, nearly everyone in the United States is now subjected to multimillion-dollar advertising campaigns by the pharmaceutical industry, and many people are further exposed to enormous amounts of misinformation over the Internet. Despite these campaigns, the facts remain that psychiatric medications in general have only small effects on the symptoms of psychiatric illnesses and that the differences in therapeutic effects between medications in the same class (for example, between different antidepressants or different antipsychotic medications) are minimal, whereas the differences in side effects are often major. Decisions to use specific medications should therefore almost always respond to preferences, and people with mental illnesses should be centrally involved in the process of shared decision making (Adams & Drake, 2006; Deegan & Drake, 2006). However, the movement toward shared decision making will require much more attention to sharing scientific information regarding medications and other treatments and will require activating both people with mental illnesses and their mental health practitioners.

Improving Medical Care

Like others in society, people with mental illnesses need regular preventive care, routine primary medical care, and specialized care for serious or chronic conditions. The usual health care system involves referrals back and forth between mental health and general medical providers, which has been termed *parallel care*. In this parallel system, a minimum of medical care is typically provided in the mental health care setting (e.g., screening for neurological side effects of medications), and clients are referred to local doctors for primary and specialty medical care. This approach has resulted in poor access and the negative outcomes reviewed above.

The literature on medical care for people with severe mental illnesses assumes that greater coordination or integration of medical and mental health care would improve each of these areas, and there is some evidence to support this view (Druss & von Esenwein, 2006). There is no consensus, however, regarding a specific approach to connecting mental health care and medical care for people with severe mental illnesses in order to improve their medical health (Bartels, 2004; Goldman, 1999). Several approaches have been suggested, and we review these next.

Care Coordinators

A common approach to linking mental health care and medical care is to rely on care coordinators. In this model, case managers or other care coordinators actively facilitate referrals and connections to general medical care. This approach has been termed the *culture broker model*, because the case manager becomes, in effect, a translator between the client's view of illness and the medical provider's perspective on the issues involved (Schwab, Drake, & Burghardt, 1988). For example, a case manager may help the person to make a list of physical health concerns to present to the physician and may even attend the appointment to ensure that the doctor understands these concerns; at the same time, the case manager can take notes and later help the person to understand the physician's explanations of the physical symptoms and recommendations for interventions. This type of translation and assistance may be particularly helpful for people who have severe neurocognitive deficits, such that attention, memory, and learning are significant barriers to communication and follow-through. People with the most severe impairments usually do have a case manager who can theoretically provide this brokering service and understand the two cultures. However, whether or not case managers, who generally have little or no medical training and who often have large caseloads and multiple responsibilities, can really provide these functions, has not been studied. Because this is the implicit model in many settings, the indirect evidence suggests that this model is not greatly effective.

One careful approach to refining the care coordinator model is to use nurses as the care coordinators. Nurses have training and experience with medical care, and they have greater authority in making linkages within the care system. In a pilot study using this approach with older adults with severe mental illnesses, the nurse care coordinator taught health care behaviors and facilitated linkages with medical providers (Bartels et al., 2004). Almost one-third of the study group had had no preventive health care or other medical visits during the 3 years prior to the study. At 1-year follow-up, 100% had received preventive health care, and one-third received care for newly detected medical disorders. However, there is a shortage of nurses in the public mental health system.

Specialized Primary Care Clinics

Another approach, which has been implemented in several large metropolitan areas, has been to establish specialized primary care clinics for people with severe mental illnesses. For example, outpatient primary care clinics staffed by internal medicine specialists in Denver serve exclusively people with severe mental illnesses (Crews et al., 1998). Case managers initiate referrals, and the internist sends a complete medical plan to the mental health staff after each visit. This model assumes that the extensive and complex medical comorbidities in this population are best treated by an internist who is interested in working with such clients. The current evidence suggests that coordination, transportation, and follow-up continue to be problematic in this arrangement, but medical care may be improved (Crews et al., 1998).

Expanded Medical Care by Mental Health Practitioners

A common way in which medical care is routinely integrated with psychiatric care involves the management of medication side effects. Psychiatrists and nurses within mental health clinics routinely monitor and manage medication side effects. Some have recommended that the psychiatrist's role should be expanded to encompass a greater amount of primary medical care, and particularly preventive medical services, such as immunizations, blood pressure checks, and interventions for obesity and smoking (Carney et al., 1998; Dobscha & Ganzini, 2001). Several pilot programs have attempted to involve psychiatrists as primary care physicians in this way (Silverman, Lu, & O'Neill, 1994; Wulsin, 1996; Shore, 1996).

The argument for this approach is that psychiatrists are often in a unique position to provide medical services to vulnerable individuals, such as those in homeless settings or institutions, who would otherwise be unlikely to receive any medical care. Barriers to this approach include psychiatrists' time constraints, inadequate reimbursement for psychiatrists in this role, psychiatrists' lack of interest and knowledge regarding medical issues, and the lack of equipment and resources in mental health clinics to address medical care. In practice, this idea has not been widely adopted because most mental health agencies providing care for persons with severe mental disorders have insufficient psychiatric time to cover basic assessment and pharmacological management carefully, and most psychiatrists are reluctant to assume primary care responsibilities. Furthermore, medical care in homeless shelters and psychiatric institutions is often provided by nonpsychiatric professionals.

Medical Care Teams within Mental Health Clinics

Another approach to integration is to colocate the medical care team and the mental health team in the same setting. Felker et al. (1998) describe a multidisciplinary primary care team located within a Veteran's Administration psychiatric clinic. In this model, the treating psychiatrist became a member of the larger medical care team. The result was excellent communication between medical staff, mental health staff, and clients; high client satisfaction; and identification of at least one new medical problem that warranted further evaluation or treatment in 56% of clients. In a separate randomized controlled trial of colocated and integrated treatment, the group receiving integrated care was more likely to receive primary care, to receive preventive interventions, to report improvements in physical health, and to avoid medical emergencies (Druss, Rohrbaugh, Levinson, & Rosenheck, 2001).

This approach to integration is common within psychiatric hospitals (e.g., many hospitals have internists, neurologists, physician's associates, nurses, and other medical staff members who attend to general medical problems while clients are in the hospital). Comprehensive medical services may, however, be difficult to establish in freestanding mental health care settings, especially smaller practices or clinics.

Public Health Nurse Outreach

An outreach approach to integration entails routine visits by general medical staff members to screen clients and link them to appropriate medical services. For example, Rosenberg, Brunette, Oxman, Marsh, Dietrich, et al. (2004b) described a model in which a public health nurse visited several community mental health centers on a regular basis to educate, screen, counsel, and link patients with medical care for blood-borne infections, such as HIV and hepatitis C. Medical treatments for these infections are complicated, and the public health nurse helped infected individuals to understand their treatment options and to link directly with infectious disease specialists, liver disease specialists (hepatologists), and other appropriate staff. This model may be particularly effective in providing expert counseling, screening, education, and linkage. The responsibility for ongoing monitoring of treatment and side effects could be shared by medical and mental health staff. A disadvantage may be a lack of appropriately trained and adequately funded public health nurses to perform these functions.

Health Care Rehabilitation

A further approach to integrated care incorporates traditional approaches to psychiatric rehabilitation, such as helping clients to take responsibility for their own medical care. Here the focus is on skills training to help people learn to pay attention to their health care needs, to make appointments and communicate clearly with medical providers, and to follow through with using medications and other health care prescriptions. As described above, Bartels and colleagues (2004) have developed and are testing an intervention for older adults with severe mental illnesses that combines health care skills training and nurse-facilitated linkage with medical care. The advantages of this approach are that the same nurse helps with skills and supports, so that skill development and autonomy can be maximized. A disadvantage may be a shortage of nurses who have all of the relevant skills and are available and affordable by community mental health centers.

Automated Systems

Information technology could enhance all approaches to integrating psychiatric and medical care. Computerized reminders for preventive and other basic medical services have been effective in primary medical clinics (Barnett & Winickoff, 1980; McDonald, Hui, & Smith, 1984; Litzelman, Dittus, & Miller, 1993). As mental health care systems move toward adopting electronic medical records and computerized decision support systems, technology can be used to improve the rates of adherence to guidelines for basic medical services. For example, computerized reminders can ensure the appropriate timing and enhance quality improvement related to a variety of health care screens and follow-ups regarding various medical appointments and procedures. The advent of client portals, which provide direct access to medical records, may also help people with mental illnesses to take greater responsibility for their own medical care.

Preventing Suicide

Although suicide rates among people with severe mental illnesses have always been high, relatively little is known about suicide prevention. Three areas of intervention are widely used: medications to address biological vulnerabilities, psychosocial interventions to address other known risk factors, and standard suicide prevention procedures. The use of medications can address biological risk factors, such as reductions in 5-hydroxy-tryptophan metabolism. There is evidence from controlled studies that some specific medications, such as lithium (Baldessarini, Tondo, & Hennen, 2003) and clozapine (Meltzer, Alphs, Green, Altamura, Anand, et al., 2003), are associated with decreased suicidal behavior or ideation in people with bipolar disorder and schizophrenia, respectively. Other medications may reduce suicide through reductions in psychotic, manic, and depressive symptoms, but do not appear to have independent effects on suicide.

Suicide risk factors for people with severe mental illnesses include previous suicidal behavior, depression, hopelessness, social isolation, and substance abuse (Caldwell & Gottesman, 1990). Those who are young, male, unmarried, who have good premorbid functioning and with high performance expectations, and who have experienced a significant loss appear to be at particularly high risk (Drake et al., 1984; Pompili et al., 2004). Thus, psychiatric rehabilitation staff members should be aware of clients' past or current suicidal ideation or behavior, monitor and address depressive symptoms, help people to develop hope by achieving success with their goals, help people to maintain social connectedness, reach out to them when they become isolated, and help them to overcome substance use disorders. These are all standard approaches to psychiatric rehabilitation described in other chapters.

Logically, standard suicide prevention techniques, such as asking people explicitly about suicidal thoughts, increasing surveillance during times of crisis, discussing their motivations and feelings, providing empathic support, and helping to remove deadly weapons from the home, may also be helpful interventions (Caldwell & Gottesman, 1990; Pompili et al., 2004). Again, however, there is little evidence that these procedures actually prevent suicides.

SUMMARY AND CONCLUSIONS

Poor physical health and threats to normal longevity are ubiquitous issues for people with severe mental illnesses. The following example illustrates how handling these issues well can affect a person's life.

People with severe mental illnesses are particularly vulnerable to poor medical health, considerable morbidity, and early mortality for a variety of reasons. To reduce these problems, four basic issues need to be addressed: (1) improving health care behaviors, such as through proper diet, exercise, smoking cessation, and preventive health care; (2) enhancing the monitoring and management of side effects related to psychiatric medications; (3) ensuring routine care from general medical providers and helping with adherence and follow-up; and (4) reducing suicide risks.

PERSONAL EXAMPLE

Mary Johnson Receives Good Medical Care

Mary Johnson, a 53-year-old woman with schizophrenia, received care at the same community mental health center through an assertive community treatment team over 25 years. In addition to regular screening for medication side effects, the nurse on the team ensured that Mrs. Johnson received regular medical care during this time and helped her to follow medical advice and regimens related to medical problems and several behaviors that posed significant risk. With the help of group support and nicotine replacement therapy, she had been able to stop smoking. The team also helped her to modify her shopping habits and diet in order to control weight gain. Her primary care doctor encouraged routine mammography, which detected early breast cancer. Mrs. Johnson subsequently received a lumpectomy and adjuvant therapy with hormonal medications. She has had no detectible cancer since surgery, and she participates faithfully in medical follow-up visits.

Although physical health has often been omitted from discussions of psychiatric rehabilitation, it is inextricably linked with mental health, functional performance, institutionalization, and quality of life. Assuming that medical health issues are separate from psychiatric rehabilitation is as naïve as earlier attempts to separate rehabilitation from mental health treatment. Holistic, integrated care is almost always more accessible and more effective than fragmented health care. Psychiatric rehabilitation staff members should be involved in helping people to obtain optimal physical health in a number of ways, as discussed throughout this chapter.

Chapter 17

Peer Services and Supports

Peer support encompasses a diversity of program models, but all share at least one common characteristic; the support is provided by an individual who has a serious mental illness and has used or is currently using mental health services and is, consequently, a peer to the subject user or participant. The premise of peer support is that individuals who have shared common experiences can provide better support and safer environments than others who have not had a history of psychiatric treatment. Peer services and supports are, by their very nature, recovery oriented, as these services and supports engender empowerment and are based on the principle of self-determination.

Although peer services and supports have been around for many years, they have grown exponentially in the last two decades (Glick & Dixon, 2002). These peer services and supports are generally categorized in the following domains: mutual support or self-help groups, consumer-operated services, consumer–professional partnership services, and consumers as employees. It is important to acknowledge that there is controversy surrounding the term *consumer* in this context, and in order to avoid conflict some writers use *consumer/survivor/ex-patient* as a means of identifying such an individual (Van Tosh & DelVecchio, 1998). The issue with the term *consumer* is the implication that mental health users have a choice when receiving mental health services, but in reality this is frequently not the situation. As a result, the term is considered a misnomer in this context. Most recently, the term *peer* has come to be considered the most neutral terminology for one who has used or is currently using mental health services. Where appropriate, this term is used in this chapter. However, because concepts like "consumer operated services" and "consumer movement" have come to be widely accepted and used in the literature, it will be difficult in some instances to retain the original meaning when altering the terminology.

This chapter begins by putting these services and supports in the historical context of the consumer movement and continues by defining and delineating peer services and supports and the theoretical basis for the peer support process. Subsequently, an elaboration of the various types of peer services and supports, including examples of peer support programs, organizations, and services is provided, along with the research on the effectiveness of the various categories of peer services and supports.

HISTORICAL CONTEXT

Persons with mental illnesses and their families protesting inhumane treatment and coming together for support and advocacy has a relatively long history. In 1845, the Alleged Lunatic's Friend Society was established in England (Frese & Davis, 1997; Van Tosh, Ralph, & Campbell, 2000). In the United States, after the Civil War, Elizabeth Packard wrote of her forced commitment by her husband and founded the Anti-Insane Asylum Society in Illinois, and Elizabeth Stone, who was institutionalized by her family for her decision to switch from her family's religion, undertook comparable activities in Massachusetts (Chamberlin, 1990; Van Tosh et al., 2000). Clifford Beers (1923), who wrote about the abuses he experienced when hospitalized for psychiatric problems in *A Mind That Found Itself*, was instrumental in founding the National Committee for Mental Hygiene which later became the National Mental Health Association (NMHA; Grob, 1994); this association has been instrumental in the promotion of peer participation in mental health advocacy, planning, and service delivery to the present.

In the 1940s two members of the staff of Rockland State Hospital in New York brought together a group of patients who were about to be discharged with the hope that these friendships might endure after their release from the hospital (Anderson, 1998). The patients formed a group, with financial support from one of these staff members, and continued to meet weekly for several years to provide support to each other. This self-help group, called the "We Are Not Alone Society" (WANA), in collaboration with professionals later formed what became Fountain House (Beard, 1978). Other self-help groups such as Recovery, Inc., founded in 1937 by Abraham Low (1950), a psychiatrist, and GROW, an international organization established in 1957 in Australia, have also been in existence for 50 years or more (Lefley, 2003). Alcoholics Anonymous (AA), not a mental health group per se, although there are dual-recovery groups today, was started in the 1930s (Wilson, 1939). There are also a number of mental health support groups that use the AA model.

However, the development of the modern American mental health consumer movement/survivor civil rights movement occurred in the early 1970s independent of these historical roots (Chamberlin, 1990; Frese & Davis, 1997). The mental health consumer movement coincided with the self-help revolution (Gartner & Riessman, 1984) and was fueled by the civil rights movement, generally, and the deinstitutionalization movement, most specifically. In 1978, the President's Commission on Mental Health noted the formation of numerous self-help groups of persons with mental and emotional problems throughout the United States (President's Commission on Mental Health, 1978).

Like other marginalized groups in the 1970s, former psychiatric patients began to realize that they were being denied basic rights, were discriminated against, and were devalued by society. Consequently, these former patients began to organize to correct some of these wrongs by regaining their rights and demonstrating that they were not powerless victims. The initial groups were the Insane Liberation Front in Oregon, the

Mental Patients' Liberation Project in New York, and the Mental Patients' Liberation Front in Boston. In 1972 the voices of these consumers began to be heard with the publication of *Madness Network News*, which terminated in 1986; the annual Conference on Human Rights and against Psychiatric Oppression started in 1973 and continued through 1985. The publication of *On Our Own: Patient-Controlled Alternatives to the Mental Health System* by Judi Chamberlin in 1978 was an important milestone for the movement, as consumers and others were able to read about the self-help movement and the development of peer-operated services in the mainstream press (Van Tosh et al., 2000).

Some of the early activists had an antipsychiatry orientation, as these consumers were angry at a system that they felt had abused and dehumanized them instead of helping them (Lefley, 2003). Hence, some called themselves "psychiatric survivors" and formed the National Association of Psychiatric Survivors (Kaufman, 1999; Lefley, 2003). This group opposed any type of involuntary commitment. Some of its members retain leadership at national consumer conferences, but the association no longer holds meetings. The more radical members formed the Support Coalition International, currently called Mindfreedom, and others went to the National Depression and Manic Depression Association (now the Depression Bipolar Support Alliance) (Mark Davis, personal communication, September 2005). Other leaders in the movement have more moderate views regarding forced treatment and the use of psychiatric medications, for they believe that without medication they would not currently be alive (Lefley, 2003). The National Mental Health Consumers Association represented those with more moderate views and took no formal position on forced treatment. This organization is no longer functioning, and some of its members have joined the National Alliance for Mental Illness (NAMI) Consumer Council (Lefley, 2003).

THE FEDERAL ROLE IN THE EXPANSION OF PEER SUPPORT INTERVENTIONS

The Community Support Program (CSP), initially at the National Institute of Mental Health (NIMH) and now at the Center for Mental Health Services (CMHS) within the Substance Abuse and Mental Health Services Administration (SAMHSA), has been a significant catalyst in the development and expansion of the consumer movement and peer services and supports (Lefley, 2003). Although the peer support programs were conceived and developed by consumers themselves, CSP had the federal financing and resources to publicize and promote these programs. CSP provided a number of initiatives, including funding for consumer-run programs, contracting and offering consultation, and technical assistance, as well as informational materials to stimulate the growth of self-help programs (Brown & Parrish, 1995). In 1985, CSP provided funds for the first national Alternatives conference. Alternatives, offered annually, is organized and planned by consumers and serves to build skills and share knowledge (Lefley, 2003; Van Tosh et al., 2000).

In 1988, CSP undertook a unique grant program to demonstrate and evaluate mental health self-help programs. This was a significant effort that helped to demonstrate how states and communities could foster the development of peer support without co-opting consumers (Brown & Parrish, 1995). Under the aegis of this program, 13 projects were funded, including employment programs, housing initiatives, and a service providing linkage between hospital and community to assist patients in transition. Furthermore, this program initiative influenced states and communities to fund similar efforts and "to employ consumers as paid workers in the mental health system" (Brown & Parrish, 1995; p. 7). The National Association of State Mental Health Program Directors (NASMHPD) in 1989 approved a position statement that recognized the significant value that consumers add to the improvement in service delivery and recommended seeking consumer delivery of services, among other contributions. Consequently, by the 1990s, 30 states had an Office of Consumer Affairs, staffed by peers (Van Tosh & DelVecchio, 1998). A national survey conducted by the Berkeley, California, Self-Help Center in conjunction with NASMHPD found that almost all states funded self-help groups (Segal et al., 1995). Most recently, CMHS funded a multisite research study, entitled Consumer Operated Services Program (COSP), to investigate the effects of consumer-operated services as an adjunct to traditional mental health services, as compared with traditional services alone, with many sites employing a randomized design (Clay, 2005; Van Tosh et al., 2000).

CMHS currently funds three consumer technical assistance centers: the National Mental Health Consumer Self-Help Clearinghouse in Philadelphia, the National Empowerment Center in Lawrence, Massachusetts, and the Consumer Organization and Networking Technical Assistance Center in West Virginia. One of these is usually the convener of Alternatives, an annual peer conference. The focus of all three centers is to provide information and assistance to develop and sustain peer support services, coalitions, and consumer networks. The third organization specifically offers leadership training that develops "politically empowered attitudes . . . the acquisition of the knowledge and skills required for advocacy" in its West Virginia Leadership Academy (Stingfellow & Muscari, 2003, p. 144). In addition to these three centers, CMHS funds two Consumer Supporter Technical Assistance Centers, one at NAMI, called the STAR (Support Technical Assistance Resource) Center, which is primarily focused on cultural outreach and adaptation of self-help to ensure availability and accessibility of self-help approaches to all cultural groups (*www.consumerstar.org*), and one at NMHA, which provides technical assistance in areas of research, information, materials, and financial aid to assist in the development and expansion of consumer initiatives. The National Consumer Supporter Technical Assistance Center (NCSTAC) of NMHA awards grants to establish and transform existing consumer programs (*www.ncstac.org*). NIMH/CSP in the 1990s also funded two research centers to examine the phenomenon of self-help, one at the University of Michigan and the other at the University of California at Berkeley, in order to increase the empirical base of peer support (Van Tosh & DelVecchio, 1998).

In addition, there have been initiatives to train peers to be providers. Paulson (1991) described an NIMH-funded program at the School of Social Work of the University of Cincinnati that includes consumers as students. The State of Georgia offers an 8-day training program that confers a certificate for peer specialists and is required for peer providers working in the Georgia mental health system (Sabin & Daniels, 2003; *www.gacps.org*, 2005). Certifying peer specialists enabled the State of Georgia to fund peer services through the Medicaid rehabilitation option (Substance Abuse and Mental Health Services Administration, 2005). Illinois has a psychiatric rehabilitation implementation manual that delineates how to recruit and retain peer providers (Schmook, 2000).

Peer services and supports now permeate much of the formal mental health system, not as a substitute, but as an adjunct to the more traditional mental health services. The surgeon general's report on mental health (1999) recognized the importance of self-help groups and consumer-operated services. In 2003, the President's New Freedom Commission on Mental Health acknowledged consumer-operated services as an "emerging best practice." Further evidence of the significance of these services and supports is their inclusion in the recent Consensus Conference in Texas that focused on the redesign of this state's mental health benefit package to ensure the provision of more psychiatric rehabilitation services (Cook, 2004; Cook, Toprac, & Shore, 2004; Solomon, 2004).

ESTIMATES OF PEER SERVICES AND SUPPORTS

With the impetus coming from these federal initiatives, peer services and supports have greatly increased to the point where current estimates of their availability are quite high in comparison to the availability of traditional mental health services. SAMHSA in 2002 funded a rigorously designed national survey of mental health support groups and self-help organizations run by and for mental health consumers and/or family members, and consumer-operated services. The survey was designed to focus, as much as possible, on those groups serving individuals with serious mental illnesses. Consequently, groups like AA and those addressing life crises like bereavement, victimization, anger management, and Alzheimer's disease were excluded. From the survey results it was estimated that there were 7,467 of these groups and organizations nationally, with 3,315 being mutual support groups (primarily providing support), 3,019 self-help organizations (education and advocacy groups that evolved from local support groups into a single network and may sponsor and/or support mutual support groups), and 1,133 consumer-operated services (including programs, businesses, or services controlled and operated by people who have received mental health services). The number of these groups eclipsed the number of traditional mental health organizations (4,546). Mutual self-help groups reported that 41,363 individuals had attended their last meetings, self-help organizations reported having a membership of 1,005,400, and consumer operated services noted serving 534,551 individuals in the past year (Goldstrom, Campbell, Rogers, Lambert, Blackow, et al., 2006). Although the finding that peer services and supports are greater in number than traditional mental health services seems quite surprising, it can been understood in the context of a geographical county. For example, in a given county there is not an excessive number of mental health agencies and organizations, but there are numerous small, local peer services and supports (Goldstrom, personal communication, August 2005; Kessler, Mickelson, & Zhao, 1997c).

In a broader context, a national comorbidity survey conducted in the 1990s found that 3.2% of respondents reported using self-help groups, accounting for more than 40% of all outpatient visits (Kessler, Zhao, Katz, Kazuzis, Frank, et al., 1999). A nationally representative telephone and mail survey conducted in 1996 by Kessler and colleagues (1997c) determined that 18% of the people in U.S. population participated in self-help groups (with no professional involvement) at some time in their lives and that 7% had done so in the past year. This translates into 25 million Americans having participated in self-help groups, excluding those organized and led by professionals, at some point in their lives (Kessler et al., 1997c). Furthermore, these investigators found dramatic growth in the number of people utilizing self-help groups for cohorts born after World War II, and they estimate a continued growth of about 8% per year into the future. Wang, Berglund, and Kessler (2000) did further analysis of this data set and found that 17.5% of those with serious mental illness had used self-help groups for mental and emotional problems in the previous 12 months. These researchers also determined that those who used self-help groups were more likely to seek professional help than those who did not use self-help groups (Kessler et al., 1997c).

Lieberman and Snowden (1994), in reviewing survey data estimating the prevalence of use of self-help groups, concluded that they had little confidence in the estimates, as the operational definition of self-help was problematic. Frequently, the definition of self-help groups relates only to those led by peers; although these researchers found the definition appealing conceptually, they noted that it did not coincide with current practice. Consequently, they concluded that without details of the self-help group and its processes, there is room for a great deal of error in these estimates. This problem of operational definition was recognized by Kessler and colleagues (1997c), as they referenced Jacobs and Goodman's (1989) research indicating that a substantial proportion of self-help groups are facilitated by professionals.

DEFINING AND DELINEATING PEER SERVICES AND SUPPORTS

It is essential to first establish what a *peer* is in the present context. There have been a variety of definitions posited, most referring to *consumer* as opposed to *peer*. Salzer and Mental Health Association of Southeastern Pennsylvania Best Practices Team (2002) have defined *consumer*, for purposes of consumer-delivered services, which is consistent with the current purpose, as "someone who has experienced, or is currently experiencing, symptoms associated with a diagnosable mental illness, and has received services to address these symptoms" (p. 336).

Copeland and Mead (2004), two consumers, elaborated as to what *peer support* is: "Peer Support is not like clinical support, and it is more than just being friends. In Peer Support we understand each other because we've 'been there,' shared similar experiences and can model for each other a willingness to learn and grow. We come together with the intention of changing unhelpful patterns, getting out of 'stuck' places, and building relationships that are respectful, mutually responsible, and potentially, mutually transforming" (p. 10). They also noted that "instead of taking care of each other and thinking of each other as 'sick,' in Peer Support we build a sense of family and community that is mutually responsible and focused on recovery and social action" (p. 10).

Peer support is emotional support, often paired with instrumental support, that is mutually provided by individuals who have a mental illness, and consequently share common experiences, who come together with the specific intent of bringing about social and personal change (Gartner & Riessman, 1984). Peer support is mutually beneficial through a reciprocal process of giving and receiving, based on the principles of "respect, shared responsibility, and mutual agreement of what is helpful" (Meade, Hilton, & Curtis, 2001). Through this system of sharing, supporting, and assisting others, feelings of rejection, discrimination, frustration, and loneliness that are common characteristics of individuals with severe mental illnesses are combated (Stroul, 1993). Usually, peer support in the traditional sense of a self-help group is voluntary, but in the context of service provision, individuals who deliver the support service are frequently compensated financially. Many of these peer support services have volunteers as well.

Within the realm of peer support are two program domains: mutual support groups or self-help groups, and peer-provided services. Mutual support or self-help groups include a recent innovation, Internet support groups; within the domain of peer-delivered services are peer-run or operated services, peer partnership services, and peer employees, individuals hired by nonpeer provider agencies or programs to provide services to other peers (Solomon, 2004). Broadly, peer-delivered services are those whereby an identified peer interacts with another identified peer for the purpose of service provision. These services are referred to as user-run or client-run (Chamberlin, Rogers, & Ellison, 1996) or consumer run alternatives (Mowbray & Moxley, 1997). These are services that are controlled, operated, and usually staffed by people who have received or are receiving mental health services. Sometimes in the literature the term *self-help services* is employed, but the operational definition of the term is not always clear. In other words, it is unclear as to whether mutual help groups are included or excluded, inasmuch as they are not services in the traditional sense (Hodges, Markward, Keele, & Evans, 2003). The term *self-help agency* has also been used to refer to agencies that are run by people with mental illness for the purpose of helping other members to gain skills and resources in order to achieve stability (Segal et al., 1995). It is difficult to make these categorical distinctions, because some groups, such as GROW, are not only support groups, but are broader organizations that offer services, such as a residential rehabilitation program to assist members in obtaining resources. Consequently, such organizations are not exclusively self-help groups, but spill over into the domain of peer support service provision. Thus, this categorization represents ideal types that do not always fit reality.

THEORETICAL BASIS FOR PEER SERVICES AND SUPPORTS

There have been a variety of psychosocial processes that are considered the theoretical bases for peer services and supports. These include social/emotional support, experiential or reciprocal learning, social learning theory, social comparison theory, and the helper-therapy principle (Salzer et al., 2002; Magura, Laudet, Mahmood, Rosenblum, Vogel, et al., 2003; see Table 17.1).

Emotional support is provided by communicating and demonstrating acceptance and approval of peers (Magura et al., 2003). It is letting others know that they are cared

---

TABLE 17.1. Social Process Theories of Peer Services and Supports

Social/emotional support

- Communication and demonstration of acceptance and approval
- Tangible materials, information, advice, feedback, resources, and companionship

Experiential/ reciprocal learning

- Specialized information and perspectives acquired through experience of coping with illness
- Practical and applicable information and strategies for problem solving

Social learning theory

- Role models through active examples and verbal instruction
- Means to cope and enhanced sense of self-efficacy in managing illness
- Reciprocal learning

Social comparison theory

- Sense of normalcy through interacting with others who share commonalities
- Upward comparison—optimism, hope, and incentive to achieve
- Downward comparison—a sense that things can be worse

Helper-therapy principle

- Help for oneself through helping others
- Sense of increased self-competency
- Enhanced self-esteem through social approval from those helped

about, valued, and loved (Sarason, Levine, Basham, & Sarasan, 1983). Two of Yalom's (1985) therapeutic factors in group psychotherapy are included in the emotional support provided by self-help groups: "universality," learning that others have similar problems and/or circumstances, and "group cohesiveness," perceiving that group members understand and accept each other (Citron et al., 1999; Llewelyn & Haslett, 1986). *Social support* means having people available who can be relied on to assist in meeting material resource and psychosocial needs (Sarason et al., 1983). Social support encompasses emotional support, which provides attachment and reassurance; instrumental support includes the provision of material goods and services; and informational support involves advice, guidance, and feedback. Thus, peer services and supports offer peer advice, acceptance, a sense of belonging, and positive feedback as to a person's self-worth (Solomon, 2004). Because of the empathic, open, and receptive nature of the peer relationship, individuals are comfortable in exploring their problems and concerns in the presence of their peers (Magura et al., 2003). Research has found that supportive relationships contribute to a person's positive adjustment, as well as buffer the stressors and adversities encountered, including those emanating from psychiatric problems (e.g., George, Blazer, Hughes, & Fowler, 1989; Gottlieb, 1981; Ell, 1996; Walsh & Connelly, 1996).

Experiential or reciprocal learning is the mechanism by which peers provide the specialized information and perspectives they have obtained through the experience of having lived with a severe psychiatric disability (Borkman, 1990). Therefore, peers who participate in self-help groups or receive services provided by a peer have an opportunity to "learn new attitudes, skills, and behaviors both through general information sharing" and by observing the role behaviors of others (Magura et al., 2003, p. 402). Experiential knowledge is practical and applicable to similar circumstances. Within a self-help group context, common elements regarding both problems and strategies for the solutions to these problems emerge from information shared by those having experienced similar problems (Schubert & Borkman, 1994). Yalom (1985) refers to this as the *identification factor*, whereby peers recognize that others share similar problems and are coping more effectively and that, consequently, their own behavioral strategies can be appropriately patterned after those of others. Through Yalom's process of "imparting information" and "guidance," in addition to direct advice given in one-on-one encounters, personal experiences are related by peers to other peers. These processes may give peers validation of their own approaches as well as provide increased confidence in their ability to cope with their disability. The peer support approach is a more active one, enabling people to cope with their disabilities and enhancing a sense of empowerment, as opposed to the more passive role that is engendered in participation in the traditional mental health services. Peer support promotes choice and self-determination (Salzer et al., 2002).

Social learning theory within the context of peer services and supports is similar to the concept of experiential learning. Peers function as competent role models, who offer a means to learning through active examples or verbal instruction. Those who are receiving or have received mental health services are credible role models for others with psychiatric disabilities, and through these interactions with their peers are more likely to experience positive behavioral changes, as well as increased self-efficacy in dealing with an illness, the sequalae of the illness, and the mental health system. Reciprocal learning is an important component of social learning. Peers who have confidence in managing their illnesses are also more optimistic about their future (Salzer et al., 2002).

Social comparison enables peers to establish a sense of normalcy through attraction to others who share commonalities with them, including the common experience of having a psychiatric disability (Festinger, 1954). There are both upward and downward comparisons. In upward comparisons, those who interact with peers whom they perceive to be doing better than themselves gain a sense of optimism and hope, as well as an incentive to strive toward improvements in themselves. In contrast, in downward comparisons, peers perceive other peers as not coping with their psychiatric disabilities as well as they are, and this offers them a perspective that circumstances can be far worse than those in their own situations (Salzer et al., 2002).

The *helper-therapy principle* maintains that in assuming a helping role with peers, one helps oneself as well (Riessman, 1965; Skovholt, 1974). This process of advising, assisting, and emotionally supporting others reinforces one's own learning of valued attitudes, skills, and behaviors (Magura et al., 2003). Thus, helpers receive as much as they give by gaining an increased sense of competence through a process of "personalized learning" (Skovholt, 1974). Furthermore, helpers gain enhanced self-esteem from the social approval and appreciation they receive from those whom they help. Roberts and colleagues (1999) tested the helper-therapy principle with a self-help group for persons with severe mental illness, GROW (a program based on Alcoholics Anonymous for persons with mental illness), and found that giving help to others improved a person's psychosocial adjustment. This was part of a larger observational study (Rappaport, Seidman, Toro, McFadden, Reischl, et al., 1985) in which two well-established measures, the Symptom Checklist-90 (SCL-90; Deragotis, Lipman, & Covi, 1973) and the Social Adjustment Scale (Weissman, & Bothwell, 1976) were administered at two time points—but not too close in time, nor for participants involved too long in the organization, that the process of change in adjustment would not be captured. Participants were found to have attended an average of 2.29 meetings per month.

MUTUAL SUPPORT OR SELF-HELP GROUPS

Self-help groups are the oldest and the most common of peer services and supports. They have been developed for individuals with a wide diversity of problems and issues, often because the formal system of care does not meet peoples' total needs (Lieberman, 1990). In the present context the focus is on groups that deal with coping with severe mental illness. Self-help groups are defined as "voluntary small group structures for mutual aid in the accomplishment of a specific purpose . . . usually formed by peers who have come together for mutual assistance in satisfying a common need, overcoming a common handicap or life disrupting problem, and bringing about desired social and/or personal change" (Katz & Bender, 1976). These do not include groups organized and led by professionals, unless the professionals are participating in the groups in a nonprofessional capacity (Goldstrom et al., 2006). Usually, these groups are free of charge, but sometimes there are dues or a nominal fee, particularly a group is an affiliate of a larger organization that needs funds to support its operations (Schubert & Borkman, 1991). Support groups offer hope, information, and an opportunity to help members themselves as well as others.

Typically, self-help groups are initiated by peers, but in some cases nonpeer providers may facilitate the development of a group and help to maintain it until a leader emerges. The most well-known examples of self-help groups for persons with severe mental illness are Recovery, Inc., GROW, Schizophrenics Anonymous, the National Depressive and Manic-Depressive Association (currently called Depression and Bipolar Support Alliance), Double Trouble groups (for persons with mental illness and substance abuse problems), and Emotions Anonymous. Other mutual support groups include NAMI–CARE (Consumers Advocating for Recovery through Empowerment) for consumers, as part of NAMI's national network. Many of these well-known support groups are quite formalized, with principles and books of readings, as they are parts of large organizational networks that have been in existence for a long time. Schubert and Borkman (1991) developed a typology of self-help groups based on internal–external dependence, locus of power, sources of leadership, and role of professionals. This typology includes unaffiliated, federated (associated with a larger organization), affiliated (subordinate to a regional or national group), managed (under professional control), and hybrid (combination of affiliated and managed). For our purposes, those managed or controlled by professionals are excluded. There are a number of support groups that are less structured, but over time they too may at least develop guiding values and a group format. For example, a certain support group, the Pink & Blues, for "people living with mental illness who are bisexual, gay, intersex, lesbian, transgender, or questioning adults," affiliated with the Depression and Bipolar Support Alliance, has guiding values that, for example, set a high priority on confidentiality and courtesy. Its literature indicates that, in regard to format, a meeting starts with brief introductions and sometimes ends with participants going to a local eatery to continue to socialize, with participation in this activity being optional (see insert values and format of the Pink & Blues Philadelphia).

Those who utilize mental health support groups tend to be white, relatively highly educated, and female (Davidson, Chinman, Kloos, Weingarten, Stagner, et al., 1999; Kurtz & Chambon, 1987). Groups such as GROW are attractive to individuals with more severe disorders, as they may feel more accepted in these groups (Kurtz & Chambon, 1987). People seek out support groups for varying reasons, including relief of symptoms, desire for a supportive community, help in recovering from or coping with their illnesses, or an opportunity to help others (Young & Williams, 1988). A generally held belief is that professionals do not make referrals to self-help groups because of their negative attitudes toward self-help. However, research has not supported this conclusion. Research has determined that a lack of knowledge about self-help and resource information is the primary reason for professionals not referring their patients to these resources (Davidson et al., 1999; Kurtz & Chambon, 1987). A recent survey of psychiatrists found that three-quarters of respondents felt knowledgeable about self-help and made referrals to such groups (Powell, Silk, & Albeck, 2000). But professionals who do not see the benefits of self-help groups are less inclined to make these referrals (Powell et al., 2000; Salzer, Rappaport, & Segre, 2001).

Until recently, a required characteristic of these groups were that their interactions be face-to-face, but with increased access to computers, Internet online support groups have emerged, which lack this face-to-face element (Gartner & Riessman, 1984; Perron, 2002). E-mail and bulletin boards are frequently utilized for communicating in Internet peer support groups, and in some instances particular software enables live interface between group members. Given the lack of in-person contact, these groups offer a high degree of anonymity, resulting in little likelihood of social repercussions (Davidson, Pennebaker, & Dickerson, 2000). This anonymity makes some individuals more comfortable about sharing embarrassing or sensitive information (Madara, 1997). Online groups also make it possible for people who have no groups in their areas, no transportation, a rare illness, or a physical disability, or who are confined to institutions, to participate (Madara, 1997). These support groups are generally public and open to anyone who would like to join; others are private and closed and require a person to make an application to the owner of the group in order to join (Perron, 2002).

PERSONAL EXAMPLE

Mark's Story of Forming the Pink & Blue Support Group

For decades the mental health consumer/survivor civil rights movement has been advocating recovery. I have been honored to work in this movement since 1985 and finally witness recovery as a psychosocial transformation goal.

Once labeled comorbid, dually diagnosed and double troubled, I am now a co-occurring person living with bipolar II, in recovery from drug and alcohol addictions and living well since diagnosed HIV positive in September 1988. This affords the label of being a person who is multiple occurring, dynamic, creative, and gifted. I am still learning how to live a recovering life.

For years I couldn't be gay in mental health treatment, advocacy, or peer groups, nor could I be out about mental illness in gay society. It was a painful duality, and peer support helped bridge this divide.

Lesbian, gay, and bisexual (LGB) are sexual identities, and transfender (T) is a gender identity, two very distinct cultural considerations. Questioning (Q) refers to coming to terms with our sexual or gender identity. Suicide is rampant in our culture. Addictions and mental illnesses are related to low self-esteem, coming-out issues, family rejection, and unhealthy social structures of being an LGBTQ person. Suicide attempts in my 20s were directly related to my shame and fear of being gay and triggered my mental illness and addictions.

Homosexuality was a mental illness until removed from the DSM [*Diagnostic and Statistical Manual*] in 1973 when I was in high school. Yet, LGBTQ people are not mentioned in the President's New Freedom Report, Co-Occurring Report to Congress, Surgeon General's Mental Health/Cultural Competency Reports, and National Strategy for Suicide Prevention. The governmental system follows a conservative moral, political agenda, disregarding research, funding, programs, policies, and competencies for sexual and gender minority health.

My passion is to share the value of peer support as a vital link to live in recovery within our cultural roots. Modeling pioneer peer-run groups scattered across the country for sexual and gender minorities, the Pink & Blue was founded in 2003. Pink represents gay culture, blue depression, and the colors assigned to our perceived birth gender. We built a safe, confidential space one step at a time.

The perks of peer support are great friends who understand, sharing recovery stories, social connections, and the stark reality of our shared experiences. I have someone to call in a time of crisis or celebration. Peer support validates past traumas, hurts, and abuse to let me become a survivor rather than a victim. My peers are my heroes.

A peer support group is a place to meet people from other sexual, gender, racial, religious, and disability roots. We are socially connected and politically enlightened. We are coming out within a coming-out movement. We openly march in pride parades and sit at tables at educational events. We have a sense of humor as "fruits and nuts" proclaim, "We're here, we're queer, and we're crazy, too."

Can I help you start Pink & Blue peer support in your community? It works for my recovery.

Mark Davis, MA
Behavioral Health System Special Needs Analyst
Philadelphia Mental Health Corporation (PMHCC)
Edits by Lynn Woodward

An Example of a Self-Help Group: GROW in Illinois

GROW is a network of structured mutual help groups that is guided by a written document, *Grow Program of Recovery and Personal Growth*. This organization was inspired by AA experience, and like AA generally meets in public venues, although in Illinois GROW rents a house in which members meet. GROW groups are open to everyone; however, most who come to them have a mental illness. Because the groups serve a diverse population in regard to need, the program is focused on recovery and personal growth, based on 12 practical steps. The meetings follow a uniform format known as the group method. These meetings include "a personal testimony, problem solving, assignment of practical tasks, reports on progress, and an educational section with a group reading of a selection from GROW literature followed by an 'attempted objective' discussion of its content" (Keck & Mussey, 2005, p. 147). GROW sponsors monthly socials, community social weekends, and leadership meetings for members who have at least 3 months of commitment and have led a minimum of three weekly meetings. The network of self-help groups is administered in an organizational structure that includes "leadership meetings, organizers' and recorders' meetings, and training events to protect, administer, and develop GROW groups, program, and community; and there are administrative teams to execute and serve the practical needs of the organization" (Keck & Mussey, 2005, p. 149). GROW stresses its voluntary nature, but does hire fieldworkers to ensure the authenticity of the groups and do outreach so that the program is available to all in need. GROW also owns a house in which it operates a residential rehabilitation program that serves about seven residents (Keck & Mussey, 2005).

Effectiveness of Mutual Support Groups

Most of the research on self-help groups has been descriptive, describing the users and the benefits perceived by participants. There has been limited research on the effectiveness of self-help groups, generally, and even less on self-help groups for persons with severe psychiatric disorders (Christensen & Jacobson, 1994; Davidson et al., 1999; DenBoer, Wiersma, & Van Den Bosch, 2004; Llewelyn & Haslett, 1986). A recent meta-analysis of self-help for emotional disorders concluded that the dearth of studies did not enable investigators to draw an evidenced-based conclusion in regard to self-help groups. Only 1 study out of 14 met the eligibility criteria for inclusion, which required randomized designs, and examined the outcomes of self-help groups, and the other 13 were on the effectiveness of bibliotherapy (DenBoer et al., 2004). The one study on self-help that was included compared a manualized cognitive-behavioral therapy (CBT) group led by professionals, with a manualized mutual help group led by paraprofessionals for persons with major depression, dysthmia, or depression not otherwise specified. Both conditions included 10 weekly sessions of 90 minutes. Participants in both groups were clinically improved at termination, but more participants in the professionally led CBT group fell within the nondepressed range on the Beck Depression Inventory than those in the self-help group (Bright, Neimeyer, & Baker, 1999). This self-help group differed from most, given that it was manualized and led by paraprofessionals.

There has been one other randomized study assessing the outcomes of self-help groups for those with severe mental illnesses. Kaufman and her colleagues (Kaufman, Shulberg, & Schooler, 1994) attempted a randomized trial of self-help group participation by individuals with severe and persistent mental illnesses, but this study failed owing to the fact that only 17% of those in both the self-help and control conditions participated in self-help groups. Consequently, the investigators could not assess the effectiveness of self-help resulting from the small number of experimental participants who utilized the self-help program and the crossover from the control condition to the experimental condition. This study points out the inherent problem with using the standards of the clinical trial paradigm to examine self-help. The intention of self-help is that it is the individual's own choice to join a self-help program and that participation cannot be dictated by the requirements of science (i.e., random assignment). Furthermore, research has found that those who choose to attend self help groups will decide to return if the match between other group members and themselves is consonant with their sociodemographic and clinical characteristics (Luke, Roberts, & Rappaport, 1993). This is consistent with research that found that dually diagnosed individuals who had more social abilities were more inclined to use self-help groups. Consequently, regular attendance was more common among those with affective disorders than those with schizophrenia (Noordsy, Schwab, Fox, & Drake, 1996). Similarly, Kelly, McKellar, and Moos (2003) determined that individuals dually diagnosed with substance abuse and major depression were less socially involved in and derived less benefit from 12-step self-help groups than those who were substance abusers only. Given the design problem with randomization, Kennedy (1989) was able to employ a quasi-experimental design to examine hospitalization outcomes of GROW participants. She found that GROW participants with recent hospitalizations matched to nonparticipants, in regard to number of prior hospitalizations and demographic characteristics, had fewer psychiatric admissions to state facilities and shorter stays when hospitalized. Similar conclusions regarding hospitalizations were reached by other investigators using weaker study designs. Both Raiff (1984) and Galanter (1988) found reductions in reported rates of hospitalization for those participating in Recovery, Inc., as did Kurtz (1988) for those in the founding chapter of National Depressive and Manic Depressive Association. A partially randomized design for patients with mood disorders determined that participation in a program of the Manic–Depressive and Depression Association (now called the Depression and Bipolar Support Alliance) resulted in improved management of the participants' illness, which included their seeking help, recognizing prodormal symptoms, and trusting professional help (Powell, Yeaton, Hill, & Silk, 2001). These behaviors require competencies that are consistent with the skills practiced in self-help groups. Research has also concluded that longer-term participants or those with more frequent attendance have better outcomes (Raif, 1984; Rappaport, 1993; Timko & Sempel, 2004). Outcomes are also better for those who are involved in or integrated into the group, as opposed to merely being attendees (Powell et al., 2001; Roberts et al., 1999).

Other positive outcomes have been reported, based on nonrandomized studies. These have included reduction in symptomatology, improved coping skills, compliance with medication, improved relationship with the physician, enhanced social networks, improved quality of life, and greater life satisfaction (Galanter, 1988; Kurtz, 1988; Raiff, 1982, 1984). The observation that support groups are frequently used in conjunction with mental health treatment, rather than as substitutes for formal care, has led researchers to conclude that participation in these groups may have the potential to reduce the number of visits to mental health professionals (Kessler et al., 1994; Kessler et al., 1999). However, the integration of self-help groups with formal treatment has resulted in some arguing that the independent effects of self-help are difficult to estimate (Kelly, 2003). The research on mutual support groups does show promise in regard to positive outcomes. However, without more systematic research, they will not achieve the level of evidenced-based practice.

PEER-PROVIDED SERVICES

Peer-provided services are delivered by persons who self-identify as individuals with mental illnesses and who are receiving or have received mental health services for their psychiatric illnesses. The primary purpose of peer-provided services is to help others with mental illnesses (Solomon, 2004; Solomon & Draine, 2001), but there is indication that peer providers also derive benefits, such as reduced hospitalizations, increased empowerment, and employment opportunities (Sherman & Porter, 1991; Yuen & Fossey, 2003). There are three categories of services that fall within this domain: peer-run or peer-operated services, peer partnership services, and peer employees. The primary distinction among these three service categories is the amount of control that persons with mental illnesses have in regard to administration and decision-making power. In peer-operated services, peers have total control over the administration and decision making in regard to providing and managing the service, whereas in partnerships peers share the administration and decision making with nonpeers. Peer partnerships are considered peer-provided services by the Center for Mental Health, in which at least 51% of the board members are consumers (Goldstrom, personal communication, August, 2005). Peer employees have no more or less control over the services than any nonpeer employees, contingent on the position held within the organization.

Peer-Operated Services

Peer-run or peer-operated services are planned, operated, administered, delivered, and evaluated by individuals with mental illnesses (Substance Abuse and Mental Health Services Administration, 1998; Stroul, 1993). These services are provided within a formal organization that is a freestanding legal entity that is directed by peers and conforms to peer values of freedom of choice and peer control. If individuals without a history of mental illness are involved in these service programs, their inclusion and supervision is under the control of persons with a history of mental illness. The size and nature of these service programs differ greatly. Examples of such services are drop-in centers, crisis services, employment services, housing programs, benefits acquisition, case management, crisis services, and psychoeducational services (Solomon, 2004; Solomon & Draine, 2001; Van Tosh & DelVecchio, 1998). In addition, peers also provide "warm lines," telephone support systems that are specifically staffed by peers, which have been found to have an advantage over the traditional mental health system by keeping crisis hotlines from being burdened by habitual noncrisis callers (Minth, 2005; Pudlinski, 2001, 2004). Peer service programs also engage in advocacy, research, education, and providing technical assistance (Van Tosh & DelVecchio, 1998). The SAMHSA Consumer Operated Services program categorized the programs into three categories: drop-in centers, peer support, and advocacy (Clay, 2005). Emerick's (1990) study of self-help/mutual aid organizations determined that the majority of those surveyed were political action-oriented agencies rather than offering social support for members. Peers have developed peer-run businesses such as bakeries, gardening services, and package delivery services. Although Emerick included peer-run businesses within consumer-operated services as does SAMHSA, for our purposes these fall within the domain of employment rather than peer support services and are not discussed in this chapter.

Peer-run services are offered by a legal entity, usually a nonprofit agency, that has a formal organizational structure. In some cases, these direct services may be only a program of an organization that also engages in advocacy, education, technical assistance, and research. Such organizations receive financial operating support from a variety of sources, including government grants, private foundations, and/or fees for service (Mowbray & Moxley, 1997).

In contrast to those who use mutual support groups, a majority of peers who utilize peer support services tend to belong to ethnic minority groups (Davidson et al., 1999; Kaufman, 1995; Mowbray & Tan, 1993; Segal et al., 1995). These programs also serve many individuals who are dually diagnosed (Segal et al., 1995). The characteristics of the recipients may have something to do with the nature of services provided, such as programs that provide assistance to homeless persons in the acquisition of resources. In addition, these services tend to attract peers who resist or have had negative experiences with the formal mental health system (Hodges et al., 2003). The utilization of peer support services has been found to encourage the appropriate use of professional services to have potential for increasing satisfaction with traditional mental health services (Hodges et al., 2003).

Effectiveness of Peer-Operated Services

Evaluations of peer-operated services have been very limited and have been basically descriptive studies focused on who uses services, characteristics of the services programs, and implementation issues (Chamberlin et al., 1996; Kaufman, Ward-Colosante, & Farmer, 1993; Mowbray, Chamberlin, Jennings, & Reed, 1988; Mowbray, Robinson, & Holter, 2002; Mowbray & Tan, 1992; Nikkel, Smith, & Edwards, 1992; Segal et al., 1995). Some studies reported on positive outcomes like improved quality of life, fewer hospitalizations, increased employment, and satisfaction with the programs (Chamberlin et al., 1996; Chinman, Weingarten, Stayner, & Davidson, 2001; Miller & Miller, 1997; Mowbray et al., 1988; Mowbray & Tan, 1992). From these studies, it can be concluded that such services can be feasibly implemented and that they generate satisfaction. One randomized investigation found that there were essentially no differences between peer-provided assertive community treatment (ACT) services and nonpeer provided ACT services in their effects on arrests, homelessness, and emergency room visits, with the exception that the number of hospitalizations and crises services were higher for those served by the non-peer-staffed ACT team (Herinckx, Kinney, Clarke, & Paulson, 1997; Clarke, Herinckx, Kinney, Paulson, Cutler, et al., 2000; see Chapter 6 for discussion of ACT).

Peer Partnership Services

Peer partnership services are interventions in which peers share responsibility in the operation of the services with nonpeers. Frequently, this means that the fiduciary responsibility for a service program lies with a nonpeer entity. Consequently, the administration and governance of the peer service is shared by peers and nonpeers, but peers have primary control over the service itself. Hence, the term *partnership* is employed to reflect the shared responsibility for the service (Solomon, 2004; Solomon & Draine, 2001). This categorization of peer partnership services in contrast to peer-run or peer-operated services is comparable to the categorization of autonomous and hybrid self-help groups: In hybrid groups professionals take a significant role, whereas in autonomous groups professionals may take a role only if invited by peers (Powell, 1985). The nature of the services provided through this partnership model is essentially no different from the type provided in peer-operated services. The major distinction between the two categories is the purity of the organizational structure in regard to peer control. Peer-run programs are nonhierarchical, whereas peer partnerships are structurally less egalitarian.

PERSONAL EXAMPLE

Lindy Functions as a Peer Support Provider

I was diagnosed with bipolar disorder in 1982, and 2 years later with alcoholism. After many hospitalizations and participation in an alcohol rehabilitation program, my illnesses stabilized. I decided I wanted to go back to school and work in the field of mental health. In 1989, I received a master's degree in Counseling Psychology. That same year I met Bob Drake and went to work for him at NH–Dartmouth Psychiatric Research Center. I was very open with Bob about my mental illness, and he hired me knowing all about it.

Over the years working at the research center, I have had the opportunity to work with several peers, and their families, using the behavioral family therapy for psychiatric disorders model. Providing services to peers was a very positive experience for me. It allowed me to share my story and my recovery with others who were struggling with issues that I had struggled with and, in some instances, continue to deal with. Sharing the negative experience of having a mental illness, as well as coping strategies and recovery strategies, with another peer turned a negative experience into a positive one. It was very empowering for me to be able to work with my peers in this capacity, increasing my self-esteem and self-confidence. Because of this, I experienced a greater stability in my own mental illness.

In working with my peers, I always respected them and saw each of them as a unique individual. While I felt empowered, I think they did too. They made choices and decisions for themselves, because even though we shared similar experiences, they needed to make choices specific to them. Many of the people with whom I worked found hope from my experience. I shared my recovery with them, and they felt as though they could move ahead too.

Although working as a professional with peers has often been a positive experience for both these consumers and me, sometimes it has had its drawbacks. For example, one person felt some discouragement in working with me. The person being counseled felt that even though we had the same illness, he could never accomplish what I had. Instead of feeling optimistic about the future, quite the opposite occurred for him. Still, I felt he could make positive changes in his life, and I continually conveyed a message of hope in the work I did with him. This person also wanted to change our relationship into a friendship. He had a hard time viewing me as a professional. It seems inevitable that this will happen from time to time.

Despite the few difficulties I have had, my work as a peer provider is very rewarding. I feel it is a reciprocal relationship with benefits to both myself and the person receiving the services.

Lindy Fox, MA, LADC
Research Associate
NH–Dartmouth Psychiatric Research Center

An Example of Peer Partnership Service: Friends Connection

Friends Connection in Philadelphia promotes the recovery of those with dual diagnoses and was established more than a decade ago in response to the closing of the state hospital serving the region. This service is a division of the local mental health association, which is a heavily consumer-run organization, with its director being a well-known consumer advocate. Although half the board members are consumers, it is not exclusively a consumer organization. Friends Connection has three components to its service: one-to-one peer support, sponsorship of group social activities, and an alumni program. Generally, referrals come from the traditional mental health services, primarily case management services. The goals of the service are to decrease substance use, decrease the number of hospitalizations, and increase satisfaction with community services, but program participants are not required to be clean and sober. Prior to entrance peers are screened by supervisory staff and the clinical manager. Entrance is based primarily on persons choosing to enter. The individual is matched with a peer support staff person who is viewed as most compatible, particularly in regard to the abused substance of choice, and the peer support person then develops an individualized personal plan of goals, objectives, and steps to achieving them. The peer support staff member helps the person to make changes in his or her life that will result in living substance free. The organization's social activities are open to anyone, and those who graduate from the program are welcome to continue with alumni support through continuing social activities (Whitecraft, Scott, Rogers, Burns-Lunch, Means, et al., 2005).

Effectiveness of Peer Partnership Services

As in the case of peer-operated services, there have been limited studies on peer partnership services, and these few were generally descriptive investigations. These studies focused on the process of implementation (Kaufman, Freund, & Wilson, 1989; Lieberman, Gowdy, & Knutson, 1991; Shelton & Ressmeyer, 1989) and the attitudes of peer and nonpeer staff (McGill & Patterson, 1990). Employing a randomized design, Kaufman (1995) assessed the outcomes of an employment program in which consumers were assigned to an experimental condition of a professional vocational rehabilitation service plus a consumer program, while the control group received only the professional vocational service. Those receiving the peer-provided program had more positive vocational outcomes, greater numbers gaining employment, higher wages, and higher vocational rehabilitation status. However, these findings are limited by the question of whether the more positive outcomes resulted from the additional service or from the delivery of the service by peers. Another randomized study comparing a team of peers providing intensive case management with a team of nonpeers found the outcomes for consumers served by the two teams to be equally effective regarding clinical, social, and quality-of-life improvements (Solomon & Draine, 1995a, 1995b). Chinman and his colleagues' (2000b) randomized case management study of peers and nonpeers had similar results. An examination utilizing a quasi-experimental design of Friends Connection found significant decreases in crisis events, improved social function and aspects of quality of life, and a reduction in substance abuse (Klien, Cnaan, & Whitecraft, 1998). The Solomon and Klien studies were conducted in the same partnership organization, and both had a number of methodological weaknesses (Solomon & Draine, 2001). These results are promising, but there is a need for further research on this service domain.

Fidelity Assessment of Peer-Operated and Peer Partnership Services

There have been two recent efforts to develop measures for assessing the fidelity of peer run services and programs, as fidelity to the intended model is an essential ingredient to determining the effectiveness of peer services and supports. As part of the Consumer Operated Services Program (COSP) of SAMHSA, there was a need to develop a measure that would capture the common ingredients of the diverse peer program models, which were conceptualized as three program models: drop-in center, peer support and mentoring services, and educational programs. Having a psychometrically sound measure would allow distinctions to be made between various peer-provided service models and between peer-provided services and traditional mental health services. The measure, Fidelity Assessment Common Ingredients Tool (FACIT), covered six factor domains: program structure, environment, belief systems, peer support, education, and advocacy. Based on preliminary studies, the measure appears to have acceptable reliability at the item level and high reliability at the total score level. The research determined that FACIT could be employed to measure the consumer orientation and consumer friendliness of programs and services (Johnsen, Teague, & Herr, 2005).

Mowbray and colleagues (Mowbray, Holter, Stark, Pfeffer, & Bybee, 2005b; Holter, Mowbray, Bellamy, MacFarlane, & Dukarski, 2004) developed a fidelity measure specifically for peer-run drop-in centers, entitled Fidelity Rating Instrument for Consumer-Run Drop-in Centers (FRI-CRDI). This measure has four domains: structure, process-beliefs systems, process-opportunity role structure, and process-social support. These researchers determined that fidelity criteria for consumer-run drop-in centers can be operationalized and measured with high reliability. They further hypothesized that this measure may well be applicable to other consumer-run services, but this requires additional testing. The preliminary work for the construction of this measure was utilized by the developers of the FACIT (Johnsen et al., 2005).

Peer Employees

Peer employees are individuals who self-identify as peers and are hired either in designated peer positions or in traditional mental health positions. Thus, peers who accept these positions must publicly acknowledge that they have a mental illness and have used or are using mental health services. Those in designated peer positions are, in some cases, in provider extender positions, such as case manager aides or peer specialists, or they may be peer counselors, peer advocates, peer case managers, or peer companions. Currently, some mental health agencies wish to hire peers in their existing positions and accept their experience of using mental health services as a substitute qualification for other requirements. The term *prosumer* is now being used for individuals with a psychiatric disorder who are mental health professionals, such as trained psychologists (Clay, 2005; Frese & Davis, 1997). However, others see this term as having application to paraprofessionals and volunteers as well (Manos, 1992, 1993).

Observations of peers as employees have delineated a number of benefits, but have also generated concerns. The positive aspects that have been noted in regard to having consumers as employees are that they are knowledgeable about a diversity of human service and health systems, have successful coping strategies, have the ability to engage with other consumers, and offer positive role models that can instill hope in others that recovery is possible (Doherty, Craig, Attafua, Boocock, & Jamieson-Craig, 2004). Consequently, peer staff have been perceived as more helpful than other staff in the mental health system (Trainor, Shepherd, Boydell, Leff, & Crawford, 1997).

However, there are some concerns in regard to having consumers as providers, such as boundary issues and dual relationships, which include fears that they will treat service recipients as friends or engage in violation of confidentiality resulting from their access to their own records and those of their associates. In addition, there are difficulties with providers accepting peers as equals, for there continues to be much prejudice against peer providers by those in the mental health system (Silver, 2004). Other concerns are that consumers may require special accommodations, such as job sharing and additional supports (Carlson, Rapp, & McDiarmid, 2001; Dixon et al., 1997, 1994; Doherty et al., 2004; Perkins & Buckfield, 1997). Peers themselves have developed methods to cope with the dual role. These coping mechanisms include support from others, participating in self-help groups, following their treatment plans, accessing supervisors for support, and attending trainings (Silver, 2004). Another issue is that some peers do not want to receive services from another peer, as they do not see them as experts who are able to help them, or they do not trust those peers who made the transition to a staff position (Mowbray, 1997). Consumers, however, have concerns that professionals intentionally or unintentionally may influence consumer employees to "adopt 'professional' beliefs and roles, thereby diminishing their unique perspective as consumers" (Resnick, Armstrong, Sperrazza, Harkness, & Rosenheck, 2004, p. 186).

Effectiveness of Peer Employees

Not unlike the case in previous areas of research on peer services and supports, there are few studies on the effectiveness of peers as employees, and most have been observational studies or process assessments rather than evaluations of outcomes. An observation frequently articulated is that peers create a more positive, less stigmatizing attitude toward persons with severe mental illnesses. In addition, peers have improved practices in serving other peers, by challenging provider prejudices and enabling providers to relate in a more genuine and personal manner (Dixon et al., 1994; Dixon et al., 1997; Doherty et al., 2004; Lyons et al., 1996; Manning & Suire, 1996; Mowbray, Moxley, Thrasher, Byvee, McCroahn, et al., 1996; Perkins & Buckfield, 1997; Segal, 1995; Sherman & Porter, 1991; Solomon, 1988b). These findings are consistent with research on employing peers as trainers for mental health providers that has found that providers receiving training from peers have more positive attitudes toward service recipients and are more recovery oriented (Cook, Jonikas, & Razzano, 1995; Young, Chinman, Forquer, Knight, Vogel, et al., 2005).

A randomized design was employed to assess whether those in the Community Network Development (CND) program, which included a consumer staff person to help recently discharged patients to adjust to the community, had more positive outcomes than those who received the usual discharge services. Those who received CND services had fewer hospitalizations, shorter lengths of stay when hospitalized, and were more able to function in the community without mental health system contact (Edmunson, Bedell, Archer, & Gordon, 1982; Edmunson, Bedell, & Gordon, 1984). A study approximating a randomized design that compared the outcomes of a team of case managers, of which one member was a peer, with the outcomes of another team that included no consumers, found no difference in crisis episodes, mental health service utilization, adherence to medication, housing stability, and substance abuse. However, the team including a consumer experienced more dropouts (Schmidt, 2005). Another randomized study of having peers as health care assistants to standard case management, as compared with standard case management, indicated that service recipients had increased service engagement, as indicated by less nonadherence to appointments, greater levels of participation in social care activities and access to benefits, and fewer unmet needs (Craig, Doherty, Jamieson-Craig, Boocock, & Attafua, 2004). A quasi-experimental study assessed whether including a peer specialist on an intensive case management team, as compared with a nonpeer specialist or no enhancement, resulted in more positive outcomes. Individuals served by the team enhanced by a peer specialist had improved quality of life, more positive self-image and outlook, gains in social support, and fewer major life problems than those in the other two conditions. Again, the evidence does support that engaging peers as employees to work with other peers produces more positive outcomes for the service recipients (Felton et al., 1995).

SUMMARY AND CONCLUSIONS

Consistent with the helper-therapy principle, peer services and supports offer many benefits, not only to consumer "service recipients," but also to the peer providers themselves and to the mental health service delivery system (Salzer & Shear, 2002). In many instances peer recipients derive the same positive outcomes from peer services and supports as from traditional mental health services, and sometimes even more positive outcomes. Peer providers have been noted to gain in enhanced recovery and self-discovery, an increased social support system, meaningful and productive ways to fill their time, professional growth toward careers, improved clinical outcomes and quality of life; hence, these are very much recovery-oriented services (Solomon, 2004). Mental health service delivery systems have gained the opportunity to fill needed positions, to serve individuals in need who would otherwise not use the system, to improve the negative attitudes of nonpeer providers who hold to a belief in the poor prognosis of individuals with severe mental illnesses, and to obtain a new creative perspective in the planning, evaluation, and development of services (Carlson et al., 2001; Solomon, 2004).

With all the pluses of these services and supports, there are also the challenges of role conflict and confusion, potential dual relationships, and risks of violations of confidentiality. These challenges are not insurmountable. However, there must be efforts directed at overcoming them. Suggested means of addressing these challenges include proper training and quality supervision of peers, an accepting and friendly consumer atmosphere, structures and opportunities for discussions among peer and nonpeer providers, use of conflict resolution methodologies, and organizational policies regarding these issues (Carlson et al., 2001).

Peer services and supports have made great strides in recent years, with everyone benefiting, not just peers themselves. Clearly, there are still challenges for these services and supports in becoming an accepted part of every mental health system. With the increasing emphasis on accountability of services generally, these services and supports have a number of barriers to overcome. The well-accepted scientific paradigm of RCT (randomized clinical trial) is not consonant with, and in many ways antithetical to peer services and supports. Less well-accepted methodological approaches, like qualitative methods and PAR (participatory action research) are far more appropriate to researching peer services and supports. Further, in the current atmosphere of budget constraints, we must not resort to the inclusion of peer services and supports for the wrong reasons to save money. These services and supports should be an integrated and accepted part of the mental health service delivery system, as another alternative and/or as a supplement, not a replacement. We must not once again abuse persons with mental illnesses by paying them less and stigmatizing them by making them feel as though their contributions are less valued because of their mental health status. Moreover, care must be taken not to employ the procrustean approach to service delivery as we have done in the past, such that we require peer services and supports to fit the model of traditional mental health services. Such an approach is likely to result in the inherent strengths of peer services and supports being lost in their inclusion and expansion. "Consumers do bring something distinctive to service encounters" (Moxley & Mowbray, 1997, p. 3), and this needs to be retained.

Chapter 18

Managing Aggressive Behavior

Contemporary models of psychiatric rehabilitation promote personal empowerment in which the person with psychiatric disability has the primary decision-making role in determining the goals of rehabilitation. Cases involving aggression define the rare times in which empowerment may have to be overruled and behavioral interventions applied to a person without that person's full approval. Managing aggressive behavior, whether turned in against the self or outward against others, is necessary to help some people return to the central decision-making role. Aggression management also prevents people from taking actions that will irrevocably harm themselves or others. Other chapters of this book have looked at self-injurious and parasuicidal behaviors as two such behaviors (e.g., see Chapter 5 on illness self-management). This chapter focuses on interpersonal aggression, how it undermines rehabilitation goals, and how interventions may help a person gain some control over it.

Research suggests that aggression related to mental illness is greatest against family members. Hence, strategies that promote family problem solving can decrease aggression against relatives. These kinds of strategies are summarized in Chapter 11. In like manner, rehabilitation strategies that help people in their homes, workplaces, or places of education can decrease aggression in these settings as well. This chapter focuses on aggression and violence that does not seem to lessen as rehabilitation goals are accomplished within various systems.

As discussed in Chapter 2, concerns about aggression and violence frequently underlie the stigma of mental illness. Rehabilitation providers need to be mindful of this prejudice when developing aggression management programs. In particular, they must make sure that any program addresses the actual problems related to aggression, rather than the biases that evolve from prejudice and discrimination.

DEFINING AGGRESSION AGAINST OTHERS

Aggression against others may show itself in many ways and has been differentiated as verbal versus physical aggression (Silver & Yudofsky, 1987; Coccaro, Harvey, Kupsaw-Lawrence, Herbert, & Bernstein, 1991). Verbal aggression may include loud and angry comments, inappropriate statements (e.g., comments that include a sexual tone), or threats. Physical aggression can be directed against others or against physical objects. Harm to others can vary from relatively mild touching to inflicting significant injury or even death. People may also throw or break things when being aggressive. At the extreme, they may trash a room in a frenzied state.

Aggression has a negative impact on almost everyone involved. Family members are often the victims of verbal or physical harm (Arboleda-Florez, 1998; Nordstroem & Kullgren, 2003). They frequently become fearful of the relative who is aggressive and want the person removed from their home. Peers in treatment programs may also be victims of aggression (Black, Compton, Wetzel, Minchin, Farber, et al., 1994; Daffern,

---

PERSONAL EXAMPLE

Harvey Kohler Can't Get Out of the Hospital

Harvey Kohler had accomplished quite a bit in his life. He had graduated from state college in accounting and met the licensing requirements of a certified public accountant. He married Simone, and together they had two children. He was settling into a comfortable career at an auditing firm. Unfortunately, when Harvey turned 30, he had the first of several bipolar episodes. During the past 5 years, Harvey experienced some unnerving psychotic symptoms that frequently led to significant anger. Violence was common when he went on a drinking binge while manic. The police were called to his home three times in the past year because of Simone's concerns about his temper.

Two months ago, Harvey was admitted to the hospital after the police were called to his home because he was shouting and threatening a neighbor. He was furious when he arrived at the hospital, arguing that the neighbor was plotting with city hall to bulldoze Harvey's home. He shouted at the admitting nurse, claiming that he could not be kept locked up like this. The nurse asked him to calm down, which only seemed to make things worse. He stood up to leave, and when she stepped in front of him, he pushed her roughly aside and headed for the unit door. The nurse activated a signal, and security from elsewhere in the hospital came to the unit to provide assistance. Unwilling to return to the unit, Harvey was wrestled to the floor by the guards, taken to seclusion, and restrained. Harvey was in and out of restraints for the next week because of angry altercations like this. At one point, he almost broke an aide's arm when she was escorting him to seclusion.

Now, 2 months after the spate of anger and seclusion, Harvey has regained control. He recognizes that his bipolar disorder and concomitant anger are significantly interfering with his life goals. Simone has asked for a trial separation, and Harvey's employer has said that Harvey must show he can come back to work calmly before the company will reinstate him. Harvey and the inpatient team believe that participation in the local rehab program may help Harvey during this transition. The team can provide support as he moves into his transitional apartment and starts a part-time job as a bookkeeper. However, the rehab team is very concerned about admitting Harvey to its program because of his potential for violence. Several members of the team want to block his admission, fearing that he may be a danger to other program participants or to staff members.

Ogloff, & Howells, 1993). Being under verbal or physical attack can significantly undermine the rehabilitation goals of peers; in these instances people may curtail their participation in an otherwise helpful program. The injury of staff members in responding to aggression is a significant and widespread on-the-job problem (Carmel & Hunter, 1993). Research studies have shown that as many as 20% of assaulted staff members required medical attention for their injuries (Bensley, Nelson, Kaufman, Silverstein, & Shields, 1995; Blow, Barry, Copeland, McCormick, Lehmann, & Ullman, 1999). The threat or presence of aggression is also a significant source of burnout for staff members (Wildgoose, Briscoe, & Lloyd, 2003; Winstanley & Whittington, 2002).

People who are aggressive also experience negative consequences themselves. They are likely to be injured when possible victims are defending themselves or when staff members are trying to place them in seclusion or in restraints (Crenshaw & Francis, 1995). They can become socially isolated because family members, peers, and staff members are afraid of them (Weisbrot & Ettinger, 2002). Being labeled aggressive can be a significant barrier to achieving rehabilitation goals. Inpatient staff members are more reluctant to discharge such individuals, and community-based programs are hesitant to admit them.

CAUSES OF AGGRESSION

Aggression may result from environmental causes, biological influences, or some interaction of the two (Barlow, Grenyer, & Ilkiw-Lavalle, 2000; Link & Stueve, 1994; McNeil, 1997; Powell, Caan, & Crowe, 1994; Reid & Parsons, 2000; Shepherd & Lavender, 1999). Developers of programs meant to decrease aggression need to be mindful of the possible biological and environmental factors. The seven types of aggression manifested by people with psychiatric disabilities, summarized in Table 18.1, are described in the following discussion.

Frustration and Aggression

People who are frustrated may become aggressive. Classic social psychological research has explained the link between blocked goals and violence (Berkowitz, 1989; Dollard, Miller, Doob, Mowrer, & Sears, 1939). That is, people who are not able to act within a specific situation to achieve a goal will likely experience frustration, which, if left unchecked, will result in aggression. The frustration–aggression link is more pronounced when the blocked goal is immediate (I was supposed to get my weekly Social Security allowance now) and the person blocking the goal is apparent (Sheila is trustee for the allowance program). The frustration–aggression link can be diminished by cognitive mediators. For example, a written note on the program director's door noting that allowances will be handed out 30 minutes late can diminish a person's frustration. In general, the more a person knows about a goal, the barriers that block it, and the means for overcoming the barriers, the less likely it is that frustration will lead to aggression.

Aggression Serving Operant Goals

Some people learn aggressive behaviors operantly, that is, in terms of the reinforcing and punishing consequences of aggression (Eichelman, 1990; Eron, 1994). According to the operant view, people who act out in specific situations and find that rewards follow are more likely to act out that way again in similar situations in the future. That is, certain

TABLE 18.1. Possible Types of Aggression Manifested by a Person with Psychiatric Disabilities

Type	Definition	Example
Frustration related	Anger and aggression are common results when a person is not able to achieve immediate goals.	Frank was told three times that staff members on the unit were not yet ready to hand out cigarettes for a smoke break. On his fourth attempt to get a cigarette, he had had enough. He threw a chair across the common area.
Operant	Sometimes being aggressive leads to a person's getting some kind of benefit.	John figured out that whenever he yelled at the people ahead of him in the lunch line, he was able to move to the front more quickly.
Nonspecific agitation	Several factors can increase a person's arousal level, which leads to agitation and aggression. These include environmental noise and ingestion of caffeine or nicotine.	Shirley was more agitated than usual at the store where she worked because the store was loud and busy during the Christmas rush. She snapped one day and yelled at a customer who asked her if a certain product was sold out.
Psychosis related	Certain delusions or hallucinations may result in a person's becoming aggressive.	Sarah hit the aide on the unit because she believed that he was part of a CIA plot that was keeping her in the hospital.
Confusion related	Some people become confused because of their illness or medication. Confusion may result in anger and violence.	Samuel came into the emergency room more confused than usual. He perceived a nurse who was trying to draw blood as a danger and hit her.
Related to loss of social support	People who lack social support are more prone to handling troubles with anger and aggression.	Stan lived with his older sister, Eileen, who tried to take care of most life demands for him. Eileen was not allowed to visit Stan during his first week on the admissions unit. Without her support, Stan got into a fight with another resident.
Intermittent explosive disorder	A syndrome marked by sudden, unprovoked, and unexplained anger.	Victor was normally a calm fellow, who rarely showed a temper. However, about a month after significant head trauma due to a car accident, he began to snap for no apparent reason. One day he unexpectedly started to scream and struck a nurse. He apologized profusely, saying that he had suddenly felt that he could no longer control his anger.

aggressive behaviors are unintentionally reinforced by family members, peers, staff members, and others; these may be viewed as bully behaviors or interpersonal extortion. Consider what happens to the bully who, after shouting that he wants to be first in the lunch line, gets the lead position and is able to pick up the freshest food and find the nicest place to sit. This person has learned that similar shouts and threats will get him first in line in the future.

Interpersonal extortion may also be understood operantly. Consider the person who pushes a peer hard against the wall and says, "Hey, I'm short on lunch money. Give me five dollars." When, out of fear, the peer hands over the money, the extortionist learns that threats and pushing can get her some money. Finally, people may be operantly aggressive in order to be left alone. Staff members and peers come to fear such people and do not make demands on them. This source of operant aggression may be especially relevant for people coming from the department of corrections or who were homeless and living on the street.

Nonspecific Agitation

Nonspecific agitation may be viewed as waking up on the wrong side of the bed. Sometimes people are angry at the world, which may be called being pan-agitated. This frequently results when a person is highly aroused and anxious. Several factors can cause this kind of arousal and agitation. Being in a noisy work or living environment can increase agitation, especially if a person has no control over the noise level (Geen & McCown, 1984). Lack of privacy or finding oneself in a crowded setting can also increase arousal and agitation. Ingesting a great amount of stimulants—for example, caffeine from coffee, soda, or chocolate or nicotine from cigarettes (Ferguson, Rule, & Lindsay, 1982)—increases arousal, as does sleep deprivation (Dennis & Crisham, 2001; Lindberg, Tani, Appelberg, Naukkarinen, Rimón, et al., 2003).

Psychosis-Related Aggression

Some psychotic symptoms may bring about aggression. Three symptoms, in particular, account for the link between mental illness and violence. Called the threat/control override symptoms, they involve either the perceived overriding of internal self-control by external factors or perceived threats from others (Link & Stueve, 1994; Monahan, 2000; Swanson, Borum, Swartz, & Monahan, 1996). Hallucinations, especially those that command a person to act in a specific way, may also increase the likelihood of violence (Kasper, Rogers, & Adams, 1996; McNeil, Eisner, & Binder, 2000).

Confusion

Psychosis may also lead to disorientation and confusion. People who are misperceiving or misunderstanding another person's intentions may respond with aggression. Confusion is not limited to psychosis. Severe mood disorders and anxiety can also yield problems related to confusion.

Loss of Social Support

The kind of interpersonal support that people get from family members and peers can help them deal with life stressors. People who are separated from their social support because of hospitalization, or because the family has decided to alienate itself, find themselves more exposed to stress. Without support, they may become more aggressive.

Intermittent Explosive Disorder

Aggression that is marked by discrete, sudden, typically severe outbursts that are unprovoked may indicate intermittent explosive disorder (Coccaro, Schmidt, Samuels, & Nestadt, 2004; Olvera, 2002). In this disorder, the degree of violence is grossly out of proportion to any provocation. The individual may describe the aggressive episodes as spells that are preceded by a sense of tension and immediately followed by a sense of relief. The individual often feels regretful after the event. Intermittent explosive disorder is often associated with neurological conditions such as migraine headaches, head injury, or periods of unconsciousness.

Other Aggression

There are additional forms of aggression that may be observed in people with psychiatric disabilities. These include psychopathy-related predatory aggression, dementia-related aggression, and aggression because of hearing impairments. These reflect the more prominent sources of aggression in people with psychiatric disabilities. Rehabilitation team members should consult the specialized research literature when they believe a person's aggression may be due to one of these causes.

INTERVENTIONS FOR AGGRESSION

In the rest of this chapter, we organize aggression management strategies into three groups: systemwide efforts, replacement strategies, and decelerative strategies (Corrigan & Mueser, 2000; see Table 18.2). Many aggressive episodes are elicited by chaotic milieus, noisy places with few rules, where some people are easily frustrated while others take advantage of the confusion by extorting weaker peers. *Systemwide* approaches can change the tenor of chaotic milieus so that rehabilitation can take place instead. *Replacement* strategies seek to teach individuals how to get their needs met without striking out at others. Aggressive behavior is replaced by skills or contingencies that promote problem solving rather than violence. Even in the best system, where the milieu is therapeutic and people have learned replacement behaviors, aggression may still occur. In these instances, *decelerative* interventions are needed; that is, strategies that calm a person sufficiently so that he or she can use replacement skills.

Two aggression management approaches are not discussed in this chapter: the use of medications and seclusion/restraints. Medications are discussed more fully in Chapter 7. Suffice it to say here that managing the biological component of aggression can be complex, given the current panoply of drugs. Although definitions of seclusion and restraint vary by state law (Rakis & Monroe, 1989; Saks, 2002), seclusion usually involves transporting a person to a quiet locked place where he or she can calm down. The use of restraints involves tying someone down, typically to a bed in a seclusion room, usually with leather straps. Most states have well-defined rules about who can prescribe seclusion or restraints, the amount of supervision needed while the person is in restraints, and built-in reevaluation periods when the team decides whether to release the person. The use of seclusion and application of restraints are not typically activities in which rehabili-

TABLE 18.2. Overview of Aggression Management

Type of intervention	Definition	Example
Systemwide	Lack of rules, ambient noise, and opportunities for bullying all lead to greater aggression. There are a variety of systemwide interventions that can help to make sure that the environment is not promoting frustration or agitation.	The token economy can set up a series of programwide contingencies that can diminish frustration and extortion. Contingencies are if-then rules: If you make your bed before breakfast, then you get 10 tokens that you can use in the program store.
Replacement	Sometimes people are aggressive because they lack the social, problem-solving, and other cognitive skills needed to deal with life demands. Replacement strategies help people acquire skills that decrease the need for aggression.	Assertiveness skills often decrease the need for anger. Instead of shouting at a roommate because he has not take out the garbage, the person can use an assertive statement like "Henry, when you don't take out the trash, I feel mad because it stinks up the house."
Decelerative	Even if systemwide and replacement programs are operating, people can become frustrated and angrily act out. Decelerative strategies constitute an intervention plan that deescalates anger or violence.	In self-controlled time out, a person takes herself out of a situation until she calms down.

tation counselors find themselves involved because of their focus on community reintegration. In fact, there is continuing debate about whether the use of seclusion and restraints should be discontinued altogether; there is a sense that when used, they represent the failings of an ineffective treatment program rather than an appropriate intervention to stop violence (Saks, 2002; Sheline & Nelson, 1993; Singh, Singh, Davis, Latham, & Ayers, 1999). Currently, seclusions and restraints are most commonly found in inpatient settings. Rehabilitation practitioners having a role in these settings who are expected to participate in secluding or restraining a person need to be fully trained in the methods in their program.

Four Primary Principles

There are four fundamental rules that guide aggression management programs. First, aggression management should reflect a plan of the entire team. Hence, all staff members working on a unit should be knowledgeable about the plan and aware of what their roles in it may be should a person become violent. Also essential to good team programs is making sure that all staff members have some influence over the aggression management program. Such a program should not be left to the behavioral expert.

Second, the quality of the relationship between a person with aggression problems and the treatment team is important for quashing violent tendencies. Research has shown, for example, that people who report a better therapeutic alliance with treatment providers are less likely to be violent (Beauford, McNiel, & Binder, 1997). Hence, the rehabilitation team needs to make sure that its antiaggression program includes efforts to promote an alliance.

Third, the person with aggression problems should have a prominent role in the aggression management program. This may seem counterintuitive, because family members or peers who have problems with an individual's aggression typically bring it to the attention of the rehabilitation team, not the aggressive person. A mother wants her son to stop shouting when she tries to wake him in the morning. A person wants his roommate to stop threatening him in order to get cigarettes. The job coach wants a person to stop slamming the door in his face when he stops by to see how the new job is going. It is typically the motivation of the victim that gets aggression into treatment planning foreground. Nevertheless, rehabilitation providers still need to help the person realize why aggression management should be a priority. How does addressing aggression in some way satisfy the aggressor's needs? Motivational interviewing is a helpful tool for this purpose (Corrigan et al., 2001c). See Chapters 4 and 5 for a fuller description of the method. The purpose of this kind of interaction, as applied to people with aggression problems, is to help them understand the costs of continuing to be aggressive as well as the benefits of their angry outbursts. The discrepancy between costs and benefits may motivate the person to work with the rehabilitation team to diminish aggression. An example is provided in the Personal Example.

Fourth, aggression management is more effective when it is preventive rather than reactive. Frequently, rehabilitation providers are called to react to an angry or violent person after he or she has already begun to shout and thrash about. At this point, the per-

---

PERSONAL EXAMPLE

John Paulsen: "What's Wrong with Yelling Sometimes?"

John Paulsen had been attending the Lincoln Clubhouse for only a month, and other clubhouse members were already expressing fear of him. John had a very tight sense of personal space. If someone sat close to him, John would mumble for the person to move back. Most times, the person could not make out what John was saying, so he had to repeat himself, which made him all the angrier. Last week, he yelled at Charlotte to stop sitting at his table. When she failed to get up quickly, John threw down the chair he was sitting on and stormed out of the room. This week, John said that Michael had cut ahead of him in the lunch line. John grabbed Michael by the back of his coat and slammed him up against the wall.

Staff members were also concerned about John's level of aggression. Just yesterday, Bonnie went to pick him up for a job interview. John said she was late and slammed the door to her car. Everyone agreed that John was bringing down the communal atmosphere they had worked so hard to develop at the Clubhouse. What could they do about it? Mort volunteered to do a motivation interview with John.

MORT: You know, John, everyone here is a little concerned about how loud and angry you can be at the Clubhouse.

JOHN: I didn't do anything wrong. It's all their fault. They get in my face and give me a hard time. They all have it coming.

M: Whoa, John. I am not here to take sides. But I am trying to get a better idea of exactly what the problem is.

J: The problem is that everyone is in my business. If they'd leave me alone, I'd leave them alone. I'd stop having to assert myself.

M: Well, you know, John, we can't always control other people's behavior. Waiting for them to change can drive a person crazy. Instead, we can look at what we have control over, and how it helps or hurts us. For example, you said you would stop having to assert yourself if they backed off. What do you mean by "having to assert yourself"?

J: You know, raising my voice, sometimes shouting, stuff like that.

M: Okay, let's get a better handle on asserting yourself like this. I am wondering, what are the costs and the benefits of shouting at other people? This is important info to figure out. Costs are the reasons why you want to give up a behavior, how yelling at others might cost you something. Benefits are the good things about yelling, reasons why you won't change. So let's make a list of both.

J: Well, the benefits are easy. People leave me alone when I shout. And sometimes maybe I get my way. Like I am able to get to the front of the line for food. But I deserve it, 'cause I am one of the newer members of the Clubhouse.

M: Okay, shouting at people guarantees that others will leave you alone . . . And sometimes it gets you special advantages. Any other benefits to raising your voice?

J: Yeah, it makes sure nosy staff don't always pry into my business so much.

M: So it keeps staff members out of your business. Okay. What about costs? Is there a downside to being angry and shouting?

J: Not really. People just learn to watch themselves around me.

M: People need to be on their toes when near you.

J: Yep. Which is a little hard for making friends.

M: People don't want to be friendly with someone who is shouting.

J: (pause) Yeah, I guess so. Sometimes I wish I had a few more friends. That's a downside to me yelling. It scares people off. But don't get me wrong. They still have it coming.

M: So let me see if I got this right. You yell at people to stop them from taking advantage of you and maybe sometimes it gives you an edge in terms of getting what you want, like ahead in line. But the downside is that it might scare off your peers a bit, making it harder to get friends.

J: Yeah, Mort, that pretty accurately sums up the problem.

M: So what if we could work together to find a way to keep people from taking advantage of you—thereby keeping down the anger—might that put you in a better position to make more friends?

J: Maybe. I am willing to give it a chance.

son's individual resources are suppressed under the weight of anger and agitation; working jointly with the person to deescalate the situation is more difficult. Reactive strategies frequently require grabbing the person in order to somehow subdue him or her; this kind of situation often ends in someone getting hurt. Preventive strategies, however, seek to avoid actual incidents of aggression that can escalate into harm. Instead, rehabilitation providers help people with aggression problems to learn skills that replace previous, aggressive tendencies. Hence, we begin this discussion by looking at those interventions that prevent aggression. They fall into two categories: systemwide strategies that help the participants in a particular milieu to have control over daily activity and strategies that seek to replace aggressive behaviors with more appropriate responses.

Systemwide Programs to Decrease Aggression

Two strategies are helpful systemwide to decrease the kind of frustration and arousal that leads to aggression: the use of a token economy and attention to ambient stress and stimulation.

The Token Economy

The use of a token economy is a behavioral approach to modifying behavior in a certain milieu through the direct manipulation of contingencies under which participants in the setting operate (Menditto, Beck, & Stuve, 2000; Paul & Menditto, 1992). In short, participants in token economies are rewarded tokens or points for performing targeted behaviors. They can then exchange these points for rewards like food, hygiene products, and stationery. Common settings for token economies include hospital wards, residential programs, and therapeutic work sites. Three steps are necessary for a rehabilitation team to set up a token economy (Corrigan, McCracken, Edwards, Kommana, & Simpatico, 1997). First, target behaviors must be defined; what prosocial or self-care behaviors must the person show to be rewarded tokens? (see Figure 18.1). Some token economies opt for token fines when a person does something that is not appropriate for the setting; for

Do's	Tokens
• Make your bed by 8:00 A.M.	3
• Take your pills before leaving for work.	5
• Cook your dinner before 4:00 P.M.	6
• Complete a problem-solving sheet when having difficulty with roommate.	7
• Start a 15-minute "pleasant" conversation with peer.	2
• Do a 30-minute recreational activity with peer.	3

Don'ts	
• Don't swear at other people.	−3
• Don't smoke in your room.	−3
• Don't come in past curfew.	−4

Exchange Rules
Store is open at 5:00 P.M.
Resident runs the store.
Store located in Apartment 6.

Store items	Cost (in tokens)
Comb	10
Cola	12
Bar of soap	5
Socks	20
Fruit	3
Tissues	10
Toothpaste	20

FIGURE 18.1. Example of elements of a token economy for a residential program.

example, a person loses five tokens when smoking out of bounds. Rehabilitation teams need to be cautious when opting for fines, because they can quickly give the token economy coercive focus in a situation where people are trying to stop antisocial behaviors. Too many fines can make a token economy aversive and thereby undermine the rehabilitative quality of the milieu.

The second step in setting up a token economy is to define the contingencies. Contingencies are if–then relationships between targeted behaviors and consequent rewards; in the token economy, rewards are secondary reinforcers (points or poker chips) that can be turned in for consumables. As shown in Figure 18.1, token values for individual target behaviors vary according to their reinforcement value. Behaviors that are more difficult to perform should earn more tokens. Difficulty can also be defined in terms of frequency. Behaviors that are not expected to be performed as often as others yield more tokens in the economy. The third step in the process is setting up the exchange rules. The value of tokens is realized when they are turned in for consumables that participants want. Hence, participants need to know when and where each day they can trade tokens for consumables. In addition, they need to know the cost of individual commodities in the store. Typically, token stores provide an array of foods, hygiene products, and stationery. Commodities and consumables that are bought more often cost more than items that are rarely purchased. Token economy price setting parallels supply-and-demand economics.

Token economies are more effective when all stakeholders participating in the program have input into the three steps (Corrigan et al., 1997). This means that each resident, as well as each staff member, in a token economy in a group home should have a voice concerning targets, contingencies, and exchange rules. This also suggests that token economies are dynamic programs. Targets, contingencies, and exchange rules regularly change to reflect the contemporary priorities of a program.

WHAT ARE THE BENEFITS OF TOKEN ECONOMIES?

Token economies decrease aggression in three ways. First, they decrease the likelihood of frustration in trying to manage a milieu. What is expected of participants is clearly laid out in the list of targets. Moreover, staff responsibilities vis-à-vis participants are also spelled out. For instance, staff members know that they are to provide x amount of tokens for behavior y and that these tokens may be cashed in once a day at the store at 4:00 P.M. Frustration occurs less frequently when expectations are clear. Second, token economies decrease confusion that may lead to aggression. Token economies attempt to define the nature of interpersonal relationships, at least in part, in terms of contingencies and exchange rules. Hence, a person who may be confused better understands when he is to make his bed, take his medications, get on the bus for work, and cook dinner at night. Third, token economies decrease operant-based aggression. It is difficult to use aggression operantly when contingencies and exchange rules are spelled out in the token economy.

Ambient Stress and Stimulation

The milieu in which rehabilitation programs operate can frequently be loud and chaotic, factors that increase arousal and lead to more aggression. Aggression can be decreased in these settings via some simple rules regarding ambient noise and clutter. Loud music and television should be discouraged. A separate music/television room should be set aside for those who want such entertainment. Noisy intercoms should not be placed in common areas or in a person's room. Simple schedules should be posted so that a person can easily determine when and where he or she should be throughout the day. Rooms should be clearly marked. Helpful reminders should be prominently displayed—for example, "Did you take your noon meds?" The less confusing the environment, the less likely a person will be agitated or frustrated. As a result, aggression can diminish.

Replacement Strategies

Sometimes people become violent because they lack the skills necessary to get their needs met. Replacement strategies attempt to proactively decrease aggression by teaching skills and otherwise replacing violent actions (Harris & Rice, 1995). Specific types of replacement strategies are explored in the following discussion.

Replace Aggression with Skills

Successfully learning three sets of skills may decrease a person's need to be violent: assertiveness, problem solving, and basic conversation (Corrigan & Mueser, 2000; Frey & Weller, 2000; Liberman, Corrigan, & Schade, 1989a). Skills training is discussed more thoroughly in Chapter 5, "Illness Self-Management." We review the three skill sets briefly here in terms of their impact on aggression. Assertiveness anchors the middle of a continuum, with submissiveness and aggressiveness at the extremes. Assertiveness is a set of skills that lets a person state his or her wants in a straightforward manner. "You know, Rob, when you turn the radio on too loud, I feel miffed, because I can't read my book." Sometimes assertiveness is sufficient—"Gee, Bill, I didn't realize my radio was bothering you; I'll turn it down." Other times, people respond to assertion with an assertive reply: "Well, why don't you go read in your bedroom?"

In the latter case, problem solving teaches a person to compromise with a peer. As discussed in Chapter 5, problem solving (D'Zurilla & Nezu, 2001) helps two people to jointly identify a problem, brainstorm solutions, evaluate how well individual solutions may resolve the problem, plan the implementation of a solution, try it out, and reevaluate. This kind of skill turns a potentially explosive situation into an opportunity for compromising in which the needs of both parties are met. Finally, some people may be aggressive because they have no social skills with which to interact with others. They do not have the simple conversational skills needed to start and maintain a dialogue. Hence, teaching people basic conversation may help them to get their interpersonal needs met and avoid being violent.

Replace Opportunity with Activity Programming

People sometimes become aggressive when they have too much unstructured time (Corrigan, Liberman, & Wong, 1993). Agitation and confusion are more likely to occur in settings that lack the cues and rewards that signal prosocial behavior. Hence, rehabilitation programs should eschew downtime. Employment programs should fill a person's 8-hour day with work. Education programs should make sure that a person is signed up for enough classes to stay busy. Psychosocial clubhouses should have ample activities that a member might engage in.

Rehabilitation teams also need to make sure that a person's day does not become overstructured (Drake & Sederer, 1986b), that is, include too many activities, which can lead to stress. It is not necessary to fill every minute of a person's day with activity. People with psychiatric disabilities are the ultimate decision makers regarding the structure of their days. They know best when there is too much downtime or too many activities. People who are especially cautious about taking on too many activities may engage in a personal trial with the support of their rehabilitation counselors. They should try adding activities to their schedules and determine their impact. Private time should also be part of the menu of activities; most people need quiet periods during the day when they can reenergize.

Replace Agitation with Control

As discussed earlier in this chapter, people sometimes become aggressive because they are agitated or otherwise overaroused in certain situations. Systematic desensitization may be a way to proactively help people decrease agitation in situations that have led to aggression in the past (Tyson, 1998; Warren & McLellarn, 1982). The effects of systematic desensitization, as used for aggression management, are based on the incompatible response hypothesis. That is, through repeated practice, people with aggression problems learn to suppress agitation in previously arousing situations, replacing it with calm. Systematic desensitization includes three components and is typically completed with the help of a rehabilitation counselor.

First, the person needs to outline a hierarchy of situations that specifically provoke agitation and aggression. This task is facilitated by developing a Subjective Units of Anger Scale (SUAS). As illustrated in Figure 18.2, a SUAS is a 100-point scale on which 100 represents a person's greatest sense of rage and 0 represents calm; 75 or above represents the point on the scale where the person needs help; 25 is running normal (i.e., no anger, mildly energized for a day's challenges). The scale is subjective because the person is asked to anchor scale points with meaningful examples from his or her own life. Figure 18.2 shows how specific examples define the scale. After learning to use the scale, the person has a simple method for signaling how upset he or she is in an anger-arousing situation.

"Wow, Jerry, you seem angry because Claudia called you a disrespectful name. Where on the SUAS does that put you?"

"Yep, I'm pretty pissed off; easily over 75, around 88."

After completing the SUAS, the person is asked to define the hierarchy of anger-arousing situations, focusing on the 75–100 portion of the scale. The person identifies several instances in which he or she gets angry and ranks them from least to most anger arousing. Figure 18.3 illustrates a sample hierarchy.

Second, individuals participating in systematic desensitization learn a relaxation technique, which they may systematically pair with each of the situations listed in Figure 18.3. There are several relaxation strategies from which a person may choose, including deep breathing, progressive muscle relaxation, calming self-statements, and imaginal relaxation. Each approach is briefly defined in Table 18.3. Typically, relaxation strategies are practiced in a quiet, private place with the person sitting or reclining and eyes closed. People should practice relaxation and not begin the third step of systematic desensitization until they are able to reduce their SUAS score to below 25 during practice.

Next, the person practices pairing each listed anger-inducing situation (see Figure 18.3) with a relaxation strategy. The goal is to start easy, so the rehabilitation counselor asks the person to imagine him- or herself in the least anger-inducing situation in the hierarchy. The person is to continue this until his or her SUAS score exceeds 75, at which

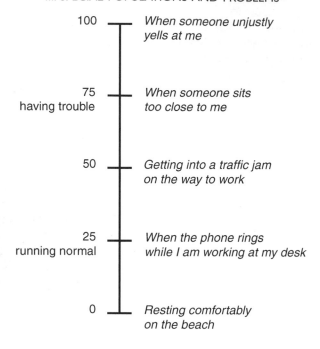

FIGURE 18.2. An example of a Subjective Units of Anger Scale.

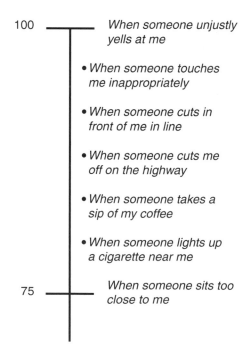

FIGURE 18.3. An example of an anger hierarchy for systematic desensitization.

TABLE 18.3. Four Relaxation Strategies

Strategy	Definition
Deep breathing	Slow, deep breaths; the person must be careful not to hyperventilate.
Progressive muscle relaxation	Alternatively tensing and relaxing muscle groups; a staff member instructs the person to notice the difference between the tension and relaxation.
Calming self-talk	Telling oneself that one is relaxed, peaceful, and at ease, in a calming voice.
Imaginal relaxation	This is a useful exercise for people who can visualize calming places. A person should imagine that he or she is at the beach, in a quiet meadow, or in any other situation that would receive a 0 on the SUAS.

time a signal is given to the counselor. At that point, the counselor instructs the person to stop imagining the stressful situation, and instead to practice the mastered relaxation exercise. Once the person's score is back down below 50, he or she is to signal the counselor, who again instructs the person to imagine the anger-inducing situation. The person and the counselor repeat this pairing until the person is able to imagine the situation without the score's exceeding 75. When this goal is met, the counselor instructs the person to imagine the next situation in the hierarchy. This kind of progressive pairing of situations and strategies ultimately helps the person to endure highly anger-inducing situations without being significantly agitated.

Relapse Prevention

Originally developed for substance abuse problems (Witkiewitz & Marlatt, 2004), relapse prevention has been extended to aggression management as a method for planning how to handle troublesome situations in the future during relatively problem-free periods (DiGiuseppe, 1999; King & Polaschek, 2003). A relapse plan (what I will do when I get angry again) is easier to make when the person is not steeped in the agitation of an anger-arousing situation. Relapse plans have two components. First, the person is asked to identify high-risk situations in which he or she is likely to be angry and aggressive. The hierarchy task used for systematic desensitization is one means of identifying high-risk situations—that is, any encounters that result in the person having trouble with anger.

Second, the person plans a way to deal with anger when these situations are encountered. Relapse plans may take one of two forms. They may be avoidance plans. That is, a person may decide to stay away from situations that provoke anger. Some situations are unavoidable because they are necessary for accomplishing another important life goal. For example, a person pursuing a regular job on the other side of town probably cannot avoid the commute, even though it makes him or her angry. In this instance, the relapse plan should include one of the replacement strategies outlined above. For example, if the situation involves another person, then the individual with anger problems may use assertiveness or problem-solving skills. If the situation involves nonspecific agitation, then relaxation learned for systematic desensitization may be warranted.

Behavioral Strategies That Decelerate Aggression

Replacement strategies can decrease, but not necessarily eliminate, aggression. Decelerative strategies are interventions that help to decrease aggression once it has occurred (Corrigan, Yudofsky, & Silver, 1993; Lennox, Miltenberger, Spengler, & Erfanian, 1988). Two aspects of decelerative approaches to aggression are reviewed here. We first discuss when decelerative approaches are most effective and then summarize specific decelerative techniques.

When to Decelerate Aggressive Behaviors

The best time to implement decelerative strategies is *before* a person loses total control and aggression is severe. The rehabilitation practitioner should partner with the person to identify preaggressive behaviors as the targets for deceleration. Many individuals engage in certain behaviors that occur just before full-blown aggression or violence. Common preaggressive behaviors include restlessness, pacing, noisily talking to oneself, in-your-face interactions, clenched fists, general loudness, and intimidating posturing or staring. Note that preaggressive behaviors are unique to the individual. Hence, what may be a signal for one person's aggression may be irrelevant for another's.

Targeting preaggression has a number of benefits. It is usually more effective to intervene with individuals when they are beginning to engage in preaggressive behaviors than after they have lost control and become fully aggressive. For example, it is easier to ask Tammy to use a coping technique or to redirect her to an activity when she first begins pacing, than it is to work with her after she has started shouting. Intervening with people when they engage in preaggressive behaviors often avoids the danger of having to intervene with them when they have become violent. It helps a person to stay in better control of his or her behavior, and it may increase that person's options.

BACKWARD CHAINING

Aggression is typically the end point of a series of behaviors, events, situations, and interactions—that is, aggression is the end point of a behavior chain. One way to identify preaggressive behaviors and prevent further incidents is to identify the sequence of events that led up to an aggressive incident (Hagopian, Farrell, & Amari, 1996; Smith, 1999). Once the elements of the behavior chain that led to an aggressive incident have been identified, the person and rehabilitation practitioner search for places in the chain where they may interdict subsequent aggressive behavior. Typically, behavior chains are easier to interrupt earlier than later in the sequence, thus derailing preaggressive behaviors.

Behavior chains are typically developed soon after an aggressive incident, when both the person and members of the rehabilitation team are in control of their behavior and emotions. The person begins by recalling all that happened during the aggressive incident and then works backward; the individual is asked to remember what occurred immediately before that incident. After describing what happened immediately preceding the incident, the person should try to remember what was going on before that, and so on, as far back as can be remembered and is relevant. The goal of behavior chaining is to identify a specific group of high-risk situations and preaggressive behaviors that can be monitored and targeted in the individual's treatment plan.

An example of a behavioral chain for Sandy is shown in Figure 18.4. The aggressive incident of concern was Sandy's hitting Pete while they were dining in the lunchroom.

Sandy admitted that she had yelled at Pete immediately prior to striking him. She yelled at him because he asked for five dollars. The example in Figure 18.4 illustrates the complexity of the chain and the high-risk factors that may have led to Sandy's ultimately hitting Pete. Relevant incidents seem to include not getting enough sleep, being disappointed by parents and by Wal-Mart, and being asked for money. These incidents can all become targets for change to head off future aggression. For example, Sandy might practice her assertion skills to handle another person's request for money and look into her evening rituals that may affect sleep.

Another important element in the behavioral chain is the events that immediately follow the targeted aggression. These events include the consequences for being aggressive. More than likely, both positive and negative consequences emerge in this aspect of the chain. A positive consequence defines the reason that the person may continue to be aggressive; that is, it indicates the reinforcer that the person received when he or she was aggressive. The negative consequence suggests the reason that the person may give up the aggressive behavior; it represents the punishing contingency that results from being aggressive. Figure 18.4 provides examples of both contingencies. Sandy taught Pete, a person she found annoying, to stay away by striking him, thereby reinforcing this behavior in the future. Sandy was assessed for hospitalization, which is a punisher and provides a reason why Sandy will learn how to avoid aggression in the future.

Figure 18.4 also illustrates the length of a behavioral chain. The person and rehabilitation provider should be sure to go back at least several hours before the aggressive incident. Failing to do that for Sandy may have missed lack of sleep as a relevant variable leading up to striking Pete. The backward chaining technique can also be used to evaluate past episodes of aggressive behavior. After several incidents are evaluated, patterns of events related to the environment and the individual should be explored. In this case, the goal is to identify a specific *group* of high-risk situations and preaggressive behaviors that can be monitored and targeted in the individual's treatment plan. The individual can be taught skills to cope with, tolerate, or avoid high-risk situations, and staff members will

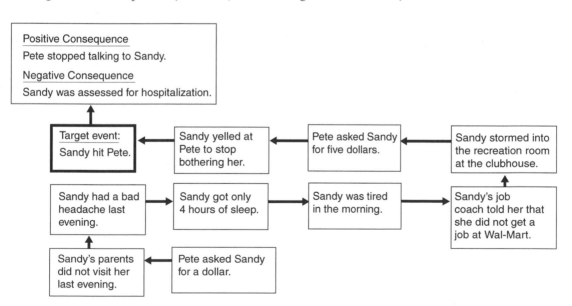

FIGURE 18.4. An example of a behavioral chain for aggression.

know to intervene and provide assistance should they become aware that one of the high-risk situations is occurring.

Techniques for Deceleration

Behavior therapists have created a hierarchy of intervention strategies designed to stop assaults, remove reinforcers, and, in some instances, provide learning opportunities for people to acquire alternative responses (Corrigan et al., 1993; Liberman & Wong, 1984). These strategies are summarized in Table 18.4. Responses in the hierarchy are ranked from least intrusive, that is, those with the least risk of physical injury or humiliation, to most intrusive, those posing greater risks. The response strategy should be decided upon ahead of the aggressive incident and reflect the person's problems and reactions to past interventions. Rehabilitation providers should select the least restrictive and intrusive intervention.

Decelerative techniques are fundamentally punitive in nature and are therefore likely to quickly reduce the frequency of targeted behaviors (Lerman & Vorndran, 2002; Mulick, 1990). Despite rapid benefits, there are several problems with using punitive strategies, which the rehabilitation provider needs to consider. Decelerative strategies will be experienced negatively. A surplus of such negative experiences can lead the person to drop out of services in order to avoid future punishment. Punishers also fail to teach the person how to handle an aggression-inducing situation. The improvements that result from decelerative techniques will be maintained only if reinforcing strategies—that teach the person coping skills that he or she may adopt in place of aggression—are paired with them. Hence, no plan for decelerative interventions should be crafted without a corresponding plan to help the person to learn coping skills.

SOCIAL EXTINCTION

Many people like to interact socially with the rehabilitation providers and peers involved in a program. Withdrawal of their attention when a person exhibits an aggressive behavior may decrease the rate of future aggression, especially if evidence suggests that the vio-

TABLE 18.4. A Hierarchy of Decelerative Interventions

Technique	Definition
Social extinction	The team ignores the aggressive behavior and pays attention to the person only when he or she is acting in a prosocial manner.
Contingent observation	The person steps out of the situation and views peers who seem to be handling demands okay.
Self-controlled time out	The person takes him- or herself out of a situation until he or she stops being angry or violent.
Overcorrection	The person makes an effort to remedy the upset in a violent situation.

Note. Techniques are ordered from least intrusive to most intrusive.

lent outburst is maintained by attention from peers or staff (Wong, Woolsey, Innocent, & Liberman, 1988). This is called social extinction, which is most commonly employed with mildly aggressive or disruptive behaviors that do not require immediate staff response (e.g., threatening gestures or loud vocalizations). Obviously, one should not ignore a person who is already showing physical aggression.

In using this technique, staff members explicitly define the target behavior and the amount of time they will ignore the person in an effort to extinguish the behavior. For example, staff members on Unit 24 decided to ignore John every time he had a tantrum when someone bumped into him in the lunchroom. They would continue to ignore him until he stopped his tantrum for 5 minutes. Effective extinction requires all staff members to ignore the designated person during the intervention. Hence, during extinction staff members should not discuss the inappropriate behavior with the person and should avoid eye contact. Members of the staff who were not present when the inappropriate behavior was exhibited should be notified that an extinction schedule has been implemented so that they will interact with the person as other providers are doing.

B.F. Skinner (1938) found that immediately after a target behavior was extinguished, the behavior *increased* in frequency before diminishing, which is known as an extinction burst. Thus, one would expect assaultive behaviors that are being extinguished by staff to initially become more severe. For example, Unit 24 staff members noticed that John's tantrums actually got worse when they first started to ignore him. Staff members need to be taught this point so that they do not prematurely relinquish the intervention strategy. If used consistently, extinction may be an effective means to diminish the rate of inappropriate behaviors (Liberman, Wallace, Teigen, & Davis, 1974).

CONTINGENT OBSERVATION

Although social extinction may decrease tantrums and threats, it does not provide an opportunity for a person to learn alternative responses to frustration and conflict. Rehabilitation practitioners using contingent observation instruct acting-out persons to sit quietly for a predefined time on the perimeter of a group (Liberman & Wong, 1984; Porterfield, Herbert-Jackson, & Risley, 1976). While sitting alone, such persons are instructed to watch peers and staff members carefully and observe alternative responses they might employ to avoid future angry responses in a similar situation. For example, Sam was instructed to sit along the wall of the snack room and watch how others dealt with the frustration of getting only one cup of coffee. Members of the staff verbally reinforce the person when he or she is quietly watching others. They also query the person about what he or she may have observed about others: "Sam, you may have noticed that Harry didn't get a second cup of coffee. How did he handle it?" The observation period continues until the person remains calm for 2 minutes, at which time he or she may return to the group.

SELF-CONTROLLED TIME OUT

Time out from reinforcement is an operant technique in which socially inappropriate and/or aggressive behaviors are decreased by separating the person from overstimulating (and perhaps reinforcing) situations (Glynn, Mueser, & Liberman, 1989). Time out is most effective for people who experience loss of social contact as punitive. For example, Mary frequently became loud and angry at clubhouse parties when the room was crowded and the radio loud. She calmed down noticeably when she stepped into her case manager's office for a few minutes' break. Time out in this case is under the person's self-control. That is, the person decides to put him- or herself into time out and decides when he or she has calmed down sufficiently to end the time out. Self-controlled time out is unlike seclusion because it evokes less resistance (Glynn et al., 1989). People have much more control over the time-out process. In this way, time out offers a less restrictive alternative to seclusion and restraints, engenders less humiliation, and involves diminished risk of injury.

To implement the procedure, people learn to enter time out on their own when they are aggressive. Staff members on an inpatient unit, for example, may tape off one corner of a quiet, low-traffic room where people learn to "time out." People learn to remain in the quiet area until they have been nonaggressive for 2 minutes. Sometimes continued aggression in the time-out area may result in a lengthy intervention. Time-out periods that are excessive (last more than an hour) become overpunitive and diminish the purpose of the intervention. People who do not comply with time-out instructions after 1 minute are told to enter the seclusion room. Hence, seclusion is used as a punisher for individuals who do not comply with a time out promptly.

OVERCORRECTION

Overcorrection combines time out and an effort requirement to reduce the rate of offensive behaviors by replacing those behaviors with more prosocial alternatives (Foxx & Azrin, 1972; Ollendick & Matson, 1978). The effort requirement compels people to restore the disturbed situation to a vastly improved condition. For example, an individual who hit another person may be required to apologize to the victim, others in the ward, and the rehabilitation staff.

Frequently, gentle physical guidance may be necessary to direct a person toward beginning the task. A person who throws soda in a meeting room may be physically guided to pick up a sponge and wash the wall thoroughly. Only the minimum force necessary to implement the overcorrection procedure should be used. Although physical guidance may at first be necessary to establish instructional control, the procedure is contraindicated for people who repeatedly refuse to participate after the initial guidance period. Extreme caution with this approach is warranted; any coercive program applied to recalcitrant individuals may escalate into incidents of staff injury or client abuse.

SUMMARY AND CONCLUSIONS

People who are aggressive can find many of their rehabilitation plans derailed. Hence, managing aggression is a priority. Seven types of aggression were reviewed in this chapter: frustration-related, operant, nonspecific agitation, psychosis related, confusion related, that related to loss of social support, and aggression related to intermittent explosive disorder. Three forms of aggression management were reviewed. Systemwide strategies are used to manage the environment so that it is not likely to be frustrating, confusing, or overarousing. Replacement strategies seek to substitute aggressive behavior with prosocial skills. Alternatively, they seek to replace a state of agitation with more calm. Finally, decelerative strategies are progressively more intrusive methods that are used when aggression does occur. Rehabilitation practitioners who have mastered the range of skills are better prepared to deal with aggression.

Part IV

SYSTEM CONSIDERATIONS

Rehabilitation makes sense only when the community in which it occurs is integrated into the rehabilitation program. The final three chapters of this book address the relevant issues. Discrimination frequently blocks a person's pursuit of his or her aspirations. Chapter 19 reviews specific strategies that help to tear down prejudicial barriers. Chapter 20 examines how rehabilitation programs are influenced by diversity. In particular, cross-cultural perspectives on rehabilitation are examined. Finally, Chapter 21 reviews the statutes and administrative decisions that influence the development of effective programs. The Americans with Disabilities Act, for example, provides certain protections for people who are seeking employment.

Chapter 19

Erasing Stigma
and Promoting Empowerment

In Chapter 2, we argued that the stigma of mental illness impedes two of the major goals of psychiatric rehabilitation: community integration and personal empowerment. Public stigma—in which the general population endorses the prejudice toward mental illness and discriminates against those with corresponding labels—prevents people from attaining such community integration goals as obtaining a good-paying job or living in comfortable housing. We distinguished between public stigma that results from individual members of the general population accepting the prejudice and that which reflects social structures that have historically developed as a result of economic and political forces. Self-stigma—in which the person with mental illness internalizes the prejudice and suffers diminished self-esteem and self-efficacy—undermines the person's sense of personal empowerment. The purpose of this chapter is to review strategies that help people with psychiatric disabilities overcome stigma and its pernicious effects. Three particular approaches are reviewed: (1) strategies that a person can use to challenge self-stigma and that promote empowerment; (2) strategies for advocates to erase public stigma and enhance community integration; and (3) strategies that replace social structures promoting discrimination with those fostering affirmative action.

CHALLENGING SELF-STIGMA

Three approaches to addressing self-stigma have been developed and researched; these are explored in the following discussion, along with some evidence about their efficacy and effectiveness.

1. Self-stigma has been framed as irrational cognitive schemas that result from internalized prejudice. Cognitive therapy has been used to challenge the irrational self-statements that emerge from these schemas.
2. Self-stigma may be influenced by a person's decision about whether to disclose his or her mental health experience. Strategic approaches to making the decision and to disclosing are reviewed.
3. Several approaches have been developed to promote personal empowerment. Individuals with greater empowerment are likely to express less self-stigma.

Each of these three strategies is reviewed more fully below.

Facilitating Change in Self-Stigmatizing Cognitive Schemas

Self-stigma may be understood as maladaptive self-statements or cognitive schemas that have developed largely as a result of socialization, whereby a person first learns mental illness prejudice and subsequently internalizes it when he or she is labeled. Interpersonal differences in cognitive schemas may help explain why, given the same social situation, one person feels significantly "stigmatized," but a second may not feel stigmatized, and a third is motivated to act against being stigmatized. The adverse effects of stigma are "located" not only in the social situation, but in the cognitive process of the stigmatized individual—that is, the way an individual perceives and understands the social situation such that disrespectful messages emerge (Crocker & Quinn, 2000).

As summarized in Chapter 12, cognitive therapy has been shown to be an effective strategy for helping people change cognitive schemas that lead to anxiety, depression, and the consequences of self-stigma. Although some readers may be concerned that people with serious psychiatric disorders might not benefit from cognitive therapy, British researchers have documented its benefits for those with psychotic disorders (Chadwick & Lowe, 1990; Tarrier, Beckett, Harwood, Baker, Yusupoff, et al., 1993; Drury, Birchwood, Cochrane, & Macmillan, 1996a; Kuipers, Garety, Fowler, Dunn, Bebbington, et al., 1997). This approach targets distressing psychotic symptoms and maladaptive understandings of mental illness, using a collaborative empirical framework. The therapist helps the client explore his or her distressing and often delusional cognitions, attempting to reframe them as beliefs rather than facts, empathically discussing how one may arrive at such beliefs (but also recognizing their emotional costs), reviewing evidence for and against the beliefs, and trying to find less distressing alternative interpretations (Chadwick et al., 1996; Garety et al., 2000).

The most promising studies in this line of research in relation to stigma were completed by David Kingdon and Douglas Turkington (1991, 1994). These researchers expanded the cognitive therapy of psychosis beyond the content of specific symptoms, also targeting the person's catastrophic interpretation of his or her symptoms and the stigma attached to mental illness generally. Following Strauss's (1969) finding that psychotic symptoms represent points on continua of function, the authors attempted to *normalize* the symptoms of therapy participants by comparing them to normal experiences such as deprivation states. Similarly, in their recent research, Garety and colleagues (2000) strive for an understanding of psychosis that promotes social functionality. Although research on cognitive therapy and psychosis is growing, more work is needed to examine the positive effects derived from using cognitive therapy to challenge beliefs consistent with self-stigma.

Deciding to Disclose

One of the distinguishing features of the stigma of mental illness is that the mark that specifically signals mental illness is frequently not apparent to the public. Unlike race and gender, for example, there are few externally manifest cues signaling that an individual belongs to this stigmatized group. One way to avoid stigma is by not disclosing one's experience with mental illness and mental health services. However, concluding that it is best to conceal one's psychiatric history suggests that disclosure yields only harm with no benefits. In reality, neither the definition of what constitutes disclosure, nor the comparative costs and benefits of disclosure, is clear. Moreover, there are not many completed studies on disclosure, either in terms of mental illness stigma or in regard to the self-prejudice experienced by other stigmatized groups. Despite this limitation, some conclusions can be drawn from the empirical literature about the nature of disclosure in other stigma groups. After a brief review of this literature, we discuss the variety of disclosure options from which a person might select, as well as the costs and benefits of these options.

Understanding the Impact of Disclosure

Individuals with a concealable stigma may vary in the ways they choose to disclose their status. One study, for example, has shown that most mothers who are HIV positive (Thampanichawat, 1999) chose to keep their status totally secret. However, most people with concealable stigma are selectively disclosing, including lesbians in the workplace (Afrank, 1999), gay men (Kennamer, Honnold, Bradford, & Hendricks, 2000), two other samples of HIV seropostive adults (Josephson, 1997; Walsh, 2000a), postsecondary school students with learning disabilities (Hoehn, 1998), and childless women (Riesmann, 2000). To whom people selectively disclose usually depends on the setting; however, frequent candidates for disclosure include family members, friends, professional helpers, and/or others with the concealable stigma (Josephson, 1997).

Several variables seem to influence selective disclosure, including overall perceptions of stigma (Hoehn, 1998) and the perceived negative consequences of disclosure, such as disappointing others, suffering their wrath, or burdening them (Chin & Kroesen, 1999). Disclosure is also associated with other demographics. One study showed that white gay men were more likely to disclose than black gay men (Kennamer et al., 2000). A second study showed that ethnicity and gender were also factors in the choice of disclosure targets (Josephson, 1997). African American and Latino gay men were more likely to disclose to their families, whereas European Americans were more likely to disclose to helpers and friends. Males were more likely to tell friends, but lesbians were more likely to inform helpers or family members (Josephson, 1997).

We found one study that examined disclosure in people with mental illness (Bradmiller, 1997). Disclosure depended on whether a person admitted his or her mental illness. "Admitters" were more likely to disclose their mental illness to a broad group of people. Deniers were more likely than their counterparts to seek community with "normals" and to not disclose their mental health status to these individuals. Interestingly, deniers also reported significantly less rejection because of their involvement with the mental health system.

PERSONAL EXAMPLE

Jon Simpson Beats Self-Stigma

Jon worked with his rehabilitation practitioner, Cindy Howard, to counter the self-statements he was making that reflected self-stigma. Before these sessions, Jon frequently felt blue and reported low self-esteem. "I'm mentally ill. People like me are never able to get good jobs or live in nice places. The mentally ill are all incapable of anything other than just getting by." Working with Cindy, he was able to challenge this belief and develop personally meaningful counters to use when self-doubt emerged again.

CINDY: So our goal today is threefold: to get a better handle on what are the self-beliefs due to stigma that are hurting you, to collect evidence that challenges these beliefs, and then to develop counters to use against those beliefs in the future. Today, we only have time for the first two tasks: identifying the beliefs and figuring out where we would find evidence to challenge them. (*pause*) Remind me, Jon, when you are beating up yourself with the stigma of mental illness, what kind of things are you thinking?

JON: That I am no good because I have a mental illness. That people like me must be weak. That we are incapable of doing anything meaningful with our lives.

C: Wow, that's quite a load—that you won't make anything of your life. How do those thoughts make you feel?

J: Low, really low. Like I am bad. Which depresses me 'cause I am trying to live a good life.

C: As we discussed, Jon, it is thoughts like these, and not facts, that bring people down. These thoughts are based on misperceptions or on false beliefs. Your job here is to collect evidence that proves this to you. And my job is to help you in the process. So let's go back and begin to tear apart these beliefs. You said something like "I'm no good because people like me, the mentally ill, are not able to live meaningful lives." Did I get that right?

J: Yep. That's right. I know that doesn't sound exactly true, but I can't help thinking that way. After all, how are mentally ill folks represented on TV? Always as homeless bums.

C: Sure, you see those things on TV, it makes you begin to wonder about yourself. But TV doesn't always get the facts right. Let's set up a little experiment for you to see what the truth is. You said, "The mentally ill are unable to live a meaningful life." So what would be a meaningful life for you?

J: Well, lots of things that adults are supposed to do . . . working for sure, and I don't mean just at a sheltered workshop, I mean a real job with a normal salary and benefits.

C: Okay, then that's our experiment. Let's get you to interview some people with serious mental illness and find out how many of them are working at real jobs. The first question is, where would you find adults with mental illness you might interview?

J: About a month ago, I started going to GROW, a self-help group, at the local church. There are about 10 regulars there who are all struggling with mental illness. I could ask them.

C: Okay, let's get a bit more specific. First, what would you ask?

J: Well, a straightforward question might be best. "Hey, Syd, do you work? What kind of job do you have?"

C: Sounds good. And now the second part. How will you analyze the information?

J: Well, I guess if everyone told me they were working in good jobs, then I would know the statement that "people with mental illness are not capable of a meaningful life" would be false.

C: Hmmm. You seem to be setting the bar a bit high. After all, not every adult I know is working, whether they have a mental illness or not. And a lot of people have jobs that are not necessarily "good."

J: Good point. I guess I just want to see if anyone is working and whether they are getting a normal wage.

C: 'Cause I guess if you find out that two or three are working, that challenges your basic assumption. Okay. Let's give it a try and see what you get, and then we can look at the data more carefully.

J: Okay, my next GROW meeting is Monday night, and I can bring what I find out to my next meeting with you on Wednesday morning.

Different Levels of Disclosure

As the aforementioned research suggests, disclosure is not a monolithic phenomenon but may actually vary in several ways. Based on a review of the limited literature (Corrigan & Lundin, 2001; Herold, 1995; Thampanichawat, 1999), we have identified five levels of disclosure, summarized in Table 19.1: social avoidance, secrecy, selective disclosure, indiscriminate disclosure, and broadcast experience. The costs and benefits of each of these types of disclosure decisions is also reviewed in the table.

SOCIAL AVOIDANCE

One way to handle disclosure is to not tell anyone. This can be accomplished by avoiding situations where the public may find out about one's mental illness. People who are victimized by stigma may choose to not socialize with, live near, or work alongside persons without disabilities. Instead, they associate only with other persons who have mental illness. This may include associating with persons with mental illness living in a therapeutic community or working in a sheltered work environment, or interacting with friends in a social club developed for people with mental illness. In this way, a person can avoid the "normal" population that may be intolerant of his or her disabilities.

In some ways, this approach is similar to the recurrent notion of *asylum* (Wasow, 1986). A few people have such severe psychiatric disabilities that they need a safe and pleasant place to live and work, a place where they can escape the pressures and disapproval of society. What was known as the "moral view of psychiatric care" originally envisioned state hospitals for this purpose (Bockoven, 1963), providing nice homes, rural settings, and supportive caretakers who help persons with extreme disabilities to escape the stresses of society and its citizens who will stigmatize them. Unfortunately, very few hospitals ever achieved this goal, in part because most state and private facilities were dominated by patients with acute symptoms, some of whom might be potentially dangerous to themselves or others. The predominant concern for protection of patients from violence frequently overrides many of the "pleasant" aspects of hospital living (Crowner, 2000). It was found that this kind of asylum could be more appropriately accomplished in community-based programs. Persons with profound disabilities, who choose not to address their community's prejudice against mental illness, could live in pleasant compounds and work in sheltered settings away from the rest of their neighbors. They could

TABLE 19.1. Five Ways to Disclose or Not Disclose

1. Social avoidance

The individual altogether avoids persons and places that may stigmatize or otherwise disrespect the person because of his or her mental illness.

Benefit: The person does not encounter others who will unfairly harm him or her.
Cost: The person loses the opportunity to meet new people who possibly may be supportive.

2. Secrecy

The individual does not tell people at places where he or she works or lives about his or her mental illness.

Benefit: As in social avoidance, the person withholds information from others he or she does not know or trust. But the person does not have to avoid important settings like work or the community in the process.
Cost: Some people feel guilty about keeping secrets.

3. Selective disclosure

The individual tells some people he or she believes will be supportive about his or her mental illness.

Benefit: The person finds a small group of people who will understand his or her experiences and provide support.
Cost: The person may disclose to some people who will hurt him or her with the information. The person may have difficulty keeping track of who does and does not know.

4. Indiscriminate disclosure

The individual is not concerned with who knows about his or her mental illness. The person tells anyone he or she encounters.

Benefit: The person does not worry about who knows about his or her problems. And the person is likely to find people who will be supportive.
Cost: The person is likely to tell people who will hurt him or her with the information.

5. Broadcast your experience

The individual purposefully communicates his or her experiences with mental illness to a large group.

Benefit: The person does not have to worry about who knows about his or her history of mental illness. He or she is promoting a personal sense of empowerment and is striking a blow against stigma.
Cost: The person can encounter people who may try to hurt him or her with this information. He or she is also going to meet people who disapprove of the political statement.

learn to cope with their symptoms or achieve their interpersonal goals in a setting relatively free of disapproving neighbors or coworkers.

Unfortunately, there are several negatives in social avoidance. Persons who choose to avoid the "normal" world lose out on all the benefits it brings: free access to a broader set of opportunities and citizens who offer support to those experiencing mental illness (Corrigan & Lundin, 2001). Moreover, social avoidance in some ways promotes stigma and discrimination. It endorses the idea that persons with mental illness should be kept away from the rest of the world. Those who choose to avoid social situations may be putting off a challenge they must eventually face. Social avoidance may be a useful strategy during times when symptoms are intense and a person needs a respite from the demands of society. But avoiding the normal world altogether will most likely prevent individuals from achieving the breadth of their life goals.

SECRECY

There is no need for a person to avoid work or community situations to keep his or her experiences with mental illness private. Many persons choose to enter these worlds without sharing their experiences with others. They keep all aspects of their psychiatric experiences—both the impact of their illness and their interactions with the mental health system—a secret. There are two parts to keeping experiences with mental illness a secret. The first part seems easy: *Do not tell anyone* (Corrigan & Lundin, 2001). A person does not share his or her history of experiences with hospitalizations, doctors, medications, or symptoms. There are several costs incurred in not talking about one's experiences, even those life events that may yield potentially harmful stigma. People may find it difficult to always have to be vigilant about what they say about themselves. This kind of vigilance may lead to resentment. Nevertheless, this simple act of keeping all or parts of their psychiatric experience to themselves may greatly open up their access to work settings and communities of other people (Afrank, 1999).

The first strategy for keeping experiences secret is an act of omission; the second is an act of commission. A person may need to fill in some gaps in his or her past and current experience. A work resume may include blanks for the years when the person was in the hospital. Consider, for example, Tamiko's experience. There were 2 years, between discharge from the Navy (she was in computer operations) and her 26th birthday, when she was in and out of hospitals for depression. Instead of leaving these years blank on her resume, she wrote, "Advanced training in computers." When asked during job interviews what this training meant, she truthfully discussed the adult education courses she completed in systems management. She did not, however, talk about how these courses were interspersed with psychiatric hospitalizations. A person must also decide how to discuss current experiences related to a mental illness. Why does he leave early to see a doctor every month? What are those medicines she takes at lunch for? Without answers to such questions, the current gaps may be of some curiosity to coworkers or neighbors.

SELECTIVE DISCLOSURE

Keeping experiences with mental illness a secret prevents a person from availing him- or herself of the support and resources of possibly empathic friends and colleagues. Hence, many people decide to disclose their experiences with mental health stigma to a selected set of people (Bradmiller, 1997). However, choosing to disclose to some people has its risks; those who find out may shun the discloser. Targets of disclosure may decide they do not want to work with, live near, or otherwise associate with a "mental patient." With the risk comes opportunity, however. Persons who disclose may find people who are supportive. Moreover, they will not have to worry about keeping a secret from those to whom they have disclosed.

There are several reasons why a person may selectively disclose. A person with mental illness may want a potential helper to know of his or her experiences. In knowing of the person's illness, the helper is better able to provide services to the person. A person may disclose because he or she seeks the support of others. This may include empathy from peers who are also struggling with mental illness but have chosen to keep their experiences a secret.

A decision to disclose to another person does not mean that one must tell everything; choosing to disclose does not have to result in giving up all privacy. Just as people must decide to whom they will disclose, they must also decide the content of their disclosures. This means making specific decisions about their experiences with mental illness as well as their *current* encounters with the mental health system. The purpose of disclosing the past is to provide others some knowledge of the extent of the mental illness, which may include diagnosis, symptoms, history of hospitalizations, and medications. Current experiences are discussed for two reasons: first, to impress upon the target that the mental illness of long ago has much less impact on the person now—that the person is able to control small problems that occur in his or her life—and second, to alert the peer that minor troubles may occur in the future for which some assistance may be needed.

INDISCRIMINATE DISCLOSURE

Selective disclosure means there are groups of people with whom information is shared and groups from whom information remains secret (Corrigan & Lundin, 2001). More than likely, the group of people who are not privy to the secret is much larger than the group of those who are informed; there remain a large number of people of whom individuals must be wary. People who choose indiscriminate disclosure abandon the secrecy. They no longer worry about who finds out about their mental illness or treatment history. A person choosing this option is relieved of the burden imposed by keeping part of his or her life underground.

Despite its benefits, indiscriminate disclosure requires a fairly hardy personality. Many people who find out about the disclosed information may react negatively to the revelations. Hence, individuals opting for indiscriminate disclosure should assess whether they can cope with the disapproval that results from bigoted reactions. One way to make this evaluation is for the person to role-play interactions that represent bigoted situations (Corrigan & Lundin, 2001; Link, Mirotznik, & Cullen, 1991). The goal of the exercise is not to practice effective replies but, rather, to monitor one's reaction; individuals who report significant feelings of shame, anxiety, sadness, or anger because of bigoted comments should ask themselves whether they want the kind of stress that is commensurate with indiscriminate disclosure.

BROADCAST EXPERIENCE

Although individuals opting for indiscriminate disclosure are no longer trying to hide their mental illness, they are not actively seeking ways to inform others about their psychiatric experiences. Broadcasting one's experience means educating people about mental illness. This kind of disclosure is much more than throwing away any notion of secret. The goal is to seek out the public and share one's history and current experiences with mental illness. Broadcasting one's experience has the same benefits as indiscriminate disclosure. One no longer needs to worry about keeping a secret. In the process, individuals who broadcast their experiences can find others who provide understanding, support, and assistance. People who choose to broadcast their experiences seem to derive an additional benefit. That is, it seems to foster their sense of power over the experience of mental illness and stigma. No longer must they cower because of feelings of inferiority (Chamberlin, 1984). This kind of consciousness raising may help them to understand that problems with mental illness are not solely a function of biological limitations; society's reactions are also to blame. Shouting this out diminishes community oppression. In fact, many people who choose to broadcast their experiences wish to surpass the limited goal of talking about their mental illness. They also express their dissatisfaction with the way they have been treated because of their mental illness (Deegan, 1990).

Broadcasting experiences can yield hostile responses, just like indiscriminate disclosure (Montini, 2000). Members of the general public hearing someone's story about mental illness frequently battle the message *and* the messenger. Civil rights leaders have experienced such reactions for decades. Challenging messages from racial groups about economic inequality and political injustice upset the status quo. In a similar manner, talking about one's mental illness and displeasure with society's reaction is disquieting to others. Citizens may rebel against the messenger with angry denials. Once again, individuals opting to broadcast their experiences need to determine whether they are able to cope with the angry response. Some persons who choose to broadcast their experiences join advocacy groups for support and guidance. The influence of these groups is discussed more fully in the section below in regard to fostering consumer empowerment.

Considering the Costs and Benefits of Disclosure

As suggested in the preceding discussion, there are both costs and benefits to disclosing one's experiences with mental illness (Chin & Kroesen, 1999; Hays, McKusick, Pollack, Hilliard, Hoff, et al., 1993). Given the positive and negative outcomes of disclosing, opting whether and how to disclose is not a transparent decision that all people stigmatized with mental illness should pursue in a standard manner. Rather, individuals should weigh their personal perceptions of the costs against the benefits to decide about disclosure. This kind of decisional comparison has been discussed extensively in both social (Ajzen & Fishbein, 1980) and clinical psychology (Miller & Rollnick, 2002) as a mechanism for opting how to proceed in terms of a specific behavioral goal.

Some people like to carefully consider all the benefits of an action (i.e., choosing to disclose one's mental illness) first, listing as many as they can think of. They then list the costs. Others just start writing down costs and benefits as they come to mind until they have them all listed. Frequently, cost and benefit columns are divided into short- and long-term sections. The impacts of costs and benefits are sometimes relatively immediate, and at other times delayed. Generally, people tend to be more influenced by short-term costs and benefits because they occur sooner. However, long-term costs and benefits frequently have greater implications for the future. Costs and benefits also vary by situation. Disclosing is significantly different at work than in one's neighborhood or with softball teammates. A person could conceivably decide to tell people at work but not people in the neighborhood, or to tell close friends but not the pastor. Hence, the costs and benefits of disclosing need to be listed separately for each setting.

Whether to disclose a mental illness is a difficult decision to make alone. Because there are so many emotion-charged factors to take into consideration, it is hard for a person to calmly and rationally weigh the pluses and minuses. Hence, some individuals may want to consider the judgment and advice of others before plunging into disclosure. Family members may be good sources of advice. They may understand the benefits of disclosure and provide emotional support throughout the process. Friends with mental illness, especially those who have disclosed, may offer positive advice or possibly a warning, depending on their experiences in disclosing a mental illness. Those who are advocates and have succeeded in organizations like the National Alliance for the Mentally Ill (NAMI) will likely advise individuals to tell. Those who have had negative experiences because of disclosure, such as loss of a job or failure of a marriage, may tell people to keep their lips sealed.

Fostering Personal Empowerment

Another approach to changing self-stigma builds on a definition of self-stigma given earlier in this chapter, that it is an internalization of the prejudice of others; personal empowerment is the opposite of self-stigma. Being empowered means having control over one's treatment and one's life (Rappaport, 1987). Persons who have a strong sense of personal empowerment can be expected to have high self-efficacy and self-esteem. They are not overwhelmed by their symptoms and psychiatric labels but have a positive outlook and take an active role in their recovery. Empowerment approaches are considered to be among the best ways to deal with self-stigma. Communities and health service providers can foster personal empowerment in mental health care consumers in a variety of ways that involve giving consumers greater control over their own treatment and integration into the community. Research findings indicate that programs that include the person with disabilities in all facets of intervention are conducive to the attainment of vocational and independent living goals (Corrigan et al., 1999a; Corrigan & Garman, 1997; Rogers, Anthony, Cohen, & Davies, 1997b).

At the most general level, fostering empowerment involves adopting a collaborative approach to treatment planning in which the consumer ceases to be merely a passive recipient of services (Corrigan et al., 1990). At the very least, programs should form a treatment partnership, seeking feedback from consumers as to their satisfaction with the services offered and their suggestions for improvement. The emphasis is on the strengths and potential of the consumer rather than his or her weaknesses (Rapp et al., 1993). Beyond this, truly empowering services promote the self-determination of consumers in relation to employment opportunities, housing, and other areas of social life. Rather than a stigmatizing and coercive removal from the community, these new approaches provide community-based support for the consumer's continuing efforts to adapt to community living. This approach can be typified in the assertive community treatment (ACT) of Stein and Test (1980). In ACT, services are brought directly to the consumer's home, workplace, or other meaningful community setting (see Chapter 6). Supported employment and supported education are also methods used to facilitate the inclusion of persons with disabilities into the fabric of society (Drake et al., 1999a; Mowbray, Collins, Bellamy, Megivern, Bybee, et al., 2005a). These approaches, which were given increased priority with the passage of the Americans with Disabilities Act in 1990, encourage the prompt placement of clients into employment and/or educational settings and provide supportive services for their continuing success in the activities involved. This approach contrasts with traditional paradigms that focus on *preparing* clients for independent social functioning before *supporting* them in actual community involvement.

Consumers can also empower themselves by becoming rehabilitation practitioners in traditional treatment programs (Mowbray, Moxley, & Collins, 1998), or they can create and operate their own services (Solomon & Draine, 2001). Services in which consumers have a central role in operation include lodges and clubhouses, as well as self-help and mutual assistance groups. The Fountain House clubhouse in New York is a paradigmatic example of consumer empowerment through mutual help. (See also discussion of Fountain House in Chapter 17.) This first clubhouse was founded in the 1940s by a group of former inpatients from Rockland State Hospital yearning for a place to gather and support one another. Fountain House, and the field of psychosocial rehabilitation that it influenced, destigmatized the recovering person by focusing on his or her strengths and by developing social competence through involvement in the very activities that constitute community integration (employment, housing, education, etc.).

The Fountain House model contrasts with traditional treatment in many ways. This program does not focus on providing "treatment" for mental illness, but rather on developing the skills and talents of its members. Participants in Fountain House are called "members," which is a much less stigmatizing and more empowering label than "patient." It also implies an element of responsibility, as members are expected to take supportive and leadership roles in groups and in teams to accomplish the tasks required to maintain the clubhouse (Beard et al., 1982; Fountain House, New York City, 1999). Members and staff have equal status and work together to serve the clubhouse community. All elements and activities are designed to ensure that each member experiences a strong sense of ownership in the clubhouse, feels expected each morning, has a sense of being wanted and needed by members and staff, and can recognize that his or her contribution is critical to the functioning of the house.

Consumer-operated services are perhaps the prototype of programs that empower people with mental illness and thereby challenge self-stigma (Clay, 2005; Weingarten, Chinman, Tworkowski, Stayner, & Davidson, 2000; Solomon & Draine, 2001). Consumer-operated services are developed *by* people with mental illness *for* people with mental illness. All facets of operation are controlled by people with mental illness. Services include mutual help programs, often in a Twelve-Step format; education programs frequently focusing on advocacy strategies; and drop-in centers (see Chapter 17).

The Paradox of Trying to Fix Self-Stigma

In trying to change self-stigma, there is a paradox of which service providers and advocates should be wary. That is, focusing on self-stigma may frame the prejudice and discrimination that results as a problem solely of people with mental illness. Like the disabilities that arise from their illness, stigma is another unfortunate result of having mental illness with which people inflicted with the disease must learn to live. This kind of perspective may ignore the responsibility of the public in creating and maintaining stigma. Although there is value in consumers of mental health services and others victimized by stigma learning how to deal with its harm for themselves, it should not release the public from its responsibility. Link and colleagues (1991) argued that because stigma is powerfully reinforced by a culture, its effects are not easily overcome by the coping actions of individuals. Citing C. Wright Mills (1967), they conclude that labeling and stigma are "social problems" that need to be addressed by public approaches, not "individual troubles" that are addressed by individual therapy. Although Link and colleagues' formulation risks being one-sided in limiting itself to interventions aimed only at society at large (research supports the conclusion that both individual-level and society-level interventions can be useful), it is true that the self-stigma experienced by some people with mental illness is less likely to thrive if the public as a whole refuses to nurture stereotypes, prejudice, and discrimination.

ERASING PUBLIC STIGMA

Whereas investigations on changing mental illness stigma are somewhat limited, social psychologists have developed a particularly rich body of research on strategies to improve intergroup attitudes related to race and ethnicity. Based on our review of this literature, we grouped the various approaches to changing public stigma of mental illness into three processes: protest, education, and contact (Corrigan & Penn, 1999).

Protest

Protest strategies highlight the injustice of specific stigmas and often lead to a moral appeal for people to stop their negative thinking: "Shame on you for holding such disrespectful ideas about people with mental illness!" Ironically, this kind of attitude suppression may yield a rebound effect so that prejudices about a group remain unchanged or actually become worse (Corrigan, River, Lundin, Penn, Uphoff-Wasowski, et al., 2001c; Macrae, Bodenhausen, Milne, & Jetten, 1994; Penn & Corrigan, 2002). Although there are both cognitive and social explanations of this kind of rebound, perhaps the simplest is the construct of psychological reactance (Brehm & Jones, 1970): "Don't tell me what to think!" Hence, protest may have a limited impact in changing public *attitudes* about people with mental illness.

This does not mean that protest has no role in affecting stigma. There is largely anecdotal evidence that protest can change some *behaviors* significantly (Wahl, 1995). For example, NAMI StigmaBusters has an e-mail alert system that notifies members about stigmatizing representations of persons with mental illness in the media and provides instructions on how to contact the offending organization and its sponsors (NAMI StigmaBusters, 2002). (See pp. 417–418 for further discussion of the role of NAMI StigmaBusters in protesting stigma.)

Research may show protest to be effective as a punishing consequence to discriminatory behavior that decreases the likelihood that people will repeat this behavior. Research may also consider other types of punishing consequences, such as legal penalties prescribed by the Americans with Disabilities Act and the Fair Housing Act. For example, what is the effect of judgments ordering punitive damages be paid by employers who discriminate in hiring individuals with mental illness or by communities that design zoning laws to keep group homes for persons with mental illness out?—though it is important to keep in mind that these are rare phenomena indeed (Stefan, 2001). Do such penalties prevent future discrimination? In like manner, research may identify reinforcing consequences of affirmative actions that undermine stigma and encourage more public opportunities for people with mental illness (e.g., government tax credits for employers who hire and provide reasonable accommodations for people with psychiatric disabilities). The importance of affirmative action is discussed more fully in the section below on addressing structural stigma and discrimination.

Education

Educational approaches to changing stigma contrast myths with facts about mental illness. Educational strategies aimed at reducing mental illness stigma have used public service announcements, books, flyers, movies, videos, and other audiovisual aids to dispel the myths and replace them with facts (Bookbinder, 1978; National Mental Health Campaign, 2002; Pate, 1988; Smith, 1990). Evidence from education studies suggests that people with a better understanding of mental illness are less likely to endorse stigma and discrimination (Brockington et al., 1993; Link & Cullen, 1986; Link et al., 1987; Roman & Floyd, 1981) and that education programs produce short-term improvements in attitudes (Corrigan et al., 2001c; Holmes, Corrigan, Williams, Canar, & Kubiak, 1999;

Keane, 1991; Morrison & Teta, 1980; Penn et al., 1994; Penn, Kommana, Mansfield, & Link, 1999). Although education can be a useful strategy, the magnitude and duration of the improvement in attitudes and behavior it produces may be limited (Corrigan et al., 2001c). Further research is needed to determine its long-term effects and to examine the implications of different mediums of delivery (e.g., public service announcements, classroom lectures, or movies) and their contents.

Research on education programs that targeted ethnic prejudice sheds some light on the mixed impact of education (Devine, 1995; Pruegger & Rogers, 1994). This research indicates that stereotypes provide a template for encoding subsequent information that may disconfirm them. Thus, if a person originally endorses the stereotype that people with mental illness are dangerous, they may be less attentive to subsequent information that these individuals are "no more dangerous than the general population" than they are to the latest news story about a violent crime committed by a person with mental illness. As a result, stereotypes may be particularly resistant to change based on new information (Fyock & Stangor, 1992; Stangor & McMillan, 1992). Despite this consistency effect, individuals may learn to inhibit these stereotypes by using more cognitively controlled personal beliefs (Devine, 1995). People can consciously override the initial stereotype and replace their reactions with those based on more accurate information indicating that most people with mental illness are not violent. Thus, although an initial reaction may activate a stereotype about a member of a stigmatized group, an individual may purposefully replace that thought with more accurate beliefs and behave accordingly.

Contact

A third strategy for reducing stigma is to have interpersonal contact with members of the stigmatized group. Contact has long been considered an effective means of reducing intergroup prejudice (Allport, 1954; Pettigrew & Tropp, 2000). In formalizing the "contact" hypothesis, Allport (1954) contended, and more recent research supports (Cook, 1985; Gaertner, Dovidio, & Bachman, 1996; Pettigrew & Tropp, 2000), that "optimal" contact interventions must contain four elements:

1. *Equal status between groups.* In a contact situation, neither the minority nor the majority group members occupy a higher status. Neither group is in charge. This differs from the type of contact certain power groups typically have with persons with mental illness (e.g., doctor/patient, landlord/ resident, employer/employee).

2. *Common goals.* Both groups should be working toward the same ends. Some studies of "optimal" contact have used contrived tasks such as completing a puzzle (Desforges, Lord, Ramsey, Mason, Van Leeuwen, et al., 1991). In more natural settings, this may include working together on a community project or solving a neighborhood problem.

3. *No competition.* The tone of the contact should indicate a joint effort, not a competitive one.

4. *Authoritative sanction for the contact.* This may mean that the contact intervention is sponsored or endorsed by management of an employment organization, or by particular community organizations (e.g., the community's board of education or the Better Business Bureau).

The benefits of this strategy are also enhanced when the contact is with a person who moderately disconfirms the stereotypes about his or her group (Johnston &

Hewstone, 1992; Reinke & Corrigan, 2002; Weber & Crocker, 1983). Individuals who highly disconfirm the prevailing stereotypes may not be believed or may be considered "special exceptions," and contact with persons who behave in ways consistent with the stereotypes about their group may reinforce stigmatizing attitudes or make them worse.

A recent meta-analysis (Pettigrew & Tropp, 2000) of more than 200 studies of intergroup contact further supports its effectiveness for reducing prejudice. The 44 studies in the meta-analysis that consisted of a structured program that maximized the "optimal" conditions listed above yielded consistently larger reductions in prejudice. In addition, the authors found that contact interventions were most effective if they involved face-to-face interactions and if they occurred in work or organizational settings. Smaller but still significant effect sizes were found for reducing prejudice against older adults and persons with mental illness. The authors noted that several of the studies on these populations included only brief contact with individuals with severe disabilities and emphasize the importance of structured contact situations that counter prevailing negative stereotypes.

Several studies specifically focusing on the effect of contact on mental illness stigma have produced promising findings. Corrigan and colleagues found that contact with a person with mental illness produced greater improvements in attitudes than protest, education, and control conditions (Corrigan et al., 2001c). In a subsequent study, contact again produced the greatest improvements in attitudes and participant willingness to donate money to NAMI (Corrigan, Rowan, Green, Lundin, River, et al., 2002). Improvements in attitude seem to be most pronounced when contact is with a person who moderately disconfirms the prevailing stereotypes (Reinke & Corrigan, 2002). Contact effects are not limited to adults. Research with schoolchildren suggests that education combined with contact leads to greater attitude improvements than education alone (Pinfold, Huxley, Thornicroft, Farmer, Toulmin, et al., 2002).

Based on these studies, contact appears to be among the best strategies for changing mental illness stigma. Although less amenable to widespread distribution than educational programs, carefully structured and strategically implemented contact interventions may have a significant impact. Future research should further elaborate factors that augment the effect of contact on stigma.

The Message Matters

Many of the existing antistigma campaigns utilize an educational approach, either by itself or in conjunction with protest or contact strategies. And many, hoping to reduce the blame associated with mental illness, have focused on a biological model of mental illness. An example is NAMI's "Mental Illness Is a Brain Disease" campaign, in which it distributed posters, buttons, and literature that provided information about the biological basis of serious mental illness. There is evidence that this type of message does reduce blame for psychiatric illness (Corrigan et al., 2002; Farina, Fisher, Getter, & Fischer, 1978; Fisher & Farina, 1979). However, framing mental illness in biological terms may increase other negative attitudes about mental illness (Mehta & Farina, 1997). For example, Farina and colleagues (1978; Fisher & Farina, 1979) found that when provided with a disease-based explanation for mental illness, subjects viewed persons labeled mentally ill as less able to help themselves than when they were provided with a psychosocial explanation for the same problems. In a later study, Mehta and Farina (1997) found that disease-based explanations for mental illness reduced blame, but also provoked harsher behavior toward an individual with mental illness.

Biological explanations of mental illness may also yield unintended consequences by supporting the benevolence stigma; namely, the belief that persons with mental illness are innocent and childlike and, as such, must be taken care of by a parental figure (Brockington et al., 1993). Although well intentioned, this type of stigma can be disempowering, leading persons with mental illness (and others) to view themselves as different from other people, less competent, and less acceptable as friends. Biological explanations may also imply that persons with mental illness have no control over their behavior and are therefore unpredictable and violent (Read & Law, 1999).

In contrast to the biological message, several studies have found that psychosocial explanations of mental illness can be effective in increasing positive images of persons with mental illness and reducing fear. Instead of arguing that mental illness is like any other medical illness, psychosocial explanations of mental illness focus on environmental stressors and trauma as causal factors. These may include childhood abuse, poverty, and job stress. The idea is to reframe psychiatric symptoms as understandable reactions to life events (Read & Law, 1999). Demythologizing seminars that present a psychosocial model of mental disorder have been shown to be effective with students and health care professionals (Morrison, 1980; Morrison, Becker, & Bourgeois, 1979; Morrison & Teta, 1979, 1980). A more recent study conducted in New Zealand also suggests that information about psychosocial causes and treatments for mental illness is effective in improving attitudes, particularly those related to dangerousness and unpredictability (Read & Law, 1999). Although the studies of educational interventions focusing on a psychosocial model did not include control or comparison groups, they do suggest that this type of message can be useful for challenging stigma. Combined with the evidence of mixed effects of interventions limited to biological explanations, this suggests an approach that frames mental illness as a disorder with both biological and psychosocial components from which people can and do recover.

Although the psychosocial model has been shown to reduce fear and perceptions of dangerousness, neither of the approaches directly addresses this particularly pervasive stigma. Other studies examined interventions for stigma change that specifically address dangerousness. Penn and colleagues (1999) found that research participants given information on the prevalence rates of violent behavior among persons with mental illness perceived individuals with mental illness as less dangerous than subjects not given this information. Another study compared educational approaches that focused on dangerousness (accurate information about the rates of violence among persons with mental illness) or that summarized causes and treatments of mental illness (Corrigan et al., 2002). Although both conditions produced improvements in perceptions of dangerousness and desired social distance, the dangerousness condition increased the blaming of the person for his or her illness.

Clearly, the content of the educational message is important and needs to be tailored to a specific component of stigma and to the group being targeted (Byrne, 2000). For example, addressing the biological causes of mental illness with a group of neighborhood residents may improve some of their attitudes about persons with mental illness. However, unless dangerousness is addressed, their unwillingness to welcome a group home to the neighborhood may go unchanged. Conversely, addressing only dangerousness with police officers may make them less likely to use undue force, but not influence their willingness to assist a victim with a mental illness.

Legislators are another group who make important decisions that may limit or expand the opportunities and resources available to persons with mental illness. For example, they decide how tax money is distributed among various types of services. Research on attributions and helping behavior indicates that people are more willing to help and give resources to people whom they do not blame for their problems (Corrigan & Watson, 2003; Skitka & Tetlock, 1992, 1993; Weiner, 1995; Zucker & Weiner, 1993). Thus, it may prove most fruitful to focus on a biological message when addressing legislators regarding funding for mental health services or health insurance parity. Including information that people with mental illness do recover and lead meaningful lives may enhance the positive effect of the message. Clearly, if time and resources allow, strategies should address multiple stereotypes. More realistically, the content of the message may have to be selectively targeted to the stereotypes most relevant to the goals of the intervention.

Existing Efforts at Changing Public Stigma

In recent years, major advocacy groups in the United States, such as the National Alliance for the Mentally Ill (NAMI) and the National Mental Health Association (NMHA), have launched antistigma campaigns. Other groups, including the National Stigma Clearinghouse and the Resource Center to Address Discrimination and Stigma Associated with Mental Illnesses, have made the stigma of mental illness its sole focus. Both federal and state governments have also joined the fray. In the past couple of years, the U.S. Substance Abuse and Mental Health Services Administration (SAMHSA) and the National Institute of Mental Health (NIMH) have supported nationwide conferences on stigma. SAMHSA produced and disseminated an antistigma kit that included posters and brochures challenging common stereotypes (see Figure 19.1). It funded the Center against Discrimination and Stigma as a national technical support center to address mental health stigma. It also sponsored the Erase the Barriers Initiative, an eight-state effort to decrease stigma using public service announcements and public education strategies. Tipper Gore and Alma Powell joined with other national leaders to form the National Mental Health Awareness Campaign, which developed a multilevel effort to challenge stigma.

Similar efforts are evident elsewhere in the world. The World Psychiatric Association has launched "Schizophrenia: Open the Doors." This program is currently active on three continents: Asia, Europe, and South America. Prominent among these demonstration projects is "Changing Minds" by the British Royal College of Psychiatrists. Like other efforts of its ilk, Changing Minds includes multiple levels of public education to change stigma about mental illness. Central to this effort is focusing on family education as key to changing stigma.

The goals and tactics of these advocacy groups neatly fall into the education, protest, and contact domains described by researchers. Many of these programs rely on public education to dispel the stigma of mental illness. Television and other media have become central vehicles for these education programs. The National Mental Health Awareness Campaign (NMHAC), for example, developed 30-second public service announcements (PSAs) concentrating on the attitudes of adolescents (National Mental Health Campaign, 2002). In an effort called "Change Your Mind," the PSAs send two messages that challenge important stereotypes: People with mental illness are not responsible for their problems and they are "just like everyone else." Being mindful of their audience, the NMHAC widely aired the PSAs on teen outlets such as MTV, as well as VH1, ESPN, ABC, Fox, and Channel One. The specific goal of the NMHAC program is to increase adolescent use of mental health services when needed. The PSAs end with a web address where interested teens can learn more about mental illness and corresponding services. Although it is difficult to determine the depth and breadth of this campaign's penetration, as of October 2001, the website reported more than 12 million hits.

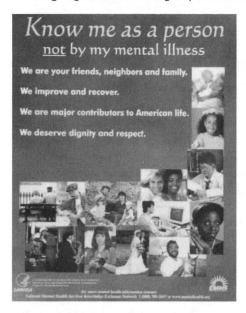

FIGURE 19.1. A frame from the "Change Your Mind" public service announcement produced by the Substance Abuse and Mental Health Services Administration.

Now numbering more than 4,000 members, NAMI StigmaBusters, as noted earlier, has been an important source of protest (NAMI StigmaBusters, 2002). Among its many efforts, StigmaBusters identifies disrespectful and inaccurate images of people with mental illness in the popular media and coordinates letter-writing campaigns to get producers of these images to stop using these disrespectful images in promoting their products. This suggests that organized protest can be a useful tool for persuading television networks, movie producers, and others to stop running stigmatizing programs, advertisements, and articles, rather than alienate an important sales demographic. See the Personal Example on p. 418 for an illustration of this kind of protest.

In 2004 NAMI developed a contact-based antistigma program called "In Our Own Voice: Living with Mental Illness." A particularly remarkable aspect of the program is its combination of carefully crafted exercises and information base that helps consumers to teach civic and other groups about the experience of mental illness. To date, it has provided the program to law enforcement agencies, schools, businesses, and other community groups.

There are also several examples of state governments using the contact strategy to diminish stigma and enhance consumer empowerment. New York (Blanch & Fisher, 1993; Knight & Blanch, 1993), Florida (Loder & Glover, 1992), and Illinois (Corrigan, Lickey, Schmook, Virgil, & Juricek, 1999b) have arranged formal dialogues between persons with mental illness and mental health care professionals as a way to change insidious attitudes in the mental health system that undermine empowerment. These dialogues provided a forum for consumers and health care professionals to exchange perspectives about mental illness and challenge latent stigmatizing attitudes. Moreover, the U.S. Center for Mental Health Services has an intramural office on consumer empowerment and funds consumer-based extramural projects that attempt to dispel stigma. Many state departments of mental health hire consumer advocates whose job, in part, includes vigilance to misrepresentations of mental health issues.

PERSONAL EXAMPLE

Stop a Stigmatizing Television Program

In the spring of 2000, ABC premiered *Wonderland*, a series about fictional Rivervue Psychiatric Hospital in New York City. Although its intent was to highlight mental health concerns as a gritty drama, *Wonderland* instead seemed to perpetuate the stigma of dangerousness associated with mental illness. In the opening scenes of the first episode, a man with schizophrenia emptied a clip from his semiautomatic pistol into a Times Square crowd. After being admitted to Rivervue's emergency room, the man stabbed a pregnant psychiatrist in the belly with a hypodermic needle.

NAMI StigmaBusters joined other advocacy groups, including the National Mental Health Association and the American Psychiatric Association, in a letter-writing campaign to express concern about the story line to the show producers and ABC management. Unfortunately, any kind of letter to a network about a new show can be viewed as positive, showing that an audience is watching the show, albeit perhaps with some disapproval. After little success with ABC and the producers of the show, StigmaBusters and other advocates began to express their disapproval to the CEOs of the show's sponsors, including Mitsubishi, Sears, and the Scott Company. Their message sought to inform these businesspeople of how *Wonderland* was stigmatizing people with mental illness as well as provide facts that countered the stigma. As a result of these efforts, ABC cancelled the show after a couple of episodes at a substantial financial loss.

This example illustrates an important power that people with mental illness and their families might utilize to reduce stigmatizing images. That is, they are an economic force that cannot be ignored by businesses. If one could muster even a small fraction of the 20% of the American population with mental illness, *and* their families, to express disapproval of a media image, commercial sponsors will take note and respond. Boycotts like this have been used effectively by people of color, women, and gays to influence the marketplace to be more sensitive to their needs. Large advocacy groups like NAMI and its StigmaBusters can organize those concerned about mental illness stigma in a like manner.

A Targeted Model of Stigma Change

These are just some of the examples of how education, protest, and contact can be used to reduce prejudice and discrimination. The reader should note the common feature of these examples that further augments the impact of a program: *Each program targets a specific group and the corresponding attitudes and behaviors for change.* The NMHAC is attempting to increase service use among *adolescents* who may be experiencing mental health-related problems. NAMI's StigmaBusters seeks to stop the *popular media* from perpetuating disrespectful images in its TV shows and movies. States are trying to change entrenched and disempowering attitudes in their *mental health systems* by pairing consumers with providers. The logic of a target-specific approach is all the more compelling when compared with the alternative, a generic effort to change the attitudes of the population as a whole. Consider, for example, a video that promotes the idea that mental illness affects 20% of the citizenry and hence is neither rare nor bizarre. Although this effort is well intentioned and poignant, such mass appeal suffers because it is not particularly relevant to specific elements of the populace. It is unclear as to who exactly is supposed to take note of this message. Moreover, the expected products of these efforts are fuzzy; it is unclear exactly how the population should change, given the highlighted stereotypes and prejudice. People may think, "Okay, so 20% of the population may be mentally ill in their lifetimes. Now, what should I do about it?"

The goal of improving attitudes about mental illness in general is laudable, yet too amorphous to achieve. A targeted approach that focuses on changing specific discriminatory behaviors of specific groups lends itself to achieving the practical attitudes outlined in Table 19.2. First, antistigma programs target specific power groups that make important decisions about the resources and opportunities available to persons with mental illness. These include employers, landlords, police officers, legislators, and media executives. Individuals acting in these power roles are significantly influenced by institutional and organizational factors (Link & Phelan, 2001; Oliver, 1992; Pincus, 1999; Scott, 1995) and may be more likely to rely on stereotypes about a group than persons in less powerful roles (Fiske, 1993). For each group, we would identify the discriminatory behavior and corresponding attitudes we would like to change. For example, we may want to address employers' unwillingness to hire persons with mental illness. The corresponding attitudes may relate to their competence and their danger to other employees.

Once the target group, behavior(s), and attitude (s) are identified, the most appropriate strategy and content can be selected. Although the effect of protest on attitudes is unclear, it seems to be useful for eliminating undesirable behaviors such as perpetuating negative images in the media and discriminatory housing and labor practices. Education appears to improve attitudes on a short-term basis and can be implemented relatively inexpensively. Contact appears to be the most promising strategy, especially when it is structured to include "optimal" conditions. This may be difficult to achieve on a broad scale unless more people become willing to disclose their illness in the workplace and other social situations. Note that antistigma campaigns may employ a combination of

TABLE 19.2. Targeting in Antistigma Programs

Targets	Discriminatory behavior	Attitudes
Employers	• Fail to hire • No reasonable accommodation	• View individuals as dangerous • View individuals as incompetent
Landlords	• Fail to lease • No reasonable accommodation	• View individuals as dangerous • View individuals as irresponsible
Criminal justice professionals	• Unnecessarily coercive • Fail to use mental health services	• View individuals as dangerous • View individuals as responsible or to blame
Policy makers	• Insufficient resource allocation • Unfriendly interpretation of regulations	• View individuals as dangerous • View individuals as responsible or to blame
The media	• Perpetuation and dissemination of stigmatizing images	• View individuals as dangerous • View individuals as responsible or to blame • View individuals as incompetent • View individuals as irresponsible

strategies to address the attitudes and behaviors of a particular group. In addition to targeting power groups, campaigns may target groups that are hesitant to access services because of stigma. Consider, for example, the NMHAC's program aimed at teens who may be struggling with mental health issues.

CHANGING SOCIAL STRUCTURES

Social scientists who have developed ideas related to institutional and structural factors conclude that individual-level strategies for stigma change—education, protest, and contact—are probably not sufficient for remediating prejudice and discrimination that are largely caused by collective variables (Pincus, 1999). Education of key power groups may have some limited impact on the kinds of intentional biases represented by institutional discrimination. For example, one way to diminish legislative actions that unjustly restrict the opportunities of people with mental illness is to educate legislators about how their actions are impinging on an important part of their constituency. More difficult, however, is altering the course of structural discrimination (see Chapter 2 for a discussion of structural stigma). Because its impact is frequently unintentional, educational and other individual-level strategies generally have no effect on structural factors. Instead, various social change strategies that fall under the rubric of affirmative action may be relevant for stopping the harm caused by structural discrimination.

Affirmative actions are a collection of government-approved activities which are meant to redress the disparities that have arisen from historical trends in prejudice and discrimination (Pincus, 1999). According to affirmative models, membership in a stigmatized group is added to considerations of an individual's skills and achievements for access to specific limited opportunities. Perhaps best known and most controversial among affirmative actions is the use of quotas; that is, a certain percentage of people given access to a limited opportunity must be from targeted ethnic or gender groups. For example, some colleges and universities have used a prospective student's minority ethnic status as an advantage in deciding admission. To our knowledge, this kind of quota has not been used in the United States as a mechanism that rectifies structural discrimination against mental illness. The Americans with Disabilities Act (ADA), however, seems to be a federal policy that mirrors affirmative goals. ADA clauses that prohibit discrimination by employers because of a person's psychiatric disability are effective for barring individual and institutional levels of discrimination. It is the ADA clause on reasonable accommodation, however, that is an affirmative action that decreases structural discrimination. That is, reasonable accommodation gives people with psychiatric disabilities (a group that has been traditionally discriminated against in job settings) an edge toward keeping their jobs. Table 19.3 provides examples of reasonable accommodations for people with psychiatric disabilities. The 1988 amendments to the Fair Housing Act provide similar guarantees to reasonable accommodations for people with psychiatric disabilities in the housing sector. Although accommodations may emerge from these statutes, neither businesses nor landlords necessarily know how to provide them. Moreover, note that there are statutory limits to reasonable accommodations. Accommodations that place an undue hardship on a business may be excluded. Rehabilitation practitioners play an important role in helping people receive these accommodations and in assisting employers in making them available. Affirmative actions like these are needed to offset the injustices that continue because of structural discrimination against people with mental illness.

TABLE 19.3. Examples of Reasonable Accommodations That May Conceivably Apply to the Needs of People with Psychiatric Disabilities

Job restructuring

- *Reallocate marginal job functions.*

    Example: As part of Sally's secretarial job, she was supposed to shred confidential documents. This was not an essential function, and the machine scared her. Therefore, this duty was given to someone else.

Sick time

- *Permit the use of accrued paid leave or unpaid leave for treatment.*

    Example: Sarah needs 3 weeks off to recover from a relapse. She has accrued 2 weeks of paid leave, so the employer will need to provide another week of unpaid leave.

Modified or part-time schedule

- *Change the work schedule.*

    Example: Harold wants to change his start time from 8:00 A.M. to 9:00 A.M. His medicine makes it hard for him to wake on time. He will still work his full 8 hours.

    Example: Shirl wants to change her full-time job as a stenographer to half-time, at least for the next 6 months. She is not able to handle the demands of a full-time job because of recurring panic attacks. Of course, she will be paid for only 4 hours of work each day.

Modified workplace

- *Provide room dividers or other soundproofing and visual barriers to decrease distractions.*

    Example: Office partitions were put around Marty's desk so that he will not be distracted by the sales room.
- *Move a person away from noisy machinery or high-traffic areas that may be distracting.*

    Example: Delores's office was moved to the back, away from the reception area, so that she will not be distracted by visitors.
- *Permit an individual to wear headphones that block out distractions.*

    Example: Molly wears headphones so that she will not be bothered by phones ringing throughout the day.
- *Allow a person to work at home.*

    Example: Emily completes much of the computer work for her job at home. In this way, she does not have to deal with the social anxiety of working with other employees.

Modified policies

- *Change work policies that govern personnel.*

    Example: Bert is permitted to take detailed notes during sales meetings even though other staff members are not.

    Example: Daniel has a soft drink at his work station for the dry mouth that results from his medication.

    Example: Stanley is permitted to have the radio on in his office. The soft music relaxes him.

(continued)

TABLE 19.3. *(continued)*

Supervision

- *Have supervisors adjust feedback style, including changes in communication and extra training materials.*

    Example: Helene receives a daily 10-minute feedback from her supervisor.

    Example: Juanita was given illustrated instructions on how to run the packing machine.
- *Provide a job coach to offer counseling and support on the job.*

    Example: Phil is visited on the job by a coach from the local rehabilitation center. The job coach provides support and counseling on work-related issues.

Reassignment

- *Provide a job reassignment to another position whose essential functions more closely parallel the skills of the employee with disabilities.*

    Example: Brunetta was moved from a clerk/typist job to a telephone/reception position because she found its required tasks easier.

Note. All these accommodations can be arranged if they do not cause *undue hardship* for the employer. From Corrigan and Lundin (2001). Copyright 2001 by Patrick W. Corrigan and Robert K. Lundin. Reprinted by permission.

SUMMARY AND CONCLUSIONS

Stigma has been portrayed as a major barrier to community integration and personal empowerment. Personal empowerment is enhanced by challenging self-stigma. The approach to diminishing self-stigma includes cognitive reframing that challenges the irrational thoughts on which self-stigma is based. Strategic decisions to disclose one's mental health history may also facilitate personal empowerment. Disclosure may include social avoidance, secrecy, selective disclosure, and indiscriminant disclosure. Psychosocial approaches that directly challenge self-stigma are also important in promoting personal empowerment. These include fostering a collaborative approach to treatment programming; community-based supported services for housing, employment, and education; consumers as providers; and consumer-operated services.

Three approaches change the public stigma of mental illness when represented as individual psychological variables. These are essential for promoting community integration—protest: appealing to a moral or economic authority to ask people to stop prejudice, education: contrasting the myths of mental illness with facts, and contact: challenging stigma by facilitating face-to-face interactions between people with mental illness and the public. Affirmative actions are necessary antistigma programs to challenge the social structures that both intentionally and unintentionally promote prejudice and discrimination. Given the various causes of stigma and the multiple approaches to diminishing it, a comprehensive program will have to combine a variety of antistigma approaches.

Chapter 20

Cultural Competence in Psychiatric Rehabilitation

The example on page 424 illustrates the role of culture in the delivery of psychiatric rehabilitation services. It suggests the challenges of assessing client needs and providing appropriate services in the face of different life experiences, languages, traditions, religious beliefs, and assumptions about the nature of mental illness and recovery. This chapter is devoted to a brief survey of perspectives on cultural factors. While recognizing the great diversity of cultural issues that must be addressed to ensure that psychiatric rehabilitation services are culturally competent, our focus in this chapter is limited primarily to cultural issues related to ethnicity and nationality.

DEFINITION OF CULTURE

Culture has been defined as group membership based on factors such as ethnicity, language, race, religion, disability, gender, age, sexual orientation, and social class (Pernell-Arnold & Finley, 1999). More specifically, individuals sharing a common culture have a shared set of beliefs, norms, and values and shared ways of thinking, feeling, acting, and perceiving the world (Siegel, Haugland, & Schore, 2005). Culture is defined by a shared group identity and not by externally defined groupings such as census categories, which mask critical differences between distinct subcultures. For example, although often presumed to be a homogeneous group, Latinos living in the mainland United States encom-

PERSONAL EXAMPLE

Issues in Helping Individuals from Southeast Asia

Southeast Asian Services, one of the programs within the Amherst H. Wilder Foundation in St. Paul, Minnesota, operates the Southeast Asian Assertive Community Treatment (SEA ACT) team. It serves Hmong, Cambodian, Vietnamese, and Laotian consumers, most of whom have a diagnosis of schizophrenia, major depression, or bipolar disorder. Many have co-occurring posttraumatic stress disorder, originating for virtually all SEA consumers in their experiences in their countries of origin and exacerbated by experiences during escape, in refugee camps, and in subsequent integration into U.S. culture. About 25% also have co-occurring substance use disorders. Substances of abuse include cocaine, methamphetamine, opium, marijuana, and alcohol. Alcohol problems tend to be identified at a late stage because of cultural customs that include the use of alcohol and because of a cultural tolerance of alcohol abuse.

Led by a European American team leader, the SEA ACT team also includes one Cambodian, one Vietnamese, and two Hmong social workers, one Hmong nurse, and a European American psychiatrist with long experience in working with SEA consumers. Language barriers are a lesser difficulty than was anticipated prior to the SEA ACT team's inception, but do frequently make it necessary for bilingual staff speaking the consumer's language to accompany other SEA ACT team staff. About a third of the SEA ACT consumers have good English skills, but others need to have bilingual workers in order to communicate comfortably and help them manage their contacts with official agencies. Typically, a care coordinator of the same culture and language is assigned to each consumer, but there have been some exceptions. However, most consumers have some contact with all members of the team.

Historical conflicts between SEA groups seem to have a very minor influence in the interactions between staff and consumers. Language matters more. In addition to their ability to communicate with consumers in their native languages, bilingual staff members understand the cultural customs and attitudes, which help them gain consumers' trust and address their needs. The integrated understanding of healing, using both Western and Asian practices, is particularly important to effectiveness.

Some SEA ACT consumers have difficulty accepting Western medications. This difficulty is partly due to the side effects of psychiatric medications. However, culturally based beliefs compound the usual reasons for not taking medications as prescribed. An example is the common Southeast Asian belief that Western medications are too strong for Asians. In addition, Southeast Asian consumers approach Western medications with different views of what causes illness and what will bring about healing and thus need more convincing to trust Western medical approaches.

Respecting and helping to integrate a consumer's beliefs about health and well-being is an important dimension of services and involves facilitating contact between ACT consumers and traditional shamans and healers as well as with Buddhist and Christian religious communities.

Because of the crucial importance of families to Southeast Asian consumers, SEA ACT has reached out extensively to family members to involve in them in the consumers' treatment. Home visits appear to be far more effective for engaging them than clinic-based family psychoeducation groups. Although some have been initially reserved in response to this outreach, families generally have been appreciative of the team's patient and persistent efforts to include them.

Despite the challenges of achieving culturally competent services, SEA ACT has achieved moderately high fidelity to the ACT model, according to state ACT standards.

pass a broad range of countries of origin, including 66% from Mexico and 9% from Puerto Rico (Vega & Lopez, 2001). Complicating this picture further is the fact that immigrant groups differ with respect to level of *acculturation*, which refers to the process of adaptation to the majority culture by learning the common language and practicing the customs of the majority culture, at least when in contact with the larger society. Even within the family unit, various family members may be at different stages of acculturation.

As the SEA ACT example suggests, refugee groups are often especially vulnerable and in need of mental health services. Understanding the history previous to immigration and the experience of immigration is paramount to understanding how to serve them better and to be sensitive to their needs.

The construct of *racial identity*, first conceptualized in regard to African American identity and later extended to other races and broadened to include *ethnic identity*, has been the subject of extensive theorizing and research (Chávez & Guido-DiBrito, 1999; Cross, 1978). Racial and ethnic identity is often "invisible" to the majority culture, although it is omnipresent for individuals from minority cultures. The historical mistreatment of African American, Native Americans, and other minorities in the United States is part of the context for these attitudes. On one hand, close identification with the traditions and rituals of one's own culture can be a source of great pride and confidence. On the other hand, individuals from a minority culture must often face prejudice and negative treatment in the general society, often resulting in distrust, anger, and self-stigma. In his original formulation of "nigrescence theory," Cross proposed four stages of racial identity among African Americans, with movement from self-hatred and idealization of "whiteness" to self-acceptance and security within one's "blackness" (Tokar & Swanson, 1991; Worrell, Cross, & Vandiver, 2001). A later version of Cross's model includes multiculturalists, who seek to build coalitions with other cultural groups (Vandiver, Cross, Worrell, & Fhagen-Smith, 2002).

Further complicating the understanding of cultural issues is the fact that individuals have multiple group identifications, any of which may be activated at a given time, often with several of these salient simultaneously. For example, the mental health issues facing women of color include those related to their ethnicity as well as gender-specific issues, such as access to child care (Coridan & O'Connell, 2001).

Cultural factors adversely affecting the provision of psychiatric rehabilitation services include language barriers, cultural misunderstandings, prejudice, and difficulties in acculturation. Poverty is common among many minority groups, leading to further inequities beyond those associated with cultural understandings. Obviously, cultural factors have a pervasive role in mental health services.

Radical shifts in national demographics highlight the need to pay attention to cultural factors. First, the U.S. population is aging. The number of Americans over 65 is expected to double by 2030 (Brock, 1998). Second, the ethnic makeup of the country is shifting. The proportion of ethnic minorities in the U.S. population increased between 1980 and 2000 (especially Asian Americans, Latinos, and Native Americans) and is expected to increase further in this century (Ton, Koike, Hales, Johnson, & Hilty, 2005). In 2000, the U.S. Latino population was 35.3 million (12.5% of the U.S. population). By 2020, the Latino population is projected to double, to 70 million, and expected to be 21% of the U.S. population (*www.hispaniconline.com/hh02/demographics_did_you_know.html*).

DEFINITIONS OF CULTURAL COMPETENCE AND CULTURAL COMPETENCY GUIDELINES

In the context of psychiatric rehabilitation, *cultural competence*, also referred to as *multiculturalism*, *cultural sensitivity*, and *cultural competencies*, refers to practitioner and organizational approaches to services that accommodate cultural differences. Cultural competence is seen as a core competency for psychiatric rehabilitation practitioners (Coursey et al., 2000b). It involves an active role for the practitioner with respect to three dimensions: (1) becoming aware of one's own preconceived notions and cultural biases, (2) seeking to understand the worldview of others without judging them, and (3) developing appropriate interventions and skills in working with culturally different consumers (Sue, Arredondo, & McDavis, 1992).

Without an organizational environment in which cultural competence is expected and valued, the efforts of individual practitioners will be diluted. To this end, the National Center for Cultural Competence (NCCC, 2006) at Georgetown University Center for Child and Human Development has identified the following organizational criteria for cultural competence.

- Have a defined set of values and principles and demonstrate behaviors, attitudes, policies and structures that enable them to work effectively cross-culturally.
- Have the capacity to (1) value diversity, (2) conduct self-assessment, (3) manage the dynamics of difference, (4) acquire and institutionalize cultural knowledge, and (5) adapt to diversity and the cultural contexts of the communities they serve.
- Incorporate the above in all aspects of policy making, administration, practice, and service delivery and involve systematically consumers, key stakeholders and communities.

To promote cultural competence, the NCCC disseminates a wide range of training curricula and technical assistance materials. Among the documents available from its website is a self-administered tool for assessing practitioner cultural competence, intended to raise practitioner awareness of the issues (Goode, 2001). Carole Siegel at the Nathan Kline Institute for Psychiatric Research in New York heads another group active in this area. She and her colleagues have developed a scale measuring cultural competence at the organizational level (Siegel et al., 2005). This scale is included in the implementation resource kits for the National Evidence-Based Practices Project (Siegel, 2002). A guiding principle is that prevalent cultural groups within a community should have representation in all aspects of organizational functioning. To this end, these groups should have input into agency programs through advisory groups and other mechanisms (Ton et al., 2005).

All of the major organizations for mental health professionals (e.g., in psychology, psychiatry, social work) and many federal agencies have guidelines advocating for the provision of culturally competent services. For example, the American Psychological Association convened the National Multicultural Conference and Summit in 1999 and endorsed a series of resolutions adopted by the association (Sue, Bingham, Porché-Burke, & Vasquez, 1999).

The multicultural guidelines established in 2001 by the Substance Abuse and Mental Health Services Administration (SAMHSA) aim at organizational-level expectations for cultural competence, including a set of recommended performance indicators and outcomes. The SAMHSA guidelines emphasize *access*:

Services shall be provided irrespective of immigration status, insurance coverage, and language. Access to services shall be individual- and family-oriented (including client-defined family) in the context of racial/ethnic cultural values. Access criteria for different levels of care shall include diagnosis, health/medical, behavior, and functioning. Criteria shall be evaluated in six areas: psychiatric, medical, spiritual, social functioning, behavior, and community support. (*www.samsha.gov*)

In 1996, the International Association of Psychosocial Rehabilitation Services (IAPSRS), now known as the United States Psychiatric Rehabilitation Association (see Chapter 21), adopted the Principles of Multicultural Psychiatric Rehabilitation Services, as shown in Table 20.1. These standards are complementary to the SAMHSA standards, in that they are focused on practitioner-level competencies.

Many of the definitions of cultural competence do not provide concrete criteria for practitioner and organizational behavior. Practice guidelines and quantitative scales are

---

TABLE 20.1. Principles of Multicultural Psychiatric Rehabilitation Services

Psychiatric rehabilitation practitioners . . .

- Accept the fact that every individual has an ethnicity, as well as a gender, sexual orientation, level of ability/disability, age, and socioeconomic status; therefore, they view every human encounter as a cross-cultural encounter.
- Study, understand, accept, and appreciate their own cultures as a basis for relating to the cultures of others.
- Recognize that differences, discrimination, and isolation continue to create unique situations in which the importance of culture may emerge. The cultures of gender, disability, or sexual orientation may also provide support, security, a sense of belonging and identity, similar to the cultures of ethnic heritage. Stigmatization, rejection, and discrimination are addressed as rights violations as well as barriers to the attainment of health.
- Recognize that people's thought patterns and behaviors are influenced by their worldviews, of which there are many.
- Show respect toward clients by accepting cultural preferences that value process or product, as well as harmony or achievement, within their lives.
- Demonstrate respect by appreciating cultural preferences that value relationships and interdependence, in addition to individuation and independence.
- Accept the idea that the solutions to problems are to be sought within consumers, their families, and their cultures.
- Apply the strengths/wellness approach to all cultures.
- Modify interventions as necessary to make them culturally syntonic, to accommodate culturally determined needs, beliefs, and behaviors, and to be compatible with family/ group patterns and structures; communication, cognitive, behavioral, and learning styles; identity development; perceptions of illness; and help-seeking behaviors.
- Recognize that discrimination and oppression exist within our society, taking many forms.
- Take responsibility for actively promoting positive intergroup relations, particularly between the consumers in their programs and the larger community.
- Engage in ongoing cultural competence training in order to increase their knowledge and skills in appropriate, effective cross-cultural interventions.
- Commit to learning about problems and issues that adversely and disproportionately affect the various cultural groups with whom they work.

Note. Adapted from the International Association of Psychosocial Rehabilitation Service (1996).

attempts to operationally define cultural competence. None of these approaches, however, have been rigorously validated.

A noteworthy feature of most cultural competence guidelines has been the effort to define general principles rather than seeking to codify specific assessment instruments, interventions, and programs for each cultural group. There have been relatively few efforts to develop guidelines for specific cultural groups (Vega & Lopez, 2001). The reason for this appears to be twofold. First, there is the matter of practicality. Given the large number of cultural groups (to say nothing of subcultures), the task of developing separate guidelines is formidable (Vega & Lopez, 2001). Second, the development of guidelines for a particular group could have the paradoxical effect of stereotyping that group, because the guidelines would by definition move toward suggesting homogeneous attitudes, customs, life experiences, and the like. In fact, cultural competence celebrates diversity and emphasizes the importance of understanding each individual in the context of his or her idiosyncratic life experiences and worldview.

WHY IS CULTURAL COMPETENCE IMPORTANT?

As the SEA ACT example at the beginning of this chapter suggests, the role of culture in psychiatric rehabilitation services is apparent when services are extended to groups representing sharply contrasting cultures from one's own. But cultural factors are always present, and their importance is greater than is usually acknowledged by individuals in the majority culture (Sue, 2004). Most consumers want cultural issues to be acknowledged by practitioners and incorporated into the services they receive (Mason, Olmos-Gallo, Bacon, McQuilken, Henley, et al., 2004).

The importance of culture is evident in many different aspects of psychiatric rehabilitation services, including the following:

1. Discrimination in the general society complicates the delivery of psychiatric rehabilitation services.
2. Assessment and diagnostic procedures developed for one cultural group may not be appropriate for others.
3. There are disparities in access to mental health care and in the quality of services provided.
4. Psychiatric rehabilitation models developed in one population may not generalize to others.

Each of these points is discussed below.

Discrimination in the General Society

As stressed throughout this book, psychiatric rehabilitation aims at community integration of individuals with severe mental illness, for example, in the workplace and in community housing. The lack of community acceptance of individuals with mental illness is a barrier to both employment and housing; however, this problem is compounded by discrimination against individuals who also differ in race, sexual orientation, age, or in other particulars. Discrimination on the basis of either mental illness or race is, of course, illegal, the former forbidden by the Americans with Disabilities Act (See Chapter 21) and the latter by the Civil Rights Act. However, de facto discrimination continues in the

United States, despite legal sanctions. For example, a national survey of labor participation found that ethnic minorities generally had lower employment rates than European Americans, and that in the presence of mental illness, the gap widened (Wewiorski & Fabian, 2004). The reasons are complex, but anecdotal evidence provides many instances in which prejudice has played a role.

Cultural Issues in Assessment and Diagnosis

Cultural biases in testing have been well documented (Leong & Lau, 2001; Suzuki, Meller, & Ponterotto, 1996). The most extensively researched areas of cultural bias involve intelligence and aptitude tests (Groth-Marnat, 2003). Such tests typically include items that assume test takers' familiarity with idioms, objects, and activities common in middle-class American culture that may be unfamiliar to members of minority cultures. To dramatize the point, tests have been devised that include idioms familiar to African Americans that are not familiar to middle-class European Americans (although MTV and other mass media may be closing this gap). Recognizing these problems, researchers have attempted to modify tests by removing obviously culturally biased items. These efforts, however, have not eliminated cultural disparities, suggesting the multidimensionality of these issues (Groth-Marnat, 2003).

Numerous studies have found different rates of diagnosis among different cultural groups. For example, many studies have suggested that African Americans are more likely to be diagnosed with schizophrenia than European Americans (Blow, Zeber, McCarthy, Valenstein, & Gillon, 2004; Snowden, 2001; Solomon, 1988a). Although these differences may reflect true variation across groups, many experts believe they are artifacts. For example, diagnostic discrepancies between African Americans and European Americans are reduced by the use of standardized research interviews (Whaley, 2004).

Beyond these statistical patterns of diagnosis are blatant deficiencies in diagnostic tools. For example, a question on the Diagnostic Interview Schedule (DIS) (Robins, Helzer, Croughan, & Ratcliff, 1981), "Do you often worry a lot about having clean clothes?" is intended to measure obsessive thoughts. However, in communities in which running water is not readily available, worrying about clean clothes is an everyday reality and does not reflect obsessive rumination at all (Rogler, 1999). Similarly, measuring manic behavior in an Amish community requires a shift in content from a DIS question about shopping sprees (which is appropriate for suburban America) to probes about behaviors considered deviant in an Amish community, such as dressing in worldly clothes (Rogler, 1999).

Symptom measures implicitly assume that the experience and expression of symptoms are universal. Yet counter examples abound, demonstrating cultural variations in the expression and experience of symptoms. As compared with European Americans, Asian Americans (especially women) tend to be stoic, self-effacing, and more reticent to disclose feelings of anxiety (Leong & Lau, 2001). Instead, Asian Americans are more likely to report somatic symptoms. Another example is the fact that there are no words for "depressed" or "anxious" in some American Indian languages (Johnson & Cameron, 2001). Latinos also differ from European Americans in the labeling and interpretation of psychological symptoms (Alverson & Vicente, 1998). In translating depression inventories into Spanish, Rogler (1999) noted the absurdity of a literal translation of the colloquial phrase, "I'm feeling blue." But an even more fundamental issue concerns the understanding of mental illness within Latino cultural groups. In an ethnographic study of Puerto Rican consumers enrolled in a supported employment program, Alverson and

Vincente (1998) concluded that "none see *nervios* or *ataques de nervios* as an inherent, essential, and largely irremediable condition of one's brain or mind" (p. 71). Their Latino informants did not interpret their social and economic condition as stemming from their nervous condition, nor did they interpret their problems within the Western biomedical framework.

These observations suggest that a cultural assessment should always be conducted before providing any services, and should examine factors such as beliefs about mental illness and its treatment, the stigma attached to mental illness, the role of the family as a support system, and the value of interdependence over independence/self-efficacy.

Mental Health Treatment Disparities

A robust literature documents ethnic disparities in all forms of health care, including mental health care. Ethnic minorities have higher rates of unmet mental health needs and lower rates of mental health treatment than do European Americans (Alegría, Canino, Rios, Vera, Calderon, et al., 2002; Barrio, Yamada, Hough, Hawthorne, Garcia, et al., 2003; Harris, Edlund, & Larson, 2005; Johnson & Cameron, 2001; Leong & Lau, 2001; Snowden, 2001; Vega & Lopez, 2001). Language is an additional barrier to treatment for those who do not speak English (Barrio et al., 2003). Asian Americans, especially immigrants who have not assimilated into the dominant culture, are reluctant to seek treatment (Leong & Lau, 2001), ostensibly because of their beliefs about the nature of psychiatric illness (Barry & Grilo, 2002), although other studies have failed to show a treatment delay (Okazaki, 2000).

Some evidence suggests that people from ethnic minority groups are less likely to receive best practices in medication management. For example, studies have found that among individuals with schizophrenia, those from ethnic minorities are more likely than European Americans to receive high doses of antipsychotics (Lehman et al., 1998b) and are less likely to be prescribed second-generation antipsychotics (Copeland, Zeber, Valenstein, & Blow, 2003; Pi & Simpson, 2005).

Disparities across cultural groups have been found regarding where people receive treatment and what services they receive. For example, when initially diagnosed with a psychotic disorder, African Americans and other minorities are more likely to be hospitalized and are less likely to be seen on an outpatient basis than are European Americans (Snowden, 2001; Snowden & Hu, 1997; Sohler, Bromet, Lavelle, Craig, & Mojtabai, 2004). Ethnic minorities are more likely to remain hospitalized for a longer time and to drop out of outpatient treatment earlier than European Americans. After discharge from a psychiatric hospital, African Americans in one survey received much less intensive psychosocial rehabilitation services from community mental health centers than European Americans (Solomon, 1988a). Various explanations have been given for such disparities. For example, Asian Americans may take care of an ill relative at home as long as they can, which can result in more serious symptoms when they do seek treatment.

Although cultural beliefs and attitudes are likely factors in explaining these disparities, other influences include level of language fluency, proximity of Medicaid services within the communities in which people live, and the ability to recognize mental health problems (Alegría et al., 2002). Another barrier is poverty; minority groups have higher percentages of individuals who are uninsured (Friedman & Clayton, 1996; Vega & Lopez, 2001).

Beyond these explanations, mental health disparities often result from distrust of the mental health system among individuals from ethnic minorities (Chen, Fryer, Phillips,

Wilson, & Pathman, 2005). This distrust often comes from their experiences with mental health services, which may include outright discriminatory practices, such as offering inferior services to those who are "different."

Cultural Issues in Psychiatric Rehabilitation Models

Although cultural competence is usually examined in reference to practitioners or organizations, one can also ask whether the principles and implementation of a psychiatric rehabilitation *model* generalize across various cultural groups. The example presented at the beginning of this chapter hints at the complexity of the question of generalizability of evidence-based practices to other cultural groups.

Evidence-based psychiatric rehabilitation practices assume the importance of individualized services and shared decision making, with close attention to consumer preferences (Drake et al., 2003c). Individualizing services certainly implies the need to incorporate the cultural context. To the extent that these principles are well understood and followed, could it not be the case that psychiatric rehabilitation practices are culturally competent?

The limitations of this view are the circumstances in which psychiatric rehabilitation principles may themselves be in conflict with cultural competence. For example, assertive outreach, often considered a fundamental principle of psychiatric rehabilitation, may be an example of a culturally insensitive intervention in certain contexts. Even though the intention behind assertive outreach is to include individuals who do not benefit from services because of their dropping out prematurely, aggressive outreach is seen as intrusive and a violation of cultural norms among Native Americans and other cultural groups (Pernell-Arnold & Finley, 1999). Phillips, Barrio, and Brekke (2001a) have speculated that "the ideology of the [psychiatric rehabilitation] interventions, based on Western behavioral models that apply values of individualism—independence, self-reliance, competitiveness, autonomous action, and emotional detachment—to persons from collectivistic sociocentric cultures, may not be culturally syntonic" (p. 679). Of course, not only should services be culturally appropriate, but also they need to be perceived as such by the cultural group (Barrio, 2000).

Moving beyond anecdotes, the critical next step is to examine the empirical literature regarding the compatibility of psychiatric rehabilitation with the cultures of various groups. Unfortunately, the answers are woefully incomplete. Although there are exceptions, the vast majority of studies on psychiatric rehabilitation programs have been conducted in European American populations. The multicultural supplement to the 1999 Surgeon General's Report on Mental Health concluded that most randomized controlled trials evaluating mental health treatments for individuals with severe mental illness have either failed to report ethnicity or reported ethnicity in the aggregate ("non-white") (U.S. Surgeon General, 2001). This same report noted that "not a single study analyzed the efficacy of the treatment by ethnicity or race" (p. 35). Johnson and Cameron (2001) have noted the total lack of mental health outcome studies of Native Americans.

Among the small handful of psychiatric rehabilitation outcome studies that have examined ethnicity, most have evaluated approaches that are not evidence-based (e.g., Cook & Razzano, 1995; Phillips et al., 2001a). Such studies are less valuable than those designed specifically to evaluate established evidence-based practices provided in samples with diverse ethnic groups.

Research on the effectiveness of evidence-based practices for specific ethnic groups is spotty. An exception is supported employment; it appears to be applicable without modification to a number of ethnic groups, including European Americans, African Americans, Latinos, and Chinese (e.g., Drake et al., 1999b; Mueser et al., 2004a; Wong et al., 2005). In contrast, family psychoeducation may require adaptations for different ethnic groups (Murray-Swank & Dixon, 2004; Telles, Karno, Mintz, Paz, Arias, et al., 1995). Unfortunately, there are relatively few psychiatric rehabilitation studies reporting separate outcome findings for two or more different ethnic groups within a single randomized controlled trial. Ethnographies have offered a vital supplement to quantitative studies for understanding differences across cultural groups (e.g., Alverson & Vicente, 1998; Quimby, Drake, & Becker, 2001).

Although many case studies of psychiatric rehabilitation programs serving specific cultural groups are reported in the literature (e.g., Wong, Chiu, Tang, Kan, Hong, et al., 2004; Yang, Law, Chow, Andermann, Steinberg, et al., 2005), few studies using control groups have evaluated the effectiveness of psychiatric rehabilitation programs designed to serve a specific cultural group. To assess the impact of culturally relevant modifications of services, the best design would be to start with an evidence-based practice and compare it with the same practice with culturally specific modifications. Unfortunately, such studies have not been conducted. Instead, the few controlled studies of practices with cultural modifications have compared their programs with weak control groups. Thus, a pilot study of a skills training program designed for older Latinos, as compared with a control group attending a conversation group (Patterson, Bucardo, McKibbin, Mausbach, Moore, et al., 2005), does not answer the critical question about the added value of the culturally specific content.

Finally, the most informative research design would consist of randomized controlled trials, with three or more groups representing different ethnicities, to partially control for social class factors (Phillips et al., 2001a). Such studies would be very expensive and complicated, and none have yet been conducted.

WHAT DO WE KNOW ABOUT CULTURAL COMPETENCE?

Do Cultural Competence Guidelines and Policies Make a Difference?

Sue (2003) has traced the history of the development of cultural competence guidelines and policies in the United States. One of the first federal reports to recognize the problem was the President's Commission on Mental Health (1978), which concluded that mental health organizations and clinicians shared the biases and racism of the mainstream culture. Since that time, Sue suggests, "remarkable progress" has been made in overcoming the barriers to adequate care among ethnic minorities. Nonetheless, a more recent federal report documents the problems that continue to exist (U.S. Surgeon General, 2001).

Acknowledging the lack of rigorous research showing the efficacy of culturally competent mental health services, Sue (2003) offers a number of explanations, including the lack of research funding and trained investigators, as well as the complexities of conducting such research. Nonetheless, he argues that the collective evidence from less rigorous studies makes the case for cultural competence "compelling." However, commenting on SAMHSA's statement that "recovery and rehabilitation are more likely to occur where managed care systems, services, and providers have and utilize knowledge and skills that are culturally competent," Vega and Lopez (2001) argue that "there are no existing data to support its validity" (p. 195).

Progress in the multicultural area also has been impeded by the failure to conduct theory-informed research (Miranda, Nakamura, & Bernal, 2003). Specifically, "population-based research," that is, studies with specific ethnic groups, is limited by the fact that researchers cannot generalize to other ethnic groups. Nor can confounding variables, such as social class, be easily ruled out.

Does Training Improve Cultural Competence?

To our knowledge, there are no published outcome studies examining training in cultural competence designed specifically for psychiatric rehabilitation practitioners. However, training in cultural competence has been examined in two systematic reviews, one of the general health care literature (Beach, Price, Gary, Robinson, Gozu, et al., 2005), and a second of multicultural education programs for mental health professionals (Smith, Constantine, Dunn, Dinehart, & Montoya, 2006).

Beach et al. (2005) identified 34 studies examining cultural competency training programs, mostly targeted at physicians or nurses. The length of the training was highly variable in this group of studies, ranging from a single 4-hour session to 30 half-day sessions spread over a year, followed by 6 weeks of full-day sessions. Curricular methods included lecture, discussion groups, case scenarios, role modeling, written assignments, field trips, cultural immersion, and interviewing members of another culture. The authors concluded that there was "excellent evidence" for knowledge acquisition and "good evidence" for improved practitioner attitudes and skills, but that these studies found meager evidence for actual impact on consumer satisfaction with treatment or consumer adherence to treatment.

Smith et al. (2006) located 45 survey studies and 37 outcome studies (mostly employing pre–post designs), most of which assessed attitudinal change after receiving multicultural counseling training. As with the Beach et al. (2005) review, these studies did suggest moderate change in attitudes, but few studies examined objective indicators of outcome.

Finally, one other study may be mentioned. It used qualitative methods to examine the challenges of providing cultural competence training for mental health practitioners (Ton et al., 2005). Practitioners reported that time limitations and language were common barriers to applying concepts from cultural competence training.

Are Culturally Competent Practitioners More Effective?

Fuertes and Brobst (2002) found strong correlations between client ratings of multicultural competence and general counselor competence and empathy. For all clients, both those who were members of ethnic minority groups and European Americans, general competence and empathy were associated with client satisfaction with counseling, as many other studies have found. In addition, ethnic minority client ratings of multicultural competence was highly related to client satisfaction, even after controlling for general counseling competence and empathy, but this pattern did not hold for European American clients. The authors concluded that mastery of general counseling skills was a necessary precondition for achieving multicultural competence. However, this study did not resolve the question of whether proficient counseling skills are sufficient to ensure culturally competent services.

Racial–Ethnic Matching Hypothesis

The racial–ethnic matching hypothesis has been labeled in various ways, including the "ethnic responsiveness hypothesis" (Gamst, Dana, Der-Karabetian, & Kremer, 2001), which is "the expectation of the beneficial effects of client–counselor ethnicity, language, and gender match variables upon clinical outcomes" (p. 58). One corollary is that clients are inevitably less trustful of counselors of a different cultural background (Whaley, 2001a, 2001b). Another corollary is that counselors are conferred more immediate credibility by clients if they are of a similar racial–ethnic background (Sue & Zane, 1987). Based on this hypothesis, researchers have predicted greater service use and longer retention in treatment, in addition to improved outcomes, for clients who have a counselor with the same ethnic background.

Assuming that racial–ethnic matching is a desirable goal, a formidable barrier to its achievement is the underrepresentation of Latinos and African Americans among mental health professionals. This underrepresentation seems likely to continue as long as these ethnic groups have lower rates of completion of postsecondary education relative to the rest of the U.S. population (Vega & Lopez, 2001). Thus, even for agencies pursuing an active strategy of ethnic matching and therefore making a good-faith effort at cultural diversity in hiring practitioners, ethnic matching is often a practical impossibility, especially in ethnically diverse communities (Ton et al., 2005). An unintended consequence of the strict application of the ethnic matching concept is that bicultural practitioners are overburdened with large caseloads, which is in fact contrary to optimal service delivery (Ton et al., 2005).

Although an intuitively plausible theory, the evidence regarding the racial–ethnic hypothesis has been mixed, both in the counseling literature, where it has been frequently examined, and in the psychiatric rehabilitation literature, where the research is sparser. Two meta-analyses document this point. One was a meta-analysis of 7 psychotherapy studies, which found that ethnic matching had a negligible effect on treatment retention

---

PERSONAL EXAMPLE

José Salinas Wants to Work

José is a 23-year-old unemployed man diagnosed with bipolar disorder who recently signed up for a supported employment program. He was born in the United States to parents who had immigrated from Mexico. He lives in a cramped household with his parents, five siblings, his grandmother, and his sister's baby. Although José speaks English, Spanish is spoken at home. His parents and grandmother hold many of the beliefs about mental illness common among Latinos, including that José is not mentally ill, but suffers from nervousness.

José's employment specialist, Ann, speaks fluent Spanish. In their initial meeting, she asks José for his language preference in discussing his employment plans. She determines that although José initially expressed a desire to work, he is now backing away from that goal. Using motivational interviewing principles, Ann does not push him to pursue work, but rather affirms his ambivalence and explores his current thinking. His family, especially his mother, is strongly opposed to his working. His mother feels that he is needed too much around the house. In addition, she does not want him to lose his Social Security benefits, which help to pay the family bills. To address these sources of resistance, Ann offers to invite José's mother to the next appointment and suggests an appointment with the benefits counselor to update his benefits situation. José also expresses the belief that most employers do not want to hire Latinos, describing the rejections he has experienced in the past with his job search. After exploring the kind of job that José is looking for, Ann suggests he look for jobs within the Latino business community and identifies several contacts she has there.

(Fuertes & Brobst, 2002). The second examined 10 studies of the ethnic matching hypothesis among African Americans and European Americans, finding no significant effects for overall functioning, treatment retention, or number of sessions attended (Maramba & Hall, 2002). Correlational studies conducted in samples of individuals with severe mental illness have been similarly unsupportive (e.g., Chinman, Rosenheck, & Lam, 2000a; Ortega & Rosenheck, 2002).

Many confounds cloud the interpretation of findings from these studies. For example, in a large clinic sample study comparing four ethnic groups (European American, African American, Latino, and Asian American), baseline functioning varied greatly between the four groups, and the outcomes varied accordingly, independent of the client–counselor matching (Gamst, Dana, Der-Karabetian, & Kremer, 2000). The authors explained the ambiguous findings for their African American group by speculating that racial matching may be important only for clients who embrace their racial identity as African Americans while disparaging European American values. With the use of a self-report measure of acculturation with Latino clients, acculturation appeared to moderate the relationship between ethnic matching and a change measure of global functioning (Gamst, Dana, Der-Karabetian, Aragón, & Kremer, 2002).

As already noted, there is an empirical basis for believing that there are, in fact, health care disparities associated with race and ethnicity. It is therefore not surprising that clients' beliefs about racism in the health care system are correlated with their preferences for the race and ethnicity of their physicians, and their satisfaction with those physicians (Chen et al., 2005).

This section examined the value of cultural competence, reviewing evidence from the practitioner level. How about from an organizational level? Are "Latino clinics," for example, better able to serve the Latino community than general community mental health centers (CMHCs) that include practitioners who are competent but isolated within a larger system that is not? In some Latino clinics, even the organization of the front desk is different from that of regular mental health centers, let alone the décor and magazines in the waiting room (Silvia Bigatti, personal communication, February 11, 2006).

SUMMARY AND CONCLUSIONS

The importance of cultural competence in psychiatric rehabilitation is widely acknowledged. Nevertheless, we do not yet have an adequate operational definition of cultural competence that differentiates it from those skills associated with general competencies of a psychiatric rehabilitation practitioner. The difficulty in defining and assessing cultural competence does not mean, however, that cultural issues can be ignored.

Disparities in services are one tangible indication that cultural issues cannot be routinely ignored. Lower rates of access, disparities in diagnosis and assessment, and discriminatory treatment recommendations for individuals from cultural backgrounds different from that of the majority are reminders of the challenges of ensuring access to evidence-based psychiatric rehabilitation services to all who need help. Unfortunately, most of the so-called evidence-based practices have themselves been validated with homogeneous European American samples, so their broad applicability to other cultures is often unknown.

To be successful in achieving cultural competence, implementation needs to occur at multiple levels, which includes training and supervising practitioners and adopting policies and procedures at the organizational level to ensure an organizational culture that supports cultural diversity. The evidence supporting the effectiveness of ethnic–racial matching is mixed. Moreover, in communities with an influx of immigrants, attempts at achieving ethnic matching may be impractical. Training and supervision in general clinical skills supplemented with culturally specific information may be the most pragmatic strategy.

An underlying issue not yet resolved is the extent to which cultural factors should be systematically and continuously addressed in providing psychiatric rehabilitation services. Multiculturalists contend that cultural factors are a primary consideration in all aspects of assessment, treatment planning, intervention, program design, and program implementation. According to their view, cultural biases are difficult to overcome, because each of us brings his or her cultural filters to interpreting and understanding the world. Thus, psychiatric rehabilitation principles must be reinterpreted to suit the cultural context, and practitioners must acquire specific cultural competency knowledge and skills to provide adequate services to cultural groups different from their own (Barrio, 2000; Pernell-Arnold & Finley, 1999).

Sometimes it is argued that cultural competence includes knowledge specific to each particular cultural group (i.e., about their customs, belief, and values). At the other extreme, the position could be taken that, properly understood, the principles of psychiatric rehabilitation are universal and require no adaptation to different cultural contexts. As summarized by Sue (2003), critics have suggested that political correctness has inhibited the critical examination of the concept of cultural competence.

Ultimately, however, the degree to which cultural factors limit the generalizability of psychiatric rehabilitation services to other cultural groups is an empirical question. It is important that theoretical debates be replaced by systematic studies to provide program planners and practitioners with tangible guidelines for action.

Chapter 21

Policy

In 1998, Illinois's state mental health authority (SMHA) launched a statewide psychosocial rehabilitation (PSR) initiative defining and funding four PSR core services (skill development, vocational, peer support, and community resource development). The SMHA also announced a psychiatric rehabilitation certificate program aimed at developing a work force with the knowledge and skills necessary to implement the PSR approaches defined in its initiative (Barton et al., 2001).

In 1999, Georgia's SMHA initiated a certified peer support training program as the centerpiece of a new emphasis on recovery-oriented psychiatric rehabilitation services. The state also received approval for a Medicaid waiver to include peer support as a Medicaid-reimbursable service (Sabin & Daniels, 2003).

In 2001, Indiana's SMHA took a different path toward implementing psychiatric rehabilitation services. State officials developed a plan to disseminate assertive community treatment (ACT) throughout the state, with the intent of eventually extending their strategy to other evidence-based practices. Their plan entailed four actions. First, a set of state standards for certification of ACT programs was adopted. Second, the SMHA funded a technical assistance center to provide education, training, and consultation to community mental health centers (CMHCs), family members, and consumers. Third, the SMHA provided incentive funding to CMHCs to develop ACT programs. Fourth, in 2004 the state obtained approval for ACT as a Medicaid-reimbursable service (Moser et al., 2004). By 2005, 20 of the 31 CMHCs in the state had ACT-certified programs.

In 2004, California voters approved Proposition 63, legislation imposing a 1% state income tax on adjusted gross income over $1 million, raising $1.8 billion (a 31% increase) in new revenues over a 3-year period to help finance new services within the state's county-operated mental health systems (Scheffler & Adams, 2005). This initiative promises to increase an emphasis on supported employment and other psychiatric rehabilitation practices.

These snapshots hint at the amazing variability in strategies states have employed to disseminate psychiatric rehabilitation services. In addition, states such as California, Oregon, Iowa, and New York are emphasizing evidence-based practices in SMHA directives and in state legislation, sometimes, however, without clear definitions of evidence-based practice. Although they are only part of the story, state and local policy decisions have important influences on the shape of psychiatric rehabilitation services in the United States. Federal legislation has also had an enduring impact. Because funding and policies regarding psychiatric rehabilitation are closely intertwined with those for mental health services, much of this chapter is devoted to mental health funding.

In this chapter we discuss the influence of policies, funding, and legislation on psychiatric rehabilitation practice, including actions taken by state and federal agencies and advocacy groups. This chapter examines (1) the roles of the federal and state governments in development of psychiatric rehabilitation; (2) the roles of advocacy groups; (3) policy barriers; and (4) costs of psychiatric rehabilitation services.

THE ROLES OF THE FEDERAL AND STATE GOVERNMENTS

Federal Legislation Affecting Psychiatric Rehabilitation

The federal bureaucracy consists of dozens of agencies with direct and indirect influence on individuals with psychiatric disabilities. These agencies are responsible for enforcing legislation, implementing policies, and providing funding either directly to individuals with psychiatric disabilities or to provider agencies that serve them. These agencies also provide leadership and funding for training, education, and research. The areas of responsibility and the associated agencies most affecting individuals with severe mental illness are as follows: *mental health*—the National Institute of Mental Health (NIMH) (*www.nimh.nih.gov/*) and the Center for Mental Health Services (CMHS) within the Substance Abuse and Mental Health Services Administration (SAMHSA) (*www.samhsa.gov/*); *financing of health care*—the Centers for Medicare and Medicaid Services (CMS) (*cms.hhs.gov/*); *vocational rehabilitation*—the Rehabilitation Services Administration (RSA) (*www.ed.gov/about/offices/list/osers/rsa/index.html*) and the National Institute of Disability and Rehabilitation Research (NIDRR) (*www.ed.gov/about/offices/list/osers/nidrr/*); *disability income support* and *welfare*—the Social Security Administration (SSA) (*www.ssa.gov/*) and Temporary Assistance for Needy Families (TANF) (*www.acf.dhhs. gov/programs/ofa/*); *housing*—the U.S. Department of Housing and Urban Development (*www.hud.gov/*); and *protection against discrimination*—the U.S. Equal Employment Opportunity Commission (EEOC) (*www.eeoc.gov/*). For each of these domains we provide a historical context and current policies and activities regarding psychiatric rehabilitation.

Not covered in this chapter is an increasingly important topic, the role of criminal justice in psychiatric rehabilitation. Criminalization of mental illness is a tragic, inhumane, but hidden policy in this country. Policy issues relevant to psychiatric rehabilitation are discussed in Chapter 13.

Mental Health

Prompted by the military's inadequate capacity to respond to psychological problems among those serving in World War II, Congress enacted the *National Mental Health Act*

(Public Law 79-487) in 1946. This Act created the NIMH, which was charged with promoting research and training in mental health and with assisting states in the use of "the most effective methods of prevention, diagnosis, and treatment of psychotic disorders."

As described in Chapter 3, the locus of mental health care in the United States shifted dramatically in the middle of the 20th century. Before 1955, psychiatric care was principally custodial and increasingly delegated to state psychiatric hospitals. Reflecting changes already occurring in state mental health systems with the growing exodus from psychiatric hospitals, the *Community Mental Health Centers Act of 1963* articulated a new vision for community-based care of people with mental illness. It also authorized funding for construction of CMHC facilities. Later legislation amending and extending the Act authorized time-limited federal funding for CMHC staff. Congress also made additional refinements regarding the role of CMHCs, adding to the list of essential services and fostering CMHC expansion to rural and inner-city areas.

CMHCs expanded dramatically during the 1970s, despite the presidencies of Nixon and Ford, who espoused opposition to the growth of the federal government's role in mental health (Cutler, Bevilacqua, & McFarland, 2003). During the Carter administration, the Community Support Program (CSP) Branch of NIMH was established and proved to be influential in redirecting CMHC efforts toward effective services for individuals with severe mental illness. At the end of the Carter administration, Congress passed the *Mental Health System Act of 1980*, which would have made many reforms, including significant expansion of mental health services to underserved populations (i.e., the young and the old, and racial and ethnic minorities).

Consistent with his philosophy of reducing the role of the federal government, President Reagan reversed several initiatives begun during the Carter administration. Notably, the Reagan administration did not implement the Mental Health System Act of 1980. One of Reagan's most far-reaching actions in mental health was a plan to gradually eliminate all direct funding to CMHCs. In its place, his administration devised the concept of a *block grant*, defined as a specific dollar amount given to each state according to a funding formula, to help it to achieve a wide range of locally defined social policy goals. Federal block grants were not merely a change in how funds were administered; the Reagan administration took this opportunity to reduce drastically the level of federal funding for social programs. In addition, block grants were not targeted to funding for CMHCs or any specific mental health initiatives, permitting state governments wide latitude on how these dollars were spent. Thus, the *Omnibus Budget Reconciliation Act of 1981* undid many of the federal mental health initiatives of the preceding 18 years. By the late 1990s, the federal block grant constituted only about 1% of public mental health funding (Hogan, 1999).

In 1992 the scientific and training/advocacy functions of NIMH were split into two separate agencies. NIMH as a federal agency responsible for mental health research was reorganized to become a part of the National Institute of Health (NIH), and a new agency, the Substance Abuse and Mental Health Services Administration (SAMHSA), was created. Within SAMHSA, CMHS was formed to continue the training/advocacy functions formerly under the purview of NIMH. Since its creation, SAMHSA has funded a number of multisite studies of psychiatric rehabilitation, including the Employment Intervention Demonstration Project (Cook, Carey, Razzano, Burke, & Blyler, 2002), two homeless outreach projects (Center for Mental Health Services, 1994; Randolph, Blasinsky, Morrissey, Rosenheck, Cocozza, et al., 2002), the Consumer-Operated Services Program Multisite Research Initiative (Holter et al., 2004), and the National Evidence-Based Practices Project (Drake et al., 2001b).

Financing of Health Care

CMS, formerly known as the Health Care Finance Administration, is the federal agency that administers the Medicaid and Medicare programs. Medicaid and Medicare were first authorized by Congress in 1965 and became incorporated as part of the Social Security Act, as described below. Medicaid is the federal–state health insurance program for people with limited incomes. A 2005 report indicated that it provided long-term care services to 52 million low-income Americans (Kaiser Commission on Medicaid and the Uninsured, 2005). Individuals who qualify for Medicaid are eligible for specific medical services, including mental health treatment, from health care providers who are reimbursed by Medicaid. To be reimbursed, a medical service must be covered by the state Medicaid plan. Covered services are established by CMS, but state-managed Medicaid programs develop and implement the state Medicaid plan, which specifies rules governing which services are covered for which patients and under what conditions. Broadly speaking, covered services are those interventions regarded by CMS as effective treatments for medical conditions. For any service to be reimbursed, *medical necessity* must be established. *Behavioral health care*, terminology often used to include mental health and substance abuse services, is a medical service covered by Medicaid. As discussed below, rehabilitation services fall in a gray area in the sense that it is difficult to partition out the medical aspect, as in the case of supported employment interventions. Each state has its own specific rules about what services are reimbursable and at what rates (Smith, Kennedy, Knipper, O'Brien, & O'Keeffe, 2005).

Medicaid is funded by a combination of federal and state dollars. The federal contribution (the *federal financial participation*) is determined by a formula based on the per capita income for a state as compared with the national average (Smith et al., 2005). The state *match* (that is, the amount paid from state sources) varies from 17 to 50 cents on the dollar. On average, the federal government pays 57% of the costs of Medicaid (Mann, 2002). To participate in Medicaid, a state must agree to cover certain groups of people (*mandatory groups*) and offer a minimum set of benefits (*mandatory benefits*). Examples of mandatory Medicaid eligibility groups include Supplemental Security Income (SSI) recipients and low-income families with children. Examples of mandatory benefits include physician visits, laboratory tests, and inpatient services. In addition, a state can choose to serve *optional groups* and to provide *optional benefits*. As of 2005, 60% of Medicaid dollars were spent on optional groups and/or services (Kaiser Commission on Medicaid and the Uninsured, 2005).

States vary widely in the percentage of the low-income nonelderly population covered by Medicaid. For example, whereas Massachusetts and Vermont covered 41% of this population in 2001, Virginia covered only 14% (Mann, 2002). Mental health costs are only a small fraction of the health care costs in the United States. In 2001, mental health costs made up 6.2% of the total health care expenditures of $1,373 billion (Mark, Coffey, McKusick, Harwood, King, et al., 2005).

When Medicaid was first enacted, it did not adequately address mental health treatment. A Medicaid rule specifically aimed at people with mental illness was the *Institutions of Mental Disease (IMD) exclusion*, which prohibits Medicaid coverage for services provided to adults ages 22–64 in psychiatric hospitals and some community-based residential facilities with 16 or more beds. This rule is still in force. In terms of community-based treatment, Medicaid did not cover mental health case management until the early 1980s (Hogan, 1999). The two main Medicaid coverages used by states to fund community mental health services are the *clinic option* and the *rehabilitation services option* (commonly referred to as the Medicaid Rehab Option, or MRO). As the label implies, the clinic option is facility based and is closely aligned with the medical model. The scope of services permissible under MRO makes it more compatible with the provision of psychiatric rehabilitation. In recent years, states have increasingly employed MRO in the provision of mental health services in lieu of the clinic option, a change that some authors argue is more compatible with psychiatric rehabilitation, because MRO is more community based, is more flexible in who provides services, and encourages active participation of patients in their own treatment (Smith et al., 2005).

Originally, Medicaid was exclusively a *fee-for-service* program, in which providers were reimbursed a flat rate for a particular unit of service. In 1982, the Medicaid reimbursement method began changing with the emergence of a mechanism known as the *Medicaid 1115 Waiver*. When approved (usually after extensive negotiation between the state Medicaid office and CMS), these waivers allowed state Medicaid programs to implement "experimental, pilot, or demonstration projects" to change federal rules for reimbursement and/or coverage. The waiver requests must be budget neutral, but they give individual states flexibility to propose creative reimbursement schemes. The most common request has been to modify the reimbursement scheme from fee-for-service to a *managed care* model. Managed care involves a range of *utilization management* techniques, such as the development of a network of providers allied with a particular approach to delivering treatment services (e.g., community mental health centers), negotiated rates, and a range of financing options that involve some sharing of risk between the first-party funder (a corporation or the government) and second-party (provider organizations), third-party (insurers), and fourth-party (managed care organizations) funders (Howard Goldman, personal communication, September 24, 2005). Managed care uses a variety of cost-containment strategies, the most common of which is known as a *capitated* approach, defined as a method of payment in which "a fixed price is paid for each enrolled client, for a specified time period, for a specific range of services" (Mechanic & Aiken, 1989). This means that providers are paid a flat rate for the care of a client regardless of the intensity of services provided. By the early 1990s, most states had either adopted or were considering adoption of some form of a capitated Medicaid system (McFarland, 1994). In 1997, Congress revised the law regarding Medicaid to give states the option to require most Medicaid beneficiaries to enroll in managed care programs (Mann, 2002). By 1998, 36 states were operating, or had received approval for a Medicaid waiver for operating, managed behavioral health care (Frank, Goldman, & Hogan, 2003).

The *Medicaid Buy-In Program* authorized by the Balanced Budget Act of 1997 and the *Ticket to Work and Work Incentives Improvement Act of 1999* have permitted state governments additional flexibility in establishing Medicaid eligibility, with the intent of reducing barriers to employment posed by the potential loss of Medicaid benefits (Golden, O'Mara, Ferrell, & Sheldon, 2000). As of 2004, 29 states had implemented new policies under this Medicaid program, expanding Medicaid eligibility with more liberal income thresholds for people with disabilities who were working (Kiernan, Halliday, & Boeltzig, 2004). States have varied widely in defining income thresholds, with Minnesota having the most liberal rules, namely, requiring no income limit. In most states, participants must pay a monthly premium of about $26 per month and/or make small copayments. In 2004, Missouri had the largest enrollment (more than 16,000) of any state in the Buy-In Program (Kiernan et al., 2004).

Medicare is the federal health insurance program covering most Americans ages 65 and older. In 1972, Medicare eligibility was expanded to individuals under age 65 with long-term disabilities receiving Social Security Disability insurance (SSDI). The rules determining what health care services are covered and what copayments apply are complicated. In general, Medicare is far less relevant to psychiatric rehabilitation than Medicaid, because the range of mental health services covered by Medicare is far more restrictive. However, Medicare is relevant to consumers with severe mental illness, including both those of ages 65 and over and those who are younger, who live in Medicare-funded nursing homes (Mechanic & McAlpine, 2000). Two national surveys reported about 100,000 individuals with schizophrenia living in nursing homes in 1995. A recurring issue has been the quality of care in nursing homes. To help maintain minimum standards of care, CMS has a certification process and has certified 17,000 nursing homes nationwide (*www.medicare.gov/Nursing*).

A new Medicare program that may impact mental health consumers in the future is a voluntary prescription drug program for low-income seniors. The *Medicare Prescription Drug, Improvement, and Modernization Act*, signed into law in 2003, established Medicare Part D, which provides a subsidy on prescription drugs for eligible seniors who voluntarily apply for this program and pay premiums of approximately $30 per month.

Vocational Rehabilitation

RSA is the federal agency that manages the federal–state program funding rehabilitation services for individuals with disabilities. This program is commonly referred to as vocational rehabilitation (VR), although state VR offices have a variety of names. Federal guidelines provide state VR offices with the basic framework; however, most of the day-to-day decision making is decentralized. Although the state VR office as well as each local VR office set policies and in many cases establish goals (e.g., number of successful closures each counselor is expected to attain for a time period), individual VR counselors have wide latitude in making decisions. Thus, VR counselors make final decisions on client eligibility for service interventions used to assist clients in achieving employment goals. Currently, new clients are presumed eligible as long as they have a diagnosable disability that interferes with getting or maintaining employment. Only in cases where "clear and convincing evidence" to the contrary is offered by the counselor can a determination of ineligibility be made owing to reasons of inability to benefit from VR in terms of employment. Nevertheless, the documentation required to achieve eligibility can be onerous and time-consuming, and clients sometimes wait weeks or longer to achieve VR approval (Noble et al., 1997).

Along with eligibility determination, the VR counselor also authorizes funding for individual clients. The VR philosophy stresses achievement of specific goals (e.g., stable employment), and therefore funding is authorized for achievement of specific outcomes. In most states, VR services are purchased from authorized *vendors*, which may include psychiatric rehabilitation agencies or CMHCs. Each state has a process for determining provider agency eligibility; in many states, vendor eligibility is determined by an external accreditation process, such as that conducted by the Commission on Accreditation of Rehabilitation Facilities (CARF).

VR services include assessment, counseling and guidance, education, training, assistance in job acquisition , and initial support on the job. In theory, VR counselors may also authorize any other services necessary to help individuals achieve their vocational goals, although this degree of latitude is seldom exercised. An important feature of the VR system is that, as a matter of practice, VR is most often limited to short-term funding. Once a VR client gains employment, VR provides funding for job support for a limited period of time (supposedly to a point where a client is "stable" in employment). After this stability is achieved (a subjective judgment of the VR counselor), then the VR case should not be closed until at least 90 days of successful, stable employment. Because of the subjectivity in judging job stability and the oft-cited pressure to close cases in the VR system, clients are often closed out as successful *rehabilitations* upon completing 90 days of employment with little regard to actual job stability. When clients are closed by VR, their VR funding ends. Moreover, if a client loses a job or wishes to change jobs, his or her re-authorization for further VR assistance is dependent on the specific circumstances. In theory, clients can be funded through VR for *post employment services* beyond the point of successful closure (Pratt, Gill, Barrett, & Roberts, 2006), and in some circumstances this occurs. One mechanism (Title VIB) permits funding of 18 months of job support, and a second (Title I, which is the core funding stream that can be used for any services to clients) permits the funding of job support for an indeterminate period of time. In practice, these mechanisms for extended support beyond the 18-month limit or as part of postemployment services are not widely used within the VR system.

VR's long history has involved numerous legislative actions progressively aimed at making its services more responsive to individuals with disabilities (Rubin & Roessler, 2001). VR had its origins in a program created after World War I to assist returning veterans who had suffered injuries that rendered them incapable of returning to their former employment. In 1920, the U.S. Congress passed the *Smith–Fess Act*, extending rehabilitation services to all citizens with physical disabilities. The *Barden–LaFollette Act* of 1943 expanded services to include individuals with psychiatric disabilities and mental retardation. However, this legislation had no immediate effect on increasing VR services to people with psychiatric disabilities. By as late as 1955, only 4% of individuals whose cases had successful VR closures had a psychiatric disability. The *1954 VR Act Amendments* (Public Law 83-565) provided impetus for expanding VR services to people with psychiatric disabilities, and by 1965, 14% of clients rehabilitated by VR had had a psychiatric disability. By 1995, 19% of clients receiving VR services had a psychiatric disability (Courtney, 2005).

By giving highest priority to persons with severe disabilities and mandating consumer involvement in the planning and delivery of services, the *Rehabilitation Act of 1973* (Public Law 93-112) reflected the political climate of the 1960s, in the context of the Civil Rights Movement and the growing consumer movement advocating for persons with disabilities. This Act also established the Individualized Written Rehabilitation Plan (IWRP), which was later mandated to be completed with each VR client. The IWRP includes a statement of long-term goals, VR services to be provided, methods to achieve the goals, and an explicit statement on how each consumer is involved in choosing the goals (Rubin & Roessler, 2001). The compatibility between the IWRP and psychiatric rehabilitation principles is apparent. In 1978, RSA and NIMH developed a collaborative agreement intended to foster coordinated and collaborative efforts at the state and local levels between mental health and VR.

The *1986 Amendments to the Rehabilitation Act* (Public Law 99-506) constituted the first federal legislation to define supported employment. In addition to establishing a new category of funds to pay for supported employment, it also allowed VR counselors to authorize regular case service funds for supported employment. Later, state regulations included a specific definition of supported employment, which included transitional employment as a form of supported employment for people with severe mental illness.

The *1992 Amendments to the Rehabilitation Act* (Public Law 102-569) contained a number of important changes to the regulations that made VR services more accommodating for people with severe mental illness. The first was an elimination of the eligibility requirement that clients have a *reasonable expectation* to benefit from VR services. Up until this time, VR counselors routinely screened out individuals they judged to be poor prospects for employment, which very often included clients with severe psychiatric disabilities. The 1992 amendments changed the language for eligibility from *reasonable expectation* to *presumption of benefit*. In essence, this shifted the burden of proof for eligibility from the individual applying for services to the VR counselor, who was now required to provide "clear and convincing evidence" that an individual is unable to work. Second, regulations following these amendments changed the minimum 20-hour-per-week requirement, originally part of the federal definition of supported employment, to a criterion number of hours based on the IWRP. The definitions for *ongoing support* were also made more flexible (e.g., allowing for contact away from the job site) to accommodate the realities of supported employment for the severely mentally ill population.

The *Workforce Investment Act of 1998* (Public Law 105-220) established a mechanism to provide universal access to "one-stop" service delivery for 60 separate federally funded job training programs. The impact of this legislation appears mixed. In theory, one-stop programs are intended to provide easy access, in a single location, to a wide array of requisite employment-related services, but in practice, these programs have not achieved this goal. Mental health advocates note that individuals with psychiatric disabilities historically have had difficulty in accessing and benefiting from generic unemployment services, which one-stop programs resemble (Courtney, 2005). Consequently, this legislation appears to have had very little impact on the population of people with severe mental illness.

In 2001, RSA announced a long overdue change in the definition of employment outcomes that would qualify in the VR system as successful closures. The revision involved limiting a successful closure to work in an integrated setting; that is, employment in a sheltered workshop or other nonintegrated settings no longer qualified (Courtney, 2005).

Disability Income Support

In response to hardships incurred during the Great Depression, the U.S. Congress passed the *Social Security Act* in 1935. It provided assistance for three groups hardest hit by the Depression—those of retirement age (many of whom had no savings), dependent children, and unemployed persons. Discussion of the Social Security retirement program is beyond the scope of this chapter. A second major program funded by the Social Security Act, originally known as *Aid to Families with Dependent Children*, was replaced in 1996, as part of welfare reform, with a new block grant program, *Temporary Assistance for Needy Families* (TANF). (TANF is not discussed in this chapter, although many individuals with psychiatric disabilities receiving TANF benefits are underserved by the mental health system.) The third program defined by the Social Security Act was an unemployment insurance program. Like other social programs described in this chapter, the unemployment program was designed as a federal–state collaboration administered by the states.

Of particular relevance to individuals with psychiatric disabilities were a number of later amendments and additions to the Social Security Act, shown in Table 21.1 (see *www.ssa.gov*). *Supplemental Security Income* (SSI) and *Social Security Disability Insurance* (SSDI) provide income support to individuals who are determined to be eligible

TABLE 21.1. Years of Passage of Important Social Security Legislation

- 1935: Social Security Old-Age Insurance; Unemployment Insurance; Public Assistance programs for needy, aged, and blind persons; and Aid to Families with Dependent Children (replaced with block grants for Temporary Assistance for Needy Families in 1996)
- 1950: Aid to the Permanently and Totally Disabled (replaced by the SSI program in 1972)
- 1956: Social Security Disability Insurance
- 1964: Food stamp program
- 1965: Medicare and Medicaid programs
- 1972: Supplemental Security Income program
- 1996: Temporary Assistance for Needy Families
- 1999: Ticket to Work and Work Incentives Improvement Act

because of a disability preventing them from engaging in substantial gainful activity (Burt & Aron, 2003). SSDI eligibility involves the accumulation of Social Security payments through FICA (Federal Insurance Contributions Act) paycheck deductions. Social Security has specific rules and formulas about the waiting period and the length of time worked to qualify for SSDI. The amount of SSDI payments depends on the amount contributed to Social Security.

Unlike SSI amounts, the amount of the monthly SSDI check is not adjusted each month by earnings. However, SSDI *status* is affected by employment earnings in the following manner. As long as a person's earnings in a given month do not exceed a specified level ($590 in 2005), his or her SSDI benefits are unaffected. In addition, SSDI beneficiaries are allowed a "trial work period" consisting of 9 months (not necessarily consecutive) in which they can earn above the specified level within a 5-year period. Once the trial work period is completed, they are subject to a *Continuing Disability Review* to determine if they are eligible for continuing SSDI status. (Regardless of work status, SSDI beneficiaries are also subject to review if there is medical improvement.) Individuals who lose their SSDI benefits and subsequently lose their jobs must reapply for SSDI status. A metaphor used in describing the plight of SSDI beneficiaries is that they are subject to "falling off a cliff" if they complete their trial work period.

SSDI beneficiaries also receive health care coverage in the form of Medicare, but only after a 24-month waiting period after starting SSDI. This waiting period puts a burden on those who do not have other forms of medical coverage.

The SSI program is a *means-tested* program (i.e., eligibility is determined by income and resources, in addition to demonstrating that the disability is severe enough to render the person unable to work for at least 12 months) and does not require prior FICA contributions to Social Security. The income test is established annually, adjusted for inflation. Each year, the SSA establishes the dollar figure for *substantial gainful activity* (SGA). Individuals who earn more than the SGA are not eligible for SSI. In 2007, the SGA for nonblind individuals with disabilities is $900 per month. Unearned income and resources also affect eligibility. The maximum amount an SSI recipient can receive monthly is called the *Federal Benefit Rate*, which is set annually (Barnett, Botrn, Katuin, Lanane, & Wong, 2005). In 2007 the amount for an individual is $623 per month. SSI recipients can work for pay without losing SSI eligibility, but the amount of SSI payments is reduced by both unearned and earned income. After certain exclusions, for every $2 in earned income, SSI payments are reduced by $1.

Individuals can qualify to receive both SSI and SSDI payments. In most (but not all) states, SSI recipients are automatically eligible for Medicaid. Some states also have state payments that are supplementary to SSI (Smith et al., 2005).

If an SSI recipient's income exceeds a certain level, he or she may be no longer eligible for SSI and consequently may be vulnerable to losing Medicaid benefits, which for some SSI recipients is more consequential than losing SSI payments. Section 1619B of the Social Security Act was designed to mitigate this disincentive to employment for SSI recipients. Section 1619B allows an individual who loses SSI eligibility because of earnings to continue to qualify for Medicaid if his or her "countable" annual income is below a threshold amount and the individual requires continuing medical coverage to maintain employment. The threshold amount is quite high in most states (e.g., $42,000 in California). Even though this provision of the Social Security Act has been available for more than two decades, it is not often used or even known by psychiatric rehabilitation practitioners.

The *Ticket to Work and Work Incentives Improvement Act of 1999* was legislation aimed at helping SSDI and SSI beneficiaries with disabilities to make informed choices about work. To accomplish this, the legislation created the *Benefits Planning, Assistance, and Outreach* (BPAO) program, which authorized the SSA to fund 116 BPAO projects throughout the United States. Located in community agencies (or in some cases within state or local government offices), these BPAO projects employed benefits specialists to provide work incentive planning and conduct outreach (*www.ssa.gov/work/ ServiceProviders/bpaofactsheet.html*). More recently, the BAAO program was renamed the Work Incentives Planning and Assistance (WIPA) program.

This legislation had other elements, as well, such as the creation of a "ticket" that SSA recipients could redeem to obtain vocational services from vocational rehabilitation providers in their community. To date, this aspect of the Ticket to Work legislation has had virtually no impact on those with psychiatric disabilities, probably because of the financial risks in participating that may be incurred by employment agencies (Rupp & Bell, 2003). According to the SSA, only 5,400 of the 9.5 million tickets issued have actually been used to access employment services (Aron, Burt, & Wittenburg, 2005).

The SSA has reason to be especially concerned about the impact of its policy on those with psychiatric disabilities, because this group is the single largest diagnostic group on the disability rolls (Kouzis & Eaton, 2000). In 1999, 34% of working-age adults receiving SSI and 27% of SSDI recipients had a psychiatric disability (McAlpine & Warner, 2000). Among SSDI/SSI recipients with psychiatric disabilities, fewer than 1% leave the disability rolls each year because of earned income exceeding eligibility criteria (Rupp & Scott, 1998). Moreover, not only are there more people with psychiatric disabilities on the disability rolls, but also, because they are generally younger and a higher proportion are female (and therefore have a longer life expectancy), they remain on rolls much longer than those with other disabilities (Aron et al., 2005; Rupp & Scott, 1996).

Housing

The Department of Housing and Urban Development (HUD) is the federal agency with the mission of increasing home/ownership, supporting community development, and increasing access to affordable housing. Congress first defined a federal role for public housing in the *U.S. Housing Act of 1937* during the height of the Depression. In 1965, HUD was elevated to a cabinet-level agency. HUD has funded construction of public housing and provided income subsidies to allow people to rent in the open housing market. Since its inception, more than 1.4 million housing units were constructed throughout the United States. In 1973, President Nixon declared a moratorium on housing and community development assistance. During the 1980s, the Reagan administration made huge cuts in federal housing subsidies for low-income groups (Youmans, 1992). In 1987, the *Stewart B. McKinney Act* authorized funding to help communities address homelessness. Congress appropriated $712 million in 1987 and 1988. Overall funding levels increased to a high of $1.49 billion in fiscal year 1995. Since that time funding has fluctuated. A 1996 amendment to the McKinney Act authorized the Shelter Plus Care program, which provides rental assistance and supportive services on a long-term basis for homeless persons with disabilities (including those with severe mental illness).

Protection against Discrimination

The Equal Employment Opportunity Commission (EEOC) is the federal agency responsible for enforcing antidiscrimination laws pertaining to employment. The federal legislation directly addressing individuals with psychiatric disabilities was the *Americans with Disabilities Act* (ADA) of 1990, which was aimed at eliminating discrimination on the basis of disability in five areas: employment, transportation, telecommunication, public accommodation, and the business of local and state governments. Its application in the workplace has important ramifications for consumers with mental illness. ADA regulations apply to employers with 15 or more employees. The ADA prohibits discrimination in all phases of employment, including the hiring process. It provides protection to "qualified individuals with disabilities," that is, individuals with disabilities who are qualified to perform the "essential functions" of an employment position. If an individual with a disability requires "reasonable accommodation" to perform the work, then employers covered under the ADA law are required to make this accommodation, provided that it does not cause "undue hardship," defined as an "action requiring significant difficulty or expense," determined on the basis of factors such as the cost of the accommodation and the employer's financial resources. Examples of psychiatric impairments requiring accommodation include difficulties in concentrating, dealing with stress, and interacting with other people. The ADA also makes it illegal during the preemployment process to ask any question about the nature or severity of a disability. So, for example, an employer cannot ask job applicants about their psychiatric history (Mancuso, 1995).

The ADA had a central role in a court case that some mental health advocates believe will ultimately have important implications for psychiatric rehabilitation. The *Olmstead case* refers to a Georgia lawsuit filed on behalf of two women with mental retardation and psychiatric disabilities who were inpatients in a state psychiatric hospital. Although hospital staff members all agreed that the women were ready for discharge, they remained hospitalized because no appropriate community placements were available. In 1999, the U.S. Supreme Court considered the case, which involved interpreting a regulation in the ADA, which states:

> A public entity shall administer services, programs, and activities in the most integrated setting appropriate to the needs of qualified individuals with disabilities. (28 C.F.R.§ 35.130(d))

The Court ruled that that the unnecessary segregation of individuals with disabilities in institutions may constitute discrimination based on disability. This decision has been interpreted as requiring the community placement of institutional residents when the state's own treating professionals have recommended such placement.

In addition to prohibiting discrimination in the workplace based on disability, federal law also prohibits discrimination in housing. Discrimination in housing is covered by the *Fair Housing Act*, which is Title VIII of the *Civil Rights Act of 1968*, which prohibits discrimination in the sale, rental, and financing of dwellings, based on a range of characteristics, including disability.

Finally, the *Protection and Advocacy for Mentally Ill Individuals Act of 1986* created an independent office in each state to investigate incidents of abuse and neglect of individuals with mental illness. Protection and Advocacy offices investigate violations of individual rights in community housing, such as board-and-care facilities, as well as violations in state psychiatric hospitals.

Court Cases and State Legislation Affecting Mental Health Treatment

In addition to the *Olmstead* case, there have been numerous court cases, and in some instances, state legislation, affecting the care of individuals with psychiatric disabilities. Often these cases have involved class action suits against the state mental health system on the grounds that the usual services are inadequate. For example, Washington and Denver are two cities that have been required under court order to institute reforms in their service systems. The cases described below are illustrative rather than a comprehensive review.

A landmark case, *Wyatt v. Stickney*, was a class action suit filed in 1970 against the Alabama SMHA (Anonymous, 2004). The lawsuit alleged that staff layoffs resulted in denial of treatment to a patient in violation of his civil rights. The U.S. District Court ruled that publicly committed patients had a constitutional right to receive treatment, and to deprive any citizen of his or her liberty would violate the fundamentals of "due process." Higher courts upheld this ruling on appeals. The significance of this case is that it established the right to treatment for persons with mental illness, along with minimal standards of treatment, within the context of a constitutional right.

Two important cases have dealt with the rights of incarcerated people with severe mental illness. In *Bowring v. Godwin* (1977), a federal appeals court ruled that a prisoner is entitled to psychological or psychiatric treatment if a health care provider concludes that the inmate has a serious mental disease and that, without treatment, he or she would suffer some harm (Hills, Siegfried, & Ickowitz, 2004). In a 2000 court case, *Brad H. v. City of New York*, the New York Supreme Court ruled that detainees with severe mental illness released from New York City jails had a right to discharge planning (Barr, 2003).

Some legislation has been passed in reaction to specific tragedies. A prominent example is the 1999 passage in New York of *Kendra's Law*, which created a mechanism for court-ordered assisted outpatient treatment to ensure that individuals with mental illness and a history of hospitalizations or violence receive intensive community-based services appropriate to their needs (New York Office of Mental Health, 2005). Kendra's Law was prompted by the death of a young woman who was pushed in front of a New York City subway train by a man with a history of mental illness and hospitalizations. Kendra's Law has been quite controversial. It has concretized the intense debate between proponents of consumer rights who argue for protection from coercion, and proponents of public safety who emphasize circumstances in which individuals are not capable of making rational decisions. One consequence of Kendra's Law for psychiatric rehabilitation is that it has been instrumental in increasing the number of intensive case management programs in New York.

Veterans Affairs

The Department of Veterans Affairs (commonly known as the VA) has a separate system of health care for military veterans, accessed by more than 650,000 veterans with psychiatric disabilities in 2004 (Rosenheck, 2005). Until a decade ago, the VA health care system was shameful: "dangerous, dirty, and scandal-ridden" (Longman, 2005). But that changed dramatically during the 1990s when the VA restructured the diffuse network of 172 hospitals and 132 nursing homes into 22 integrated systems, each responsible for providing integrated care. The VA also modernized its computer system, introducing effective electronic medical records and electronic decision support systems focusing on outcomes (Gaul, 2005).

Some of these changes have been reflected in improvement in psychiatric rehabilitation services. In years past, VA psychiatric rehabilitation services lagged behind their non-VA counterparts in terms of incorporating principles of recovery and emerging research. Recently, many of the innovations used outside the VA are finding their way into the VA. For example, in many VA hospitals, day treatment services based on the medical model are being converted to incorporate psychiatric rehabilitation principles. Initiatives are under way to increase peer services, for example, through *Vet-to-Vet* programs (Resnick et al., 2004). Changes are also under way in the primary VA program for vocational rehabilitation, *Compensated Work Therapy* (CWT), which historically involved set-aside jobs within VA hospitals (Drebing, Rosenheck, & Penk, 2001). A recent VA initiative has led to a plan for wide-scale adoption of evidence-based supported employment, with the goal of ensuring that all VA CWT programs will have staff dedicated to providing supported employment services (Anonymous, 2005). An adaptation of ACT known as *Mental Health Intensive Case Management* (formally known as Intensive Psychiatric Community Care) has been widely implemented throughout the VA (Rosenheck et al., 1995).

Federal Reports on Mental Health

Presidential leadership, or in some cases, lack of leadership, has played an important role in shaping mental health policy. In 1854, President Pierce vetoed the *Indigent Insane Bill* for fear that it would cost too much, and it took more than a century to return to the idea of a federal role in mental health care. In 1963, the CMHC Act would not have passed without President Kennedy's leadership. He took a personal interest because of his experience in growing up with a sister with mental retardation who was institutionalized for most of her life. President Carter was another strong mental health advocate, appointing his wife to head his President's Commission on Mental Health. This commission recommended increased mental health funding and major reforms, including priority given to vulnerable populations and the restructuring of federal mental health funding to the states (Cutler et al., 2003). President Reagan's view of a limited role for the federal government in social programs has been described above. During the Clinton administration, the influential Surgeon General's Report on Mental Health (U.S. Department of Health and Human Services, 1999) documented the fact that most individuals with severe mental illness failed to receive treatment congruent with widely accepted treatment recommendations (Lehman et al., 1998a). In 1999 mental health advocates were invited to a White House Conference at which President Clinton directed the Health Care Financing Administration (i.e., now CMS), to authorize ACT as a Medicaid-reimbursable treatment (News & Notes, 1999).

TABLE 21.2. Goals Identified by the President's New Freedom Commission on Mental Health

- *Goal 1.* Americans understand that mental health is essential to overall health.
- *Goal 2.* Mental health care is consumer and family driven.
- *Goal 3.* Disparities in mental health services are eliminated.
- *Goal 4.* Early mental health screening, assessment, and referral to services are common practice.
- *Goal 5.* Excellent mental health care is delivered and research is accelerated.
- *Goal 6.* Technology is used to access mental health care and information.

Because it is so recent, the impact of President Bush's New Freedom Commission on Mental Health (2003) report is uncertain. However, many observers have praised its emphasis on evidence-based practice (Azrin & Goldman, 2005) and its far-reaching vision. This report identified six broad goals for mental health system change, as shown in Table 21.2. These goals are congruent with the principles of psychiatric rehabilitation described throughout this book. In addition, the report specifically recommended that individuals with severe mental illness should have access to evidence-based practices. For example, the report recommended that supported employment should be made widely available, noting, "Every adult served in the mental health system and every young person with serious emotional disturbances making the transition from school to work must have access to supported employment services if they are to participate fully in society" (p. 48). Similarly, the report recommended making housing with supports widely available.

Fundamental questions regarding the role and responsibility of government at all levels in the provision of health care and social programs continue to be debated. Federal, state, and local elections, as well as appointments of federal judges, have a palpable impact on the character of the service system.

State and Local Roles in Psychiatric Rehabilitation

Although federal agencies and presidential commissions have had some impact on the general direction of psychiatric rehabilitation services, the state role in implementing policies is enormous. States have always varied greatly in their implementation of mental health policies, as suggested by a series of state-by-state surveys conducted during the 1980s (Torrey et al., 1990). The researchers concluded that a state's per capita spending for mental health, its geographic size, and its leadership were three factors influencing the quality of care. But even state-level analyses do not tell the full story. Hogan (1999) has noted a process of "devolution," which is "the transfer of responsibility for social programs (such as welfare) from the state and especially local governments" (p. 107), which has led to transferring responsibility for mental health care to county-level organizations in about half the states with three-fourths of the total population. The memorable phrase of Tip O'Neill, former U.S. Speaker of the House, "All politics are local," applies to community mental health services.

The SMHA is the agency responsible for providing leadership, setting priorities, and administering state funding for mental health services, although a number of other state agencies also have important roles in establishing and maintaining the quality of psychiatric rehabilitation services. Policies and actions taken by state Medicaid offices frequently have ramifications for mental health. As the Medicaid role has enlarged, the monitoring and regulatory role historically played by SMHAs has been shifting to state Medicaid offices (Frank et al., 2003). Unfortunately, "the dynamics of Medicaid's role in funding public mental health systems are complex, poorly understood, and frequently problematic" (Hogan, 1999, pp. 108–109). Clearly, whoever decides what services are funded and at what level, as well as the structure for funding these services (e.g., fee-for-service, cost reimbursement, milestone, etc.), has a major influence on the type of service system provided. Although sufficient funding does not ensure high-quality programs, the lack of sufficient funding for psychiatric services is a clear deterrent to providing full access to those services (Becker et al., 2006).

Historically, one reason for the central role of SMHAs in establishing psychiatric rehabilitation policy was that state dollars were the single largest source of funding for public mental health (Hogan, 1999). This situation has changed dramatically, as both the absolute dollar amounts and the proportion of state funds for mental health have diminished. One report concluded that funding administered by SMHAs declined 6% in real dollars between 1981 and 1997 (Kotler, 2002). The decline was explained by reductions in hospital expenditures, while state funding for community-based services actually increased. However, the major dramatic change in mental health financing has been the ever-increasing role of Medicaid. As compared with 1985, when Medicaid accounted for one-third of the funding for all state and locally administered mental health services, by 1997, Medicaid's share was more than half, according to a Center for Mental Health Services report (Kotler, 2002). Unless reversed (e.g., prompted by budget deficits in light of spending on the Gulf area reconstruction and military action), the proportion of mental health treatment paid for by Medicaid is expected to increase even further. A federal report on national expenditures for mental health services documents these trends (Mark et al., 2005). In 2001, the United States spent $85 billion on mental health treatment. An estimated $53.6 billion (63%) of the mental health treatment expenditures were by public sources, as follows: Medicaid (44%), Medicare (12%), other federal sources (7%), state and local sources (37%). Mental health expenditures grew from $49 billion in 1991 to $85 billion in 2001, a 3.7% annual growth (adjusted for inflation), as compared with 4.4% for health care overall. During this decade, the percentage paid by state and local governments for public mental health declined from 47% to 37%, and Medicaid increased in share from 33% to 44%. During this period there were dramatic changes as well in the allocation of funding for different treatment categories. There was a continuing shift away from inpatient expenditures, from 38% of total mental health expenditures in 1991 to 22% in 2001. In contrast, expenditures for prescription medications grew from 7% in 1991 to 21% in 2001. In fact, between 1991 and 2000, Medicaid expenditures for psychotropic drugs increased 12-fold, with even greater rates of increase for antidepressants and antipsychotics (Frank et al., 2003).

To be successful in shaping positive psychiatric rehabilitation policy, SMHAs must juggle the competing demands of complying with Medicaid regulations and meeting the expectations of state legislators. From the standpoint of promoting evidence-based psychiatric rehabilitation, the obvious general strategies are to reduce or eliminate funding for practices that are not evidence-based and to increase funding for those that are. Lynde (2005) describes the implementation of this strategy in one state as seen through the eyes of a frontline practitioner and CSP director. Unfortunately, in most states, Medicaid does not specifically cover most evidence-based psychiatric rehabilitation practices (Azrin & Goldman, 2005). Moreover, even when evidence-based services do qualify for Medicaid, provider agencies often do not understand how to bill Medicaid. At the local level, the fear of Medicaid audits can be a great deterrent to incorporating new practices into routine practice, even when these innovations are well established on a scientific basis.

Despite a potentially diminished role for SMHAs with the growth of Medicaid regulation, SMHA leadership continues to have a crucial role in the development of effective psychiatric rehabilitation services, as suggested by case studies (Moser et al., 2004; Rapp, Bond, Becker, Carpinello, Nikkel, et al., 2005). SMHAs have shown creativity in using Medicaid waivers to fund psychiatric rehabilitation programs, such as Minnesota's coverage of services for Living and Social Skills, Nebraska's Residential Services coverage, and Maine's coverage of in-home support (Smith et al., 2005).

These examples notwithstanding, given the categorical nature of Medicaid funding and the requirement for state dollars to be dedicated to ensuring a Medicaid match, SMHAs (and provider agencies) often do not have much flexibility in changing mental health policy. A small source of funding that SMHAs can use flexibly to effect change is block grant money (Azrin & Goldman, 2005).

Finally, a critical and salient characteristic of SMHAs is frequent turnover in leadership, prompted in part by gubernatorial elections. A 1991 report noted that the average tenure of an SMHA director was less than 2 years (Cohen, Shore, & Mazade, 1991), and it appears that this same instability in leadership continues to the present. Until 2007, Ohio was a noteworthy exception, with Mike Hogan as the longtime SMHA director. Only a handful of states have maintained stability in leadership that has made it possible to sustain momentum in state initiatives to develop community-based programs (Hogan, 1992).

ADVOCACY ORGANIZATIONS

National Association of State Mental Health Program Directors

As its name suggests, the National Association of State Mental Health Program Directors (NASMHPD) is an organization for SMHA leaders (*www.nasmhpd.org*). It was founded in 1959 and is based in Alexandria, Virginia. NASMHPD advocates for SMHAs at the federal level and disseminates information on issues regarding the delivery of high-quality mental health services, through various publications and two annual meetings. NASMHPD networks with other advocacy organizations and with federal agencies such as SAMHSA. In 2002, NASMHPD conducted a survey of all the SMHAs in the United States regarding the dissemination of evidence-based psychiatric rehabilitation practices (Ganju, 2003).

NAMI

Since its formation in 1979, NAMI (recently renamed the National Alliance on Mental Illness) has been a "grassroots, self-help, support and advocacy organization" for families of individuals with severe mental illness as well as consumers and other supporters (*www.nami.org*). With 1,200 local affiliates, NAMI has a membership exceeding 130,000. NAMI has persistently advocated for more federal money for research on mental illness. In particular, in the 1980s NAMI leaders concluded that NIMH would have more scientific credibility if it were part of the National Institutes of Health (NIH). Consequently, NAMI played a major role in lobbying for the shift of the NIMH to the NIH.

For the early part of its history, NAMI took the organizational position that it would not advocate for any specific psychiatric rehabilitation models. However, in a major reversal of this policy in the 1990s, NAMI embraced the Program for Assertive Community Treatment and became a major force in promoting the national dissemination of ACT. NAMI has an ACT technical assistance center disseminating information on the ACT model.

Another major function of NAMI has been its long-standing antistigma campaigns. NAMI has provided strong support to U.S. senators in the passage of legislation congruent with its agenda, such as parity in health insurance. NAMI also provides psychoeducation through its Family-to-Family program, which reports an annual graduation rate of 12,000, its peer-to-peer recovery education course, and more recently, a provider education program.

Consumer Advocacy Groups

Scores of national, state, and local consumer-run advocacy organizations dedicated to the recovery of individuals with severe mental illness have been developed since the 1980s (Chamberlin et al., 1989). One such group, the National Mental Health Consumers Association (NMHCA), was one of the most influential during the 1980s and 1990s (Frese et al., 2001). Its mission statement identified employment, housing, benefits, service choice, and the end of discrimination and abuse as primary issues.

Bazelon Center for Mental Health Law

The Bazelon Center for Mental Health Law (*www.bazelon.org/*) is an advocacy organization that disseminates information on mental health policy, particularly in the areas of housing and Medicaid.

United States Psychiatric Rehabilitation Association

The United States Psychiatric Rehabilitation Association (USPRA) is an organization for psychiatric rehabilitation agencies, practitioners, and others dedicated to promoting, supporting, and strengthening community-oriented rehabilitation services. In addition to its advocacy role, USPRA organizes an annual conference, disseminates technical reports, and provides education and certification of practitioners. USPRA was founded in 1975 and has a membership of almost 1,500 members (*www.uspra.org*). It was known as the International Association of Psychosocial Rehabilitation Services until 2003, when Canadian members formed their own separate organization.

POLICY BARRIERS
TO IMPLEMENTING PSYCHIATRIC REHABILITATION

The intricate set of federal, state, and local rules and policies affecting people with psychiatric disabilities are not, and have never been, perfectly aligned with the goal of providing high-quality, evidence-based services promoting the recovery of this population. Two recent federal reports (President's New Freedom Commission on Mental Health, 2003; U.S. Department of Health and Human Services, 1999) echo many themes found in federal reports dating back to the 1950s. Azrin and Goldman (2005) note "a discouragingly long list of rules, regulations, and policies that serve as barriers to implementation of

EBPs [evidence-based practices] in routine mental health care" (p. 77). They list four main barriers: lack of a trained work force, lack of financing, lack of a comprehensive research base on effective practices and on effective implementation, and a lack of an infrastructure to support dissemination. Other barriers they identify include short-term horizons for policy planning (a problem exacerbated by the relatively short tenures of SMHA directors) and competing priorities.

In this section we review some of the major policies that inhibit development of psychiatric rehabilitation in the United States. Some are specific to particular federal or state agencies, and others are broader in scope. Policy barriers include lack of access to health care, rehabilitation, housing, and other rehabilitation services; inadequate coverage for many who do have access; evidence-based psychiatric services that are often difficult to fund through existing funding systems; and fragmentation and lack of coordination between different governmental agencies. We discuss the policy barriers associated with each of the areas outlined above (mental health, vocational rehabilitation, disability income support and welfare, housing, and protection against discrimination).

Policy Barriers in Mental Health

A broad failing of the U.S. health care/rehabilitation system is the lack of universal coverage. This issue is, of course, broader than the issue of coverage for mental health care, with more than 40 million Americans without any health care coverage at all (Cutler et al., 2003). In principle, Medicaid and Medicare are the means for ensuring health care coverage for individuals who do not have private insurance, but there remains a large group of Americans with severe mental illness with neither Medicaid/Medicare nor private insurance. With respect to community mental health, one unfortunate unintended consequence of the growth of Medicaid has been the increasing allocation of state mental health dollars to the Medicaid match, thereby reducing the availability of state dollars to serve those not covered by Medicaid (Frank et al., 2003).

A second problem that is very apparent in the mental health arena concerns the artificial divisions in the funding and administration of services, even when integrated services are known to be more effective (see e.g., Cook et al., 2005). For example, in most states, the state administrative structures for financing, regulation, and licensing for treatment of addictions and for mental health services are completely separate, even though integrated treatment and rehabilitation is the most effective approach for individuals with co-occurring mental illness and substance use disorders (Drake et al., 2001a). Such divisions are seen between mental health and the areas of criminal justice, substance abuse treatment, vocational rehabilitation, and housing (as well as between each of these areas and the others).

A third problem has been the restrictions in funding for effective psychiatric rehabilitation services, given the current funding mechanisms (Mechanic, 2003). Because Medicaid has become the primary source of funding for mental health services, a key challenge for psychiatric rehabilitation programs is to ensure that the services provided are reimbursable under Medicaid. Assertive outreach, family interventions, and treatment team meetings are three key components of psychiatric rehabilitation practices for which, providers note, it is difficult to secure Medicaid reimbursement in a fee-for-service arrangement. Medicaid funding for supported employment—even for those service elements that advocates argue do fit the Medicaid service definitions—has been problematic. Conversely, day treatment has historically been handsomely reimbursed through Medicaid, even though it is not evidence-based.

Advocacy groups have taken the position that the Medicaid IMD exclusion has been discriminatory toward individuals with severe mental illness (NASMHPD, 2000). Because of the IMD exclusion, SMHAs have not pursued the Medicaid waiver program known as home and community-based services. The hope that the New Freedom Commission on Mental Health (2003) recommendations would prompt repeal of this exclusion has not yet been realized (NAMI E-News, 2002).

As noted above, many states have adopted managed care approaches to mental health care. This wide-scale shift is a potential opportunity for obtaining waivers to fund evidence-based practices as Indiana has done for ACT (Moser et al., 2004). But, clearly, managed care has been no panacea. In the 1990s a number of studies of managed behavioral health care were conducted, including studies in New York, Minnesota, Utah, Colorado, and Oregon (Bloom, Hu, Wallace, Cuffel, Hausman, et al., 2002; McFarland, 1994). Some of these studies used randomized controlled trials, increasing the credibility of the results. Nonetheless, the conclusions have been complicated and confusing, partly because so many different variations of managed care have been implemented (e.g., in regard to what organization is responsible for administering the health care program, whether mental health is part of general health care or "carved out," what the capitation rates are). A general finding is that managed behavioral health care usually has saved money, typically by shifting costs from inpatient to outpatient treatment (Frank et al., 2003). However, in some instances, psychiatric rehabilitation services have worsened under managed care, with Tennessee's system being a prime example (Chang, Kiser, Bailey, Martins, Gibson, et al., 1998). In other instances, managed care organizations have withdrawn from state contracts. Agencies offering psychiatric rehabilitation services have been required to make drastic changes in terminology, paperwork, and services provided (Jacobs & Moxley, 1993). Individuals with severe mental illness, especially those who are high-intensity service recipients, generally have not fared well under managed behavioral health care (Mechanic, 2003).

Because Medicaid spending involves both the federal budget and the state match, both levels of government have a stake controlling these costs. Even before Hurricane Katrina, rising Medicaid costs were of increasing concern as the federal government and many states faced large deficits. In August 2005, a federal commission charged with cutting Medicaid costs made a number of recommendations that would dramatically affect mental health services by changing the funding formulas for the MRO and for targeted case management (NAMI E-News, 2005). Also in August 2005, CMS denied Colorado's State Medicaid Plan Amendment, noting that Colorado's MRO plan was out of compliance with federal law, and that 35 other states were also out of compliance, apparently signaling a major shift in CMS policy. The implications of these actions are not yet known.

Many observers of the mental health financing systems are pessimistic. Mechanic (2003) summarizes the problems as follows:

> Barriers exist at all levels and are extraordinarily difficult to eliminate. Reimbursement often distorts behavior; the incentives are often wrong and counterproductive; professionals fight over turf; teams rarely work effectively together; and the relevant organizational structures are often bureaucratic and not accountable. Our chaotic overall health insurance framework simply adds to the confusion and dysfunctions. (p. 1231)

Policy Barriers in VR

Historically, even though VR is the federal agency responsible for vocational services for people with disabilities, federal funding for VR has never been sufficient to serve more than a tiny proportion (perhaps 5%) of the population in need (Wehman, 1988). Moreover, many observers have raised doubts about whether this funding has been used wisely. VR expenditures have been disproportionately devoted to administration and to assessment and other preemployment activities (Noble et al., 1997), and VR agencies continue to allocate minimal funding for supported employment services (Wehman & Kregel, 1995). Despite amendments to the Rehabilitation Act embracing supported employment, VR continued to approve funding for sheltered work up until the 2001 revision of the VR regulations. Prior to this change, VR funding continued to facilitate the maintenance of the status quo regarding sheltered workshop options, to the dismay of supported employment advocates (Mank, 1994; Wehman, Revell, & Brooke, 2003).

There have been a number of reports critical of VR, particularly regarding the lack of access to services by individuals with psychiatric disabilities. As evidence of this lack, a widely cited 1990 study found that consumers with psychiatric disabilities seeking VR services were half as likely as those with physical disabilities to obtain VR eligibility (Marshak et al., 1990). A more optimistic view was voiced in a recent article noting that RSA data from 2001 suggest recent improvements in the direction of a smaller discrepancy between cases of individuals with psychiatric disabilities and the total VR caseload, with respect to those closed without an employment outcome (32% vs. 25%, respectively) and closed without services (25% vs. 20%, respectively) (Farkas, Kilbury, McNulty, Wireman, Cochran, et al., 2005). Even today, however, state VR agencies are outcome-oriented, with VR counselors expected to achieve high rates of successful closures, which sometimes translates into negative attitudes toward individuals with psychiatric disabilities.

NAMI has been especially harsh in its criticism of VR in a 1997 report recommending that "vocational rehabilitation funds targeted for people with severe mental illnesses should be separated from state vocational rehabilitation programs" (Noble et al., 1997, p. 77). A subsequent NAMI survey noted the lack of access to supported employment and other evidence-based practices (Hall et al., 2003). The inadequacies of time-limited funding for people with severe disabilities have been noted for many years (U.S. General Accounting Office, 1993). The President's New Freedom Commission on Mental Health (2003) also expressed concern about access and the time-limited funding limitations of VR, as well as the limitations of Medicaid as a source of financing for employment services. This report recommended restructuring state and federal programs to pay for evidence-based practices, including supported employment.

Another pervasive barrier has been the fragmentation of services. As discussed in Chapter 9, VR has historically been partitioned off from mental health services, to the great detriment of consumers pursuing vocational goals (Drake et al., 2003a). The 1978 collaborative agreement between RSA and NIMH was a federal effort to address the problem of lack of coordination between mental health and VR agencies found widely at the federal, state, local, and program levels. The degree of cooperation and communication between these two worlds continues to vary widely at all levels. The evidence suggests that a close working relationship between VR and mental health fosters better employment outcomes (Drake et al., 1998a). A recent Johnson & Johnson initiative has demonstrated that a high degree of cooperation between mental health and VR at the state and local levels is feasible (Becker et al., 2006).

Of all the areas of federal policy, VR has had perhaps the most problematic relationship with psychiatric rehabilitation. In part, this emanates from the fact that employment is so central to the mission of psychiatric rehabilitation, making VR a natural source for both intellectual leadership and funding for psychiatric rehabilitation services. Philosophically, many of the core values of RSA are closely aligned with psychiatric rehabilitation: priority for those with the most severe disabilities, an emphasis on consumer choice, and an emphasis on outcomes. Other core principles from the VR perspective are decidedly not compatible: time-limited services and a narrow focus on rehabilitation to the exclusion of treatment. In addition, according to its critics, VR regulations and procedures have often handcuffed VR counselors and dismayed those who would seek help. For example, achieving VR eligibility may take a matter of weeks, yet sometimes vocational programs help applicants achieve employment in the interim. In some instances, achieving employment disqualifies an applicant for receiving VR assistance.

Policy Barriers Related to Social Security

The limitations of SSI and SSDI include the meager income beneficiaries receive under these programs. As discussed in Chapter 8, housing costs are often not affordable for individuals whose sole source of income is SSI (McCabe et al., 1993). The second major problem concerns the disincentives to returning to work for a person who is receiving SSI or SSDI (Averett, Warner, Little, & Huxley, 1999; Polak & Warner, 1996; Walls, Dowler, & Fullmer, 1990). An obvious disincentive is the reduction in SSI income if a person is employed. A second disincentive concerns the "implicit tax" in the form of lost subsidies in other areas (food stamps, housing subsidies, utility supplements, and transportation subsidies) (Polak & Warner, 1996). The greatest concern, however, is usually not the potential loss of disability income but rather the perception that medical benefits may be lost with the change in disability income status (MacDonald-Wilson, Rogers, Ellison, & Lyass, 2003). An added concern is the challenge of reinstatement if a consumer subsequently loses his or her job. SSA has recognized these disincentives (both those that are real and those based on misinformation) and appointed a task force to study such problems for SSDI recipients (Aron et al., 2005). The good news is that the provision of systematic, individualized benefits counseling leads to improved employment outcomes for consumers with severe mental illness (Tremblay, Smith, Xie, & Drake, 2004).

Disability income support poses a challenge to individuals in their recovery process. To qualify for SSI or SSDI, consumers must attest to their disability, inability to work, and need for financial support. The double message of these requirements has been oft noted.

Policy Barriers Related to Housing

During the Johnson administration in the late 1960s, the federal government made a strong commitment to public housing, but this approach was severely curtailed during the Reagan administration (Youmans, 1992). The main barrier in the housing area is a lack of federal commitment to funding Section 8 certificates (housing subsidies, described in Chapter 8) and other programs that address the poverty associated with psychiatric disabilities. Although it is now well established that providing Section 8 vouchers is an effective way to get people housed (Hurlburt et al., 1996), the waiting lists for such vouchers is 5 years or more in most communities, essentially eliminating them as a viable solution to housing problems.

As discussed in Chapter 8, adequate housing is an essential requirement for recovery. At present, governmental response to this need is inadequate in most communities.

Policy Barriers Related to Discrimination Protection

Although the ADA is rightfully regarded as important legislation for combating discrimination, any legislation is only as useful as its actual enforcement. As mentioned earlier, the ADA was cited in the *Olmstead* decision, which has promised to improve services in Georgia, as well as in other states. If we look at the ADA in terms of application in individual cases, the picture is unclear. During the first 6 years after the ADA was enacted, a total of 145,000 discrimination cases were filed with the EEOC or local Fair Employment Practice Agencies (Moss, Ullman, Starrett, Burris, & Johnsen, 1999). Only 377 (0.3%) involved individuals with schizophrenia. Moreover, only a small proportion of all cases resulted in benefits (e.g., financial compensation) or a finding of reasonable cause. On the basis of more recent data, this research group further concluded that "claimants with psychiatric disabilities were also significantly less likely to benefit from their claims" (Ullman, Johnsen, Moss, & Burris, 2001, p. 644). This low rate of enforcement, however, does not measure the indirect impact of the ADA, in the form of compliance to avoid legal action.

Another indicator of the impact of the ADA is the extent to which clients receive reasonable accommodations. A 1994 survey examining the effects of the ADA found that respondents with psychiatric disabilities were less likely than people with other disabilities to report receiving such accommodations (Zwerling, Whitten, Sprince, Davis, Wallace, et al., 2003). Nonetheless, some observers believe that the ADA's impact on job retention through reasonable accommodation appears greater than its impact on job acquisition (J. Marrone, personal communication, October 8, 2005).

A provocative analysis of the impact of the ADA on employment rates for individuals with disabilities examined employment trends before and after the ADA went into effect (Acemoglu & Angrist, 2001). The authors found a sharp decrease in employment rates for individuals with disabilities that could not be explained by other causes. Moreover, this decline was larger for medium-sized companies than for small firms, consistent with the target of ADA enforcement. In addition, the decline in employment rates among individuals with disabilities was larger in states with more ADA-related discrimination charges.

In sum, the impact of the ADA is unclear. The full implications may take years to realize, and during this time further refinement of the regulations may occur. The broader question is the degree to which societal attitudes and behaviors can be influenced through legislation. In the 1960s, leaders of the civil rights movement held that societal mores could be changed though laws and through determined advocacy. For people with severe mental illness, these strategies have been adopted at a modest level of commitment, with mixed results (J. Marrone, personal communication, October 8, 2005).

Strategies to Overcome Policy Barriers

Although we have cataloged a long list of formidable policy barriers to implementing evidence-based psychiatric rehabilitation practices in routine settings, it is also true that SMHAs and other groups described in this chapter have made strides in overcoming them. States that have made progress typically have had a long-term commitment and vision that included strategic planning, stakeholder involvement, and a focus on outcomes that consumers value (Rapp et al., 2005). Some of the specific strategies used by SMHAs include encouraging academic institutions to train students in the competencies needed for the psychiatric rehabilitation field (Hoge et al., 2005), promoting collaboration between various state agencies responsible for psychiatric rehabilitation, such as mental health and VR (Becker et al., 2006), providing incentives for achieving improved consumer outcomes (Rapp, Huff, & Hansen, 2003), aligning policies and regulations to be compatible with evidence-based practice (Rapp et al., 2005), defining standards and certifying programs meeting these standards (Moser et al., 2004), and funding technical assistance centers to provide training and consultation to agencies implementing evidence-based practices (Moser et al., 2004).

COSTS OF PSYCHIATRIC REHABILITATION SERVICES

Throughout this chapter we have emphasized the role of financing as an influence on psychiatric rehabilitation practice. Therefore, a fundamental question is, what do these services cost? And further, what is their cost-effectiveness? Answers to both of these basic questions are very difficult to find. Certainly, costs of services are variable, depending on what service components are included in the estimates, as well as local economic conditions, including wage scales for mental health professionals, costs of housing, and other obvious factors.

A step toward answering the question of costs is to examine typical costs for specific psychiatric rehabilitation services. According to Phillips and Burns (2002), a ballpark figure for ACT program costs is $9,000 to $12,000 per year per person, but estimates depend heavily on the extent to which the multidisciplinary team concept is followed, as well as salary scales within a community. A detailed template for estimating the costs of ACT in a given community has been developed (Lewin Group, 2001).

A 2004 multistate study estimated the average annual agency cost for high-fidelity supported employment services (excluding mental health treatment costs) to be $2,500 per client (Latimer et al., 2004). As is common in such studies, the cost estimates varied widely; the primary determinant of cost was caseload size. From the standpoint of VR expenditures, the cost of supported employment services is relatively modest. According to an RSA database for 2003, which included more than 100,000 clients with mental illness, the mean cost per VR case closure was $1,775 per client with mental illness (as compared with a mean cost for all VR clients of $2,161), whereas the corresponding costs for successful case closures was $3,502 for 31,000 clients with mental illness (as compared with a mean cost for all VR clients of $4,008) (Institute for Community Inclusion, 2005). VR costs, however, are short-term expenses, so these figures do not include long-term follow-along expenditures, which in some instances are funded through Medicaid.

SUMMARY AND CONCLUSIONS

This chapter has described policies and regulations at the state and federal levels influencing the development of psychiatric rehabilitation services. In some cases, policies do in fact promote psychiatric rehabilitation practices; in other cases, the policies are relatively neutral, but with ingenuity can be used to promote psychiatric rehabilitation. In still other cases, psychiatric rehabilitation programs have been implemented despite policies that are in opposition to their promotion. Some legislation, such as the ADA and the Workforce Investment Act, has not achieved the benefits for individuals with severe mental illness intended by those who worked for its passage. Other legislation has had unintended negative consequences, such as the disincentives apparent in SSI and SSDI. Unfortunately, governmental policies and inaction also have often encouraged practices that do not facilitate the recovery of individuals with severe mental illness, for example, when they have fostered institutionalized care, indifference to homelessness and incarceration, episodic clinic-based treatment, brokered case management, day treatment, and sheltered work.

At the federal level, a historical review of policy affecting psychiatric rehabilitation mirrors a broader debate between conservative and liberal viewpoints regarding the role of government in providing welfare, health care, housing subsidies, rehabilitation, and other social programs that directly affect individuals with severe mental illness.

An obvious conclusion is the need to change many policies to make them more congruent with evidence-based psychiatric rehabilitation. Clearly, this is often a difficult path, especially in the case of major legislation, such as Medicaid and Social Security, in which there are many stakeholders, of which people with mental illness are a small group, or at least perceived as such.

Interestingly, it is often not the actual policies that have been barriers to implementing evidence-based psychiatric rehabilitation, but rather the implementation of policies. For example, in the area of VR services, VR counselors could in theory be key allies in implementing all of the principles of supported employment, including zero exclusion, focus on competitive employment, and long-term support. The actual VR regulations make provision for tremendous flexibility, and the language of the Rehabilitation Act strongly advocates consumer choice. Yet, at the individual counselor level, a host of factors strongly influence the day-to-day decision making: state directives regarding substance abuse, limited funds, personal experiences with mental health practitioners and with consumers, and pressures to increase one's closure rates—and these factors weigh more heavily than the broader evidence-based principles that are implied in the actual policies.

References

Abram, K., & Teplin, L. (1991). Co-occurring disorders among mentally ill detainees: Implications for public policy. *American Psychologist, 46*, 1036–1045.

Abramowitz, I., & Coursey, R. (1989). Impact of an educational support group on family participants who take care of their schizophrenic relatives. *Journal of Counseling and Clinical Psychology, 57*, 632–636.

Abramson, M. F. (1972). The criminalization of mentally disordered behavior: Possible side-effects of a mental health law. *Hospital and Community Psychiatry, 23*, 101–105.

Acemoglu, D., & Angrist, J. (2001). Consequences of employment protection? The case of the Americans with Disabilities Act. *Journal of Political Economy, 109*, 915–957.

Adams, J. R., & Drake, R. E. (2006). Shared decision making and evidence-based practice. *Community Mental Health Journal, 42*, 87–105.

Adams, N., & Grieder, D. (2004). *Treatment planning for person-centered care: The road to mental health and addiction recovery.* Amsterdam: Elsevier Academic Press.

Addington, J., & Addington, D. (1993). Premorbid functioning, cognitive functioning, symptoms and outcome in schizophrenia. *Journal of Psychiatry and Neuroscience, 18*, 19–23.

Addington, J., & Addington, D. (1999). Neurocognitive and social functions of schizophrenia. *Schizophrenia Bulletin, 25*, 173–182.

Afrank, J. S. (1999). Lesbian identity management in the workplace. Unpublished doctoral dissertation, Wichita State University, Wichita, Kansas.

Aguilera, R., Anderson, A., Gabire, E., Merlo, M., Paredes, T., & Pastrana, R. (1999). A clinical impact evaluation of integrated and disease specific substance abuse program models in Honduras. *Psychiatric Services, 3*, 97–167.

Ajzen, I., & Fishbein, M. (1980). *Understanding attitudes and predicting social behavior.* Englewood Cliffs, NJ: Prentice-Hall.

Alegría, M., Canino, G., Rios, R., Vera, M., Calderon, J., Rusch, D., et al. (2002). Inequalities in use of specialty mental health services among Latinos, African Americans, and non-Latino whites. *Psychiatric Services, 53*, 1547–1555.

Allebeck, P. (1989). Schizophrenia: A life-threatening disease. *Schizophrenia Bulletin, 15*, 81–89.

Allison, D. B., Mentore, J. L., & Heo, M. (1999). Antipsychotic-induced weight gain: A comprehensive research synthesis. *American Journal of Psychiatry, 156*, 1686–1696.

Allport, G. W. (1954). *The nature of prejudice.* Cambridge, MA: Addison-Wesley.

Allport, G. W. (1979). *The nature of prejudice.* New York: Doubleday Anchor Books.

Alverson, H., Alverson, M., & Drake, R. E. (2000). An ethnographic study of the longitudinal course of substance abuse among people with servere mental illness. *Community Mental Health Journal, 36,* 557–569.

Alverson, H., & Vicente, E. (1998). An ethnographic study of vocational rehabilitation for Puerto Rican Americans with severe mental illness. *Psychiatric Rehabilitation Journal, 22*(1), 69–72.

Amador, X. F., & David, A. S. (Eds.). (1998). *Insight and psychosis.* Oxford, UK: Oxford University Press.

Amador, X. F., Flaum, M., Andreasen, N. C., Strauss, D. H., Yale, S. A., Clark, S., et al. (1994). Awareness of illness in schizophrenia and schizoaffective and mood disorders. *Archives of General Psychiatry, 51*(10), 826–836.

Amador, X. F., Strauss, D. H., Yale, S. A., Flaum, M. M., Endicott, J., & Gorman, J. M. (1993). Assessment of insight in psychosis. *American Journal of Psychiatry, 150*(6), 873–879.

Amador, X. F., Strauss, D., Yale, S., & Gorman, J. M. (1991). Awareness of illness in schizophrenia. *Schizophrenia Bulletin, 17,* 113–132.

American Diabetes Association, American Psychiatric Association, American Association of Clinical Endocrinologists, & North American Association for the Study of Obesity. (2004). Consensus development conference on antipsychotic drugs and obesity and diabetes. *Diabetes Care, 27,* 596–601.

American Psychiatric Association. (1987). *Diagnostic and statistical manual of mental disorders* (3rd ed., rev.). Washington, DC: Author.

American Psychiatric Association. (1994). *Diagnostic and statistical manual of mental disorders* (4th ed.). Washington, DC: Author.

American Psychiatric Association. (1997). Practice guidelines for the treatment of patients with schizophrenia. *American Journal of Psychiatry, 154*(Suppl.), 1–63.

American Psychiatric Association. (2000). *Diagnostic and statistical manual of mental disorders* (4th ed., text rev.). Washington, DC: Author.

American Psychological Association. (1989). *Psychiatric services in jails and prisons.* Washington, DC: American Psychological Association.

Anderson, A. (1999). Comparative impact evaluation of two therapeutic programs for mentally ill chemical abusers. *International Journal of Psychosocial Rehabilitation, 4,* 11–26.

Anderson, C. M., Reiss, D. J., & Hogarty, G. E. (1986). *Schizophrenia and the family.* New York: Guilford Press.

Anderson, S. B. (1998). *We are not alone: Fountain House and the development of the Clubhouse culture.* New York: Fountain House.

Andreasen, N. C. (1984). *Modified Scale for the Assessment of Negative Symptoms.* Bethesda, MD: U.S. Department of Health and Human Services.

Andreasen, N. C., Flaum, M., & Arndt, S. (1992). The Comprehensive Assessment of Symptoms and History (CASH): An instrument for assessing diagnosis and psychopathology. *Archives of General Psychiatry, 48,* 615–623.

Andreasen, N. C., Flaum, M., Swayze, V. W., Tyrrell, G., & Arndt, S. (1990). Positive and negative symptoms in schizophrenia: A critical reappraisal. *Archives of General Psychiatry, 47*(7), 615–621.

Andreasen, N. C., & Olsen, S. A. (1982). Negative v. positive schizophrenia: Definition and validation. *Archives of General Psychiatry, 39*(7), 789–794.

Andrews, H., Barker, J., Pittman, J., Mars, L., Struening, E., & LaRocca, N. (1992). National trends in vocational rehabilitation: A comparison of individuals with physical disabilities and individuals with psychiatric disabilities. *Journal of Rehabilitation, 58,* 7–16.

Angell, B. (2003). Contexts of social relationship development among assertive community treatment clients. *Mental Health Services Research, 5,* 13–25.

Angermeyer, M. C., & Kuehn, L. (1988). Gender differences in age at onset of schizophrenia: An overview. *European Archives of Psychiatry and Clinical Neuroscience, 237*(6), 351–364.

Angermeyer, M. C., & Matschinger, H. (2003). The stigma of mental illness: Effects of labelling on public attitudes towards people with mental disorder. *Acta Psychiatrica Scandinavica, 108,* 304–309.

Angst, J., Gamma, A., Bennazzi, F., Ajdacic, V., Eich, D., & Rossler, W. (2003). Toward a redefinition of subthreshold bipolarity: Epidemiology and proposed criteria for bipolar-II, minor bipolar disorders and hypomania. *Journal of Affective Disorder, 73,* 133–146.

Anonymous. (2004). Historic *Wyatt* case ends. *Central Office Outlook,* First Quarter FY-04, 1–3.

Anonymous. (2005). Federal partner spotlight: U.S. Department of Veterans Affairs. *Mental Health Transformation Trends, 1*(2), 4.

Anthony, W. A. (1977). Psychological rehabilitation: A concept in need of a method. *American Psychologist, 32,* 658–662.

Anthony, W. A. (1982). Explaining "psychiatric rehabilitation" by an analogy to "physical rehabilitation." *Psychosocial Rehabilitation Journal, 5*(1), 61–65.

Anthony, W. A. (1993). Recovery from mental illness: The guiding vision of the mental health service system in the 1990s. *Psychosocial Rehabilitation Journal, 16*(4), 11–23.

Anthony, W. A. (1994). Whither the "Boston University model"? *Psychosocial Rehabilitation Journal, 17*(4), 169–170.

Anthony, W. A., & Blanch, A. (1989). Research on community support services: What have we learned? *Psychosocial Rehabilitation Journal, 12*(3), 55–81.

Anthony, W. A., Buell, G. J., Sharratt, S., & Althoff, M. E. (1972). The efficacy of psychiatric rehabilitation. *Psychological Bulletin, 78,* 447–456.

Anthony, W. A., Cohen, M. R., & Farkas, M. D. (1982). A psychiatric rehabilitation program: Can I recognize one when I see one? *Community Mental Health Journal, 18,* 83–96.

Anthony, W. A., Cohen, M., Farkas, M. D., & Gagne, C. (2002). *Psychiatric rehabilitation* (2nd ed.). Boston: Center for Psychiatric Rehabilitation.

Anthony, W., Forbess, R., & Cohen, M. (1993). Rehabilitation-oriented case management. In M. Harris & H. Bergman (Eds.), *Case management for mentally ill patients: Theory and practice* (pp. 99–118). Langhorne, PA. Harwood Academic Publishers.

Anthony, W. A., & Liberman, R. P. (1986). The practice of psychiatric rehabilitation. *Schizophrenia Bulletin, 12,* 542–559.

Anthony, W. A., & Liberman, R. P. (1992). Principles and practice of psychiatric rehabilitation. In R. P. Liberman (Ed.), *Handbook of psychiatric rehabilitation* (pp. 1–29). New York: Macmillan.

Applebaum, P. S. (1994). *Almost a revolution: Mental health law and the limits of change.* New York: Oxford University Press.

Appelbaum, P. S., Grisso, T., Frank, E., O'Donnell, S., & Kupfer, D. J. (1999). Competence of depressed patients for consent to research. *American Journal of Psychiatry, 156,* 1380–1384.

Appleby, L., & Desai, P. (1987). Residential instability: A perspective on system imbalance. *American Journal of Orthopsychiatry, 57,* 515–524.

Arata, C. M. (2002). Child sexual abuse and sexual revictimization. *Clinical Psychology: Science and Practice, 9,* 135–164.

Arboleda-Florez, J. (1998). Mental illness and violence: An epidemiological appraisal of the evidence. *Canadian Journal of Psychiatry, 43,* 989–996.

Arboleda-Florez, J., Holley, H., & Crisanti, A. (1998). Understanding causal paths between mental illness and violence. *Social Psychiatry and Psychiatric Epidemiology, 33,* S38–S46.

Arns, P. G., & Linney, J. A. (1993). Work, self, and life satisfaction for persons with severe and persistent mental disorders. *Psychosocial Rehabilitation Journal, 17,* 63–79.

Arns, P. G., & Linney, J. A. (1995). Relating functional skills of severely mentally ill clients to subjective and societal benefits. *Psychiatric Services, 46,* 260–265.

Aron, L. Y., Burt, M. R., & Wittenburg, D. (2005). *Recommendations to the Social Security Administration on the design of the mental health treatment study.* Washington, DC: Urban Institute.

Arseneault, L., Moffitt, T. E., Caspi, A., Taylor, P. J., & Silva, P. A. (2000). Mental disorders and violence in a total birth cohort. *Archives of General Psychiatry, 57,* 979–986.

Åsberg, M., Montgomery, S. A., Perris, C., Schalling, D., & Sedvall, G. (1978). A comprehensive psychopathological rating scale. *Acta Psychiatrica Scandanavia* (Suppl. 271), *58,* 5–27.

Ascher-Svanum, H., & Krause, A. A. (1991). *Psychoeducational groups for patients with schizophrenia: A guide for practitioners.* Gaithersburg, MD: Aspen.

Ascher-Svanum, H., Lafuze, J., Barrickman, P., Van Dusen, C., Fompa-Loy, J., et al. (1997). Education needs of families of mentally ill adults. *Psychiatric Services, 48,* 1072–1074.

ASPE Research Notes. (1993). *Licensed board and care homes: Preliminary findings from the 1991 National Health Provider Inventory.* Office of the Assistant Secretary for Planning and Evaluation. Retrieved July 17, 2005, from *aspe.hhs.gov/daltcp/reports/rn06.htm.*

Atkinson, J. M., Coia, D. A., Gilmour, W. H., & Harper, J. P. (1996). The impact of education groups for people with schizophrenia on social functioning and quality of life. *British Journal of Psychiatry, 168,* 199–204.

Atkinson, R. C., & Shiffrin, R. M. (1968). Human memory: A proposed system and its control processes. In K. W. Spence & J. T. Spence (Eds.), *The Psychology of Learning and Motivation* (Vol. 2, pp. 89–195). New York: Academic Press.

Atkinson, S. (1994). Grieving and loss in parents with a schizophrenic child. *American Journal of Psychiatry, 151,* 1137–1139.

Aubrey, T., Cousins, B., LaFerriere, D., & Wexler, A. (2003). *Evaluation of concurrent disorders group treatment program: Outcome evaluation report*. Ottawa: Center for Research on Community Services, Faculty of Social Sciences, University of Ottawa.

Augoustinos, M., Ahrens, C., & Innes, J. (1994). Stereotypes and prejudice: The Australian experience. *British Journal of Social Psychology, 33,* 125–141.

Averbach, E., & Coriell, A. S. (1961). Short-term memory in vision. *Bell Systems Technical Journal, 40,* 309–328.

Averett, S., Warner, R., Little, J., & Huxley, P. (1999). Labor supply, disability benefits and mental illness. *Eastern Economic Journal, 25,* 279–288.

Aviram, U., & Segal, S. P. (1973). Exclusion of the mentally ill: Reflection on an old problem in a new context. *Archives of General Psychiatry, 29,* 126–131.

Axelrod, S., & Wetzler, S. (1989). Factors associated with better compliance with psychiatric aftercare. *Hospital and Community Psychiatry, 40,* 397–401.

Axelson, G., & Wahl, O. (1992). Psychotic versus non-psychotic misdemeanants in a county jail: An analysis of pre-trial treatment by the legal system. *International Journal of Law and Psychiatry, 15,* 379–386.

Ayanian, J. Z., & Epstein, A. M. (1991). Differences in the use of procedures between women and men hospitalized for coronary heart disease. *New England Journal of Medicine, 325,* 221–225.

Ayanian, J. Z., Udvarhelyi, I. S., Gatsonis, C. A., Pashos, C. L., & Epstein, A. M. (1993). Racial differences in the use of revascularization procedures after coronary angiography. *Journal of the American Medical Association, 269,* 2642–2646.

Ayllon, T., & Azrin, N. H. (1968). *The token economy: A motivational system for therapy and rehabilitation.* New York: Appleton-Century-Crofts.

Azrin, N. H., & Teichner, G. (1998). Evaluation of an instructional program for improving medication compliance for chronically mentally ill outpatients. *Behaviour Research and Therapy, 36,* 849–861.

Azrin, S. T., & Goldman, H. H. (2005). Evidence-based practice emerges. In R. E. Drake, M. R. Merrens, & D. W. Lynde (Eds.), *Evidence-based mental health practice* (pp. 67–93). New York: Norton.

Babor, T. F., De La Fuente, J. R., Saunders, J., & Grant, M. (1989). *The Alcohol Use Disorders Identification Test: Guidelines for use in primary health care.* Paper presented at the World Health Organization, Geneva.

Bachrach, L. L. (1988). The chronic patient: On exporting and importing model programs. *Hospital and Community Psychiatry, 39,* 1257–1258.

Bachrach, L. L. (1989). Case management: Toward a shared definition. *Hospital and Community Psychiatry, 40,* 883–884.

Bachrach, L. L. (1992). Psychosocial rehabilitation and psychiatry in the care of long-term patients. *American Journal of Psychiatry, 149,* 1455–1463.

Bailey, E., Ricketts, S., Becker, D. R., Xie, H., & Drake, R. E. (1998). Conversion of day treatment to supported employment: One-year outcomes. *Psychiatric Rehabilitation Journal, 22,* 24–29.

Baker, A., Lewin, T., Reichler, H., Clancy, R., Carr, V., Garrett, R., et al. (2002). Motivational interviewing among psychiatric in-patients with substance use disorders. *Acta Psychiatrica Scandinavica, 106,* 233–240.

Baker, A. W., & Duncan, S. P. (1985). Child sexual abuse: A study of prevalence in Great Britain. *Child Abuse and Neglect, 9,* 457–467.

Baker, F., & Intagliata, J. (1992). Case management. In R. P. Liberman (Ed.), *Handbook of psychiatric rehabilitation* (pp. 213–244). Boston: Allyn & Bacon.

Baldessarini, R. J., Tondo, L., & Hennen, J. (2003). Lithium treatment and suicide risk in major affective disorders: Update and new findings. *Journal of Clinical Psychiatry, 64*(Suppl. 5), 44–52.

Balint, M. (1957). *The doctor, the patient, and his illness.* London: Tavistock.

Bandura, A. (1969). *Principles of behavior modification.* New York: Holt, Rinehart and Winston.

Bandura, A. (1977). Self-efficacy: Toward a unifying theory of behavioral change. *Psychological Review, 84,* 191–215.

Bandura, A. (1989). Regulation of cognitive processes through perceived self-efficacy. *Developmental Psychology, 25,* 729–735.

Banks, S., McHugo, G. J., Williams, V., Drake, R. E., & Shinn, M. (2002). A prospective meta-analytic approach to a multisite study of homelessness prevention. In J. M. Herrell & R. B. Straw (Eds.), *New directions for evaluation* (Vol. 94, pp. 45–59). San Francisco: Jossey-Bass.

Barbee, J. G., Clark, P. D., Craqanzano, M. S., Heintz, G. C., & Kehoe, C. E. (1989). Alcohol and substance abuse among schizophrenic patients presenting to an emergency service. *Journal of Nervous and Mental Disease, 177,* 400–407.

Barker, S., Barron, N., & McFarlane, B. (1994). *Multnomah Community Ability Scale: Users manual*. Portland, OR: Western Mental Health Research Center, Oregon Health Sciences University.

Barlow, D. H. (2002). *Anxiety and its disorders: The nature and treatment of anxiety and panic* (2nd ed.). New York: Guilford Press.

Barlow, K., Grenyer, B., & Ilkiw-Lavalle, O. (2000). Prevalence and precipitants of aggression in psychiatric inpatient units. *Australian and New Zealand Journal of Psychiatry, 34*, 967–974.

Barnett, B., Born, D., Katuin, C. H., Lanane, C. T. S., & Wong, L. (2005). *Work, benefits, and you*. Anderson, IN: Supported Employment Consultation and Training Center.

Barnett, G. O., & Winickoff, R. N. (1980). Quality assurance and computer-based patient records. *American Journal of Public Health, 80*, 527–528.

Barofsky, I. (1978). Compliance, adherence, and the therapeutic alliance: Steps in the development of self-care. *Social Science and Medicine, 12*, 369–376.

Baronet, A. M. (1999). Factors associated with caregiver burden in mental illness: A critical review of the research literature. *Clinical Psychology Review, 19*, 819–841.

Baronet, A. M., & Gerber, G. (1998). Psychiatric rehabilitation: Efficacy of four models. *Clinical Psychology Review, 18*, 189–228.

Barr, H. (2003). Transitional institutionalization in the courts: *Brad H. v. the City of New York* and the fight for discharge planning for people with psychiatric disabilities leaving Rikers Island. *Crime and Delinquency, 49*, 97–123.

Barrio, C. (2000). The cultural relevance of community support programs. *Psychiatric Services, 51*, 879–884.

Barrio, C., Yamada, A. M., Hough, R. L., Hawthorne, W., Garcia, P., & Jeste, D. V. (2003). Ethnic disparities in use of public mental health case management services among patients with schizophrenia. *Psychiatric Services, 54*, 1264–1270.

Barrowclough, C., Haddock, G., Tarrier, N., Lewis, S. W., Moring, J., O'Brien, R., et al. (2001). Randomized controlled trial of motivational interviewing, cognitive behavior therapy, and family intervention for patients with comorbid schizophrenia and substance use disorders. *American Journal of Psychiatry, 158*, 1706–1713.

Barrowclough, C., & Hooley, J. (2003). Attributions and expressed emotion: A review. *Clinical Psychology Review, 23*, 849–880.

Barrowclough, C., Johnston, M., & Tarrier, N. (1994). Attributions, expressed emotion, and

patient relapse: An attributional model of relatives' response to schizophrenic illness. *Behavior Therapy, 25*, 67–88.

Barrowclough, C., & Tarrier, N. (1990). Social functioning in schizophrenic patients: I. The effects of expressed emotion and family intervention. *Social Psychiatry and Psychiatric Epidemiology, 25*, 125–129.

Barrowclough, C., & Tarrier, N. (1992). *Families of schizophrenic patients: Cognitive behavioural intervention*. London: Chapman & Hall.

Barrowclough, C., & Tarrier, N. (1998). Social functioning and family interventions. In K. T. Mueser & N. Tarrier (Eds.), *Handbook of social functioning in schizophrenia* (pp. 327–341). Boston: Allyn & Bacon.

Barry, D. T., & Grilo, C. M. (2002). Cultural, psychological, and demographic correlates of willingness to use psychological services among East Asian immigrants. *Journal of Nervous and Mental Disease, 190*, 32–39.

Bartels, S. J. (2004). Caring for the whole person: Integrated health care for older adults with severe mental illness and medical comorbidity. *Journal of the American Geriatric Society, 52*, S249–S257.

Bartels, S. J., Drake, R. E., & McHugo, G. (1992). Alcohol abuse, depression, and suicidal behavior in schizophrenia. *American Journal of Psychiatry, 149*, 394–395.

Bartels, S. J., Forester, B., Mueser, K. T., Dums, A. R., Pratt, S. I., Sengupta, A., et al. (2004). Enhanced skills training and health care management for older persons with severe mental illness. *Community Mental Health Journal, 40*, 75–90.

Barton, R., Steiner, L., & Giffort, D. (2001). Competency development in a statewide initiative to implement psychiatric rehabilitation (PSR) services: Mechanisms and choices. *Psychiatric Rehabilitation Skills, 5*, 290–320.

Basco, M. R., & Rush, A. J. (2005). *Cognitive-behavioral therapy for bipolar disorder* (2nd ed.). New York: Guilford Press.

Basto, P. M., Pratt, C. W., Gill, K. J., & Barrett, N. M. (2000). The organizational assimilation of consumer providers: A quantitative examination [Special issue]. Employment programs for persons with serious mental illness. *Psychiatric Rehabilitation Skills, 4*(1), 105–119.

Battaglino, L. (1987). Family empowerment through self-help groups. In A. Hatfield (Ed.), *Families of the mentally ill meeting the challenges* (pp. 43–51). San Francisco: Jossey-Bass.

Baucom, D., Meuser, K., Shoham, U., Daiuto, A., & Stickle, T. (1998). Empirically supported couple and family interventions for marital distress and adult mental health problems. *Journal of Counseling and Clinical Psychology, 66,* 53–88.

Baxter, D. N. (1996). The mortality experience of individuals on the Salford case register: I. All-cause mortality. *British Journal of Psychiatry, 168,* 772–779.

Bazelon Center. (1999). Available at *www.bazelon .org/issues/disability rights/resources/olmstead/.*

Beach, M. C., Price, E. G., Gary, T. L., Robinson, K. A., Gozu, A., Palacio, A., et al. (2005). Cultural competence: A systematic review of health care provider educational interventions. *Medical Care, 43,* 356–373.

Beale, V., & Lambric, T. (1995). *The recovery concept: Implementation in the mental health system: A report by the Community Support Program Advisory Committee.* Columbus, OH: Department of Mental Health, Office of Consumer Services.

Beard, J. H. (1978). The rehabilitation services of Fountain House. In L. Stein & M. Test (Eds.), *Alternatives to Mental Hospital Treatment.* New York: Plenum Press.

Beard, J. H., Malamud, T. J., & Rossman, E. (1978). Psychiatric rehabilitation and long-term rehospitalization rates: The findings of two research studies. *Schizophrenia Bulletin, 4,* 622–635.

Beard, J. H., Propst, R. N., & Malamud, T. J. (1982). The Fountain House model of rehabilitation. *Psychosocial Rehabilitation Journal, 5*(1), 47–53.

Beauford, J., McNiel, D., & Binder, R. (1997). Utility of the initial therapeutic alliance in evaluating psychiatric patients' risk of violence. *American Journal of Psychiatry, 154,* 1272–1276.

Bebbington, P., & Kuipers, L. (1992). Life events and social factors. In D. J. Kavanagh (Ed.), *Schizophrenia: An overview and practical handbook* (pp. 126–144). London: Chapman & Hall.

Bebbington, P., Wilkins, S., Jones, P. B., Foerster, A., Murray, R., & Toone, B. (1993). Life events and psychosis: Initial results from the Camberwell Collaborative Psychosis Study. *British Journal of Psychiatry, 162,* 72–79.

Beck, A. (1976). *Cognitive therapy and the emotional disorders.* New York: New American Library.

Beck, A. T., Rush, A. J., Shaw, B. F., & Emery, G. (1979). *Cognitive therapy of depression.* New York: Guilford Press.

Beck, A. T., Steer, R. A., & Brown, G. K. (1996). *Manual for the Beck Depression Inventory–II.* San Antonio, TX: Psychological Corporation.

Beck, A. T., Steer, R. A., & Garbin, M. G. (1988).

Psychometric properties of the Beck Depression Inventory: Twenty-five years of evaluation. *Clinical Psychology Review, 8,* 77–100.

Beck, A. T., Wright, F. D., Newman, C. F., & Liese, B. S. (1993). *Cognitive therapy of substance abuse.* New York: Guilford Press.

Beck, J. C., & van der Kolk, B. A. (1987). Reports of childhood incest and current behavior of chronically hospitalized psychotic women. *American Journal of Psychiatry, 144,* 1474–1476.

Beck, J. S. (1995). *Cognitive therapy: Basics and beyond.* New York: Guilford Press.

Becker, D., Whitley, R., Bailey, E., & Drake, R. E. (2007). A long-term follow-up of adults with psychiatric disabilities who receive supported employment. *Psychiatric Services, 58,* 922–928.

Becker, D. R., & Bond, G. R. (Eds.). (2002). *Supported employment implementation resource kit.* Rockville, MD: Center for Mental Health Services, Substance Abuse and Mental Health Services Administration.

Becker, D. R., Bond, G. R., McCarthy, D., Thompson, D., Xie, H., McHugo, G. J., et al. (2001a). Converting day treatment centers to supported employment programs in Rhode Island. *Psychiatric Services, 52,* 351–357.

Becker, D. R., & Drake, R. E. (2003). *A working life for people with severe mental illness.* New York: Oxford University Press.

Becker, D. R., Drake, R. E., Farabaugh, A., & Bond, G. R. (1996). Job preferences of clients with severe psychiatric disorders participating in supported employment programs. *Psychiatric Services, 47,* 1223–1226.

Becker, D. R., Drake, R. E., & Naughton, W. (2005). Supported employment for people with co-occurring disorders. *Psychiatric Rehabilitation Journal, 28,* 332–338.

Becker, D. R., Smith, J., Tanzman, B., Drake, R. E., & Tremblay, T. (2001b). Fidelity of supported employment programs and employment outcomes. *Psychiatric Services, 52,* 834–836.

Becker, D. R., Xie, H., McHugo, G. J., Halliday, J., & Martinez, R. A. (2006). What predicts supported employment program outcomes? *Community Mental Health Journal, 42,* 303–313.

Bedell, J., Cohen, N., & Sullivan, A. (2000). Case management: The current best practices and the next generation of innovation. *Community Mental Health Journal, 36,* 179–194.

Beeler, J., Rosenthal, A., & Cohler, B. (1999). Patterns of family caregiving and support provided to older psychiatric patients in long-term care. *Psychiatric Services, 50,* 1222–1224.

Beers, C. W. (1923). *A mind that found itself.* Garden City, NY: Doubleday.

Belcher, J. K. (1988). Are jails replacing the mental health system for the homeless mentally ill? *Community Mental Health Journal, 24*, 185–95.

Bell, M., Bryson, G., & Wexler, B. E. (2003). Cognitive remediation of working memory deficits: Durability of training effects in severely impaired and less severely impaired schizophrenia. *Acta Psychiatrica Scandinavica, 108*, 101–109.

Bell, M. D., Bryson, G., Greig, T. C. C., & Wexler, B. E. (2001). Neurocognitive enhancement therapy with work therapy: Effects on neurocognitive test performance. *Archives of General Psychiatry, 58(8)*, 763–768.

Bellack, A. S. (2004). Skills training for people with severe mental illness. *Psychiatric Rehabilitation Journal, 27*, 375–391.

Bellack, A. S. (2006). Psychometric characteristics of role play assessments of social skill in schizophrenia. *Behavior Therapy, 37*, 339–352.

Bellack, A. S., Bennet, M. E., & Gearon, J. S. (2006a). *Behavioral treatment for substance abuse in people with serious and persistent mental illness.* New York: Taylor & Francis.

Bellack, A. S., Bennet, M. E., Gearon, J. S., Brown, C. H., & Yang, Y. (2006b). A randomized clinical trial of a new behavioral treatment for drug abuse in people with severe and persistent mental illness. *Archives of General Psychiatry, 63*, 426–432.

Bellack, A. S., & DiClemente, C. C. (1999). Treating substance abuse among patients with schizophrenia. *Psychiatric Services, 50*, 75–80.

Bellack, A. S., Gold, J. M., & Buchanan, R. W. (1999). Cognitive rehabilitation for schizophrenia: Problems, prospects, and strategies. *Schizophrenia Bulletin, 25(2)*, 257–274.

Bellack, A. S., Morrison, R. L., Mueser, K. T., Wade, J. H., & Sayers, S. L. (1990a). Role play for assessing the social competence of psychiatric patients. *Psychological Assessment, 2*, 248–255.

Bellack, A. S., Morrison, R. L., Wixted, J. T., & Mueser, K. T. (1990b). An analysis of social competence in schizophrenia. *British Journal of Psychiatry, 156*, 809–818.

Bellack, A. S., & Mueser, K. T. (1993). Psychosocial treatment for schizophrenia. *Schizophrenia Bulletin, 19*, 317–336.

Bellack, A. S., Mueser, K. T., Gingerich, S., & Agresta, J. (1997). *Social skills training for schizophrenia: A step-by-step guide.* New York: Guilford Press.

Bellack, A. S., Mueser, K. T., Gingerich, S., & Agresta, J. (2004). *Social skills training for schizophrenia: A step-by-step guide* (2nd ed.). New York: Guilford Press.

Bellack, A. S., Sayers, M., Mueser, K. T., & Bennett, M. (1994). Evaluation of social problem solving in schizophrenia. *Journal of Abnormal Psychology, 103*, 371–378.

Bellus, S., Kost, P., Vergo, J., Gramse, R., & Weiss, K. (1999). The effects of shaping classes on academic skills, self care skills and on-ward behavior with persons who are cognitively impaired and chronic psychiatric inpatients. *Psychiatric Rehabilitation Skills, 3(1)*, 23–40.

Bengtsson-Tops, A., & Hansson, L. (1999). Clinical and social needs of schizophrenic outpatients living in the community: The relationship between needs and subjective quality of life. *Social Psychiatry and Psychiatric Epidemiology, 34*, 513–518.

Bensley, L., Nelson, N., Kaufman, J., Silverstein, B., & Shields, J. W. (1995). Patient and staff views of factors influencing assaults on psychiatric hospital employees. *Issues in Mental Health Nursing, 16*, 433–446.

Bentall, R. P. (1994). Cognitive biases and abnormal beliefs: Towards a model of persecutory delusions. In A. S. David & J. C. Cutting (Eds.), *The neuropsychology of schizophrenia* (pp. 337–360). Hove, UK: LEA.

Bentall, R. P. (2001). Social cognition and delusional beliefs. In P. W. Corrigan & D. L. Penn (Eds.), *Social cognition and schizophrenia.* Washington, DC: American Psychiatric Association.

Bentall, R. P., Kinderman, P., & Kaney, S. (1994). The self, attributional processses and abnormal beliefs: Towards a model of persecutory delusions. *Behaviour Research and Therapy, 32*, 331–341.

Bentall, R., & Slade, P. (1985). Reality testing and auditory hallucinations: A signal detection analysis. *British Journal of Clinical Psychology, 24*, 59–169.

Bentley, K. J., Rosenson, M. K., & Zito, J. M. (1990). Promoting medication compliance: Strategies for working with families of mentally ill people. *National Association of Social Workers*, pp. 274–277.

Benton, M. K., & Schroeder, H. E. (1990). Social skills training with schizophrenics: A meta-analytic evaluation. *Journal of Consulting and Clinical Psychology, 58*, 741–747.

Ben-Yishay, Y. (1996). Reflections on the evolution of the therapeutic milieu concept. *Neuropsychological Rehabilitation, 6(4)*, 327–343.

Berk, M. L., Schur, C. L., & Cantor, J. C. (1995). Ability to obtain health care: Recent estimates from the Robert Wood Johnson Foundation National Access to Care Survey. *Health Affairs, 14*, 139–146.

Berkowitz, L. (1989). *Advances in experimental social psychology*. San Diego: Academic Press.

Bernheim, K. (1982). Supportive family counseling. *Schizophrenic Bulletin, 8,* 634–648.

Bernheim, K., & Lehman, A. (1985). *Working with families of the mentally ill.* New York: Norton.

Bernheim, K., & Switalski, T. (1988). The Buffalo Family Support Project: Promoting institutional change to meet families' needs. *Hospital and Community Psychiatry, 39,* 663–665.

Besio, S. W., & Mahler, J. (1993). Benefits and challenges of using consumer staff in supported housing services. *Hospital and Community Psychiatry, 44,* 490–491.

Bhugra, D. (1989). Attitudes towards mental illness: A review of the literature. *Acta Psychiatrica Scandinavica, 80,* 1–12.

Biegel, D., Milligan, S., Putnam, P., & Song, L. (1994). Predictors of burden among lower socio-economic status caregivers of persons with chronic mental illness. *Community Mental Health Journal, 30,* 473–494.

Biegel, D., & Yamatani, H. (1986). Self-help groups for families of the mentally ill: Research perspectives. In M. Z. Goldstein (Ed.), *Family involvement in the treatment of schizophrenia* (pp. 57–80), Washington, DC: American Psychological Press.

Bigelow, D., Bloom, J., Williams, M., & McFarland, B. (1999). An administrative model for close monitoring and managing high risk individuals. *Behavioral Sciences and the Law, 17,* 227–235.

Birchwood, M., Mason, R., MacMillian, F., & Healy, J. (1993). Depression, demoralization and control over psychotic illness: A comparison of depressed and non-depressed patients with a chronic psychosis. *Psychological Medicine, 23,* 387–395.

Birchwood, M., Smith, J., Cochrane, R., Wetton, S., & Copestake, S. (1990). The Social Functioning Scale: The development and validation of a new scale of social adjustment for use in family intervention programmes with schizophrenic patients. *British Journal of Psychiatry, 157,* 853–859.

Bisson, J. I., Ehlers, A., Matthews, R., Pilling, S., Richards, D., & Turner, S. (2007). Psychological treatments for chronic posttraumatic stress disorder: Systematic review and meta-analysis. *British Journal of Psychiatry, 190,* 97–104.

Bittner, E. (1967). Police discretion in emerging apprehension of mentally ill persons. *Social Problems, 14,* 278–292.

Black, K. J., Compton, W. M., Wetzel, M., Minuchin, S., Farber, N. B., & Rastogi-Cruz, D. (1994). Assaults by patients on psychiatric residents at three training sites. *Hospital and Community Psychiatry, 45,* 706–710.

Blackwell, B. (1973). Drug therapy—patient compliance. *New England Journal of Medicine, 289*(5), 249–252.

Blackwood, D. H. R., Fordyce, A., Walker, M. T., St. Clair, D. M., Porteous, D. J., & Muir, W. J. (2001). Schizophrenia and affective disorders—cosegregation with a translocation at chromosome 1q42 that directly disrupts brain-expressed genes: Clinical and P300 finding in a family. *American Journal of Human Genetics, 69,* 428–433.

Blake, D. D., Weathers, F. W., Nagy, L. M., Kaloupek, D. G., Charney, D. S., & Keane, T. M. (1995). *Clinician administered PTSD Scale for DSM-IV.* Boston: National Center for Posttraumatic Stress Disorder.

Blanch, A., & Fisher, D. (1993). Consumer-practitioners and psychiatrists share insights about recovery and coping. *Disability Studies Quarterly, 13,* 17–20.

Blanchard, E. P., Jones-Alexander, J., Buckley, T. C., & Forneris, C. A. (1996). Psychometric properties of the PTSD Checklist. *Behavior Therapy, 34,* 669–673.

Blanchard, J. J., & Neale, J. M. (1992). Medication status of participants in psychopathology research: Selective review of current reporting practices. *American Psychological Association, 101*(4), 732–734.

Blank, A., Draine, J., & Solomon, P. (2003, November). *Diversion vs. in-jail services: Enhancing surveillance?* Paper presented at the meeting of the American Society of Criminology Annual Conference, Denver, CO.

Blankertz, L. E., & Cnaan, R. A. (1994). Assessing the impact of two residential programs for dually diagnosed homeless individuals. *Social Service Review, 68,* 536–560.

Blankertz, L. E., & Robinson, S. E. (1996). Who is the psychosocial rehabilitation worker? *Psychiatric Rehabilitation Journal, 19*(4), 3–13.

Blazer, D. G., Kessler, R. C., McGonagle, K. A., & Swartz, M. S. (1994). The prevalence and distribution of major depression in a national community sample: The National Comorbidity Survey. *American Journal of Psychiatry, 151*(7), 979–986.

Bleuler, E. (1911/1950). *Dementia praecox or the group of schizophrenias* (J. Zinken, Trans.). New York: International University Press.

Bleuler, M. (1978). *The schizophrenic disorders: Long-term patient and family studies* (S. M. Clemens, Trans.). New Haven, CT: Yale University Press.

Bloom, B. L. (1984). *Community mental health: A general introduction.* Monterey, CA: Brooks/Cole.

Bloom, J. R., Hu, T.-W., Wallace, N., Cuffel, B., Hausman, J. W., Sheu, M.-L., et al. (2002). Mental health costs and access under alternative capitation systems in Colorado. *Health Services Research, 37,* 315–340.

Bloom, J., Williams, M., & Bigelow, D. (2000). The forensic psychiatric system in the United States. *International Journal of Law and Psychiatry, 23,* 605–613.

Blow, F. C., Barry, K. L., Copeland, L. A., McCormick, R. A., Lehmann, L. S., & Ullman, E. (1999). Repeated assaults by patients in VA hospital and clinic settings. *Psychiatric Services, 50,* 390–394.

Blow, F. C., Zeber, J. E., McCarthy, J. F., Valenstein, E. M., Gillon, L., & Bingham, C. R. (2004). Ethnicity and diagnostic patterns in veterans with psychoses. *Social Psychiatry and Psychiatric Epidemiology, 39,* 841–851.

Blumenthal, D., Mort, E., & Edwards, J. (1995). The efficacy of primary care for vulnerable population groups. *Health Services Research, 30,* 253–273.

Boccaccini, M., Christy, A., Poythress, N., & Kershaw, D. (2005). Rediversion in two post-booking jail diversion programs in Florida. *Psychiatric Services, 56,* 835–839.

Bockian, N. R. (2002). *New hope for people with borderline personality disorder.* New York: Prima.

Bockoven J. S. (1963). *Moral treatment in American psychiatry.* New York: Springer.

Boczkowski, J., Zeichner, A., & DeSanto, N. (1985). Neuroleptic compliance among chronic schizophrenic outpatients: An intervention outcome report. *Journal of Consulting and Clinical Psychology, 53,* 666–671.

Bogart, T., & Solomon P. (1999). Procedures to share treatment information among mental health providers, consumers, and families. *Psychiatric Services, 50,* 1321–1325.

Bohus, M., Haaf, B., Simms, T., Limberger, M. F., Schmahl, C., Unckel, C., et al. (2004). Effectiveness of inpatient dialectical behavioral therapy for borderline personality disorder: A controlled trial. *Behaviour Research and Therapy, 42,* 487–499.

Bolton, E. E., Mueser, K. T., & Rosenberg, S. D. (2006). Symptom correlates of posttraumatic stress disorder in clients with borderline personality disorder. *Comprehensive Psychiatry, 47,* 357–361.

Bond, G., McGrew, J., & Fekete, D. (1995c). Assertive outreach for frequent users of psychiatric hospitals: A meta-analysis. *Journal of Mental Health Administration, 22,* 4–16.

Bond, G. R. (1991). Variations in an assertive outreach model. *New Directions for Mental Health Services, 52,* 65–80.

Bond, G. R. (1992). Vocational rehabilitation. In R. P. Liberman (Ed.), *Handbook of psychiatric rehabilitation* (pp. 244–275). New York: MacMillan.

Bond, G..R. (2004a). Supported employment: Evidence for an evidence-based practice. *Psychiatric Rehabilitation Journal, 27,* 345–359.

Bond, G. R. (2004b, December 14). *Critical ingredients of supported employment: Research evidence.* Paper presented at the University of North Carolina/Duke Mental Health Seminar, Durham, NC.

Bond, G. R., Becker, D. R., Drake, R. E., Rapp, C. A., Meisler, N., Lehman, A. F., et al. (2001a). Implementing supported employment as an evidence-based practice. *Psychiatric Services, 52,* 313–322.

Bond, G. R., Becker, D. R., Drake, R. E., & Vogler, K. M. (1997). A fidelity scale for the Individual Placement and Support model of supported employment. *Rehabilitation Counseling Bulletin, 40,* 265–284.

Bond, G. R., & Dietzen, L. L. (1993). Predictive validity and vocational assessment: Reframing the question. In R. L. Glueckauf, L. B. Sechrest, G. R. Bond, & E. C. McDonel (Eds.), *Improving assessment in rehabilitation and health* (pp. 61–86). Newbury Park, CA: Sage.

Bond, G. R., Dietzen, L., McGrew, J., & Miller, L. (1995a). Accelerating entry into supported employment for persons with severe psychiatric disabilities. *Rehabilitation Psychology, 40,* 91–111.

Bond, G. R., Dietzen, L. L., Vogler, K. M., Katuin, C. H., McGrew, J. H., & Miller, L. D. (1995b). Toward a framework for evaluating costs and benefits of psychiatric rehabilitation: Three case examples. *Journal of Vocational Rehabilitation, 5,* 75–88.

Bond, G. R., Drake, R. E., & Becker, D. R. (1998). The role of social functioning in vocational rehabilitation. In K. T. Mueser & N. Tarrier (Eds.), *Handbook of social functioning in schizophrenia* (pp. 372–390). Boston, MA: Allyn & Bacon.

Bond, G. R., Drake, R. E., Becker, D. R., & Mueser, K. T. (1999). Effectiveness of psychiatric rehabilitation approaches for employment of people with severe mental illness. *Journal of Disability Studies, 10,* 18–52.

Bond, G. R., Drake, R. E., Mueser, K. T., & Latimer, E. (2001b). Assertive community treatment for people with severe mental illness: Critical ingredients and impact on patients. *Disease Management and Health Outcomes, 9,* 141–159.

Bond, G. R., Evans, L., Salyers, M. P., Williams, J., & Kim, H. K. (2000a). Measurement of fidelity in psychiatric rehabilitation. *Mental Health Services Research, 2,* 75–87.

Bond, G. R., & Friedmeyer, M. H. (1987). Predictive validity of situational assessment at a psychiatric rehabilitation center. *Rehabilitation Psychology, 32,* 99–112.

Bond, G. R., McDonel, E. C., Miller, L. D., & Pensec, M. (1991). Assertive community treatment and reference groups: An evaluation of their effectiveness for young adults with serious mental illness and substance abuse problems. *Psychosocial Rehabilitation Journal, 15,* 31–43.

Bond, G. R., & Resnick, S. G. (2000). Psychiatric rehabilitation. In R. G. Frank & T. Elliott (Eds.), *Handbook of rehabilitation psychology* (pp. 235–258). Washington, DC: American Psychological Association.

Bond, G. R., Resnick, S. G., Drake, R. E., Xie, H., McHugo, G. J., & Bebout, R. R. (2001c). Does competitive employment improve nonvocational outcomes for people with severe mental illness? *Journal of Consulting and Clinical Psychology, 69,* 489–501.

Bond, G. R., Salyers, M. P., Rollins, A. L., Rapp, C. A., & Zipple, A. M. (2004). How evidence-based practices contribute to community integration. *Community Mental Health Journal, 40,* 569–588.

Bond, G. R., Williams, J., Evans, L., Salyers, M., Hea-won, K., Sharpe, H., et al. (2000b). *Psychiatric rehabilition fidelity toolkit.* Cambridge, MA: The Evaluation Center at HSRI.

Bond, G. R., Witheridge, T. F., Wasmer, D., Dincin, J., McRae, S. A., Mayes, J., et al. (1989). A comparison of two crisis housing alternatives to psychiatric hospitalization. *Hospital and Community Psychiatry, 40,* 177–183.

Bonovitz, J., & Guy, E. (1979). Impact of restrictive civil commitment procedures on a prison psychiatric service. *American Journal of Psychiatry, 136,* 1045–1048.

Bonovitz, J. C., & Bonovitz, J. (1981). Diversion of the mentally ill into the criminal justice system: The police intervention perspective. *American Journal of Psychiatry, 138,* 973–976.

Bookbinder, S. (1978) *Mainstreaming: What every child needs to know about disabilities.* Providence, RI: Easter Seal Society.

Boothroyd, R., Mercado, C., Poythress, N. Christy, A., & Petrila, J. (2005). Cinical outcomes of defendants in mental health courts. *Psychiatric Services, 56,* 829–834.

Boothroyd, R., Poythress, N., McGaha, A., & Petrila, J. (2003). The Broward Mental Health Court: Process, outcomes, and service utilization. *International Journal of Law and Psychiatry, 26,* 55–71.

Bordieri, J. E., & Drehmer, D. E. (1986). Hiring decisions for disabled workers: Looking at the cause. *Journal of Applied Social Psychology, 16,* 197–208.

Bordin, E. S. (1976). The generalizability of the psychoanalytic concept of the working alliance. *Psychotherapy: Theory, Research and Practice, 16,* 252–260.

Borkman, T. (1990). Experimental, professional, and lay frames of reference. In T. J. Powell (Ed.), *Working with self-help groups* (pp. 3–30). Silver Springs, MD: NASW Press.

Borum, R. (2000). Improving high risk encounters between people with mental illness and police. *Journal of the American Academy of Psychiatry and the Law, 28,* 332–337.

Borum, R., Deane, M. W., Steadman, H., & Morrissey, J. (1998). Police perspectives to responding to mentally ill people in crisis: Perceptions of program effectiveness. *Behavioral Sciences and the Law, 16,* 393–405.

Bowden, C. L., Schoenfeld, L. S., & Adams, R. L. (1980). Mental health attitudes and treatment expectations as treatment variables. *Journal of Clinical Psychology, 36,* 653–657.

Bowen, L., Wallace, C. J., Glynn, S. M., Nuechterlein, K. H., Lutzker, J. R., & Kuehnel, T. G. (1994). Schizophrenic individuals' cognitive functioning and performance in interpersonal interactions and skills training procedures. *Journal of Psychiatric Research, 28,* 289–301.

Boye, B., Bentsen, H., Notland, T., Munkvold, O., Lersbryggen, A., Oskarson, K., et al. (1999). What predicts the course of expressed emotion in relatives of patients with schizophrenia or related psychosis? *Social Psychiatry and Psychiatric Epidemiology, 34,* 35–43.

Boyer, S. L., & Bond, G. R. (1999). Does assertive community treatment reduce burnout?: A comparison with traditional case management. *Mental Health Services Research, 1,* 31–45.

Brad, H v. City of New York, 712 N.Y.S. 2d 336 2000 N.Y. Misc. 2 exds. 305(2000).

Bradley, R., Greene, J., Russ, E., Dutra, L., & Westen, D. (2005). A multidimensional meta-analysis of psychotherapy for PTSD. *American Journal of Psychiatry, 162,* 214–227.

Bradmiller, M. A. (1997). Consumer models of long-term mental illness. Unpublished doctoral dissertation, University of Maryland College Park.

Brady, K. T., Sonnes, A. R., & Ballenger, J. C.

(1995). Valproate in the treatment of acute bipolar affective episodes complicated by substance abuse: A pilot study. *Journal of Clinical Psychology, 56,* 118–121.

Braginsky, B. M., Braginsky, D. D., & Ring, K. (1969). *The mental hospital as a last resort.* New York: Holt, Rinehart & Winston.

Breakey, W. R., Fischer, P. J., Kramer, M., Nestadt, G., Romanoski, A., Ross, A., et al. (1989). Health and mental health problems of homeless men and women in Baltimore. *Journal of the American Medical Association, 262,* 1352–1357.

Breen, R., & Thornhill, J. T. (1998). Noncompliance with medication for psychiatric disorders. *CNS Drugs, 9,* 457–471.

Brehm, J. W. (1966). *A theory of psychological reactance.* San Diego: Academic Press.

Breier, A., Schreiber, J. L., Dyer, J., & Pickar, D. (1991). National Institute of Mental Health longitudinal study of chronic schizophrenia. *Archives of General Psychiatry, 48,* 239–246.

Brekke, J. S. (1988). What do we really know about community support programs?: Strategies for better monitoring. *Hospital and Community Psychiatry, 39,* 946–952.

Brekke, J. S., Raine, A., Ansel, M., Lencz, T., & Bird, L. (1997). Neuropsychological and psychophysiological correlates of psychosocial functioning in schizophrenia. *Schizophrenia Bulletin, 23,* 19–28.

Brekke, J. S., & Test, M. A. (1987). An empirical analysis of services delivery in a model community support program. *Psychosocial Rehabilitation Journal, 10,* 51–61.

Brennan, P. A., Mednick, S. A., & Hodgins, S. (2000). Major mental disorders and criminal violence in a Danish birth cohort. *Archives of General Psychiatry, 57,* 494–500.

Brenner, H. D., Hodel, B., Roder, V., & Corrigan, P. (1992). Treatment of cognitive dysfunctions and behavioral deficits in schizophrenia. *Schizophrenia Bulletin, 18*(1), 21–26.

Brenner, H. D., Roder, V., Hodel, B., Kienzle, N., Reed, D., & Liberman, R. P. (1994). *Integrated psychological therapy for schizophrenic patients.* Seattle: Hogrefe & Huber.

Breslau, N., Davis, G. C., & Andreski, P. (1995). Risk factors for PTSD-related traumatic events: A prospective analysis. *American Journal of Psychiatry, 152,* 529–535.

Breslau, N., Davis, G. C., Andreski, P., & Peterson, E. (1991). Traumatic events and posttraumatic stress disorder in an urban population of young adults. *Archives of General Psychiatry, 48,* 216–222.

Breslau, N., Davis, G. C., Andreski, P., Peterson, E.

L., & Schultz, L. R. (1997). Sex differences in posttraumatic stress disorder. *Archives of General Psychiatry, 54,* 1044–1048.

Brett-Jones, J. R., Garety, P. A., & Hemsley, D. R. (1987). Measuring delusional experiences: A method and its application. *British Journal of Clinical Psychology, 26,* 257–265.

Brewin, C., MacCarthy, B., Duda, K., & Vaughn, C. (1991). Attribution and expressed emotion in the relatives of patients with schizophrenia. *Journal of Abnormal Psychology, 157,* 221–227.

Briere, J., Woo, R., McRae, B., Foltz, J., & Sitzman, R. (1997). Lifetime victimization history, demographics, and clinical status in female psychiatric emergency room patients. *Journal of Nervous and Mental Disease, 185,* 95–101.

Bright, J., Neimeyer, R., & Baker, K. (1999). Professional and paraprofessional group treatments for depression: A comparison of cognitive-behavioral and mutual support interventions. *Journal of Consulting and Clinical Psychology, 67*(4), 491–501.

Broadbent, D. E. (1958). *Perception and communication.* Oxford, UK: Pergamon.

Broadbent, D. E. (1977). The hidden pre-attentive process. *American Psychologist, 32,* 109–118.

Brock, J. N. (1998). The evolution of the aging population. *State of Business, 11*(3). (Retrieved January 13, 2006, from *www.cba.gsu.edu/magazine/aging.html*).

Brockington, I. F., Hall, P., Levings, J., & Murphy, C. (1993). The community's tolerance of the mentally ill. *British Journal of Psychiatry, 162,* 93–99.

Broen, W. E. J., & Storms, L. H. (1966). Lawful disorganization: The process underlying a schizophrenic syndrome. *Psychological Review, 73*(4), 265–279.

Broner, N., Nguyen, H., Swern, A., & Goldfinger, S. (2003). Adapting a substance abuse court diversion model for felony offenders with co-occurring disorders: Initial implementation. *Psychiatric Quarterly, 74,* 361–385.

Brooker, C., Falloon, I., Butterworth, A., Goldberg, D., Graham-Hole, V., & Hillier, V. (1994). The outcome of training community psychiatric nurses to deliver psychosocial intervention. *British Journal of Psychiatry, 165,* 222–230.

Brothers, L. (1990). The neural basis of primate social communication. *Motivation and Emotion, 14,* 81–91.

Brown, D. (1997). Excess mortality of schizophrenia: A meta-analysis. *British Journal of Psychiatry, 171,* 502–508.

Brown, G., Monck, E., Carstairs, G., & Wing, J.

(1962). The influence of family life on the course of schizophrenic illness. *British Journal of Preventive and Social Medicine, 16,* 55–68.

Brown, G., & Rutter, M. (1966). The measurement of family activities and relationships. *Human Relations, 19,* 241–263.

Brown, G. W., Birley, J. L., & Wing, J. K. (1972). Influence of family life on the course of schizophrenic disorders: A replication. *British Journal of Psychiatry, 121,* 241–258.

Brown, G. W., Carstairs, G., & Topping, G. (1958). The post-hospital adjustment of chronic mental patients. *Lancet, 2,* 685–689.

Brown, G. W., & Harris, T. O. (1978). *Social origins of depression.* London: Tavistock.

Brown, N., & Parrish, J. (1995). CSP champion of self-help. *Journal of the California Alliance for the Mentally Ill, 6*(3), 6–7.

Brown, N. W. (2003). *Loving the self-absorbed: How to create a more satisfying relationship with a narcissistic partner.* Oakland, CA: New Harbinger.

Brown, S., Birtwistle, J., Roe, L., & Thompson, C. (1999). The unhealthy lifestyle of people with schizophrenia. *Psychological Medicine, 29,* 697–701.

Brown, S., Inskip, H., & Barraclough, B. (2000). Causes of the excess mortality of schizophrenia. *British Journal of Psychiatry, 177,* 212–217.

Browne, A., & Finkelhor, D. (1986). Impact of child sexual abuse: A review of the research. *Psychological Bulletin, 99,* 66–77.

Brunette, M. F., Drake, R. E., Marsh, B. J., Torrey, W. C., Rosenberg, S. D., & Five-Site Health and Risk Study Research Committee. (2003a). Responding to blood-borne infections among persons with severe mental illness. *Psychiatric Services, 54,* 860–865.

Brunette, M. F., Drake, R. E., Woods, M., & Hartnett, T. (2001). A comparison of long-term and short-term residential treatment programs for dual diagnosis patients. *Psychiatric Services, 52,* 526–528.

Brunette, M. F., Mueser, K. T., & Drake, R. E. (2004a). A review of research on residential problems for people with severe mental illness and co-occurring substance use disorders. *Drug and Alcohol Review, 23,* 471–481.

Brunette, M. F., Noordsy, D. L., Buckley, P., & Green, A. I. (2005). Pharmacologic treatments for co-occurring substance use disorders in patients with schizophrenia: A research review. *Journal of Dual Diagnosis, 1,* 41–55.

Brunette, M. F., Noordsy, D. L., Xie, H., & Drake, R. E. (2003b). Benzodiazepine use and abuse among patients with severe mental illness and co-occurring substance use disorders. *Psychiatric Services, 54,* 1395–1401.

Brunette, M. F., Richardson, F., White, L., Bemis, G., & Eelkema, R. (2004b). Integrated family treatment for parents with severe psychiatric disabilities. *Psychiatric Rehabilitation Journal, 28,* 177–179.

Buchanan, J. (1995). Social support and schizophrenia: A review of the literature. *Archives of Psychiatric Nursing, 9,* 68–76.

Buchanan, R. W., Holstein, C., & Breier, A. (1994). The comparative efficacy and long-term effect of clozapine treatment on neuropsychological test performance. *Biological Psychiatry, 36,* 717–725.

Buckley, P., McCarthy, M., Chapman, P., Richman, C., & Yamamoto, B. (1999). Clozapine treatment of comorbid substance abuser in patients with schizophrenia. *Schizophrenia Research, 36,* 272.

Buda, M., Tsuang, M. T., & Fleming, J. A. (1988). Causes of death in DSM-III schizophrenics and other psychotics (atypical): A comparison with the general population. *Archives of General Psychiatry, 45,* 283–285.

Budd, R., & Hughes, I. (1997). What do relatives of people with schizophrenia find helpful about family interventions? *Schizophrenia Bulletin, 23,* 341–347.

Budney, A. J., Sigmons, S. C., & Higgins, S. T. (2001). Contingency management: Using science to motivate change. In R. H. Coombs (Ed.), *Addiction recovery tools: A practical handbook* (pp. 147–170). Thousand Oaks, CA: Sage.

Budson, R. D. (1978). *The psychiatric halfway house: A handbook of theory and practice.* Pittsburgh: University of Pittsburgh Press.

Bulger, M., Wanderman, A., & Goldman, G. (1993). Burdens and gratifications of caregiving: Appraisal of parental care of adults with schizophrenia. *Journal of Orthopsychiatry, 63,* 255–265.

Burland, J. (1998). Family-to-family: A trauma-and-recovery model of family education. In H. Lefley (Ed.), *Family coping with mental illness: The cultural context* (pp. 33–41). San Francisco: Jossey-Bass.

Burnam, M. A., Morton, S. C., McGlynn, E. A., Petersen, L. P., Stecher, B. M., Hayes, C., et al. (1995). An experimental evaluation of residential and nonresidential treatment for dually diagnosed homeless adults. *Journal of Addictive Diseases, 14,* 111–134.

Burnam, M. A., Stein, J. A., Golding, J. M., Siegel, J. M., Sorenson, S. B., Forsythe, A. B., et al. (1988). Sexual assault and mental disorders in a community population. *Journal of Consulting and Clinical Psychology, 56,* 843–850.

Burns, B., & Santos, A. (1995). Assertive community treatment: An update of randomized trials. *Psychiatric Services, 46,* 669–675.

Burns, D. D. (1980). *Feeling good: The new mood therapy.* New York: Avon.

Burns, T., Catty, C., Becker, T., Drake, R. E., Fioritti, A., Lauber, C., et al. (in press). Supported employment for people with severe mental illness: A European multi-centre controlled trial. *Lancet.*

Burt, M. R., & Aron, L. Y. (2003). *Promoting work among SSI/DI beneficiaries with serious mental illness.* Washington, DC: Urban Institute.

Burt, M. R., Duke, A., & Hargreaves, W. A. (1998). The Program Environment Scale: Assessing client perceptions of community-based programs for the severely mentally ill. *American Journal of Community Psychology, 26,* 853–879.

Bustillo, J. R., Lauriello, J., Horan, W. P., & Keith, S. J. (2001). The psychosocial treatment of schizophrenia: An update. *American Journal of Psychiatry, 158,* 163–175.

Butcher, J. N., Dahlstrom, W. G., Graham, J. R., Tellegen, A., & Kaemmer, B. (1989). *Manual for the administration and scoring of the MMPI-2.* Minneapolis: University of Minnesota Press.

Butler, R. W., Mueser, K. T., Sprock, J., & Braff, D. L. (1996). Positive symptoms of psychosis in posttraumatic stress disorder. *Biological Psychiatry, 39,* 839–844.

Butterfield, F. (1998, March 5). Persons replace hospitals for the nation's mentally ill. *New York Times,* p. A1.

Butzlaff, R. L., & Hooley, J. M. (1998). Expressed emotion and psychiatric relapse. *Archives of General Psychiatry, 55*(6), 547–552.

Byerly, M., Fisher, R., & Rush, A. J. (2002, December). *Comparison of clinician vs. electronic monitoring of antipsychotic adherence in schizophrenia.* Paper presented at the 41st annual meeting of the American College of Neuropsychopharmacology, San Juan, Puerto Rico.

Byrne, P. (2000). The stigma of mental illness and ways of diminishing it. *Advances in Psychiatric Treatment, 6,* 65–72.

Calabrese, J. D., & Corrigan, P. (2004). Beyond dementia praecox: Findings from long-term follow-up studies. In R. Ralph & P. Corrigan (Eds.), *Recovery and mental illness: Consumer visions and research paradigms.* Washington, DC: American Psychological Association.

Caldwell, C. B., & Gottesman, I. I. (1990). Schizophrenics kill themselves too: A review of risk factors for suicide. *Schizophrenia Bulletin, 16,* 571–589.

Calhoun, P. S., Beckham, J. C., & Bosworth, H. B. (2002). Caregiver burden and psychological distress in partners of veterans with chronic posttraumatic stress disorder. *Journal of Traumatic Stress, 15,* 202–212.

Callaghan, P., & Morrissey, J. (1993). Social support and health: A review. *Journal of Advanced Nursing, 18,* 203–210.

Callan, A. F. (1999). Schizophrenia in Afro-Caribbean immigrants. *Journal of the Royal Society of Medicine, 89,* 253–256.

Campbell, J. (1989). *The Well Being Project: Mental health clients speak for themselves* (Vol. 6). Sacramento: California Network of Mental Health Clients.

Campbell, J. (1997). How consumers/survivors are evaluating the quality of psychiatric care. *Evaluation Review, 21,* 357–363.

Campbell, M., Donaldson, L., Roberts, S., & Smith, J. (1996). A prescribing incentive scheme for non-fundholding general practices: An observational study. *British Medical Journal, 313,* 535–538.

Candido, C. L., & Romney, D. M. (1990). Attributional style in paranoid vs. depressed patients. *British Journal of Medical Psychology, 63*(4), 355–363.

Cannon, T. D., van Erp, T. G., & Glahn, D. C. (2002). Elucidating continuities and discontinuities between schizotypy and schizophrenia in the nervous system. *Schizophrenia Research, 54*(1–2), 151–156.

Cannon-Spoor, E., Potkin, S. G., & Wyatt, R. J. (1982). Measurement of premorbid adjustment in chronic schizophrenia. *Schizophrenia Bulletin, 8,* 470–484.

Carey, K. (1996). Substance use reduction in the context of outpatient psychiatric treatment: A collaborative, motivational, harm reduction approach. *Community Mental Health Journal, 32,* 291–306.

Carey, K., Maisto, S. A., Carey, M. P., & Purnine, D. M. (2001). Measuring readiness-to-change substance misuse among psychiatric outpatients: I. Reliability and validity of self-report measures. *Journal of Studies on Alcohol, 62,* 79–88.

Carey, K. B., & Correia, C. J. (1998). Severe mental illness and addictions: Assessment considerations. *Addictive Behaviors, 23,* 735–748.

Carey, M. P., Carey, K. B., & Kalichman, S. C. (1997). Risk for human immunodeficiency virus (HIV) infection among persons with severe mental illnesses. *Clinical Psychology Review, 17,* 271–291.

CARF. (2000). *2000 behavioral standards manual.* Tuscon, AZ: CARF, Rehabilitation Accreditation Commission.

Carkhuff, R. R. (1972). *The art of helping.* Amherst, MA: Human Resource Development Press.

Carling, P. J. (1988). Directions for the 1990s. *Switzer Monograph* (pp. 25–47). Alexandria, VA: National Rehabilitation Association.

Carling, P. J. (1990). Major mental illness, housing, and supports. *American Psychologist, 45,* 969–975.

Carling, P. J. (1993). Housing and supports for persons with mental illness: Emerging approaches to research and practice. *Hospital and Community Psychiatry, 44,* 439–449.

Carling, P. J. (1994). Supports and rehabilitation for housing and community living. In L. Spaniol & Publications Committee (Eds.), *An introduction to psychiatric rehabilitation* (pp. 89–110). Columbia, MD: International Association of Psychosocial Rehabilitation Services.

Carling, P. J. (1995). *Return to community: Building support systems for people with psychiatric disabilities.* New York: Guilford Press.

Carlson, L. S., Eichler, M., Huff, S., & Rapp, C. A. (2003). *A tale of two cities: Best practices in supported education.* Lawrence: University of Kansas School of Social Welfare.

Carlson, L., Rapp, C., & McDiarmid, D. (2001). Hiring consumer-providers: Barriers and alternative solutions. *Community Mental Health Journal, 37*(3), 199–213.

Carmel, H., & Hunter, M. (1993). Staff injuries from patient attack: Five years' data. *Bulletin of the American Academy of Psychiatry and the Law, 21,* 485–493.

Carmen, E., Rieker, P. P., & Mills, T. (1984). Victims of violence and psychiatric illness. *American Journal of Psychiatry, 141,* 378–383.

Carmichael, D., Tackett-Gibson, M., & Dell, O. (1998). *Texas Dual Diagnosis Project evaluation report 1997–1998.* College Station: Texas A&M University, Public Policy Research Institute.

Carney, C. P., Allen, J., & Doebbing, B. N. (2002). Receipt of clinical preventive medical services among psychiatric patients. *Psychiatric Services, 53,* 1028–1030.

Carney, C. P., Yates, W. R., Goerdt, C. J., & Doebbeling, B. N. (1998). Psychiatrists' and internists' knowledge and attitudes about delivery of clinical preventive medical services. *Psychiatric Services, 49,* 1594–1600.

Carpenter, W. T., Heinrichs, D. W., & Wagman, A. M. I. (1988). Deficit and nondeficit forms of schizophrenia: The concept. *American Journal of Psychiatry, 145,* 578–583.

Carpentier, N., Lesage, A., Goulet, I., Lalonde, P., & Renaird, M. (1992). Burden of care of families not living with young schizophrenic relatives. *Hospital and Community Psychiatry, 43,* 38–43.

Carroll, J., & Lurigio, A. (1984). Conditional release on probation and parole: Implications for provision of mental health services. In L. Teplin (Ed.), *Mental Health and Criminal Justice* (pp. 297–315). Beverly Hills, CA: Sage.

Casarino, J. P., Wilner, M., & Maxey, J. T. (1982). American Association for Partial Hospitalization (AAPH) standards and guidelines for partial hospitalization. *International Journal of Partial Hospitalization, 1,* 5–21.

Cascardi, M., Mueser, K. T., DeGiralomo, J., & Murrin, M. (1996). Physical aggression against psychiatric inpatients by family members and partners: A descriptive study. *Psychiatric Services, 47,* 531–533.

Casper, E. S., & Oursler, J. D. (2003). The Psychiatric Rehabilitation Beliefs, Goals, and Practices Scale: Sensitivity to change. *Psychiatric Rehabilitation Journal, 26,* 311–314.

Castle, D. J., Wessely, S., & Murray, R. M. (1993). Sex and schizophrenia: Effects of diagnostic stringency, and associations with premorbid variables. *British Journal of Psychiatry, 162,* 658–664.

Catapano, L., & Castle, D. (2004). Obesity in schizophrenia: What can be done about it? *Australasian Psychiatry, 12,* 23–25.

Caton, C. (1981). The new chronic patient and the system of community care. *Hospital and Community Psychiatry, 32,* 475–478.

Caton, C., Cournos, F., & Dominiquez, B. (1999). Parenting and adjustments in schizophrenia. *Psychiatric Services, 50,* 232–243.

Caton, C., Shrout, P., Eagle, P., Opler, L., Felix, A., & Dominguez, B. (1994). Risk factors for homelessness among schizophrenic men: A case-control study. *American Journal of Public Health, 84,* 265–270.

Center for Mental Health Services. (1994). *Making a difference: Interim status report of the McKinney Demonstration Program for Homeless Adults with Serious Mental Illness.* Rockville, MD: Substance Abuse and Mental Health Services Administration.

Chadwick, P. D., Birchwood, M. J., & Trower, P. (Eds.). (1996). *Cognitive therapy for delusions, voices and paranoia.* Chichester, UK: Wiley.

Chadwick, P. D., & Lowe, C. F. (1990). Measure and modification of delusional beliefs. *Journal of Consulting Clinical Psychology, 58*(2), 225–232.

Chafetz, L., White, M. C., Collins-Bride, G.,

Nickens, J., & Cooper, B. A. (2006). Predictors of physical functioning among adults with severe mental illness. *Psychiatric Services, 57,* 225–231.

Chamberlain, F., & Rapp, C. (1991). A decade of case management: A methodological review of outcome research. *Community Mental Health Journal, 27,* 171–188.

Chamberlain, J. (1990). The ex-patient's movement: Where we've been and where we're going. *Journal of Mind and Behavior, 11,* 323–336.

Chamberlain, J., Rogers, E., & Ellison, M. (1996). Self-help programs: A description of their characteristics and their members. *Psychiatric Rehabilitation Journal, 19,* 33–42.

Chamberlin, J. (1978). *On our own: Patient-controlled alternatives to the mental health system.* New York: Hawthorne.

Chamberlin, J. (1984). Speaking for ourselves: An overview of the ex-psychiatric inmates' movement. *Psychosocial Rehabilitation Journal, 3*(2), 323–336.

Chamberlin, J., Rogers, J. A., & Sneed, C. S. (1989). Consumers, families, and community support systems. *Psychosocial Rehabilitation Journal, 12*(3), 93–106.

Chandler, D., Meisel, J., Hu, T., McGowen, M., & Madison, K. (1997). A capitated model for a cross-section of severely mentally ill clients: Employment outcomes. *Community Mental Health Journal, 33,* 501–516.

Chandler, D. W., & Spicer, G. (in press). Integrated treatment for jail recidivists with co-occurring psychiatric and substance use disorders. *Community Mental Health Journal, 42,* 405–425.

Chang, C. F., Kiser, L. J., Bailey, J. E., Martins, M., Gibson, W. C., Schaberg, K. A., et al. (1998). Tennessee's failed managed care program for mental health and substance abuse services [see comment]. *Journal of the American Medical Association, 279,* 864–869.

Chávez, A. F., & Guido-DiBrito, F. (1999). Racial and ethnic identity and development. *New Directions for Adult and Continuing Education, 84,* 39–47.

Chen, F. M., Fryer, G. E., Phillips, R. L., Wilson, E., & Pathman, D. E. (2005). Patients' beliefs about racism, preferences for physician race, and satisfaction with care. *Annals of Family Medicine, 3,* 138–143.

Chien, W., & Chan, S. (2004). One-year follow-up of a multiple-family group intervention for Chinese families of patients with schizophrenia. *Psychiatric Services, 55,* 1276–1284.

Chin, D., & Kroesen, K. W. (1999). Disclosure of HIV infection among Asian/Pacific Islander American women: Cultural stigma and support. *Cultural Diversity and Ethnic Minority Psychology, 5*(3), 222.

Chinman, M., Rosenheck, R., Lam, L., & Davidson, L. (2000b). Comparing consumer and nonconsumer provided case management services for homeless persons with serious mental illness. *Journal of Nervous and Mental Disease, 188,* 446–453.

Chinman, M., Weingarten, R., Stayner, D., & Davidson, L. (2001). Chronicity reconsidered: Improving person–environment fit through a consumer-run service. *Community Mental health Journal, 37,* 215–229.

Chinman, M., Young, A. S., Rowe, M., Forquer, S., Knight, E., & Miller, A. (2003). An instrument to assess competencies of providers treating severe mental illness. *Mental Health Services Research, 5,* 97–108.

Chinman, M. J., Rosenheck, R. A., & Lam, J. A. (2000a). Client–case manager racial matching in a program for homeless persons with serious mental illness. *Psychiatric Services, 51,* 1265–1272.

Chou, K. R., Chen, R., Lee, J. F., Ku, C. H., & Lu, R. B. (2004). The effectiveness of nicotine-patch therapy for smoking cessation in patients with schizophrenia. *International Journal of Nursing Studies, 41,* 321–330.

Christenson, A., & Jacobson, N. (1994). Who (or what) can do psychotherapy: The status and challenge of nonprofessional therapists. *Psychological Science, 5,* 8–14.

Chue, P. (2004). The assessment and management of antipsychotic associated metabolic disturbances from a psychiatric perspective. *Canadian Journal of Psychiatry, 49,* 200–207.

Cimpean, D., Torrey, W. C., & Green, A. I. (2005). Schizophrenia and co-occurring general medical illness. *Psychiatric Annals, 35,* 71–81.

Ciompi, L. (1980). Catamnestic long-term study on the course of life and aging of schizophrenia. *Schizophrenia Bulletin, 6,* 606–618.

Citron, M., Solomon, P., & Draine, J. (1999). Self-help groups for families of persons with mental illness: Perceived benefits of helpfulness. *Community Mental Health Journal, 35,* 15–30.

Clark, C., & Rich, A. R. (2003). Outcomes of homeless adults with mental illness in a housing program and in case management only. *Psychiatric Services, 54,* 78–83.

Clark, D. A. (2004). *Cognitive-behavioral therapy for obsessive–compulsive disorder.* New York: Guilford Press.

Clark, R. (2001). Family support and substance use outcomes for persons with mental illness and substance use disorders. *Schizophrenia Bulletin, 27,* 93–101.

Clark, R. E. (1998). Supported employment and managed care: Can they coexist? *Psychiatric Rehabilitation Journal, 22*(1), 62–68.

Clarke, G., Herinckx, H., Kinney, R., Paulson, R., Cutler, D., & Oxman, E. (2000). Psychiatric hospitalizations, arrests, emergency room visits, and homelessness of clients with serious and persistent mental illness: Findings from a randomized trial of two ACT programs vs. usual care. *Mental Health Services Research, 2*, 155–164.

Clarkin, J. F., Carpenter, D., Hull, J., Wilner, P., & Glick, I. (1998). Effects of psychoeducational intervention for married patients with bipolar disorder and their spouses. *Psychiatric Services, 49*, 531–533.

Clausen J., & Yarrow, M. (1955). The impact of mental illness on the family. *Journal of Social Issues, 11*, 3–64.

Clay, S. (Ed.). (2005). *On our own, together: Peer programs for people with mental illness.* Nashville: Vanderbilt University Press.

Cleckley, H. (1976). *The mask of sanity* (fifth ed.). St. Louis, MO: Mosby.

Cloitre, M., Koenen, K. C., Cohen, L. R., & Han, H. (2002). Skills training in affective and interpersonal regulation followed by exposure: A phase-based treatment for PTSD related to childhood abuse. *Journal of Consulting and Clinical Psychology, 70*, 1067–1074.

Cnaan, R. A., Blankertz, L., & Aunders, M. (1992). Perceptions of consumers, practitioners, and experts regarding psychosocial rehabilitation principles. *Psychosocial Rehabilitation Journal, 16*(1), 95–119.

Cnaan, R. A., Blankertz, L., Messinger, K. W., & Gardner, J. R. (1988). Psychosocial rehabilitation: Toward a definition. *Psychosocial Rehabilitation Journal, 11*(4), 61–77.

Cnaan, R. A., Blankertz, L., Messinger, K. W., & Gardner, J. R. (1989). Psychosocial rehabilitation: Toward a theoretical base. *Psychosocial Rehabilitation Journal, 13*(1), 33–55.

Cnaan, R. A., Blankertz, L., Messinger, K. W., & Gardner, J. R. (1990). Experts' assessment of psychosocial rehabilitation principles. *Psychosocial Rehabilitation Journal, 13*(3), 59–73.

Coccaro, E. F., Harvey, P. D., Kupsaw-Lawrence, E., Herbert, J. L., & Bernstein, D. D. (1991). Development of neuropharmacologically based behavioral assessments of impulsive aggressive behavior. *Journal of Neuropsychiatry and Clinical Neurosciences, 3*, S44–S51.

Coccaro, E. F., Schmidt, C. A., Samuels, J. F., & Nestadt, G. (2004). Lifetime and 1-month prevalence rates of intermittent explosive disorder in a community sample. *Journal of Clinical Psychiatry, 65*, 820–824.

Cohen, A. (2001). *The effectiveness of mental health services in primary care: The view from the developing world.* Geneva: World Health Organization.

Cohen, C. I., Sichel, W. R., & Berger, D. (1977). The use of a mid-Manhattan hotel as a support system. *Community Mental Health Journal, 13*, 76–83.

Cohen, M. D., Shore, M. F., & Mazade, N. A. (1991). Development of a management training program for state mental health program directors. *Administration and Policy in Mental Health, 18*, 247–256.

Coldham, E. L., Addington, J., & Addington, D. (2002). Medication adherence of individuals with a first episode of psychosis. *Acta Psychiatrica Scandinavica, 106*, 286–290.

Colom, F., Vieta, E., Martinez-Aran, A., Reinares, M., Goikolea, J. M., Benabarre, A., et al. (2003). A randomized trial on the efficacy of group psychoeducation in the prophylaxis of recurrences in bipolar patients whose disease is in remission. *Archives of General Psychiatry, 60*, 402–407.

Cometa, M. S., Morrison, J. K., & Ziskoven, M. (1979). Halfway to where?: A critique of research on psychiatric halfway houses. *Journal of Community Psychology, 7*, 23–27.

Community Residences Information Services Program. (1986). *"There goes the neighborhood . . . "* White Plains, NY: Author.

Condelli, W., Bradigan, B., & Holanchock, H. (1997). Intermediate care programs to reduce risk and better manage inmates with psychiatric disorders. *Behavioral Sciences and the Law, 15*, 459–467.

Condelli, W., Dvoskin, J., & Holanchock, H. (1994). Intermediate care programs for inmates with psychiatric disorders. *Bulletin of the American Academy of Psychiatry and the Law, 22*, 63–70.

Connors, K. A., Graham, R. S., & Pulso, R. (1987). Playing the store: Where is the vocational in psychiatric rehabilitation? *Psychosocial Rehabilitation Journal, 10*(3), 21–33.

Cook, J. (2004). Blazing New Trials: Using evidence-based practice and stakeholder consensus to enhance psychosocial rehabilitation services in Texas. *Psychiatric Rehabilitation Journal, 27*, 305–306.

Cook, J., Jonikas, J., & Razzano, L. (1995). A randomized evaluation of consumer versus nonconsumer training of state and mental health service providers. *Community Mental Health Journal, 31*, 229–238.

Cook, J., Toprac, M., & Shore, S. (2004). Combining evidence-based practice with stakeholder consensus to enhance psychosocial rehabilitation services in the Texas benefit design initiative. *Psychiatric Rehabilitation Journal, 27,* 307–318.

Cook, J. A. (2002, August 8). *Employment and income supports.* Paper presented at the President's New Freedom Commission on Mental Health, Washington, DC.

Cook, J. A., Carey, M. A., Razzano, L. A., Burke, J., & Blyler, C. R. (2002). The pioneer: The Employment Intervention Demonstration Project. *New Directions for Evaluation, 94,* 31–44.

Cook, J. A., & Hoffschmidt, S. J. (1993). Comprehensive models of psychosocial rehabilitation. In R. W. Flexer & P. L. Solomon (Eds.), *Psychiatric rehabilitation in practice* (pp. 81–97). Boston: Andover.

Cook, J. A., Lehman, A. F., Drake, R., McFarlane, W. R., Gold, P. B., Leff, H. S., et al. (2005). Integration of psychiatric and vocational services: A multisite randomized, controlled trial of Supported employment. *American Journal of Psychiatry, 162,* 1948–1956.

Cook, J. A., & Razzano, L. (1995). Discriminant function analysis of competitive employment outcomes in a transitional employment program for persons with severe mental illness. *Journal of Vocational Rehabilitation, 5,* 127–140.

Cook, S. W. (1985). Experimenting on social issues: The case of school desegregation. *American Psychologist, 40,* 452–460.

Cooper, B. (1961). Social class and prognosis in schizophrenia. *British Journal of Preventive and Social Medicine, 15,* 14–41.

Copeland, L. A., Zeber, J. E., Valenstein, M., & Blow, F. C. (2003). Racial disparity in the use of atypical antipsychotic medications among veterans. *American Journal of Psychiatry, 160,* 1817–1812.

Copeland, M. E. (1997). *Wellness Recovery Action Plan.* Brattleboro, VT: Peach Press.

Copeland, M. E. (1999). *Winning against relapse: A workbook of action plans for recurring health and emotional problems.* Oakland, CA: New Harbinger.

Copeland, M. E. (2001). *Wellness Recovery Action Plan (WRAP) for dual diagnosis.* Dummerston, VT: Peach Press.

Copeland, M. E., & Mead, S. (2004). *Wellness Recovery Action Plan and peer support: Personal, group and program development.* Dummerston, VT: Peach Press.

Corcoran, R. (2001). Theory of mind and schizophrenia. In P. W. Corrigan & D. L. Penn (Eds.), *Social cognition and schizophrenia.* Washington, DC: American Psychological Association.

Coridan, C., & O'Connell, C. (2001). *Meeting the challenge: Ending treatment disparities for women of color.* Retrieved January 12, 2006, from *www.nasmhpd.org/publications.cfm#cultcomp.*

Corrigan, P. W. (1991). Social skills training in adult psychiatric populations: A meta-analysis. *Journal of Behavior Therapy and Experimental Psychiatry, 22,* 203–210.

Corrigan, P. W. (1996). Models of "normal" cognitive functioning. In P. W. Corrigan & S. C. Yudofsky (Eds.), *Cognitive rehabilitation for neuropsychiatric disorders* (pp. 3–51). Washington, DC: American Psychiatric Press.

Corrigan, P. W. (1998). The impact of stigma on severe mental illness. *Cognitive and Behavioral Practice, 5,* 201–222.

Corrigan, P. W. (2000). Mental health stigma as social attribution: Implications for research methods and attitude change. *Clinical Psychology-Science and Practice, 7,* 48–67.

Corrigan, P. W. (2001). Place-then-train: An alternative service paradigm for persons with psychiatric disabilities. *Clinical Psychology-Science and Practice, 8,* 334–349.

Corrigan, P. W. (2002). Adherence to anti-psychotic medications and health behavior theories. *Journal of Mental Health, 11,* 243–254.

Corrigan, P. W. (2004). How stigma interferes with mental health care. *American Psychologist, 59,* 614–625.

Corrigan, P. W., Buican, B., & McCracken, S. (1995a). The Needs and Resources Assessment Interview for severely mentally ill adults. *Psychiatric Services, 46,* 504–505.

Corrigan, P. W., & Calabrese, J. D. (2005). Strategies for assessing and diminishing self-stigma. In P. W. Corrigan (Ed.), *On the stigma of mental illness: Practical strategies for research and social change* (pp. 239–256). Washington, DC: American Psychological Association.

Corrigan, P. W., Faber, D., Rashid, F., & Leary, M. (1999a). The construct validity of empowerment among consumers of mental health services. *Schizophrenia Research, 38,* 77–84.

Corrigan, P. W., & Garman, A. N. (1997). Considerations for research on consumer empowerment and psychosocial interventions. *Psychiatric Services, 48,* 347–352.

Corrigan, P. W., Green, A., Lundin, R., Kubiak, M. A., & Penn, D. L. (2001a). Familiarity with and social distance from people who have serious mental illness. *Psychiatric Services, 52,* 953–958.

Corrigan, P. W., Green, M. F., & Toomey, R. (1994). Cognitive correlates to social cue perception in schizophrenia. *Psychiatry Research, 53,* 141–151.

Corrigan, P. W., & Holmes, E. P. (1994). Patient identification of "street skills" for a psychosocial training module. *Hospital and Community Psychiatry, 45,* 273–276.

Corrigan, P. W., Larson, J., Watson, A. C., Barr, L., & Boyle, M. (2006). Solutions to discrimination in work and housing identified by people with mental illness. *Journal of Nervous and Mental Disease, 194*(9), 716–718.

Corrigan, P. W., Liberman R. P., & Engel, J. D. (1990). From non-compliance to collaboration in the treatment of schizophrenia. *Hospital and Community Psychiatry, 41*(11), 1203–1211.

Corrigan, P. W., Liberman, R. P., & Wong, S. E. (1993). Recreational therapy and behavior management on inpatient units: Is recreational therapy therapeutic? *Journal of Nervous and Mental Disease, 181,* 644–646.

Corrigan, P. W., Lickey, S. E., Schmook, A., Virgil, L., & Juricek, M. (1999b). Dialogue among stakeholders of severe mental illness. *Psychiatric Rehabilitation Journal, 23,* 62–65.

Corrigan P. W., & Lundin R. K. (2001). *Don't call me nuts! Coping with the stigma of mental illness.* Tinley Park, IL: Recovery Press.

Corrigan, P. W., MacKain, S. J., & Liberman, R. P. (1994). Skills training modules: A strategy for dissemination and utilization of a rehabilitation innovation. In J. Rothman & E. J. Thomas (Eds.), *Intervention research: Design and development for human service* (pp. 317–352). New York: Haworth Press.

Corrigan, P. W., McCorkle, B., Schell, B., & Kidder, K. (2003). Religion and spirituality in the lives of people with serious mental illness. *Community Mental Health Journal, 39,* 487–500.

Corrigan, P. W., McCracken, S. G., Edwards, M., Kommana, S., & Simpatico, T. (1997). Staff training to improve implementation and impact of behavioral rehabilitation programs. *Psychiatric Services, 48,* 1336–1338.

Corrigan, P. W., McCracken, S. G., & Holmes, E. (2001b). Motivational interviews as goal assessment for persons with psychiatric disability. *Community Mental Health Journal, 37,* 113–122.

Corrigan, P. W., & Mueser, K. T. (2000). Behavior therapy for aggressive psychiatric patients. In M. L. Crowner (Ed.), *Understanding and treating violent psychiatric patients: Progress in psychiatry* (pp. 69–85). Washington, DC: American Psychiatric Press.

Corrigan, P. W., Nugent-Hirschbeck, J., & Wolfe, M. (1995b). Memory and vigilance training to improve social perception in schizophrenia. *Schizophrenia Research, 17,* 257–265.

Corrigan, P. W., & Penn, D. L. (1995). The effects of antipsychotic and antiparkinsonian medication on psychosocial skill learning. *Clinical Psychology-Science and Practice, 2,* 251–262.

Corrigan, P. W., & Penn, D. L. (1999). Lessons from social psychology on discrediting psychiatric stigma. *American Psychologist, 54,* (9) 765.

Corrigan, P. W., & Penn, D. L. (2001). *Social cognition and schizophrenia* (Vol. 16). Washington, DC: American Psychological Association.

Corrigan P. W., River, L. P., Lundin, R. K., Penn, D. L., Uphoff-Wasowski, K., Campion, J., et al. (2001c). Three strategies for changing attributions about severe mental illness. *Schizophrenia Bulletin, 27*(2), 187–195.

Corrigan, P. W., Rowan, D., Green, A., Lundin, R., River, P., Uphoff-Wasowski, K., et al. (2002). Challenging two mental illness stigmas: Personal responsibility and dangerousness. *Schizophrenia Bulletin, 28,* 293–310.

Corrigan, P. W., Salzer, M., Ralph, R., Sangster, Y., & Keck, L. (2004a). Examining the factor structure of the Recovery Assessment Scale. *Schizophrenia Bulletin, 30,* 1035–1041.

Corrigan, P. W., & Stephenson, J. A. (1994). Information processing and clinical psychology. In V. S. Ramachandran (Ed.), *Encyclopedia of human behavior* (Vol. 2). Orlando, FL: Academic Press.

Corrigan, P. W., & Toomey, R. (1995). Interpersonal problem solving and information processing in schizophrenia. *Schizophrenia Bulletin, 21*(3), 395–403.

Corrigan, P. W., Wallace, C. J., Schade, M. L., & Green, M. F. (1994). Learning medication self-management skills in schizophrenia: Relationships with cognitive deficits and psychiatric symptoms. *Behavior Therapy, 25,* 5–15.

Corrigan, P. W., & Watson, A. C. (2003). Factors that explain how policy makers distribute resources to mental health services. *Psychiatric Services, 54,* 501–507.

Corrigan, P. W., & Watson, A. C. (2005). Findings from the National Comorbidity Survey on the frequency of dangerous behavior in individuals with psychiaric disorders. *Psychiatry Research, 136,* 153–162.

Corrigan, P. W., Watson, A. C., & Miller, F. E. (2004b). The impact of mental illness and substance abuse stigma on family members. *Journal of Family Psychology.* Manuscript submitted for publication.

Corrigan, P. W., Yudofsky, S. C., & Silver, J. M. (1993). Pharmacological and behavioral treatments for aggressive psychiatric inpatients. *Hospital and Community Psychiatry, 44,* 125–133.

Corse, S. J., Hirschinger, N. B., & Zanis, D. (1995). The use of the Addiction Severity Index with people with severe mental illness. *Psychiatric Rehabilitation Journal, 19,* 9–18.

Cosden, M., Ellens, J., Schnell, J., Yasmeen, Y., & Wolfe, M. (2003). Evaluation of a mental health treatment court with assertive community treatment. *Behavioral Sciences and the Law, 21,* 415–427.

Cosoff, S. J., & Hafner, R. (1998). The prevalence of comorbid anxiety in schizophrenia, schizoaffective disorder and bipolar disorder. *Australian and New Zealand Journal of Psychiatry, 32*(1), 67–72.

Costa, P. T., Jr., & McCrae, R. R. (1992). *Revised NEO Personality Inventory (NEO-PI-R) and NEO Five-Factor Inventory (NEO-FFI).* Odessa, FL: Psychological Assessment Resources.

Cournos, F., & McKinnon, K. (1997). HIV seroprevalence among people with severe mental illness in the United States: A critical review. *Clinical Psychology Review, 17,* 159–169.

Coursey, R., Curtis, L., Marsh, D., Campbell, J., Harding, C., Spaniol, L., et al. (2000a). Competencies for direct service staff members who work with adults with severe mental illness in outpatient public mental health managed care systems. *Psychiatric Rehabilitation Journal, 23,* 370–377.

Coursey, R. D., Curtis, L., Marsh, D. T., Campbell, J., Harding, C., Spaniol, L., et al. (2000b). Competencies for direct services staff members who work with adults with severe mental illnesses: Specific knowledge, attitudes, skills, and bibliography. *Psychiatric Rehabilitation Journal, 23*(4), 378–392.

Courtney, C. (2005). History. In D. W. Dew & G. M. Alan (Eds.), *Innovative methods for providing VR services to individuals with psychiatric disabilities* (Institute on Rehabilitation Issues Monograph 30) (pp. 27–45). Washington, DC: George Washington University Center for Rehabilitation Counseling Research and Education. (*www.gwu.edu/%7Eiri/publications.htm*)

Covell, N. H., Jackson, C. T., Evans, A. C., & Essock, S. M. (2002). Antipsychotic prescribing practices in Connecticut's public mental health system: Rates of changing medications and prescribing styles. *Schizophrenia Bulletin, 28,* 17–29.

Cowell, A., Broner, N., & Dupont, R. (2004). The cost-effectiveness of criminal justice diversion programs in people with serious mental illness co-occurring with substance abuse. *Journal of Contemporary Criminal Justice, 20,* 292–315.

Craig, T., Doherty, I., Jamieson-Craig, R., Boocock, A., & Attafua, A. (2004). The consumer-employee as a member of a Mental Health Assertive Outreach Team: I. Clinical and social outcomes. *Journal of Mental Health, 13,* 59–69.

Craine, L. S., Henson, C. E., Colliver, J. A., & MacLean, D. G. (1988). Prevalence of a history of sexual abuse among female psychiatric patients in a state hospital system. *Hospital and Community Psychiatry, 39,* 300–304.

Cramer, J. A., & Rosenheck, R. (1999). Enhancing medication compliance for people with serious mental illness. *Journal of Nervous and Mental Disease, 187,* 53–55.

Crane-Ross, D., Roth, D., & Lauber, B. G. (2000). Consumers' and case managers' perceptions of mental health and community support service needs. *Community Mental Health Journal, 36,* 161–178.

Crawford, M., deJonge, E., Freeman, G., & Weaver, T. (2004). Providing continuity of care for people with severe mental illness. *Social Psychiatry and Psychiatric Epidemiology, 39,* 265–272.

Creed, R., Black, D., & Anthony, P. (1989). Day-hospital and community treatment for acute psychiatric illness: A critical appraisal. *British Journal of Psychiatry, 154,* 300–310.

Crenshaw, W. B., & Francis, P. S. (1995). A national survey on seclusion and restraint in state psychiatric hospitals. *Psychiatric Services, 46,* 1026–1031.

Crews, C., Batal, H., Elasy, T., Casper, E. S., & Mehler, P. S. (1998). Primary care for those with severe and persistent mental illness. *Western Journal of Medicine, 169,* 245–250.

Crisanti, A. S., & Love, E. J. (2002). From one legal system to another?: An examination of the relationship between involuntary hospitalization and arrest. *International Journal of Law and Psychiatry, 25,* 581–597.

Crocetti, G., Spiro, H. R., & Siassi, I. (1971). Are the ranks closed?: Attitudinal social distance and mental illness. *American Journal of Psychiatry, 127,* 1121–1127.

Crocker, A. G., Mueser, K. T., Clark, R. E., McHugo, G. J., Ackerson, T., & Alterman, A. I. (2005). Antisocial personality, psychopathy and violence in persons with dual disorders: A longitudinal analysis. *Criminal Justice and Behavior, 32,* 452–476.

Crocker, J., & Lawrence, J. S. (1999). Social stigma and self-esteem: The role of contingencies. In D. A. Prentice & D. T. Miller (Eds.), *Cultural divides: Understanding and overcoming group conflict* (pp. 364–392). New York: Russell Sage Foundation.

Crocker, J., & Major, B. (1989). Social stigma and self-esteem: The self-protective properties of stigma. *Psychological Review, 96,* 608–630.

Crocker, J., Major, B., & Steele, C. (1998). Social stigma. In D. T. Gilbert, S. Fiske, & G. Lindzey (Eds.), *The handbook of social psychology* (Vol. 2, 4th ed., pp. 504–553). New York: McGraw-Hill.

Crocker, J., & Quinn, D. M. (2000). Social stigma and the self: Meaning, situations and self-esteem. In T. F. Heatherton, R. E. Kleck, M. R. Hebl, & J. G. Hull (Eds.), *The social psychology of stigma* (pp. 153–183). New York: Guilford Press.

Cross, W. E. (1978). The Thomas and Cross models of psychological nigrescence: A review. *Journal of Black Psychology, 5*, 13–31.

Crow, T. (1982). Two syndromes in schizophrenia? *Trends in Neurosciences, 5*(10), 351–354.

Crow, T. (1986). The continuum of psychosis and its implication for the structure of the gene. *British Journal of Psychiatry, 149*, 419–429.

Crow, T. (1995). Brain changes and negative symptoms in schizophrenia. *Psychopathology, 28*(1), 18–21.

Crow, T. (2003). Obstetric complications and schizophrenia. *American Journal of Psychiatry, 130*(5), 1011–1012.

Crowner, M. L. (Ed.). (2000). Understanding and treating violent psychiatric patients. Washington, DC: American Psychiatric Press.

Cuffel, B. J., Alford, J., Fischer, E. P., & Owen, R. R. (1996). Awareness of illness in schizophrenia and outpatient treatment adherence. *Journal of Nervous and Mental Disease, 184*(11), 653–659.

Cuijpers, P. (1999). The effects of family interventions on relatives' burden: A meta-analysis. *Journal of Mental Health, 8*, 275–285.

Curran, H. V. (1995). Antidepressant drugs, cognitive function and human performance. In A. P. Smith & D. M. Jones (Eds.), *Handbook of human performance* (Vol. 2, pp. 319–336). Boston: Academic Press.

Cusack, K. J., Frueh, B. C., & Brady, K. T. (2004). Trauma history screening in a community mental health center. *Psychiatric Services, 55*, 157–162.

Cutler, D. H., Bevilacqua, J., & McFarland, B. H. (2003). Four decades of community mental health: A symphony in four movements. *Community Mental Health Journal, 39*, 381–398.

Daffern, M., Ogloff, J., & Howells, K. (1993). Aggression in an Australian forensic psychiatric hospital. *British Journal of Forensic Practice, 5*, 18–28.

Dalack, G. W., Healy, D. J., & Meador-Woodruff, J. H. (1998). Nicotine dependence in schizophrenia: Clinical phenomena and laboratory findings. *American Journal of Psychiatry, 155*, 1490–1501.

Danley, K. S., & Anthony, W. A. (1987). The Choose-Get-Keep Model: Serving severely disabled psychiatrically disabled people. *American Rehabilitation, 13*(4), 6–9, 27–29.

Daumit, G. L., Pratt, L. A., Crum, R. M., Powe, N. R., & Ford, D. E. (2002). Characteristics of primary care visits for individuals with severe mental illness in a national sample. *General Hospital Psychiatry, 24*, 391–395.

Davidson, K., Pennebacker, J., & Dickerson, S. (2000). Who talks?: Social psychology of illness support groups. *American Psychologist, 55*, 215–217.

Davidson, L. (1992). Developing an empirical-phenomenological approach to schizophrenia research. *Journal of Phenomenological Psychology, 23*, 3–15.

Davidson, L., Chinman, M., Kloos, B., Weingarten, R., Stagner, D., & Tebes, J. (1999). Peer support among individuals with severe mental illness: A review of the evidence. *Clinical Psychology Science and Practice, 6*, 165–187.

Davidson, L., Shahar, G., Stayner, D. A., Chinman, M. J., Rakfeldt, J., & Tebes, J. K. (2004). Supported socialization for people with psychiatric disabilities: Lessons from a randomized controlled trial. *Journal of Community Psychology, 32*, 453–477.

Davidson, L., Stayner, D., & Haglund, K. E. (1998). Phenomenological perspectives on the social functioning of people with schizophrenia. In K. T. Mueser & N. Tarrier (Eds.), *Handbook of social functioning in schizophrenia* (pp. 97–120). Boston: Allyn & Bacon.

Davies-Netzley, S., Hurlburt, M. S., & Hough, R. (1996). Childhood abuse as a precursor to homelessness for homeless women in severe mental illness. *Violence and Victims, 11*, 129–142.

Davis, D., & Schultz, C. (1998). Grief parenting and schizophrenia. *Social Science and Medicine, 46*, 369–379.

Davis, J. M. (1980). Antipsychotic drugs. In H. I. Kaplan, A. M. Freedman, & B. J. Sadock (Eds.), *Comprehensive textbook of psychiatry* (Vol. 3, pp. 2257–2289). Baltimore: Williams & Wilkins.

Davis, J. M., Barter, J. T., & Kane, J. M. (1989). Antipsychotic drugs. In H. I. Kaplan & B. J. Sadock (Eds.), *Comprehensive textbook of psychiatry* (Vol. 5, pp. 1591–1626). Baltimore: Williams & Wilkins.

Davis, J. M., Chen, N., & Glick, I. D. (2003). A meta-analysis of the efficacy of second-generation antipsychotics. *Archives of General Psychiatry, 60*, 553–564.

Dazord, A., Astolfl, F., Guisti, P., Rebetez, M.,

Mino, A., Terra, J., et al. (1998). Quality of life assessment in psychiatry: The subjective quality of life profile (SQLP): First results of a new instrument. *Community Mental Health Journal, 34*, 525–535.

De Leon, G., Sacks, S., Staines, G., & McKendrick, K. (2000). Modified therapeutic community for homeless mentally ill chemical abusers: Treatment outcomes. *American Journal of Drug and Alcohol Abuse, 26*, 461–480.

Deane, M., Steadman, H., Borum, R., Veysey, B., & Morrissey, J. (1999). Emerging partnerships between mental health and law enforcement. *Psychiatric Services, 50*, 99–101.

DeChillo, N., Matorin, S., & Hallahan, C. (1987). Children of psychiatric patients: Rarely seen or heard. *Health and Social Work, 12*, 296–302.

Deegan, P. E. (1990). Spirit breaking: When the helping professionals hurt. *Humanistic Psychologist, 18*(3), 301–313.

Deegan, P. E. (2005). The importance of personal medicine: A qualitative study of resilience in people with psychiatric disabilities. *Scandinavian Journal of Public Health, 33*, 29–35.

Deegan, P. E., & Drake, R. E. (2006). Shared decision-making and medication management in the recovery process: From compliance to alliance. *Psychiatric Services, 57*, 1636–1639.

Dekle, D., & Christensen, L. (1990). Medication management [Letter to the editor]. *Hospital and Community Psychiatry, 41*, 96–97.

Delespaul, P. A., & deVries, M. W. (1987). The daily life of ambulatory chronic mental patients. *Journal of Nervous and Mental Disease, 175*, 537–544.

DenBoer, P., Wiersma, D., & Van Den Bosch, R. (2004). Why is self-help neglected in the treatment of emotional disorders?: A meta-analysis. *Psychological Medicine, 34*, 959–971.

Dennis, J. L., & Crisham, K. P. (2001). Chronic assaultive behavior improved with sleep apnea treatment. *Journal of Clinical Psychiatry, 62*, 571–572.

Derogotis, L., Lipman, R., Covi, L. (1973). Symtom Checklist-90: An outpatient psychiatric rating scale preliminary report. *Psychopharmacology Bulletin, 9*, 13–17.

Derogatis, L. R. (1977). *Symptom Checklist-90* (rev.). Baltimore, MD: Johns Hopkins University School of Medicine.

Derogatis, L. R. (1993). *Brief Symptom Inventory (BSI): Administration, scoring, and procedures manual* (3rd ed.). Minneapolis, MN: National Computer Systems.

DeRubeis, R. J., Gelfand, L. A., Tang, T. Z., & Simons, A. D. (1999). Medications versus cognitive behavior therapy for severely depressed outpatients: Mega-analysis of four randomized comparisons. *American Journal of Psychiatry, 156*, 1007–1013.

Desai, M. M., Rosenheck, R. A., Druss, B. G., & Perlin, J. B. (2002). Mental disorders and quality of care among postacute myocardial infarction outpatients. *Journal of Nervous and Mental Disease, 190*, 51–53.

Desai, R. (2003). Jail diversion services for people with mental illness: What do we really know? *Community-based Interventions for Criminal Offenders with Severe Mental Illness, 12*, 99–121.

Desforges, D. M., Lord, C. G., Ramsey, S. L., Mason, J. A., Van Leeuwen, M. D., West, S. C., et al. (1991). Effects of structured cooperative contact on changing negative attitudes toward stigmatized social groups. *Journal of Personality and Social Psychology, 60*, 531–544.

DeSisto, M. J., Harding, C. M., McCormick, R. V., Ashikaga, T., & Brooks, G. W. (1995). The Maine and Vermont three-decade studies of serious mental illness. *British Journal of Psychiatry, 167*, 331–342.

Detrick, A., & Stiepock, V. (1992). Treating persons with mental illness, substance abuse, and legal problems: The Rhode Island experience. In L. I. Stein (Ed.), *Innovative community mental health programs: New directions for mental health services* (Vol. 56, pp. 65–77). San Francisco: Jossey-Bass.

Devine, P. G. (1988). *Stereotype assessment: Theoretical and methodological issues*. Madison: University of Wisconsin-Madison.

Devine, P. G. (1989). Stereotypes and prejudice: Their automatic and controlled components. *Journal of Personality and Social Psychology, 56*, 5–18.

Devine, P. G. (1995). Prejudice and out-group perception. In A. Tessor (Ed.), *Advanced social psychology* (pp. 467–524). New York: McGraw-Hill.

Diamond, R. (1996). Coercion and tenacious treatment in the community. In D. L. Dennis & J. Monahan (Eds.), *Coercion and aggressive community treatment* (pp. 51–72). New York: Plenum Press.

Diamond, R. J. (1983). Enhancing medication use in schizophrenic patients. *Journal of Clinical Psychiatry, 44*, 7–14.

Diamond, R. J. (1998). *Instant psychopharmacology: A guide for the nonmedical mental health professional*. New York: Norton.

Dickerson, F. B. (2000). Cognitive behavioral psychotherapy for schizophrenia: A review of recent empirical studies. *Schizophrenia Research, 43*, 71–90.

Dickerson, F. B., McNary, S. W., Brown, C. H., Kreyenbuhl, J., Goldberg, R. W., & Dixon, L. (2003). Somatic healthcare utilization among adults with serious mental illness who are receiving community psychiatric services. *Medical Care, 41,* 560–570.

Dickey, B., & Azeni, H. (1996). Persons with dual diagnosis of substance abuse and major mental illness: Their excess costs of psychiatric care. *American Journal of Public Health, 86,* 973–977.

Dickey, B., Norman, S.-L., Weiss, R. D., Drake, R. E., & Azeni, H. (2002). Medical morbidity, mental illness, and substance use disorders. *Psychiatric Services, 53,* 861–867.

Dickstein, L. J., & Hinz, L. D. (1992). The stigma of mental illness for medical students and residents. In P. J. Fink & A. Tasman (Eds.), *Stigma and mental illness.* Washington DC: American Psychiatric Press.

DiGiuseppe, R. (1999). End piece: Reflections on the treatment of anger. *Journal of Clinical Psychology, 55,* 365–379.

Dilk, M. N., & Bond, G. R. (1996). Meta-analytic evaluation of skills training research for individuals with severe mental illness. *Journal of Consulting and Clinical Psychology, 64,* 1337–1346.

Dincin, J. (1975). Psychiatric rehabilitation. *Schizophrenia Bulletin, 1,* 131–147.

Dincin, J. (1988). A crucial dimension. *Switzer Monograph* (25–47). Alexandria, VA: National Rehabilitation Association.

Dincin, J. (1995a). Core programs in the Thresholds approach. *New Directions for Mental Health Services, 68,* 33–54.

Dincin, J. (1995b). A pragmatic approach to psychiatric rehabilitation: Lessons from Chicago's Thresholds program [Special issue]. *New Directions for Mental Health Services, 68.*

Dincin, J., Selleck, V., & Streicker, S. (1978). Reconstructing parental attitudes: Working with parents of adult mentally ill. *Schizophrenia Bulletin, 4,* 597–608.

Dincin, J., & Witheridge, T. F. (1982). Psychiatric rehabilitation as a deterrent to recidivism. *Hospital and Community Psychiatry, 33,* 645–650.

Ditton, P. J. (1999). *Bureau of Justice Statistics Special Report: Mental Health Treatment of Inmates and Probationers.* Washington, DC: U.S. Department of Justice.

Dixon, L. (1999). Providing services to families of persons with schizophrenia: Present and future. *Journal of Mental Health Policy and Economics, 2,* 3–8.

Dixon, L., Adams, C., & Lucksted, A. (2000a). Update on family psychoeducation for schizophrenia. *Schizophrenia Bulletin, 26,* 5–20.

Dixon, L., Goldman, H., & Hirad, A. (1999a). State policy and funding of services to families of adults with serious and persistent mental illness. *Psychiatric Services, 50,* 631–643.

Dixon, L., Hackman, A., & Lehman, A. (1997). Consumers as staff in assertive community treatment programs. *Administration and Policy in Mental Health, 25,* 99–208.

Dixon, L., Krauss, N., & Lehman, A. (1994). Consumers as service providers: The promise and challenge. *Community Mental Health Journal, 30,* 615–625.

Dixon, L., & Lehman, A. (1995). Family interventions for schizophrenia. *Schizophrenia Bulletin, 21,* 631–643.

Dixon, L., Lucksted, A., Stewart, B., Burland, J., Brown, C., Postrado, L., et al. (2004). Outcomes of the peer-taught 12 week family-to-family education program for severe mental illness. *Acta Psychiatrica Scandinavica, 109,* 207–215.

Dixon, L., Lyles, A., Scott, J., Lehman, A., & McGlynn, E. (1999b). Services to families of adults with schizophrenia: From treatment recommendations to dissemination. *Psychiatric Services, 50,* 233–238.

Dixon, L., McFarlane, W., Lefley, H., Lucksted, A., Cohen, C., Falloon, I., et al. (2001a). Evidence-based practices for services to family members of people with psychiatric disabilities. *Psychiatric Services, 52,* 903–910.

Dixon, L., Postrado, L., Delahanty, J., Fischer, P. J., & Lehman, A. (1999c). The association of medical comorbidity in schizophrenia with poor physical and mental health. *Journal of Nervous and Mental Disease, 187,* 496–502.

Dixon, L., Stewart, B., Burland, J., Delahanty, J., Lucksted, A., & Hoffman, M. (2001b). Pilot study of the effectiveness of the Family-to-Family Education Program. *Psychiatric Services, 52,* 965–967.

Dixon, L., Stewart, B., Krauss, N., Robbins, J., Hackman, A., & Lehman, A. (1998). The participation of families of homeless persons with severe mental illness in an outreach intervention. *Community Mental Health Journal, 34,* 251–259.

Dixon, L., Weiden, P. J., Delahanty, J., Goldberg, R., Postrado, L., Lucksted, A., et al. (2000b). Prevalence and correlates of diabetes in national schizophrenia samples. *Schizophrenia Bulletin, 26,* 904–912.

Dobscha, S. K., & Ganzini, L. (2001). A program for teaching psychiatric residents to provide integrated psychiatric and primary medical care. *Psychiatric Services, 52,* 1651–1653.

Doherty, I., Craig, T., Attafua, G., Boocock, A., & Jamieson-Craig, R. (2004). The consumer-employee as a member of Mental Health Assertive Outreach Team: II. Impressions of consumer-employees and other team members. *Journal of Mental Health, 13,* 71–81.

Dohrenwend, B. P., Levav, I., Shrout, P. E., Schwartz, S., Naveh, G., Link, B. G., et al. (1992). Socioeconomic status and psychiatric disorders: The causation-selection issue. *Science, 255,* 946–952.

Dohrenwend, B. P., Levav, I., Shrout, P. E., Schwartz, S., Naveh, G., Link, B. G., et al. (1998). Ethnicity, socioeconomic status, and psychiatric disorders: A test of the social causation-social selection issue. In B. P. Dohrenwend (Ed.), *Adversity, stress, and psychopathology* (pp. 285–318). New York: Oxford University Press.

Dolder, C. R., Larco, J. P., & Dunn, L. B. (2002). Antipsychotic medication adherence: Is there a difference between typical and atypical agents? *American Journal of Psychiatry, 159,* 103–108.

Dolder, C. R., Lacro, J. P., Warren, K. A., Golshan, S., Perkins, D. O., & Jeste, D. V. (2004). Brief evaluation of medication influences and beliefs: Development and testing of a brief scale for medication adherence. *Journal of Clinical Psychopharmacology, 24,* 404–409.

Dollard, J., Miller, N. E., Doob, L. W., Mowrer, O. H., & Sears, R. R. (1939). *Frustration and aggression.* New Haven, CT: Yale University Press.

Donahoe, C. P., Carter, M. J., Bloem, W. D., Hirsch, A., Laasi, N., & Wallace, C. W. (1990). Assessment of interpersonal problem-solving skills. *Psychiatry, 53,* 329–339.

Donahoe, C. P. J., & Driesenga, S. A. (1988). A review of social skills training with chronic mental patients. In M. Hersen, R. M. Eisler, & P. M. Miller (Eds.), *Progress in behavior modification* (Vol. 24, pp. 131–164). Newbury Park, CA: Sage.

Doornbos, M. (2001). The 24-7-52 job: Family caregiving for young adults with serious and persistent mental illness. *Journal of Family Nursing, 7,* 328–344.

Doughtery, R. J. (1997). Naltrexone in the treatment of alcojol dependent dual diagnosed patients. *Journal of Addictive Diseases, 16,* 107.

Draine, J. (2003). Where is the "illness" in the criminalization of mental illness? *Community-based Interventions for Criminal Offenders with Mental Illness, 12,* 9–21.

Draine, J., Blank, A., Kottsieper, P., & Solomon, P. (2005). Contrasting jail diversion and in-jail services for mental illness and substance abuse: Do they serve the same clients? *Behavioral Science and the Law, 23,* 171–181.

Draine, J., Salzer, M. S., Culhane, D. P., & Hadley, T. R. (2002). Role of social disadvantage in crime, joblessness, and homelessness among persons with serious mental illness. *Psychiatric Services, 53,* 565–573.

Draine, J., & Solomon, P. (1994). Jail recidivism and the intensity of case management services among homeless persons with mental illness leaving jail. *Journal of Psychiatry and the Law, 4,* 39–49.

Draine, J., & Solomon, P. (1999). Describing and evaluating jail diversion services for persons with serious mental illness. *Psychiatric Services, 50,* 56–61.

Drake, R. E., Becker, D. R., Biesanz, J. C., Torrey, W. C., McHugo, G. J., & Wyzik, P. F. (1994). Rehabilitative day treatment vs. supported employment: I. Vocational outcomes. *Community Mental Health Journal, 30,* 519–532.

Drake, R. E., Becker, D. R., Biesanz, J. C., Wyzik, P. F., & Torrey, W. C. (1996a). Day treatment versus supported employment for persons with severe mental illness: A replication study. *Psychiatric Services, 47,* 1125–1127.

Drake, R. E., Becker, D. R., Bond, G. R., & Mueser, K. T. (2003a). A process analysis of integrated and non-integrated approaches to supported employment. *Journal of Vocational Rehabilitation, 18,* 51–58.

Drake R. E., Becker D. R., Clark R. E., & Mueser K. T. (1999a). Research on the individual placement and support model of supported employment. *Psychiatric Quarterly, 70*(4), 289–301.

Drake, R. E., Becker, D. R., Goldman, H. H., & Martinez, R. A. (2006a). The Johnson & Johnson-Dartmouth Community Mental Health Program: Best practices in disseminating an evidence-based practice. *Psychiatric Services, 57,* 302–304.

Drake, R. E., & Brunette, M. F. (1998). Complications of severe mental illness related to alcohol and other drug use disorders. In M. Galanter (Ed.), *Recent developments in alcoholism: Consequences of alcoholism* (Vol. 14, pp. 285–299). New York: Plenum Press.

Drake, R. E., Essock, S. M., Shaner, A., Carey, K. B., Minkoff, K., Kola, L., et al. (2001a). Implementing dual diagnosis services for clients with severe mental illness. *Psychiatric Services, 52*(4), 469–476.

Drake, R. E., Fox, T. S., Leather, P. K., Becker, D. R., Musumeci, J. S., Ingram, W. F., et al. (1998a). Regional variation in competitive employment for persons with severe mental illness. *Administration and Policy in Mental Health, 25,* 493–504.

Drake, R. E., Gates, C., Cotton, P. G., & Whitaker, A. (1984). Suicide among schizophrenics: Who is at risk? *Journal of Nervous and Mental Disease, 172,* 613–617.

Drake, R. E., Goldman, H. H., Leff, H. S., Lehman, A. F., Dixon, L., Mueser, K. T., et al. (2001b). Implementing evidence-based practices in routine mental health service settings. *Psychiatric Services, 52,* 179–182.

Drake, R. E., Green, A. I., Mueser, K. T., & Goldman, H. H. (2003b). The history of community mental health treatment and rehabilitation for persons with severe mental illness. *Community Mental Health Journal, 39,* 427–440.

Drake, R. E., McHugo, G. J., Bebout, R. R., Becker, D. R., Harris, M., Bond, G. R., et al. (1999b). A randomized clinical trial of supported employment for inner-city patients with severe mental illness. *Archives of General Psychiatry, 56,* 627–633.

Drake, R. E., McHugo, G. J., Becker, D. R., Anthony, W. A., & Clark, R. E. (1996b). The New Hampshire Study of Supported Employment for people with severe mental illness: Vocational outcomes. *Journal of Consulting and Clinical Psychology, 64,* 391–399.

Drake, R. E., McHugo, G. J., & Biesanz, J. C. (1995). The test–retest reliability of standardized instruments among homeless persons with substance use disorder. *Journal of Alcohol Studies, 56,* 161–167.

Drake, R. E., McHugo, G. J., Clark, R. E., Teague, G. B., Xie, H., Miles, K., et al. (1998b). Assertive community treatment for patients with co-occurring severe mental illness and substance use disorder: A clinical trial. *American Journal of Orthopsychiatry, 68,* 201–215.

Drake, R. E., McHugo, G., & Noordsy, D. L. (1993). Treatment of alcoholism among schizophrenic outpatients: Four-year outcomes. *American Journal of Psychiatry, 150,* 328–329.

Drake, R. E., McHugo, G. J., Xie, H., Fox, M., Packard, J., & Helmstetter, B. (2006b). Ten-year recovery outcomes for clients with co-occurring schizophrenia and substance use disorder. *Schizophrenia Bulletin, 32,* 464–473.

Drake, R. E., Mercer-McFadden, C., Mueser, K. T., McHugo, G. J., & Bond, G. R. (1998c). Review of integrated mental health and substance abuse treatment for patients with dual disorders. *Schizophrenia Bulletin, 24,* 589–608.

Drake, R. E., Merrens, M. R., & Lynde, D. W. (Eds.). (2005a). *Evidence-based mental health practice: A textbook.* New York: Norton.

Drake, R. E., Morrissey, J., & Mueser, K. T. (2006c). The challenge of treating forensic dual diagnosis clients. *Community Mental Health Journal, 42,* 427–432.

Drake, R. E., Mueser, K. T., Brunette, M., &

McHugo, G. J. (2004). A review of treatments for people with severe mental illness and co-occurring substance use disorder. *Psychiatric Rehabilitation Journal, 27,* 360–374.

Drake, R. E., Mueser, K. T., Torrey, W. C., Miller, A. F., Lehman, A. F., Bond, G. R., et al. (2000a). Evidence-based treatment of schizophrenia. *Current Psychiatry Reports, 2,* 393–397.

Drake, R. E., O'Neal, E. L., & Wallach, M. A. (in press). A systematic review of psychosocial interventions for people with co-occurring substance use and severe mental disorders. *Journal of Substance Abuse Treatment.*

Drake, R. E., Osher, F. C., Noordsy, D. L., Hurlbut, S. C., Teague, G. B., & Beaudett, M. S. (1990). Diagnosis of alcohol use disorders in schizophrenia. *Schizophrenia Bulletin, 16,* 57–67.

Drake, R. E., Osher, F. C., & Wallach, M. A. (1991). Homelessness and dual diagnosis. *American Psychologist, 46,* 1149–1158.

Drake, R. E., Rosenberg, S. D., Teague, G. B., Bartels, S. J., & Torrey, W. C. (2003c). Fundamental principles of evidence-based medicine applied to mental health care. *Psychiatric Clinics of North America, 24,* 811–820.

Drake, R. E., & Sederer, L. I. (1986a). The adverse effects of intensive treatment of chronic schizophrenia. *Comprehensive Psychiatry, 27,* 313–326.

Drake, R. E., & Sederer, L. I. (1986b). Inpatient psychosocial treatment of chronic schizophrenia: Negative effects and current guidelines. *Hospital and Community Psychiatry, 37,* 897–901.

Drake, R. E., & Wallach, M. A. (1989). Substance abuse among the chronic mentally ill. *Hospital and Community Psychiatry, 40,* 1041–1046.

Drake, R. E., Wallach, M. A., Alverson, H. S., & Mueser, K. T. (2002). Psychosocial aspects of substance abuse by clients with severe mental illness. *Journal of Nervous and Mental Disease, 190,* 100–106.

Drake, R. E., Wallach, M. A., & McGovern, M. P. (2005b). Preventing relapses to substance use disorder among clients with severe mental illnesses: What do we know and what do we do next? *Psychiatric Services, 56,* 1297–1302.

Drake, R. E., Xie, H., McHugo, G. J., & Green, A. I. (2000b). The effects of clozapine on alcohol and drug use disorders among schizophrenic patients. *Schizophrenia Bulletin, 26,* 441–449.

Drake, R. E., Yovetich, N. A., Bebout, R. R., Harris, M., & McHugo, G. J. (1997). Integrated treatment for dually diagnosed homeless adults. *Journal of Nervous and Mental Disease, 185,* 298–305.

Drebing, C. E., Rosenheck, R., & Penk, W. (2001).

Compensated Work Therapy National Survey: Summary of project director responses. Bedford, MA: New England Mental Illness Research, Education and Clinical Center.

Drebing, C. E., Van Ormer, E. A., Krebs, C., Rosenheck, R., Rounsaville, B., Herz, L., et al. (2005). The impact of enhanced incentives on vocational rehabilitation outcomes for dually diagnosed veterans. *Journal of Applied Behavior Analysis, 38,* 359–372.

Drury, V., Birchwood, M., Cochrane, R., & Macmillan, F. (1996a). Cognitive therapy and recovery from acute psychosis: A controlled trial: I. Impact on psychotic symptoms. *British Journal of Psychiatry, 169,* 593–601.

Drury, V., Birchwood, M., Cochrane, R., & MacMillan, F. (1996b). Cognitive therapy and recovery from acute psychosis: A controlled trial: II. Impact on recovery time. *British Journal of Psychiatry, 169,* 602–607.

Druss, B. G., Allen, H. M., & Bruce, M. L. (1998). Physical health, depressive symptoms, and managed care enrollment. *American Journal of Psychiatry, 155,* 878–882.

Druss, B. G., Bradford, D. W., Rosenheck, R. A., Radford, M. J., & Krumholz, H. M. (2000a). Mental disorders and use of cardiovascular procedures after myocardial infarction. *Journal of the American Medical Association, 283,* 506–511.

Druss, B. G., Marcus, S. C., Rosenheck, R. A., Olfson, M., Tanielian, T., & Pincus, H. A. (2000b). Understanding disability in mental and general medical conditions. *American Journal of Psychiatry, 157*(9), 1485–1491.

Druss, B. G., Rohrbaugh, R. M., Levinson, C. M., & Rosenheck, R. A. (2001). Integrated medical care for patients with serious psychiatric illness: A randomized trial. *Archives of General Psychiatry, 58,* 861–868.

Druss, B. G., & Rosenheck, R. A. (1997). Use of medical services by veterans with mental disorders. *Psychosomatics, 38,* 451–458.

Druss, B. G., & Rosenheck, R. A. (1998). Mental disorders and access to medical care in the United States. *American Journal of Psychiatry, 155,* 1775–1777.

Druss, B. G., Rosenheck, R. A., & Desai, M. M. (2002). Quality of preventive medical care for patients with mental disorders. *Medical Care, 40,* 129–136.

Druss, B. G., & von Esenwein, S. A. (2006). Improving general medical care for persons with mental and addictive disorders: Systematic review. *General Hospital Psychiatry, 28,* 145–153.

Dube, S. R., Anda, R. F., Felitti, V. J., Chapman, D. P., Williamson, D. F., & Giles, W. H. (2001). Childhood abuse, household dysfunction, and the risk of attempted suicide throughout the life span: Findings from the Adverse Childhood Experiences Study. *Journal of the American Medical Association, 286,* 3089–3096.

Durell, J., Lechtenberg, B., Corse, S., & Frances, R. (1993). Intensive case management of persons with chronic mental illness who abuse substances. *Hospital and Community Psychiatry, 44,* 415–416.

Dyck, D. G., Short, R. A., Hendryx, M. S., Norell, D., Myers, M., Patterson, T., et al. (2000). Management of negative symptoms among patients with schizophrenia attending multiple-family groups. *Psychiatric Services, 51,* 513–519.

D'Zurilla, T. J., & Nezu, A. M. (2001). Problem-solving therapies. In K. S. Dobson (Ed.), *Handbook of cognitive-behavioral therapies* (p. 446). New York: Guilford Press.

Eagly, A. H., Ashmore, R. D., Makhijani, M. G., & Longo, L. C. (1991). What is beautiful is good, but . . . : A meta-analytic review of research on the physical attractiveness stereotype. *Psychological Bulletin, 110,* 109–128.

Eagly, A. H., & Chaiken, S. (1993). *The psychology of attitudes.* Fort Worth, TX: Harcourt Brace Jovanovich.

Eaton, W. W., Jr. (1994). Residence, social class, and schizophrenia. *Journal of Health and Social Behavior, 15,* 289–299.

Eckman, T. A., Liberman, R. P., Phipps, C. C., & Blair, K. E. (1990). Teaching medication management skills to schizophrenic patients. *Journal of Clinical Psychopharmacology, 10,* 33–38.

Eckman, T. A., Wirshing, W. C., Marder, S. R., Liberman, R. P., Johnston-Cronk, K., Zimmermann, K., et al. (1992). Technique for training schizophrenic patients in illness self-management: A controlled trial. *American Journal of Psychiatry, 149,* 1549–1555.

Edens, J., Peters, R., & Hills, H. (1997). Treating prison inmates with co-occurring disorders: An integrative review of existing programs. *Behavioral Sciences and the Law, 15,* 439–457.

Edmunson, E., Bendell, J., Archer, R., & Gordon, R. (1982). Integrating skill building and peer support in mental health treatment: The Early Intervention and Community Network Development Projects. In R. Jergert-Slotnick (Ed.), *Community mental health and behavioral ecology* (pp. 127–139). New York: Plenum Press.

Edmunson, E. Bendell, J., Archer, R., & Gordon, R. (1984). The Community Network Development Project. In A. Gartner & F. Riesman (Eds.), *The self-help revolution* (pp. 195–215). New York: Human Sciences Press.

Edwards, J., & McGorry, P. D. (2002). *Imple-*

menting early intervention in psychosis. London: Martin Dunitz.

Ehlers, A., & Clark, D. M. (2000). A cognitive model of posttraumatic stress disorder. *Behaviour Research and Therapy, 38,* 319–345.

Eichelman, B. S. (1990). Neurochemical and psychopharmacologic aspects of aggressive behavior. *Annual Review of Medicine, 41,* 149–158.

Eichler, M., Gowdy, E. A., & Etzel-Wise, D. (2004). *I'm in my home and I'm happy: Effective housing practices in Kansas.* Lawrence: University of Kansas School of Social Welfare.

Eilenberg, J., Fullilove, M. T., Goldman, R. G., & Mellman, L. (1996). Quality and use of trauma histories obtained from psychiatric outpatients through mandated inquiry. *Psychiatric Services, 47,* 165–169.

Eisen, S. V., Dill, D. L., & Grob, M. C. (1994). Reliability and validity of a brief patient-report instrument for psychiatric outcome evaluation. *Hospital and Community Psychiatry, 45,* 242–247.

Eisenthal, S., Emery, R., & Lazare, A. (1979). Adherence and the negotiated approach to patienthood. *Archives of General Psychiatry, 36,* 393–398.

el-Bayoumi, G., Borum, M. L., & Haywood, Y. (1998). Domestic violence in women. *Medical Clinics of North America, 82,* 391–401.

Ell, K. (1996). Social networks, social support, and coping with serious mental illness: The family connection. *Social Science and Medicine, 42,* 173–183.

Ellis, A. (1962). *Reason and emotion in psychotherapy.* New York: Lyle Stuart.

Ellis, A. (1977). Rational-emotive therapy: Research data that supports the clinical and personality hypotheses of RET and other modes of cognitive-behavior therapy. *Counseling Psychologist, 7*(1), 2–42.

Ellison, M. L., Rogers, E. S., Sciarappa, K., Cohen, M., & Forbess, R. (1995). Characteristics of mental health case management: Results of a national survey. *Journal of Mental Health Administration, 22,* 101–112.

Emerick, R. (1990). Self-help groups for former patients: Relations with mental health professionals. *Hospital and Community Psychiatry, 41,* 401–407.

Endicott, J., Hertz, M. I., & Gibbon, M. (1978). Brief versus standard hospitalization: The differential costs. *American Journal of Psychiatry, 135,* 707–712.

Endicott, J., Nee, J., Harrison, W., & Blumenthal, R. (1993). Quality of Life Enjoyment and Satisfaction Questionnaire: A new measure. *Psychopharmacology Bulletin, 29,* 321–326.

Endicott, J., & Spitzer, R. L. (1978). A diagnostic interview: The Schedule of Affective Disorders and Schizophrenia. *Archives of General Psychiatry, 35,* 837–844.

Engel, G. (1960). A unified concept of health and disease. *Perspectives on Biology and Medicine, 3,* 459–485.

Engel, R. S., & Silver, E. (2001). Policing mentally disordered suspects: A re-examination of the criminalization hypothesis. *Criminology, 39,* 225–252.

Enger, C., Weatherby, L., Reynolds, R. F., Glasser, D. B., & Walker, A. M. (2004). Serious cardiovascular events and mortality among patients with schizophrenia. *Journal of Nervous and Mental Disease, 192,* 19–27.

Engstrom, K., Brooks, E. B., Jonikas, J. A., Cook, J. A., & Witheridge, T. F. (1992). *Creating community linkages: A guide to assertive outreach for homeless persons with severe mental illness.* Chicago: Thresholds.

Erickson, D. H., Beiser, M., Iacono, W. G., Fleming, J. A. E., & Lin, T. (1989). The role of social relationships in the course of first-episode schizophrenia and affective psychosis. *American Journal of Psychiatry, 146,* 1456–1461.

Erikson, E. H. (1956). The problem of ego identity. *Journal of the American Psychoanalytic Association, 4,* 56–121.

Eron, L. D. (1994). Theories of aggression: From drives to cognitions. In L. Huesmann (Ed.), *Aggressive behavior: Current perspectives* (pp. 3–11). New York: Plenum Press.

Eronen, M., Angermeyer, M., & Schulze, B. (1998). The psychiatric epidemiology of violent behavior. *Social Psychiatry and Psychiatric Epidemiology, 33,* S13–S23.

Esses, V. M., Haddock, G., & Zanna, M. P. (1994). The role of mood in the expression of intergroup stereotypes. In M. P. Zanna & J. M. Olson (Eds.), *The psychology of prejudice: Ontario Symposium on Personality* (Vol. 7, pp. 77–101). Hillsdale, NJ: Erlbaum.

Essock, S. M., Goldman, H. H., Van Tosh, L., Anthony, W. A., Appell, C. R., Bond, G. R., et al. (2003). Evidence-based practices: Setting the context and responding to concerns. *Psychiatric Clinics of North America, 26,* 919–938.

Essock, S. M., Mueser, K. T., Drake, R. E., Covell, N. H., McHugo, G. J., Frisman, L. K., et al. (2006). Assertive community treatment versus standard case management for patients receiving integrated treatment for co-occurring severe mental illness and substance use disorder. *Psychiatric Services, 57,* 185–196.

Estroff, S. (1989). Self, identity, and subjective experiences of schizophrenia: In search of the subject. *Schizophrenia Bulletin, 15*, 189–196.

Estroff, S., Zimmer, C., Lachecotte, W., & Benoit, J. (1994). The influence of social networks and social support on violence by persons with severe mental illness. *Hospital and Community Psychiatry, 45*, 669–679.

Estroff, S. E. (1995). Whose story is it anyway? Authority, voice, and responsibility in narratives of chronic illness. In S. K. Toombs, D. Barnard, R. A. Carson, et al. (Eds.), *Chronic illness: From experience to policy. Medical ethics series* (pp. 77–102). Bloomington: Indiana University Press.

Everett, B., & Nelson, A. (1992). We're not cases and you're not managers: An account of a client/professional partnership developed in response to the "borderline" diagnosis. *Psychosocial Rehabilitation Journal, 15*, 49–60.

Evins, A. E., Cather, C., Deckersbach, T., Freudenreich, O., Culhane, M. A., Olm-Shipman, C. M., et al. (2005). A double-blind placebo-controlled trial of bupropion sustained-release for smoking cessation in schizophrenia. *Journal of Clinical Psychopharmacology, 25*, 218–225.

Evins, A. E., & Mayes, V. K. (2001). A pilot trial of bupropion added to cognitive behavioral therapy for smoking cessation in schizophrenia. *Nicotine and Tobacco Research, 3*, 397–403.

Fabian, E. S. (1989). Work and the quality of life. *Psychosocial Rehabilitation Journal, 12*, 39–49.

Fabian, E. S. (1992). Supported employment and the quality of life: Does a job make a difference? *Rehabilitation Counseling Bulletin, 36*, 84–97.

Fadden, G., Bebbington, P., & Kuipers, L. (1987). Caring and its burdens: A study of the spouses of depressed patients. *British Journal of Psychiatry, 151*, 660–667.

Fairweather, G. W. (1980). The Fairweather lodge: A twenty-five year retrospective [Special issue]. *New Directions for Mental Health Services, 7*.

Fairweather, G. W., Sanders, D., Cressler, D., & Maynard, H. (1969). *Community life for the mentally ill: An alternative to hospitalization.* Chicago: Aldine.

Fakhoury, W. K., Murray, A., Shepherd, G., & Priebe, S. (2002). Research in supported housing. *Social Psychiatry and Psychiatric Epidemiology, 37*, 301–315.

Falconer, D. S. (1965). The inheritance of liability to certain diseases estimated from the incidence among relatives. *Annals of Human Genetics, 29*, 51–76.

Falloon, I. R. H., Boyd, J. L., & McGill, C. W. (1984). *Family care of schizophrenia: A problem-solving approach to the treatment of mental illness.* New York: Guilford Press.

Falloon, I. R. H., Held, T., Coverdale, J., Roncone, R., & Laidlaw, T. (1999). Family interventions for schizophrenia: A review of long-term benefits of international studies. *Psychiatric Rehabilitation Skills, 3*, 268–290.

Falloon, I. R. H., McGill, C. W., Boyd, J. L., & Pederson, J. (1987). Family management in the prevention of morbidity of schizophrenia: Social outcome of a two-year longitudinal study. *Psychological Medicine, 17*, 59–66.

Falloon, I. R. H., & Talbot, R. E. (1981). Persistent auditory hallucinations: Coping mechanisms and implications for management. *Psychological Medicine, 11*, 329–339.

Fallot, R. D., & Harris, M. (2001). A trauma-informed approach to screening and assessment. *New Directions for Mental Health Services, 89*, 23–31.

Fallot, R. D., & Harris, M. (2002). The Trauma Recovery and Empowerment Model (TREM): Conceptual and practical issues in a group intervention for women. *Community Mental Health Journal, 38*, 475–485.

Fallot, R. D., McHugo, G. J., & Harris, M. (2005). *Preliminary studies of the Trauma Recovery and Empowerment Model (TREM).* Unpublished manuscript.

Farina, A., & Felner, R. D. (1973). Employment interviewer reactions to former mental patients. *Journal of Abnormal Psychology, 82*, 268–272.

Farina, A., Felner, R. D., & Boudreau, L. A. (1973). Reactions of workers to male and female mental patient job applicants. *Journal of Consulting and Clinical Psychology, 41*, 363–372.

Farina, A., Fisher, J. D., Getter, H., & Fischer, E. H. (1978). Some consequences of changing people's views regarding the nature of mental illness. *Journal of Abnormal Psychology, 87*, 272–279.

Farina, A., Thaw, J., Lovern, J. D., & Mangone, D. (1974). People's reactions to a former mental patient moving to their neighborhood. *Journal of Community Psychology, 2*, 108–112.

Farkas, M., & Anthony, W. (1993). Rehabilitation case management research. In M. Harris & H. Bergman (Eds.), *Case management for mentally ill patients: Theory and practice* (pp. 119–141). Langhorne, PA. Hardwood Academic.

Farkas, M., Kilbury, R. F., McNulty, K. C., Wireman, K. R., Cochran, W. A., & Taylor, S. P. (2005). People. In D. W. Dew & G. M. Alan (Eds.), Innovative methods for providing VR services to individuals with psychiatric disabilities. *Monographs of the Institute on Rehabilitation Issues, 30*, 9–23. Washington, DC: George

Washington University Center for Rehabilitation Counseling Research and Education.

Farkas, M. D., & Anthony, W. A. (1989). *Psychiatric rehabilitation programs: Putting theory into practice*. Baltimore: Johns Hopkins University Press.

Faulkner, G., Soundy, A. A., & Lloyd, K. (2003). Schizophrenia and weight management: A systematic review of interventions to control weight. *Acta Psychiatrica Scandinavica, 108*, 324–332.

Federal Register. (1987). Final Regulations, State Supported Employment Services Program, 34 CFR § 363, V 52 (157).

Federal Task Force on Homelessness and Severe Mental Illness. (1992). *Outcasts on Main Street: A report of the Federal Task Force on Homelessness and Severe Mental Illness*. Delmar, NY: National Resource Center on Homelessness and Mental Illness.

Fekete, D., Bond, G., McDonel, E., Salyers, M., Chen, A., & Miller, L. (1998). Rural intensive case management: A controlled study. *Psychiatric Rehabilitation Journal, 21*, 371–379.

Feldman, S., Bachman, J., & Bayer, J. (2002). Mental health parity: A review of research and a bibliography. *Administration and Policy in Mental Health, 29*, 215–228.

Felker, B., Workman, E., Stanley-Tilt, C., Albanese, R., & Short, D. (1998). The psychiatric primary care team: A new program to provide medical care to the chronically mentally ill. *Medicine and Psychiatry 1*, 36–41.

Felker, B., Yazel, J., & Short, D. (1996). Mortality and medical comorbidity among psychiatric patients: A review. *Psychiatric Services, 47*, 1356–1363.

Felton, C. J., Stastny, P., Shern, D. L., Blanch, A., Donahue, S. A., Knight, E., et al. (1995). Consumers as peer specialists on intensive case management teams: Impact on client outcomes. *Psychiatric Services, 46*, 1037–1044.

Fennell, M. J. (1989). Depression. In K. Hawton, P. Salkovskis, J. Kirk, & D. M. Clark (Eds.), *Cognitive behavioural therapy for psychiatric problems* (pp. 169–234). Oxford, UK: Oxford University Press.

Fenton, W. S. (2003). Shared decision making: A model for the physician–patient relationship in the 21st century? *Acta Psychiatrica Scandinavica, 107*, 401–402.

Fenton, W. S., Blyler, C. R., & Heinssen, R. K. (1997). Determinants of medication compliance in schizophrenia: Empirical and clinical findings. *Schizophrenia Bulletin, 23*, 637–651.

Ferguson, T. J., Rule, B. G., & Lindsay, R. C. (1982). The effects of caffeine and provocation on aggression. *Journal of Research in Personality, 16*, 60–71.

Festinger, L. (1954). A theory of social comparison processes. *Human Relations, 7*, 117–140.

Fields, S. (1990). The relationship between residential treatment and supported housing in a community system of services. *Psychosocial Rehabilitation Journal, 13*(4), 105–113.

Figueroa, E. F., Silk, K. R., Huth, A., & Lohr, N. E. (1997). History of childhood sexual abuse and general psychopathology. *Comprehensive Psychiatry, 38*, 23–30.

Fine, M. J., & Caldwell, T. E. (1967). Self evaluation of school related behavior of educable mentally retarded children: A preliminary report. *Exceptional Children, 33*, 324.

Finn, P., & Sullivan, M. (1998, January). Police response to special populations: Handling the mentally ill public inebriate and the homeless. *National Institute of Justice: Research in Action Series*. Washington, DC: U.S. Department of Justice, National Institute of Justice, National Office of Justice Programs.

First, M. B., Frances, A., & Pincus, H. (1997a). *DSM-IV-TR handbook of differential diagnosis*. Washington, DC: American Psychiatric Association.

First, M. B., Spitzer, R. L., Gibbon, M., & Williams, J. B. W. (1997b). *Structured clinical interview for DSM-IV*. New York: Biometrics Research Department, New York State Psychiatric Institute.

Fischer, P. J. (1988). Criminal activity among the homeless: A study of arrests in Baltimore. *Hospital and Community Psychiatry, 39*, 46–51.

Fishbein, M., & Ajzen, I. (1975). Misconception about the Fisbein model: Reflections on a study by Songer-Nocks. *Journal of Experimental Social Psychology, 12*, 579–584.

Fishbein, S. M. (1988). Partial care as a vehicle for rehabilitation of individuals with severe psychiatric disability. *Rehabilitation Psychology, 33*, 57–64.

Fisher, G., Benson, P., & Tessler, R. (1990). Family response to mental illness: Developments since deinstitutionalization. *Research in Community and Mental Health, 8*, 203–236.

Fisher, J. D., & Farina, A. (1979). Consequences of beliefs about the nature of mental disorders. *Journal of Abnormal Psychology, 88*, 320–327.

Fisher, W., Packer, I., Banks, S., Smith, D., Simon, L., & Roy-Bujnowski, K. (2002a). Self-reported lifetime psychiatric hospitalization histories of jail detainees with mental disorders: Comparison with a non-incarcerated national sample. *Journal of Behavioral Health Services and Research, 29*, 458–465.

Fisher, W., Packer, I., Simon, L., & Smith, D. (2000b). Community mental health services and the prevalence of severe mental illness in local jails: Are they related? *Administration and Policy in Mental Health, 27*, 371–382.

Fisher, W., Wolff, N., & Roy-Bujnowski, K. (2003). Community mental health services and criminal justice involvement among persons with mental illness. *Community-based Intervention for Criminal Offenders with Severe Mental Illness, 12*, 25–51.

Fiske, S. T. (1993). Controlling other people: The impact of power on stereotyping. *American Psychologist, 48*, 621–628.

Flegal, K. M., Carroll, M. D., Ogden, C. L., & Johnson, C. L. (2002). Prevalence and trends in obesity among U.S. adults, 1999–2000. *Journal of the American Medical Association, 288*, 1723–1727.

Flexer, R. W., & Solomon, P. L. (1993). Introduction. In R. W. Flexer & P. L. Solomon (Eds.), *Psychiatric rehabilitation in practice* (pp. xiii–xvii). Boston: Andover Medical Publishers.

Foa, E. B., Cashman, L., Jaycox, L. H., & Perry, K. J. (1997). The validation of a self-report measure of posttraumatic stress disorder: The Posttraumatic Diagnostic Scale. *Psychological Assessment, 9*, 445–451.

Foa, E. B., Ehlers, A., Clark, D. M., Tolin, D. F., & Orsillo, S. M. (1999). The Posttraumatic Cognitions Inventory (PTCI): Development and validation. *Psychological Assessment, 11*, 303–314.

Foa, E. B., Keane, T. M., & Friedman, M. J. (Eds.). (2000). *Effective treatments for PTSD*. New York: Guilford Press.

Foa, E. B., & Rothbaum, B. O. (1998). *Treating the trauma of rape: Cognitive-behavioral therapy for PTSD*. New York: Guilford Press.

Foa, E. B., & Wilson, R. (2001). *Stop obsessing! How to overcome your obsessions and compulsions* (rev. ed.). New York: Bantam.

Fogarty, J. S. (1997). Reactance theory and patient noncompliance. *Social Science and Medicine, 45*, 1277–1288.

Foley, S. R., Kelly, B. D., Clarke, M., McTigue, O., Gervin, M., Kamali, M., et al. (2005). Incidence and clinical correlates of aggression and violence at presentation in patients with first episode psychosis. *Schizophrenia Research, 72*, 161–168.

Folsom, D. P., McCahill, M., Bartels, S. J., Lindamer, L. A., Ganiats, T. G., & Jeste, D. V. (2002). Medical comorbidity and receipt of medical care by older homeless people with schizophrenia or depression. *Psychiatric Services, 53*, 1456–1460.

Folstein, M. F., Folstein, S. E., & McHugh, P. R. (1975). Mini-mental state: A practical method for grading the cognitive state of patients for the clinician. *Journal of Psychiatric Research, 12*, 189–198.

For mentally ill, death and misery. (2002, April 28). *New York Times*.

Fountain House, New York City. (1999). *The wellspring of the clubhouse model for social and vocational adjustment of persons with serious mental illness*. Center City, MN: Hazelden Press.

Fowler, D., Garety, P., & Kuipers, E. (1995). *Cognitive behaviour therapy for psychosis: Theory and practice*. Chichester: Wiley.

Fox, J. W. (1990). Social class, mental illness, and social mobility: The social selection-drift hypothesis for serious mental illness. *Journal of Health and Social Behavior, 31*, 344–353.

Foxx, R., & Azrin, N. H. (1972). The elimination of self-stimulatory behavior of autistic and retarded children by overcorrection. *Proceedings of the Annual Convention of the American Psychological Association, 7*, 761–762.

Frame, L., & Morrison, A. P. (2001). Causes of posttraumatic stress disorder in psychotic patients. *Archives of General Psychiatry, 58*, 305–306.

Frank, A. F., & Gunderson, J. G. (1990). The role of the therapeutic alliance in the treatment of schizophrenia. *Archives of General Psychiatry, 47*, 228–236.

Frank, R. G., Goldman, H. H., & Hogan, M. (2003). Medicaid and mental health: Be careful what you ask for. *Health Affairs, 22*, 101–113.

Frankel, A., White, T., Wilzor, J., Lamon, S., & McAuliffe, N. (1998). The evaluation of a successful community-based program for forensic MICA clients. *The Justice Professional, 11*, 423–436.

Freeman, A., & Davis, D. D. (1990). Cognitive therapy of depression. In A. S. Bellack & M. Hersen (Eds.), *International handbook of behavior modification and therapy* (2nd ed., pp. 333–352). New York: Plenum Press.

Freeman, D. W. (2001). Trauma-informed services and case management. In M. Harris & R. D. Fallot (Eds.), *Using trauma theory to design service systems* (Vol. 89, pp. 75–82). San Francisco: Jossey-Bass.

Frese, F. J., & Davis, W. W. (1997). The consumer-survivor movement, recovery, and consumer professionals. *Professional Psychology: Research and Practice, 28*, 243–245.

Frese, F. J., Stanley, J., Kress, K., & Vogel-Scibilia, S. (2001). Integrating evidence-based practices and the recovery model. *Psychiatric Services, 52*, 1462–1468.

Frey, R. E. C., & Weller, J. (2000). Behavioral management of aggression through teaching interpersonal skills. *Psychiatric Services, 51,* 607–609.

Friday, J. C., & McPheeters, H. L. (1985). *Assessing and improving the performance of psychosocial rehabilitation staff.* Atlanta: Southern Regional Education Board.

Friedman, C. A., & Clayton, R. J. (1996). Multiculturalism and neuropsychological assessment. In L. A. Suzuki, P. J. Meller, & J. G. Ponterotto (Eds.), *Handbook of multicultural assessment: Clinical, psychological, and educational applications* (pp. 291–318). San Francisco: Jossey-Bass.

Frith, C. D. (1994). Theory of mind in schizophrenia. In A. S. David & J. C. Cutting (Eds.), *The neuropsychology of schizophrenia* (pp. 147–161). Hillsdale, NJ: Erlbaum.

Frith, C. D. (1999). Commentary on Garety & Freeman II: Cognitive approaches to delusions: A critical review of theories and evidence. *British Journal of Clinical Psychology, 38*(3), 319–321.

Frith, C. D., & Corcoran, R. (1996). Exploring "theory of mind" in people with schizophrenia. *Psychological Medicine, 26,* 521–530.

Frueh, B. C., Buckley, T. C., Cusack, K. J., Kimble, M. O., Grubaugh, A. L., Turner, S. M., et al. (2004). Cognitive-behavioral treatment for PTSD among people with severe mental illness: A proposed treatment model. *Journal of Psychiatric Practice, 10,* 26–38.

Frueh, B. C., Cousins, V. C., Hiers, T. G., Cavanaugh, S. D., Cusack, K. J., & Santos, A. B. (2002). The need for trauma assessment and related clinical services in a state public mental health system. *Community Mental Health Journal, 38,* 351–356.

Fuertes, J. N., & Brobst, K. (2002). Clients' ratings of counselor multicultural competency. *Cultural Diversity and Ethnic Minority Psychology, 8,* 214–233.

Fyock, J., & Stangor, C. (1992). The role of memory biases in stereotype maintenance. *British Journal of Social Psychology, 33,* 331–343.

Gabbard, G. O., & Gabbard, K. (1992). Cinematic stereotypes contributing to the stigmatization of psychiatrists. In P. J. Fink & A. Tasman (Eds.), *Stigma and mental illness* (pp. 113–126). Washington, DC: American Psychiatric Press.

Gaertner, S. L., Dovidio, J. F., & Bachman, B. A. (1996). Revisitng the contact hypothesis: The induction of a common ingroup identity. *International Journal of Intercultural Relations, 20,* 271–290.

Galanter, M. (1988). Zealous self-help groups as adjuncts to psychiatric treatment: A study of recovery. *American Journal of Psychiatry, 145,* 1248–1253.

Gallo, J. J., Marino, S., Ford, D., & Anthony, J. C. (1995). Filters on the pathway to mental health care: II. Sociodemographic factors. *Psychological Medicine, 25*(6), 1149–1160.

Gallo, K. M. (1994). First person account: Self-stigmatization. *Schizophrenia Bulletin, 20,* 407–410.

Gamache, G., Tessler, R., & Nicholson, J. (1995). Childcare as a neglected dimension of family burden research. *Research in Community and Mental Health, 8,* 63–90.

Gamst, G., Dana, R. H., Der-Karabetian, A., Aragón, M., & Kremer, T. (2002). Effects of Latino acculturation and ethnic identity on mental health outcomes. *Hispanic Journal of Behavioral Sciences, 24,* 479–504.

Gamst, G., Dana, R. H., Der-Karabetian, A., & Kremer, T. (2000). Ethnic match and client ethnicity effects on global assessment and visitation. *Journal of Community Psychology, 28,* 547–564.

Gamst, G., Dana, R. H., Der-Karabetian, A., & Kremer, T. (2001). Asian American mental health clients: Effects of ethnic match and age on global asssessment and visitation. *Journal of Mental Health Counseling, 23,* 57–71.

Ganju, V. (2003). Implementation of evidence-based practices in state mental health systems: Implications for research and effectiveness studies. *Schizophrenia Bulletin, 29,* 125–131.

Ganju, V. (2004). *Evidence-based practice and mental health system transformation.* Paper presented at the 2004 National Statistics Conference, Washington, DC.

Garety, P. A., Fowler, D., & Kuipers, E. (2000). Cognitive-behavioral therapy for medication-resistant symptoms. *Schizophrenia Bulletin, 26*(1), 73–86.

Garety, P. A., & Freeman, D. (1999). Cognitive approaches to delusions: A critical review of theories and evidence. *British Journal of Clinical Psychology, 38,* 113–154.

Garety, P. A., & Hemsley, D. R. (1994). *Delusions: Investigations into the psychology of delusional reasoning.* Oxford, UK: Oxford University Press.

Garety, P. A., Kuipers, E., Fowler, D., Chamberlain, F., & Dunn, G. (1994). Cognitive behavior therapy for drug resistant psychosis. *British Journal of Medical Psychology, 67,* 259–271.

Gartner, A., & Riessman, F. (1977). *Self-help in the human services.* San Francisco: Jossey-Bass.

Gartner, A., & Riessman, F. (Eds.). (1984). *The self help revolution.* New York: Human Sciences Press.

Gaul, G. M. (2005). Revamped veterans' health care now a model. *The Washington Post,* p. A01.

Gearon, J. S., & Bellack, A. S. (1999). Women with schizophrenia and co-occurring substance use disorders: An increased risk for violent victimization and HIV. *Community Mental Health Journal, 35,* 401–419.

Geen, R. G., & McCown, E. J. (1984). Effects of noise and attack on aggression and physiological arousal. *Motivation and Emotion, 8,* 231–241.

Gehrs, M., & Goering, R. (1994). The relationship between the working alliance and rehabilitation outcomes of schizophrenia. *Psychosocial Rehabilitation Journal, 18*(2), 43–54.

Geller, J. L. (2000). The last half-century of psychiatric services as reflected in *Psychiatric Services. Psychiatric Services, 51,* 41–67.

Gellis, Z., Kim, J., & Hwang, S. (2004). New York State case management survey: Urban and rural differences in job activities, job stress, and job satisfaction. *Journal of Behavioral Health Services and Research, 31,* 430–440.

George, L., Blazer, D., Hughes, D., & Fowler, N. (1989). Social support and the outcome of major depression. *British Journal of Psychiatry, 154,* 478–485.

George, T. P., Sernyak, M. J., Ziedonis, D. M., & Wood, S. M. (1995). Effects of clozapine on smoking in chronic schizophrenic outpatients. *Journal of Clinical Psychiatry, 56,* 344–346.

Gerace, L., Camilleri, D., & Ayers, L. (1993). Sibling perspectives on schizophrenia and the family. *Schizophrenia Bulletin, 19,* 637–647.

Gerber, G., & Prince, P. (1999). Measuring client satisfaction with assertive community treatment. *Psychiatric Services, 50,* 546–550.

Gerbner, G. (1985). Dreams that hurt: Mental illness in the mass media. In *Proceedings of the first Rosalyn Carter symposium on mental health policy: Stigma and mental illness.* Atlanta, GA: Emory University School of Medicine.

Gervey, R., & Bedell, J. R. (1994). *Supported employment in vocational rehabilitation in psychological assessment and treatment of persons with severe mental disorders.* Washington, DC: Taylor & Francis.

Gibbs, J. J. (1983). Problems and priorities: Perceptions of jail custodians and social service providers. *Journal of Criminal Justice, 1,* 327–349.

Gift, T. E., & Harder, D. W. (1985). The severity of psychiatric disorder: A replication. *Psychiatry Research, 14*(2), 163–173.

Gill, K. J., Pratt, C. W., & Barrett, N. (1997). Preparing psychiatric rehabilitation specialists through undergraduate education. *Community Mental Health Journal, 33,* 323–329.

Gilmer, T. P., Dolder, C. R., Lacro, J. P., Folsom, D. P., Lindamer, L., Garcia, P., et al. (2004). Adherence to treatment with antipsychotic medication and health care costs among Medicaid beneficiaries with schizophrenia. *American Journal of Psychiatry, 161,* 692–699.

Gingerich, S., & Mueser, K. T. (2005). Illness management and recovery. In R. E. Drake, M. R. Merrens, & D. W. Lynde (Eds.), *Evidence-based mental health practice: A textbook* (pp. 395–424). New York: Norton.

Glick, I., & Dixon, C. (2002). Patient and family support organization services should be included as part of treatment for the severely mentally ill. *Journal of Psychiatric Practice, 8,* 63–69.

Gloaguen, V., Cottraux, J., Cucherat, M., & Blackburn, I. M. (1998). A meta-analysis of the effects of cognitive therapy in depressed patients. *Journal of Affective Disorders, 62,* 59–72.

Glynn, S. M. (1998). Psychopathology and social functioning in schizophrenia. In K. T. Mueser & N. Tarrier (Eds.), *Handbook of social functioning in schizophrenia* (pp. 66–78). Boston: Allyn & Bacon.

Glynn, S. M., Marder, S. R., Liberman, R. P., Blair, K., Wirshing, W. C., Wirshing, D. A., et al. (2002). Supplementing clinic-based skills training with manual-based community support sessions: Effects on social adjustment of patients with schizophrenia. *American Journal of Psychiatry, 159,* 829–837.

Glynn, S. M., Mueser, K. T., & Liberman, R. P. (1989). The behavioral approach. In A. Lazere (Ed.), *Outpatient psychiatry: Diagnosis and treatment* (2nd ed., 59–68). Baltimore: Williams & Wilkins.

Godley, S. H., Finch, M., Dougan, L., McDonnell, M., McDermit, M., & Carey, A. (2000). Case management for dually diagnosed individuals involved in the criminal justice system. *Journal of Substance Abuse Treatment, 18,* 137–148.

Godley, S. H., Hoewing-Roberson, R., & Godley, M. D. (1994). *Final MISA report.* Bloomington, IL: Lighthouse Institute.

Goering, P. N., & Stylianos, S. K. (1988). Exploring the helping relationship between the schizophrenic client and rehabilitation therapist. *American Journal of Orthopsychiatry, 58,* 271–278.

Goering, P. N., Wasylenki, D. A., Farkas, M. D., Lancee, W. J., & Ballantyne, R. (1988). What difference does case management make? *Hospital and Community Psychiatry, 39,* 272–276.

Goff, D. C., Brotman, A. W., Kindlon, D., Waites, M., & Amico, E. (1991). Self-reports of childhood abuse in chronically psychotic patients. *Psychiatry Research, 37,* 73–80.

Goffman, E. (1963). *Stigma: Notes on the management of spoiled identity.* Englewood Cliffs, NJ: Prentice-Hall.

Gold, J. M. (2004). Cognitive deficits as treatment targets in schizophrenia. *Schizophrenia Research, 72,* 21–28.

Gold, J. M., Queern, C., Iannone, V. N., & Buchanan, R. W. (1999). Repeatable battery for the assessment of neuropsychological status as a screening test in schizophrenia: II. Convergent/discriminant validity and diagnostic group comparisons. *American Journal of Psychiatry, 156,* 1944–1950.

Gold, M., & Marrone, J. (1998). Mass Bay Employment Services (a service of Bay Care Human Services, Inc.): A story of leadership, vision, and action resulting in employment for people with mental illness. *Roses and Thorns from the Grassroots, 1,* 1–4.

Gold, P. B., Meisler, N., Santos, A. B., Carnemolla, M. A., Williams, O. H., & Kelleher, J. (2006). Randomized trial of supported employment integrated with assertive community treatment for rural adults with severe mental illness. *Schizophrenia Bulletin, 32,* 378–395.

Golden, T. P., O'Mara, S., Ferrell, C., & Sheldon, J. R. (2000). A theoretical construct for benefits planning and assistance in the Ticket to Work and Work Incentive Improvement Act. *Journal of Vocational Rehabilitation, 14,* 147–152.

Goldfinger, S. M., Schutt, R. K., Tolomiczenko, G. S., Seidman, L., Penk, W. E., Turner, W., et al. (1999). Housing placement and subsequent days homeless among formerly homeless adults with mental illness. *Psychiatric Services, 50,* 674–679.

Goldkamp, J., & Irons-Guynn, C. (2000, April). *Emerging judicial strategies for the mentally ill in criminal caseload: Mental health courts in Fort Lauderdale, Seattle, San Bernadino, and Anchorage;* Crime and Justice Research Institute, Philadelphia PA. U.S. Department of Justice, Office of Justice Programs (NCJ-NCJ 182504). Washington, DC: U.S. Government Printing Office.

Goldman H. (1982). Mental illness and family burden: A public health perspective. *Hospital and Community Psychiatry, 33,* 557–559.

Goldman, H., Skodol, A., & Lave, T. (1992). Revising Axis V for DSM-IV: A review of measures of social functioning. *American Journal of Psychiatry, 149,* 1148–1156.

Goldman, H. H. (1984). Epidemiology. In J. A. Talbott (Ed.), *The chronic mental patient: Five years later* (pp. 15–31). Orlando, FL: Grune & Stratton.

Goldman, H. H., & Morrissey, J. P. (1985). The alchemy of mental health policy: Homelessness and the fourth cycle of reform. *American Journal of Public Health, 75,* 727–731.

Goldman, L. A. (1999). Medical illness in patients with schizophrenia. *Journal of Clinical Psychiatry, 6*(Suppl. 21), 10–15.

Goldman, M. B., Blake, L., Marks, R. C., Hedeker, D., & Luchins, D. J. (1993). Association of nonsuppression of cortisol on the DST with primary polydipsia in chronic schizophrenia. *American Journal of Psychiatry, 150,* 653–655.

Goldstein, M. (1995). Psychoeducational and relapse prevention. *International Clinical Psychopharmacology, 9*(Suppl. 5), 59–69.

Goldstrom, I., Campbell, J., Rogers, J., Lambert, D., Blaklow, B., Henderson, M., et al. (2006). National estimates for mental health mutual support groups, self-help organizations, and consumer-operated services. *Administration and Policy in Mental Health and Mental Health Services Research, 33,* 92–103.

Golomb, S. L., & Kocsis, A. (1988). *The halfway house: On the road to independence.* New York: Bruner/Mazel.

Gomory, T. (1999). Programs of assertive community treatment (PACT): A critical review. *MADNation.* Retrieved December 1, 1999 from *www.madnation.org.*

Gomory, T. (2001). A critique of the effectiveness of assertive community treatment. *Psychiatric Services, 52,* 1394.

Gonzalez-Pinto, A., Gonzalez, C., Enjuto, S., Fernandez de Corres, B., Lopez, P., Palomo, J., et al. (2004). Psychoeducation and cognitive-behavioral therapy in bipolar disorder: An update. *Acta Psychiatrica Scandinavica, 109,* 83–90.

Goode, T. (2001). The role of self-assessment in achieving cultural competence. *Cultural Competence Exchange.* Retrieved January 16, 2006 from *gucchd.georgetown.edu/nccc/products.html,* 1.

Goodman, L. A., Dutton, M. A., & Harris, M. (1995). Physical and sexual assault prevalence among episodically homeless women with serious mental illness. *American Journal of Orthopsychiatry, 65,* 468–478.

Goodman, L. A., Rosenberg, S. D., Mueser, K. T., & Drake, R. E. (1997). Physical and sexual assault history in women with serious mental illness: Prevalence, correlates, treatment, and future research directions. *Schizophrenia Bulletin, 23,* 685–696.

Goodman, L. A., Salyers, M. P., Mueser, K. T., Rosenberg, S. D., Swartz, M., Essock, S. M., et al. (2001). Recent victimization in women and men with severe mental illness: Prevalence and correlates. *Journal of Traumatic Stress, 14,* 615–632.

Goodman, L. A., Thompson, K. M., Weinfurt, K., Corl, S., Acker, P., Mueser, K. T., et al. (1999). Reliability of reports of violent victimization and PTSD among men and women with SMI. *Journal of Traumatic Stress, 12,* 587–599.

Goodman, S. H., Sewell, D. R., Cooley, E. L., & Leavitt, N. (1993). Assessing levels of adaptive functioning: The Role Functioning Scale. *Community Mental Health Journal, 29,* 119–131.

Goodwin, D. W., Alderson, P., & Rosenthal, R. (1971). Clinical significance of hallucinations in psychiatric disorders: A study of 116 hallucinatory patients. *Archives of General Psychiatry, 24,* 76–80.

Goodwin, F. K., & Jamison, K. R. (2007). *Manic depressive illness* (2nd ed.). New York: Oxford University Press.

Goodwin, R. D., Hoven, C. W., Murison, R., & Hotopf, M. (2003). Childhood abuse and risk of gastrointestinal disorders and migraine during adulthood. *American Journal of Public Health, 93,* 1065–1067.

Goodwin, R. D., & Stein, M. B. (2004). Association between childhood trauma and physical disorders among adults in the United States. *Psychological Medicine, 34,* 509–520.

Gorey, K., Leslie, D., Morris, T., Carruthers, W. V., Lindsay, J., & Chacko, J. (1998). Effectiveness of case management with severely and persistently mentally ill people. *Community Mental Health Journal, 34,* 241–250.

Gottlieb, B. (Ed.). (1981). *Social networks and social support.* Beverly Hills, CA: Sage.

Gould, R. A., Mueser, K. T., Bolton, E., Mays, V., & Goff, D. (2001). Cognitive therapy for psychosis in schizophrenia: An effect size analysis. *Schizophrenia Research, 48,* 335–342.

Gournay, K., & Thornicroft, G. (2000). Comments on the UK700 case management trial. *British Journal of Psychiatry, 177,* 371.

Gove, W. (1975). The labeling theory and mental illness: A reply to Scheff. *American Sociological Review, 40,* 242–248.

Gove, W. (1980). *Labeling deviant behavior.* Newbury Park, CA: Sage.

Gove, W. R. (1982). Labeling theory's explanation of mental illness: An update of recent evidence. *Deviant Behavior: An Interdisciplinary Journal, 3,* 307–327.

Gove, W. R., & Fain, T. (1973). The stigma of mental hospitalization: An attempt to evaluate its consequences. *Archives of General Psychiatry, 28,* 494–500.

Graeber, D. A., Moyers, T. B., Griffiths, C., Guajardo, E., & Tonigan, S. (2003). A pilot study comparing motivational interviewing and an educational intervention in patients with schizophrenia and alcohol use disorders. *Community Mental Health Journal, 39,* 189–202.

Graham, H. L., Copello, A., Birchwood, M. J., Mueser, K. T., Orford, J., McGovern, D., et al. (2004). *Cognitive-behavioural integrated treatment (C-BIT): A treatment manual for substance misuse in people with severe mental health problems.* Chichester: Wiley.

Green, A. I., Burgess, E. S., Dawson, R., Zimmet, S. V., & Strous, R. D. (2003). Alcohol and cannabis use in schizophrenia: Effects of clozapine vs. risperidone. *Schizophrenia Research, 60,* 81–85.

Green, A. I., Patel, J. K., Goisman, R. M., Allison, D. B., & Blackburn, G. (2000). Weight gain from novel antipsychotic drugs: Need for action. *General Hospital Psychiatry, 22,* 224–235.

Green, B. L. (1996a). Trauma History Questionnaire. In B. H. Stamm (Ed.), *Measurement of stress, self-report trauma, and adaptation* (pp. 366–368). Lutherville, MD: Sidran Press.

Green, M. F. (1996b). What are the functional consequences of neurocognitive deficits in schizophrenia? *American Journal of Psychiatry, 153,* 321–330.

Green, M. F. (1998). *Schizophrenia from a neurocognitive perspective.* Needham Heights, MA: Allyn & Bacon.

Green, M. F. (1999). Interventions for neurocognitive deficits. *Schizophrenia Bulletin, 25,* 197–200.

Green, M. F., Ganzell, S., Satz, P., & Vaclav, J. F. (1990). Teaching the Wisconsin Card Sorting Test to schizophrenic patients. *Archives of General Psychiatry, 47,* 91–92.

Green, M. F., Kern, R. S., Braff, D. L., & Mintz, J. (2000). Neurocognitive deficits and functional outcome in schizophrenia: Are we measuring the "right stuff"? *Schizophrenia Bulletin, 26,* 119–136.

Green, M. F., & Nuechterlein, K. H. (1999). Should schizophrenia be treated as a neurocognitive disorder? *Schizophrenia Bulletin, 25,* 309–318.

Greenberg, J. (1995). The other side of caring: Adult children with mental illness as supports to their mothers in later life. *Social Work, 40,* 414–423.

Greenberg, J., Greenley, J., & Kim, H. W. (1995). The provision of mental health services to families of persons with severe mental illness. *Research in Community and Mental Health, 8,* 181–204.

Greenberg, J., Kim, H., & Greenley, J. (1997). Factors associated with subjective burden in siblings of adults with severe mental illness. *American Journal of Orthopsychiatry, 67*, 231–241.

Greenfield, S. F., Strakowski, S. M., Tohen, M., Batson, S. C., & Kolbrener, M. L. (1994). Childhood abuse in first-episode psychosis. *British Journal of Psychiatry, 164*, 831–834.

Greenfield, S. F., Weiss, R. D., & Tohen, M. (1995). Substance abuse and the chronically mentally ill: A description of dual diagnosis treatment services in a psychiatric hospital. *Community Mental Health Journal, 31*, 265–278.

Greenley, J. R. (1984). Social factors, mental illness, and psychiatric care: Recent advances from a sociological perspective. *Hospital and Community Psychiatry, 35*, 813–820.

Grella, C., & Grusky, O. (1989). Families of the seriously mentally ill and their satisfaction with services. *Hospital and Community Psychiatry, 40*, 831–835.

Grob, G. (1966). *The state and the mentally ill.* Chapel Hill: University of North Carolina Press.

Grob, S. (1983). Psychosocial rehabilitation centers: Old wine in a new bottle. In I. Barofsky & R. D. Budson (Eds.), *The chronic patient in the community: Principles of treatment* (pp. 265–280). Jamaica, NY: Spectrum.

Grobe, G. (1994). Mad, homeless, and unwanted: A history of the care of the chronically mentally ill in America. *Psychiatric Clinician of North America, 17*, 541–558.

Groff, A., Burns, B., Swanson, J., Swartz, M., Wagner, H., & Tompson, M. (2004). Caregiving for persons with mental illness: The impact of outpatient commitment on caregiving strain. *Journal of Nervous and Mental Disease, 192*, 554–562.

Groth-Marnat, G. (2003). *Handbook of psychological assessment* (4th ed.). Hoboken, NJ: Wiley.

Guardiano, J., & von Brook, P. (2001). *Highlights of the 2000 Institute on Psychiatric Services, 52*, 37–42.

Guarnaccia, P. (1998). Multicultural experiences in family caregiving: A study of African American, European American, and Hispanic American families. *New Directions for Mental Health Services, 77*, 45–61.

Gunderson, J. G., Frank, A. F., Katz, H. M., Vannicelli, M. L., Frosch, J. P., & Knapp, P. H. (1984). Effects of psychotherapy in schizophrenia: II. Comparative outcome of two forms of treatment. *Schizophrenia Bulletin, 10*, 564–596.

Gunderson, J. G., & Zanarini, M. C. (1992). *Revised Diagnostic Interview for Borderlines (DIB-R).* Boston: Harvard Medical School.

Guyatt, G., & Rennie, D. (Eds.). (2002). *Users' guides to the medical literature.* Chicago: American Medical Association.

Haddock, G., Barrowclough, C., Tarrier, N., Moring, J., O'Brien, R., Schofield, N., et al. (2003). Cognitive-behavioural therapy and motivational intervention for schizophrenia and substance misuse. *British Journal of Psychiatry, 183*, 418–426.

Haddock, G., Bentall, R., & Slade, P. (1996). Psychological treatment of auditory hallucinations: Focusing or distraction? In G. Haddock & P. Slade (Eds.), *Cognitive-behavioral interventions with psychiatric disorders* (pp. 45–70). London: Routledge.

Haddock, G., Tarrier, N., Morrison, A., Hopkins, R., Drake, R., & Lewis, S. (1999). A pilot study evaluating the effectiveness of individual inpatient cognitive-behavioural therapy in early psychosis. *Social Psychiatry and Psychiatric Epidemiology, 34*, 254–258.

Häfner, H. (2000). Onset and early course as determinants of the further course of schizophrenia. *Acta Psychiatrica Scandinavica, 102*(Suppl. 407), 44–48.

Häfner, H., & an der Heiden, W. (2003). Course and outcome of schizophrenia. In S. R. Hirsch & D. R. Weinberger (Eds.), *Schizophrenia* (2nd ed., pp. 101–141). Oxford, UK: Blackwell Scientific.

Hagopian, L. P., Farrell, D. A., & Amari, A. (1996). Treating total liquid refusal with backward chaining and fading. *Journal of Applied Behavior Analysis, 29*, 573–575.

Hails, J., & Borum, R. (2003). Police training and specialized approaches to people with mental illness. *Crime and Delinquency, 49*, 52–61.

Haimowitz, S. (2004). Slowing the revolving door: Community re-entry of offenders with mental illness. *Psychiatric Services, 55*, 373–375.

Halbreich, U., & Kahn, L. (2003). Hormonal aspects of schizophrenias: An overview. *Psychoneuroendocrinology, 28*(Suppl. 2), 1–16.

Halford, W. K., & Hayes, R. (1991). Psychological rehabilitation of chronic schizophrenic patients: Recent findings on social skills and family psychoeducation. *Clinical Psychology Review, 23*, 23–44.

Hall, L. L., Graf, A. C., Fitzpatrick, M. J., Lane, T., & Birkel, R. C. (2003). *Shattered lives: Results of a national survey of NAMI members living with mental illness and their families.* Arlington, VA: National Alliance for the Mentally Ill/Treatment/Recovery Information and Advocacy Data Base.

Halweg, K., Goldstein, M., Nuechterlein, K., Magana, A., Mintz, J., Doane, J., et al. (1989). Expressed emotion and patient–relative interaction in families of recent onset schizophrenia. *Journal of Consulting and Clinical Psychology, 57,* 11–18.

Hamann, J., Leucht, S., & Kissling, W. (2003). Shared decision making in psychiatry. *Acta Psychiatrica Scandinavica, 107,* 403–409.

Hamilton, D. L., & Sherman, J. W. (1994). Stereotypes. In R. S. Wyer & T. K. Srull (Eds.), *Handbook of social cognition* (Vol. 2, 2nd ed., pp. 1–68). Hillsdale, NJ: Erlbaum.

Hamilton, M. (1960). A rating scale for depression. *Journal of Neurology, Neurosurgery, and Psychiatry, 23,* 56–62.

Hamilton, T., & Sample, P. (1994). *The twelve steps and dual recover: A framework of recovery for those of us with addiction and an emotional or psychiatric illness.* Center City, MN: Hazelden.

Hamner, M. B. (1997). Psychotic features and combat-associated PTSD. *Depression and Anxiety, 5,* 34–38.

Hamre, P., Dahl, A. A., & Malt, U. F. (1994). Public attitudes to the quality of psychiatric treatment, psychiatric patients, and prevalence of mental disorders. *Nordic Journal of Psychiatry, 48,* 275–281.

Hansen, T. E., Goetz, R. R., Bloom, J. D., & Fenn, D. S. (1998). Changes in questions about psychiatric illness asked on medical licensure applications between 1993 and 1996. *Psychiatric Services, 49,* 202–206.

Hanson, J., & Rapp, C. (1992). Families' perceptions of community mental health programs for their relatives with a severe mental illness. *Community Mental Health Journal, 28,* 181–197.

Hanson, R. W. (1986). Physician–patient communication and compliance. In K. E. Gerber & A. M. Nehemkis (Eds.), *Compliance: The dilemma of the chronically ill* (pp. 182–212). New York: Springer.

Harding, C. M., Brooks, G. W., Ashikaga, T., Strauss, J. S., & Breier, A. (1987a). The Vermont longitudinal study of persons with severe mental illness: I. Methodology, study sample, and overall status 32 years later. *American Journal of Psychiatry, 144*(6), 718–726.

Harding, C. M., Brooks, G. W., Ashikaga, T., Strauss, J. S., & Breier, A. (1987b). The Vermont longitudinal study of persons with severe mental illness: II. Long-term outcome of subjects who retrospectively met DSM-III criteria for schizophrenia. *American Journal of Psychiatry, 144*(6), 727–735.

Harding, C. M., Strauss, J., Hafez, H., & Liberman, P. (1987c). Work and mental illness: I. Toward an integration of the rehabilitation process. *Journal of Nervous and Mental Disease, 175,* 317–326.

Hare, R., Clark, D., Gramm, M., & Thorton, D. (2000). Psychopathy and the predictive validity of the PCL-R: An international perspective. *Behavioral Science and the Law, 18,* 623–645.

Hare, R. D. (1991). *The Hare Psychopathy Checklist—Revised Manual.* North Tonawanda, NY: Multi-Health Systems.

Harkness, J., Newman, S., Galster, G., & Reschovsky, J. (2004). The financial viability of housing for the mentally ill. *Housing Policy Debate, 15*(11). Retrieved June 30, 2007, from *www.knowledgeplex.org/.*

Harris, E. C., & Barraclough, B. (1997). Suicide as an outcome for mental disorders: A meta-analysis. *British Journal of Psychiatry, 170,* 205–228.

Harris, G. T., & Rice, M. E. (1995). The effectiveness of therapeutic communities for psychopaths. *Therapeutic Communities: International Journal for Therapuetic and Supportive Organizations, 16,* 147–149.

Harris, G. T., Rice, M., & Quinsey, V. (1993). Violent recidivism of mentally disordered offenders: The development of a statistical prediction instrument. *Criminal Justice and Behavior, 20,* 315–335.

Harris, K. M., Edlund, M. J., & Larson, S. (2005). Racial and ethnic differences in the mental health problems and use of mental health care. *Medical Care, 43,* 775–784.

Harris, M. (1994). Modifications in service delivery and clinical treatment for women diagnosed with severe mental illness who are also the survivors of sexual abuse trauma. *Journal of Mental Health Administration, 21,* 397–406.

Harris, M. (1998). *Trauma recovery and empowerment: A clinician's guide for working with women in groups.* New York: Free Press.

Harris, M., & Bergman, H. (1987). Case management with the chronically mentally ill: A clinical perspective. *American Journal of Orthopsychiatry, 57,* 296–302.

Harris, M., & Bergman, H. (Eds.). (1993). *Case management for mentally ill patients.* Langhorne, PA., Harwood.

Harris, M., & Fallot, R. D. (2001a). Envisioning a trauma-informed service system: A vital paradigm shift. *New Directions for Mental Health Services, 89,* 3–22.

Harris, M., & Fallot, R. D. (2001b). Trauma-informed inpatient services. *New Directions for Mental Health Services, 89,* 33–46.

Harris, M., & Jeste, D. V. (1988). Late-onset schizophrenia: An overview. *Schizophrenia Bulletin, 14*(1), 39–55.

Harrison, G., Hopper, K., Craig, T., Laska, E., Siegel, C., Wanderling, J., et al. (2001). Recovery from psychotic illness: A 15- and 25-year international follow-up study. *British Journal of Psychiatry, 178,* 506–517.

Harry, B., & Steadman, H. (1988). Arrest rates of patients treated at a community mental health center. *Hospital and Community Psychiatry, 39,* 862–866.

Hartwell, S. (2003). Short-term outcomes for offenders with mental illness released from incarceration. *International Journal of Offender Therapy and Comparative Criminology, 47,* 145–158.

Hartwell, S., Friedman, D., & Orr, K. (2001). From correctional custody to community: The Massachusetts Forensic Transition Program. *New England Journal of Public Policy, 19,* 73–81.

Harvey, P. D., Davidson, M., Mueser, K. T., Parrella, M., White, L., & Powchik, P. (1997). Social-Adaptive Functioning Evaluation (SAFE): A rating scale for geriatric psychiatric patients. *Schizophrenia Bulletin, 23,* 131–145.

Hasher, L., & Zacks, R. T. (1979). Automatic and effortful processes in memory. *Journal of Experimental Psychology: General, 108,* 356–388.

Hasher, L., & Zacks, R. T. (1984). Automatic processing of fundamental information: The case of frequency of occurrence. *American Psychologist, 39,* 1372–1388.

Hasson-Ohayon, I., Roe, D., & Kravetz, S. (in press). The effectiveness of the Illness Management and Recovery Program: A randomized controlled trial. *Psychiatric Services.*

Hatfield, A. (1983). What families want of family therapy. In W. McFarlane (Ed.), *Family therapy in schizophrenia* (pp. 41–65). New York: Guilford Press.

Hatfield, A. (1987a). Coping and adaptation: a conceptual framework for understanding families. In A. Hatfield & H. Lefley (Eds.), *Families of the mentally ill.* New York: Guilford Press.

Hatfield, A. (1987b). Systems resistance to effective family coping. In A. T. Myerson (Ed.), *Barriers to treating the chronic mentally ill: Vol. 33. New directions for mental health services* (pp. 51–61). San Francisco: Jossey-Bass.

Hatfield, A. (1990). *Family education in mental illness.* New York: Guilford Press.

Hatfield, A. (1994a). Family education theory and practice. In A. Hatfield (Ed.), *Family interventions in mental illness: Vol. 62. New directions for mental health services* (pp. 3–11). San Francisco: Jossey-Bass.

Hatfield, A. (1994b). Developing collaborative relationships with families. In A. Hatfield (Ed.), *Family interventions in mental illness: Vol. 62. New directions for mental health services* (pp. 51–59). San Francisco: Jossey-Bass.

Hatfield, A. (1997). Families of adults with severe mental illness: New directions in research. *American Journal of Orthopsychiatry, 6,* 254–260.

Hatfield, A., & Lefley, H. (2000). Helping elderly caregivers plan for the future care of a relative with mental illness. *Psychiatric Rehabilitation Journal, 24,* 103–107.

Hatfield, A., Spaniol, L., & Zipple, A. (1987). Expressed emotion: A family perspective. *Schizophrenia Bulletin, 13,* 221–226.

Hawthorne, W. B., Green, E. E., Lohr, J. B., Hough, R., & Smith, P. G. (1999). Comparison of outcomes of acute care in short-term residential treatment and psychiatric hospital settings. *Psychiatric Services, 50,* 401–406.

Hays, R. B., McKusick, L., Pollack, L., Hilliard, R., Hoff, C., & Coates, T. J. (1993). Disclosing HIV seropositivity to significant others. *AIDS, 7,* 425–431.

Hayward, P., & Bright, J. A. (1997). Stigma and mental illness: A review and critique. *Journal of Mental Health, 6,* 345–354.

Haywood, T. W., Kravitz, H. M., Grossman, L. S., Cavanaugh, J. L., Davis, J. M., & Lewis, D. A. (1995). Predicting the "revolving door" phenomenon among patients with schizophrenic, schizoaffective, and affective disorders. *American Journal of Psychiatry, 152*(6), 856–861.

Healey, A., Knapp, M., Astin, J., Beecham, J., Kemp, R., Kirov, G., et al. (1998). Cost-effectiveness evaluation of compliance therapy for people with psychosis. *British Journal of Psychiatry, 172,* 420–424.

Healey, K. (1999, February). Case management in the criminal justice system. *National Institute of Justice: Research in Action Series.* Washington, DC: U.S. Department of Justice, Office of Justice Programs.

Health, N. I. o. M. (1975). Abnormal Involuntary Movement Scale (AIMS). *Psychopharmacology, 4,* 3–6.

Heaton, R., Paulsen, J. S., McAdams, L. A., Kuck, J., Zisook, S., Braff, D., et al. (1994). Neuropsychological deficits in schizophrenics: Relationship to age, chronicity, and dementia. *Archives of General Psychiatry, 51,* 469–476.

Heimberg, R. G., & Becker, R. E. (2002). *Cognitive-behavioral group therapy for social phobia.* New York: Guilford Press.

Hein, D. A., Cohen, L. R., Miele, G. M., Litt, L. C., & Capstick, C. (2004). Promising treatments for women with comorbid PTSD and substance use disorders. *American Journal of Psychiatry, 161,* 1426–1432.

Heinrichs, D. W., Hanlon, T. E., & Carpenter, W. T. J. (1984). The Quality of Life Scale: An instrument for rating the schizophrenia deficit syndrome. *Schizophrenia Bulletin, 10*, 388–396.

Heinrichs, R. W., & Zakzanis, K. K. (1998). Neurocognitive deficit in schizophrenia: A quantitative review of the evidence. *Neuropsychology, 12*, 426–445.

Heinssen, R. K., Liberman, R. P., & Kopelowicz, A. (2000). Psychosocial skills training for schizophrenia: Lessons from the laboratory. *Schizophrenia Bulletin, 26*, 21–46.

Heller, T., Roccoforte, J., Hsieh, K. Cook, J., & Pickett, S. (1997). Benefits of support groups for families of adults with severe mental illness. *American Journal of Orthopsychiatry, 62*, 187–198.

Hellerstein, D. J., Rosenthal, R. N., & Miner, C. R. (1995). A prospective study of integrated outpatient treatment for substance-abusing schizophrenic patients. *American Journal on Addictions, 42*, 33–42.

Helzer, J. E., & Robins, L. N. (1988). The Diagnostic Interview Schedule: Its development, evolution, and use. *Social Psychiatry and Psychiatric Epidemiology, 23*, 6–16.

Hemmens, C., Miller, M., Burton, V. S., & Milner, S. (2002). The consequences of official labels: An examination of the rights lost by the mentally ill and the the mentally incompetent ten years later. *Community Mental Health Journal, 38*, 129–140.

Henderson, D. C., Cagliero, E., Copeland, P. M., Borba, C. P., Evins, E., Hayden, D., et al. (2005). Glucose metabolism in patients with schizophrenia treated with atypical antipsychotic agents: A frequently sampled intravenous glucous tolerance test and minimal model analysis. *Archives of General Psychiatry, 62*, 19–28.

Herbert, J. D., Lilienfeld, S. O., Lohr, J. M., Montgomery, R. W., O'Donohue, W. T., Rosen, G. M., et al. (2000). Science and pseudoscience in the development of Eye Movement Densitization and Reprocessing: Implications for clinical psychology. *Clinical Psychology Review, 20*, 945–971.

Herbert, J. D., & Mueser, K. T. (1992). Eye movement desensitization: A critique of the evidence. *Journal of Behavior Therapy and Experimental Psychiatry, 23*, 169–174.

Herbert, P. B., & Young, K. A. (1999). The Americans with Disabilities Act and deinstitutionalization of the chronically mentally ill. *Journal of the American Academy of Psychiatry and the Law, 27*(4), 603–613.

Herdelin, A., & Scott, D. (1999). Experimental studies of the Program of Assertive Community Treatment (PACT). *Journal of Disability Policy Studies, 10*, 53–89.

Herinckx, H., Kinney, R., Clarke, G., & Paulson, R. (1997). Assertive community treatment versus usual care in engaging and retaining clients with severe mental illness. *Psychiatric Services, 48*, 1297–1306.

Herinckx, H., Swart, J., Ama, S., Dolezal, C., & King, S. (2005). Rearrest and linkage to mental health service among clients of the Clark County Mental Health Court program. *Psychiatric Services, 56*, 853–857.

Herman, J. L. (1992). *Trauma and recovery*. New York: Basic Books.

Herold, K. P. P. (1995). *The effects of an interviewee's self disclosure and disability on selected perceptions and attitudes of interviewers.* Unpublished doctoral dissertation, University of Southern Mississippi.

Hersen, M., & Turner, S. M. (Eds.). (2004). *Diagnostic interviewing* (3rd ed.). New York: Plenum Press.

Hertzman, M. (2002). Divalproex sodium to treat concomitant abuse and mood disorders. *Journal of Substance Abuse Treatment, 18*, 371–372.

Herz, M. (1985). Prodromal symptoms and prevention of relapse in schizophrenia. *Journal of Clinical Psychiatry, 46*, 22–25.

Herz, M. I. (1984). Recognizing and preventing relapse in patients with schizophrenia. *Hospital and Community Psychiatry, 35*, 344–349.

Herz, M. I., Glazer, W., Mirza, M., Mostert, M. A., & Hafez, H. (1989). Treating prodromal episodes to prevent relapse in schizophrenia. *British Journal of Psychiatry, 155*(Suppl. 5), 123–127.

Herz, M. I., Lamberti, J. S., Mintz, J., Scott, R., O'Dell, S. P., McCartan, L., et al. (2000). A program for relapse prevention in schizophrenia: A controlled study. *Archives of General Psychiatry, 57*, 277–283.

Hiday, V. (1999). Mental illness and criminal justice system. In A. Horwitz & T. Scheid (Eds.), A handbook for the study of mental health. Cambridge, UK: Cambridge University Press.

Hiday, V. (2006). Putting community risk in perspective: A look at correlations, causes and controls. *International Journal of Psychiatry and Law, 29*, 316–331.

Hiday, V. A., Swartz, M. S., Swanson, J. W., Borum, R., & Wagner, H. R. (1999). Criminal victimization of persons with severe mental illness. *Psychiatric Services, 50*, 62–68.

Higgins, S. T., Alessi, S. M., & Dantona, R. I. (2002). Voucher-based incentives: A substance abuse treatment innovation. *Addictive Behaviors, 27*, 887–910.

Hill, P. C., Pargament, K. I., Hood, R. W., McCullough, M. E., Swyers, J. P., Larson, D. B., et al. (2000). Conceptualizing religion and spirituality: Points of commonality, points of departure. *Journal for the Theory of Social Behaviour,* *30*(1), 51–77.

Hills, H., Siegfried, C., & Ickowitz, A. (2004). *Effective prison mental health services: Guidelines to expand and improve treatment* (NIC Accession Number 018604). Washington, DC: National Institute of Corrections, U.S. Department of Justice. *www.nicic.org.*

Hilton, J. L., & von Hippel, W. (1996). Stereotypes. *Annual Review of Psychology, 47,* 237–271.

Himmelhoch, S., Lehman, A., & Kreyenbuhl, J. (2004). Prevalence of chronic obstructive pulmonary disease among those with serious mental illness. *American Journal of Psychiatry, 161,* 2317–2319.

Ho, A. P., Tsuang, J. W., Liberman, R. P., Wang, R., Wilkins, J. N., Eckman, T. A., et al. (1999). Achieving effective treatment of patients with chronic psychotic illness and comorbid substance dependence. *American Journal of Psychiatry, 156,* 1765–1770.

Ho, B.-C., & Andreasen, N. C. (2001). Positive symptoms, negative symptoms, and beyond. In A. Breier, P. V. Tran, J. M. Herrea, G. D. Tollefson, & F. P. Bymaster (Eds.), *Current issues in the psychopharmacology of schizophrenia* (pp. 407–416). Philadelphia: Lippincott Williams & Wilkins.

Hodge, M., & Giesler, L. (1997). *Case management practice guidelines for adults with severe and persistent mental illness.* Ocean Ridge, FL: The National Association of Case Management and the Community Support Program, Division of Knowledge Development and Systems Change, Center for Mental Health Services, Substance Abuse and Mental Health Services Administration.

Hodges, J., Markward, M., Keele, C., & Evans, C. (2003). Use of self-help services and consumer satisfaction with professional mental health services. *Psychiatric Services, 54,* 1161–1163.

Hoehn, S. C. (1998). *Relationships between self-perception of disability and help-seeking behaviors of postsecondary students with learning disabilities.* Unpublished doctoral dissertation, University of California, Los Angeles.

Hoelter, J. W. (1983). Factorial invariance and self-esteem: Reassessing race and sex differences. *Social Forces, 61,* 834–846.

Hoenig, J., & Hamilton, M. (1966). The schizophrenic patient in the community and his effect on the household. *International Journal of Social Psychiatry, 12,* 165–176.

Hoff, A. L., Harris, D., Faustman, W. O., Beal, M.,

DeVilliers, D., Mone, R. D., et al. (1996). A neuropsychological study of early onset schizophrenia. *Schizophrenia Research, 20*(1–2), 21–28.

Hogan, M. F. (1992). New futures for mental health care: The case of Ohio. *Health Affairs, 11,* 69–83.

Hogan, M. F. (1999). Public-sector mental health care: New challenges. *Health Affairs, 18*(5), 106–111.

Hogan, R. (1985a). *Gaining community support for group homes.* Unpublished manuscript.

Hogan, R. (1985b). *Not in my town: Local government in opposition to group homes.* Unpublished manuscript.

Hogan, T. P., Awad, A. G., & Eastwood, R. (1983). A self-report scale predictive of drug compliance in schizophrenics: Reliability and discriminitive validity. *Psychological Medicine, 13,* 177–183.

Hogarty, G. E. (1995). Schizophrenia and modern mental health services. *Decade of the Brain, 6*(1), 3–6.

Hogarty, G. E. (2002). *Personal therapy for schizophrenia and related disorders: A guide to individualized treatment.* New York: Guilford Press.

Hogarty, G. E., & Flesher, S. (1999). Practice principles of cognitive enhancement therapy for schizophrenia. *Schizophrenia Bulletin, 25,* 693–708.

Hogarty, G. E., Flesher, S., Ulrich, R., Carter, M., Greenwald, D., Pogue-Geile, M., et al. (2004). Cognitive enhancement therapy for schizophrenia: Effects of a 2-year randomized trial on cognition and behavior. *Archives of General Psychiatry, 61,* 866–876.

Hogarty, G. E., & Goldberg, S. C. (1973). Drug and sociotherapy in the aftercare of schizophrenia patients: One-year relapse rates. *Archives of General Psychiatry, 28,* 54–64.

Hogarty, G. E., Goldberg, S., & Schooler, N. R. (1974). Drug and sociotherapy in the aftercare of schizophrenia patients: III. Adjustment of nonrelapsed patients. *Archives of General Psychiatry, 31,* 797–805.

Hogarty, G. E., Greenwald, D., Ulrich, R. F., Kornblith, S. J., DiBarry, A. L., Cooley, S., et al. (1997a). Three year trials of personal therapy among schizophrenic patients living with or independent of family: II. Effects of adjustment on patients. *American Journal of Psychiatry, 154,* 1514–1524.

Hogarty, G. E., Kornblith, S. J., Greenwald, D., DiBarry, A. L., Cooley, S., Flesher, S., et al. (1995). Personal therapy: A disorder-relevant psychotherapy for schizophrenia. *Schizophrenia Bulletin, 21,* 379–393.

Hogarty, G. E., Kornblith, S. J., Greenwald, D.,

DiBarry, A. L., Cooley, S., Ulrich, R. F., et al. (1997b). Three year trials of personal therapy among schizophrenic patients living with or independent of family: I. Description of study and effects on relapse rates. *American Journal of Psychiatry, 154*, 1504–1513.

Hogarty, G. E., Schooler, N. R., Ulrich, R. F., Mussare, F., Herron, E., & Ferro, P. (1979). Fluphenazine and social therapy in the aftercare of schizophrenic patients: Relapse analysis of a two-year controlled study of fluphenazine decanoate and fluphenazine hydrocholoride. *Archives of General Psychiatry, 36*, 1283–1294.

Hoge, M. A., Jacobs, S., Belitsky, R., & Migdole, S. (2002). Graduate education and training for contemporary behavioral health practice. *Administration and Policy in Mental Health, 29*, 335–357.

Hoge, M. A., Morris, J. A., Daniels, A. S., Huey, L. Y., Stuart, G. W., Adams, N., et al. (2005). Report of recommendations: The Annapolis Coalition Conference on Behavioral Health Work Force Competencies. *Administration and Policy in Mental Health, 32*, 651–663.

Hoge, M. A., Paris, M., Adger, H., Collins, F. L., Finn, C. V., Fricks, L., et al. (2005). Workforce competencies in behavioral health: An overview. *Administration and Policy in Mental Health, 32*, 593–631.

Holley, H. L., Hodges, P., & Jeffers, B. (1998). Moving psychiatric patients from hospital to community: Views of patients, providers, and families. *Psychiatric Services, 49*, 513–517.

Holloway, F. (1991). Case management for the mentally ill: Looking at the evidence. *International Journal of Social Psychiatry, 37*, 2–13.

Holloway, F., Oliver, N., Collins, E., & Carson, J. (1995). Case management: A critical review of outcome literature. *European Psychiatry, 10*, 113–128.

Holmes, E., Corrigan, P. W., Williams, P., Canar, J., & Kubiak, M. A. (1999). Changing attitudes about schizophrenia. *Schizophrenia Bulletin, 25*, 447–456.

Holmes, P., & River, L. P. (1998). Individual strategies for coping with the stigma of severe mental illness. *Cognitive and Behavioral Practice, 5*, 231–239.

Holter, M. C., Mowbray, C. T., Bellamy, C. D., MacFarlane, P., & Dukarski, J. (2004). Critical ingredients of consumer run services: Results of a national survey. *Community Mental Health Journal, 40*, 47–63.

Holzinger, A., Loffler, W., Muller, P., Priebe, S., & Angermeyer, M. C. (2002). Subjective illness theory and antipsychotic medication compliance by patients with schizophrenia. *Journal of Nervous and Mental Disease, 190*, 597–603.

Honigfeld, G., & Klett, C. J. (1976). Nurses Observation Scale for Inpatient Evaluation (NOSIE). In W. Guy (Ed.), *ECDEU assessment manual for psychopharmacology* (rev. ed., pp. 265–273). Rockville, MD: U.S. National Institute of Health, Psychopharmacology Research Branch.

Honkonen, T., Henriksson, M., Koivisto, A.-M., Stengård, E., & Salokangas, R. K. R. (2004). Violent victimization in schizophrenia. *Social Psychiatry and Psychiatric Epidemiology, 39*, 606–612.

Hooley, J., Richters, J., Weintraub, S., & Neal, J. (1987). Psychopathology and marital distress: The positive side of positive symptoms. *Journal of Abnormal Psychology, 96*, 27–33.

Hopper, K., & Barrow, S. M. (2003). Two genealogies of supported housing and their implications for outcome assessment. *Psychiatric Services, 54*, 50–54.

Hornung, W. P., Feldman, R., Klingberg, S., Buchkremer, G., & Reker, T. (1999). Long-term effects of a psychoeducational psychotherapeutic intervention for schizophrenic outpatients and their key-persons: Results of a five-year follow-up. *European Archives of Psychiatry and Clinical Neuroscience, 249*, 162–167.

Horowitz, A. (1993). Adult siblings as sources of social support for seriously mentally ill: A test of the serial model. *Journal of Marriage and the Family, 55*, 623–632.

Horowitz, A., & Reinhard, S. (1995). Ethnic differences in caregiving duties and burden among parents and siblings of persons with severe mental illness. *Journal of Health and Social Behavior, 36*, 138–150.

Horowitz, A., Tessler, R., Fisher, G., & Gamache, G. (1992). The role of adult siblings in providing social support to the severely mentally ill. *Journal of Marriage and the Family, 54*, 233–241.

Horowitz, M. D., Wilner, N., & Alvarez, W. (1979). Impact of Event Scale: A measure of subjective stress. *Psychosomatic Medicine, 41*, 209–218.

Horowitz, M. J. (1986). *Stress response syndromes* (2nd ed.). New York: Jason Aronson.

Howard, R., Almeida, O. P., & Levy, R. (1994). Phenomenology, demography and diagnosis in late paraphrenia. *Psychology and Medicine, 24*, 397–410.

Howgego, I. M., Owen, C., Meldrum, L., Yellowlees, P., Dark, F., & Parslow, R. (2005). Posttraumatic stress disorder: An exploratory study examining rates of trauma and PTSD and its effect on client outcomes in community mental health. *BMC Psychiatry, 5*(21).

Howgego, I. M., Yellowlees, P., Owen, C., Meldrum, L., & Dark, F. (2003). The therapeutic alliance: The key to effective patient outcome? A descriptive review of the evidence in community mental health case management. *Australian and New Zealand Journal of Psychiatry, 37*, 169–183.

Howie the Harp. (1990). Independent living with support services: The goals and future for mental health consumers. *Psychosocial Rehabilitation Journal, 13*(4), 85–89.

Hromco, J., Lyons, J., & Nikkel, R. (1995). Mental health case management, characteristic, job function, and occupational stress. *Community Mental Health Journal, 31*, 11–125.

Hu, T.-W., Snowden, L. R., Jerrell, J. M., & Nguyen, T. D. (1991). Ethnic populations in public mental health: Services choice and level of use. *American Journal of Public Health, 81*(11), 1429–1434.

Huber, G., Gross, G., Schuttler, R., & Linz, M. (1980). Longitudinal studies of schizophrenic patients. *Schizophrenia Bulletin, 6*, 592–605.

Huffine, C. L., & Clausen, J. A. (1979). Madness and work: Short- and long-term effects of mental illness on occupational careers. *Social Forces, 57*, 1049–1062.

Hughes, R., & Clement, J. (1999, March 1). Time to end the model wars. *IAPSRS Connection, 1*, 1.

Hughes, R., & Weinstein, D. (1997b). Introduction. In R. Hughes & D. Weinstein (Eds.), *Best practices in psychosocial rehabilitation* (pp. vi–xvi). Columbia, MD: International Association of Psychosocial Rehabilitation.

Hughes, R., & Weinstein, D. (Eds.). (1997a). *Best practices in psychosocial rehabilitation*. Columbia, MD: International Association of Psychosocial Rehabilitation.

Hull, C. L. (1952). *A behavior system*. New Haven: Yale University Press.

Hurlburt, M. S., Hough, R. L., & Wood, P. A. (1996). Effects of substance abuse and housing stability of homeless mentally ill persons in supported housing. *Psychiatric Services, 47*, 731–736.

Hutchings, P. S., & Dutton, M. A. (1993). Sexual assault history in a community mental health center clinical population. *Community Mental Health Journal, 29*, 59–63.

Huxley, N. A., Rendall, M., & Sederer, L. (2000). Psychosocial treatments in schizophrenia: A review of the past 20 years. *Journal of Nervous and Mental Disease, 188*, 187–201.

Huxley, P. (1998). Quality of life. In K. T. Mueser & N. Tarrier (Eds.), *Handbook of social functioning in schizophrenia* (pp. 52–65). Needham Heights, MA: Allyn & Bacon.

Iacono, W. G., & Beiser, M. (1992). Are males more likely than females to develop schizophrenia? *American Journal of Psychiatry, 149*(8), 1070–1074.

Ingram, R. E., & Kendall, P. C. (1986). Cognitive clinical psychology: Implications of an information processing perspective. In R. E. Ingram (Ed.), *Information processing approaches to clinical psychology* (pp. 3–21). San Diego: Academic Press.

Institute for Community Inclusion. (2005). What do vocational rehabilitation (VR) services cost? *Data Note, 1*. Retrieved June 30, 2007, from *statedata.info/datanotes/datanote1. php*.

Institute of Medicine. (2001). *Crossing the quality chasm: A new health system for the 21st century*. Washington DC: National Academy Press.

Intagliata, J. (1982). Improving the quality of community care for chronically mentally disabled: The role of case management. *Schizophrenia Bulletin, 8*, 655–673.

Intagliata, J., Willer, B., & Egri, G. (1986). Role of the family in case management of the mentally ill. *Schizophrenia Bulletin, 12*, 699–708.

International Association of Psychosocial Rehabilitation Services. (1990). *A national directory: Organizations providing psychosocial rehabilitation and related community support services in the United States*. Columbia, MD: Author.

International Association of Psychosocial Rehabilitation Services. (1996). *Principles of multicultural psychiatric rehabilitation services*. Retrieved February 11, 2006, from *www.uspra. org/i4a/pages/Index.cfm?pageid=3384*.

Jablensky, A., Sartorius, N., Ernberg, G., Anker, M., Korten, A., Cooper, J. E., et al. (1992). Schizophrenia: Manifestations, incidence and course in different cultures: A World Health Organization ten-country study. *Psychological Medicine Monograph Supplement*(20), pp. 1–97.

Jackson, C., Knott, C., Skeate, A., & Birchwood, M. (2004). The trauma of first episode psychosis: The role of cognitive mediation. *Australian and New Zealand Journal of Psychiatry, 38*, 327–333.

Jackson, H., McGorry, P., Edwards, J., Hulbert, C., Henry, L., Francey, S., et al. (1998). Cognitively oriented psychotherapy for early psychosis (COPE): Preliminary results. *British Journal of Psychiatry, 172*, 93–100.

Jacobs, D. R., & Moxley, D. P. (1993). Anticipating managed mental health care: Implications for psychosocial rehabilitation agencies.

Psychosocial Rehabilitation Journal, 17(2), 15–31.

Jacobs, M., & Goodman, G. (1989). Psychology and self help groups: Predictions on a partnership. *American Psychologist, 42,* 536–545.

Jacobson, A. (1989). Physical and sexual assault histories among psychiatric outpatients. *American Journal of Psychiatry, 146,* 755–758.

Jacobson, A., & Herald, C. (1990). The relevance of childhood sexual abuse to adult psychiatric inpatient care. *Hospital and Community Psychiatry, 41,* 154–158.

Jacobson, A., & Richardson, B. (1987). Assault experiences of 100 psychiatric inpatients: Evidence of the need for routine inquiry. *American Journal of Psychiatry, 144,* 508–513.

Jaeger, J., & Douglas, E. (1992). Neuropsychiatric rehabilitation for persistent mental illness. *Psychiatric Quarterly, 63,* 71–94.

James, W., Preston, N. J., Koh, G., Spencer, C., Kisely, S. R., & Castle, D. J. (2004). A group intervention which assists patients with dual diagnosis reduce their drug use: A randomised controlled trial. *Psychological Medicine, 34,* 983–990.

Janoff-Bulman, R. (1989). Assumptive worlds and the stress of traumatic events: Applications of the schema construct. *Social Cognition, 7,* 113–136.

Jeffers, S. (1992). *Feel the fear and do it anyway.* New York: Fawcett Books.

Jemelka, R., Trupin, E., & Chiles, J. A. (1989). The mentally ill in prisons: A review. *Hospital and Community Psychiatry, 40,* 481–491.

Jennings, A. (2004). *Models for developing trauma-informed behavioral health systems and trauma-specific services.* Alexandria, VA: National Technical Assistance Center for State Mental Health Planning, National Association of State Mental Health Program Directors.

Jennings, A. F. (1994). On being invisible in the mental health system. *Journal of Mental Health Administration, 21,* 374–387.

Jensen, G. F., White, C. S., & Gelleher, J. M. (1982). Ethnic status and adolescent self-evaluations: An extention of research on minority self-esteem. *Social Problems, 30,* 226–239.

Jerrell, J. M., & Ridgely, M. S. (1995). Comparative effectiveness of three approaches to serving people with severe mental illness and substance use disorders. *Journal of Nervous and Mental Disease, 183,* 566–576.

Jerrell, J. M., & Ridgely, M. S. (1999). Impact of robustness of program implementation on outcomes of clients in dual diagnosis programs. *Psychiatric Services, 50,* 109–112.

Jeste, D. V., Gilbert, P. L., McAdams, L. A., & Harris, M. (1995). Considering neuroleptic maintenance and taper on a continuum: Need for individual rather than dogmatic approach. *Archives of General Psychiatry, 52*(3), 209–212.

Jeste, D. V., Gladsjo, J. A., Lindamer, L. A., & Lacro, J. P. (1996). Medical comorbidity in schizophrenia. *Schizophrenia Bulletin, 22,* 413–430.

Johnsen, M., Teague, G., & Herr, M. E. (2005). Common ingredients as a fidelity measure for peer-run programs. In S. Clay (Ed.), *On our own, together: Peer programs for people with mental illness* (pp. 213–238). Nashville: Vanderbilt University Press.

Johnson, E. (2000). Differences among families with serious mental illness: A qualitative analysis. *American Journal of Orthopsychiatry, 70,* 126–134.

Johnson, J. L., & Cameron, M. C. (2001). Barriers to providing effective mental health services to American Indians. *Mental Health Services Research, 3,* 215–223.

Johnson, P., & Rubin, A. (1983). Case management in mental health: A social work domain? *Social Work, 28,* 49–55.

Johnson, S., Salkeld, G., Sanderson, K., Issakidis, C., Teesson, M., & Buhrich, N. (1998). Intensive case management: A cost effectiveness analysis. *Australian and New Zealand Journal of Psychiatry, 32,* 551–559.

Johnston, L., & Hewstone, M. (1992). Cognitive models of stereotype change: III. Subtyping and the perceived typicality of disconfirming group members. *Journal of Experimental Social Psychology, 28,* 360–386.

Johnstone, E., Frith, C., Lang, F., & Owens, D. (1995). Determinants of the extremes of outcome in schizophrenia. *British Journal of Psychiatry, 167,* 604–609.

Johnstone, E., Owens, D., Bydder, G., & Colter, N. (1989). The spectrum of structural brain changes in schizophrenia: Age of onset as a predictor of cognitive and clinical impairments and their cerebral correlates. *Psychological Medicine, 19*(1), 91–103.

Johnstone, E. C., Macmillan, J. F., Frith, C. D., Benn, D. K., & Crow, T. J. (1990). Further investigation of the predictors of outcome following first schizophrenic episodes. *British Journal of Psychiatry, 157,* 182–189.

Joint Commission on Accreditation of Healthcare Organizations. (1997). Comprehensive accreditation manual for hospitals, and the comprehensive manual for behavioral care. Chicago: Author.

Jones, D. R., Macias, C., Barreira, P. J., Fisher, W. H., Hargreaves, W. A., & Harding, C. M. (2004). Prevalence, severity, and co-occurrence of chronic physical health problems of persons with serious mental illness. *Psychiatric Services, 55,* 1250–1257.

Jones, E. E., Farina, A., Hastorf, A. H., Markus, H., Miller, D. T., & Scott, R. A. (1984). *Social stigma: The psychology of marked relationships.* New York: W. H. Freeman.

Jones, R. A., & Brehm, J. W. (1970). Persuasiveness of one- and two-sided communications as a function of awareness: There are two sides. *Journal of Experimental Social Psychology, 6,* 47–56.

Jones, S., Roth, D., & Jones, P. (1995). Effect of demographic and behavioral variables on burden of caregivers of chronic mentally ill persons. *Psychiatric Services, 46,* 141–145.

Jonikas, J. A. (1994). *Staff competencies for service delivery staff in psychosocial rehabilitation programs: A review of the literature.* Chicago: UIC National Research and Training Center on Psychiatric Disability.

Jordan, K., Schlenger, W., Fairbank, J., & Caddell, J. (1996). Prevalence of psychiatric disorders among incarcerated women: Convicted felons entering prison. *Archives of General Psychiatry, 53,* 513–519.

Josephson, S. B. (1997). Correlates of HIV/AIDS disclosure: Psychosocial stresses; demographics; social support; coping; and quality of life. Unpublished doctoral dissertation, Columbia University, New York.

Judd, C. M., & Park, B. (1993). Definition and assessment of accuracy in social stereotypes. *Psychological Review, 100,* 109–128.

Jungbauer, J., & Angermeyer, M. (2002). Living with a schizophrenic patient: A comprehensive study of burden as it affects parents and spouses. *Psychiatry, 65,* 110–123.

Jungbauer, J., Wittmund, B., Dietrich, S., & Angermeyer, M. (2004). The disregarded caregivers: Subjective burden in spouses of schizophrenia patients. *Schizophrenia Bulletin, 30,* 665–675.

Jussim, L., Nelson, T. E., Manis, M., & Soffin, S. (1995). Prejudice, stereotypes, and labeling effects: Sources of bias in person perception. *Journal of Personality and Social Psychology, 68,* 228–246.

Kaas, M., Lee, S., & Peitzman, C. (2003). Barriers to collaboration between mental health professionals and families in the care of persons with severe mental illness. *Issues in Mental Health Nursing, 24,* 741–756.

Kahn, M. W., Obstfeld, L., & Heiman, E. (1979).

Staff conceptions of patients' attitudes toward mental disorder and hospitalization as compared to patients' and staff's actual attitudes. *Journal of Clinical Psychology, 35,* 415–420.

Kaiser Commission on Medicaid and the Uninsured. (2005). *Medicaid: An overview of spending on "mandatory" vs. "optional" populations and services* (Issue Paper #7331). Menlo Park, CA: Kaiser Family Foundation. Retrieved June 30, 2007, from *www.kff.org/medicaid/7331.cfm.*

Kalichman, S. C., Sikkema, K., Kelly, J. A., & Bulto, M. (1996). Use of a brief behavioral skills intervention to prevent HIV infection among chronically mentally ill adults. *Psychiatric Services, 46,* 275–280.

Kamali, M., Kelly, L., Gervin, M., Browne, S., Larkin, C., & O'Callaghan, E. (2001). Insight and comorbid substance misuse and medication compliance among patients with schizophrenia. *Psychiatric Services, 52,* 161–166.

Kanter, J. (1989). Clinical case management: Definition, principles, components. *Hospital and Community Psychiatry, 40,* 361–368.

Kanter, J. (1996). Case management with long term patients: A comprehensive approach. In S. M. Soreff (Ed.), *Handbook for the treatment of the seriously mentally ill* (pp. 257–277). Ashland, OH: Hogrefe & Huber.

Karmel, M. (1969). Total institution and self-mortification. *Journal of Health and Social Behavior, 10,* 134–141.

Karras, A. (1962). The effects of reinforcement and arousal on the psychomotor performance of chronic schizophrenics. *Journal of Abnormal and Social Psychology, 65,* 104–111.

Karras, A. (1968). Choice reaction time of chronic and acute psychiatric patients under primary or secondary aversive stimulation. *British Journal of Social and Clinical Psychology, 7,* 270–279.

Kasper, M. E., Rogers, R., & Adams, P. A. (1996). Dangerousness and command hallucinations: An investigation of psychotic inpatients. *Bulletin of the American Academy of Psychiatry and the Law, 24,* 219–224.

Kasprow, W. J., Rosenheck, R., Frisman, L., & DiLella, D. (1999). Residential treatment for dually diagnosed homeless veterans: A comparison of program types. *American Journal on Addictions, 8,* 34–43.

Kaufman, A. (1998). Older patients who care for adult children with serious mental illness. *Journal of Gerontological Social Work, 29,* 35–55.

Kaufman, C. (1995). The self-help employment center: Some outcomes from the first year. *Psychosocial Rehabilitation Journal, 18,* 145–162.

Kaufman, C. (1999). An introduction to the mental health consumer movement. In A. Horowitz & T. Scheid (Eds.), *A handbook for the study of mental health* (pp. 493–507). New York: Cambridge University Press.

Kaufman, C., Freund, P., & Wilson, J. (1989). Self help in mental health system: A model for consumer–provider collaboration. *Psychosocial Rehabilitation Journal, 13,* 5–21.

Kaufman, C., Shulberg, H., & Schooler, N. (1994). Self-help group participation among people with severe mental illness. *Prevention in Human Services, 11,* 315–33.

Kaufman, C., Ward-Colosante, C., & Farmer, J. (1993). Development and evaluation of drop-in centers operated by mental health consumers. *Hospital and Community Psychiatry, 44,* 675–678.

Kavanagh, D. J., Young, R., White, A., Saunders, J. B., Wallis, J., Shocklewy, N., et al. (2004). A brief motivational intervention for substance misuse in recent-onset psychosis. *Drug and Alcohol Review, 23,* 151–155.

Kay, S. R., Opler, L. A., & Fiszbein, A. (1987). The Positive and Negative Syndrome Scale (PANSS) for schizophrenia. *Schizophrenia Bulletin, 13,* 261–276.

Kay, S. R., Wolkenfeld, F., & Murrill, L. M. (1988). Profiles of aggression among psychiatric patients: I. Nature and prevalence. *Journal of Nervous and Mental Disease, 176,* 539–546.

Keane, C. (1991). Socioenvironmental determinants of community formation. *Environment and Behavior, 23,* 27–46.

Keane, T. M., Fairbank, J. A., Caddell, J. M., & Zimering, R. T. (1989). Implosive (flooding) therapy reduces symptoms of PTSD in Vietnam combat veterans. *Behavior Therapy, 29,* 245–260.

Keck, L., & Mussey, C. (2005). GROW in Illinois. In S. Clay (Ed.), *On our own, together: Peer programs for people with mental illness* (pp. 14–158). Nashville: Vanderbilt University Press.

Keefe, R. S., Goldberg, T. E., Harvey, P. D., Gold, J. M., Poe, M. P., & Coughenour, L. (2004). The Brief Assessment of Cognition in Schizophrenia: Reliability, sensitivity, and comparison with a standard neurocognitive battery. *Schizophrenia Research, 68,* 283–297.

Keefe, R. S., Silva, S. G., Perkins, D. O., & Lieberman, J. A. (1999). The effects of atypical antipsychotic drugs on neurocognitive impairment in schizophrenia: A review and meta-analysis. *Schizophrenia Bulletin, 25,* 201–222.

Kelly, A. E., & McKillop, K. J. (1996). Consequences of revealing personal secrets. *Psychological Bulletin, 120,* 450–465.

Kelly, G. R., & Scott, J. E. (1990). Medication compliance and health education among outpatients with chronic mental disorders. *Medical Care, 28,* 1181–1197.

Kelly, J. (2003). Self-help for substance-use disorders: History, effectiveness, knowledge gaps, and research opportunities. *Clinical Psychology Review, 23,* 639–663.

Kelly, J., McKeller, J., & Moos, R. (2003). Major depression in patients with substance use disorders: Relationship to 12-step self help involvement and substance use outcomes. *Addiction, 98,* 499–508.

Kemp, R., & David, A. (1995). Insight and compliance. In B. Blackwell (Ed.), *Compliance and the treatment alliance in serious mental illness.* Newark, NJ: Gordon and Breach.

Kemp, R., Hayward, P., Applewhaite, G., Everitt, B., & David, A. (1996). Compliance therapy in psychotic patients: Randomised controlled trial. *British Medical Journal, 312,* 345–349.

Kemp, R., Kirov, G., Everitt, B., Hayward, P., & David, A. (1998). Randomised controlled trial of compliance therapy: 18-month follow-up. *British Journal of Psychiatry, 173,* 271–272.

Kendall, P. C. (1982). Cognitive processes and procedures in behavior therapy. *Annual Review of Behavior Therapy: Theory and Practice, 8,* 120–155.

Kendler, K. S., Bulik, C. M., Silberg, J., Hettema, J. M., Myers, J., & Prescott, C. A. (2000). Childhood sexual abuse and adult psychiatric and substance abuse disorders in women: An epidemiological and cotwin control analysis. *Archives of General Psychiatry, 57,* 953–959.

Kendler, K. S., & Diehl, S. R. (1993). The genetics of schizophrenia: A current, genetic-epidemiologic perspective. *Schizophrenia Bulletin, 19*(2), 261–285.

Kendler, K. S., Gruenberg, A. M., & Tsuang, M. T. (1985). Psychiatric illness in first-degree relatives of schizophrenic and surgical control patients: A family study using DSM-III criteria. *Archives of General Psychiatry, 42,* 770–779.

Kendler, K. S., Kuhn, J. W., & Prescott, C. A. (2004). Childhood sexual abuse, stressful life events and risk for major depression in woman. *Psychological Medicine, 34,* 1475–1482.

Kendler, K. S., McGuire, M., Gruenberg, A. M., Spellman, M., & Walsh, D. (1993). The Roscommon Family Study: II. The risk of nonschizophrenic nonaffective psychoses in relatives. *Archives of General Psychiatry, 50*(8), 645–652.

Kennamer, D. J., Honnold, J., Bradford, J., & Hendricks, M. (2000). Differences in disclosure of sexuality among African American and white gay/bisexual men: Implications for HIV/AIDS prevention. *AIDS Education and Prevention, 12*(6), 519–532.

Kennedy, M. (1989, June 23). *Psychiatry hospitalizations of GROWers.* Paper presented at the Biennial Conference on Community Research and Action, East Lansing, Michigan.

Kern, R. S., Green, M. F., & Satz, P. (1992). Neuropsychological predictors of skills training for chronic psychiatric patients. *Psychiatry Research, 43,* 223–230.

Kern, R. S., Liberman, R. P., Kopelowicz, A., Mintz, J., & Green, M. F. (2002). Applications of errorless learning for improving work performance in persons with schizophrenia. *American Journal of Psychiatry, 159,* 1921–1926.

Kessler, R., McGonagle, K., Zhao, S., Nelson, C., Hughes, M., Eshlenon, S., et al. (1994). Lifetime and 12-month prevalence of DSM-III-R psychiatry disorders in the United States. *Archives of General Psychiatry, 51,* 8–19.

Kessler, R., Michelson, F., & Zhao, S. (1997c). Patterns and correlates of self-help group membership in the United States. *Social Policy, 27,* 27–46.

Kessler, R., Zhao, S., Katz, S., Kauzis, A., Frank, R., Edlund, M., et al. (1999). Past-year use of outpatient services for psychiatric problems in the National Comorbidity Survey. *American Journal of Psychiatry, 156,* 115–123.

Kessler, R. C. (2000). Gender differences in major depression: Epidemiological findings. In E. Frank (Ed.), *Gender and its effects on psychopathology American Psychopathological Association series* (pp. 61–84). Washington, DC: American Psychiatric Association.

Kessler, R. C., Berglund, P. A., Bruce, M. L., Koch, R., Laska, E. M., Leaf, P. J., Menderscheid, R. W., et al. (2001). The prevalence and correlates of untreated serious mental illness. *Health Services Research, 36,* 987–1007.

Kessler, R. C., Borges, G., & Walters, E. E. (1999). Prevalence of and risk factors for lifetime suicide attempts in the National Comorbidity Survey. *Archives of General Psychiatry, 56*(7), 617–626.

Kessler, R. C., Crum, R. M., Warner, L. A., Nelson, C. B., Schulenberg, J., & Anthony, J. C. (1997a). Lifetime co-occurrence of DSM-III-R alcohol abuse and dependence with other psychiatric disorders in the National Comorbidity Survey. *Archives of General Psychiatry, 54,* 313–321.

Kessler, R. C., Davis, C. D., & Kendler, K. S. (1997b). Childhood adversity and adult psychiatric disorder in the U.S. National Comorbidity Survey. *Psychological Medicine, 27,* 1101–1119.

Kessler, R. C., DuPont, R. L., Berglund, P., & Wittchen, H.-U. (1999). Impairment in pure and comorbid generalized anxiety disorder and major depression at 12 months in two national surveys. *American Journal of Psychiatry, 156*(12), 1915–1923.

Kessler, R. C., Nelson, C. B., McGonagle, K. A., Edlund, M. J., Frank, R. G., & Leaf, P. J. (1996). The epidemiology of co-occurring addictive and mental disorders: Implications for prevention and service utilization. *American Journal of Orthopsychiatry, 66*(1), 17–31.

Kessler, R. C., Sonnega, A., Bromet, E., Hughes, M., & Nelson, C. B. (1995). Posttraumatic stress disorder in the National Comorbidity Survey. *Archives of General Psychiatry, 52,* 1048–1060.

Kiernan, R. J., Mueller, J., Langston, J. W., & Van Dyke, C. (1987). The Neurobehavioral Cognitive Screening Examination: A brief but quantitative approach to cognitive assessment. *Annals of Internal Medicine, 107,* 481–485.

Kiernan, W. E., Halliday, J. F., & Boeltzig, H. (2004). *Economic engagement: An avenue to employment for individuals with disabilities: A preliminary report of a panel of experts on employment systems.* Boston: Institute for Community Inclusion. Retrieved June 30, 2007, from *www.communityinclusion.org.*

Kinderman, P., & Bentall, R. P. (1997). Causal attributions in depression and paranoia: Internal, personal and situational attributions for negative events. *Journal of Abnormal Psychology, 106,* 341–345.

Kinderman, P., Dunbar, R., & Bentall, R. P. (1998). Theory-of-mind deficits and causal attributions. *British Journal of Psychology, 89,* 191–204.

King, L. L., & Polaschek, D. (2003). The abstinence violation effect: Investigating lapse and relapse phenomena using the Relapse Prevention Model with domestically violent men. *New Zealand Journal of Psychology, 32,* 67–75.

Kingdon, D., & Turkington, D. (1991). The use of cognitive behavior therapy with a normalizing rationale in schizophrenia: A preliminary report. *Journal of Nervous and Mental Disease, 179,* 207–211.

Kingdon, D. G., & Turkington, D. (2004). *Cognitive Therapy of Schizophrenia.* New York: Guilford Press.

Kinsella, K., Anderson, R., & Anderson, W. (1996). Coping skills, strengths, and needs as perceived by adult offspring and siblings of people with mental illness: A retrospective study. *Psychiatric Rehabilitation Journal, 20,* 24–32.

Klien, A., Cnaan, R., & Whitecraft, J. (1998). Significance of peer social support for dually-diagnosed clients: Findings from a pilot study. *Research on Social Work Practice, 8,* 529–551.

Klinkenberg, W., & Calsyn, R. J. (1997). The moderating effects of race on return visits to the psychiatric emergency room. *Psychiatric Services, 48*(7), 942–945.

Knight, E., & Blanch, A. (1993). *A dialogue on recovery: Tips for structuring a recipient dialogue.* Albany: New York State Office of Mental Health.

Koegel, L. (1992). Assessment of assertiveness and social skills of adolescents. In I. G. Fodor (Ed.), *Adolescent assertiveness and social skills training: A clinical handbook* (pp. 43–61). New York: Springer.

Koh, S. D. (1978). Remembering of verbal materials by schizophrenic young adults. In S. Schwartz (Ed.), *Language and cognition in schizophrenia* (pp. 59–69). Hillsdale, NJ: Erlbaum.

Koh, S. D., Grinker, R. R., Marusarz, T. Z., & Forman, P. L. (1981). Affective memory and schizophrenia anhedonia. *Schizophrenia Bulletin, 7*, 292–307.

Kohler, C. G., Turner, T., Bilker, W. B., Brensinger, C. M., Siegel, S. J., Kanes, S. J., et al. (2003). Facial emotion recognition in schizophrenia: Intensity effects and error pattern. *American Journal of Psychiatry, 160*, 1768–1774.

Koons, C. R., Robins, C. J., Tweed, J. L., Lynch, T. R., Gonzalez, A. M., Morse, J. Q., Bishop, G. K., et al. (2001). Efficacy of dialectical behavior therapy in women veterans with borderline personality disorder. *Behavior Therapy, 32*, 371–390.

Kopelowicz, A., & Liberman, R. P. (1994). Self-management approaches for seriously mentally ill persons. *Directions in Psychiatry, 14*(17), 1–7.

Koranyi, E. (1979). Morbidity and rate of undiagnosed physical illnesses in a psychiatric clinic population. *Archives of General Psychiatry, 36*, 414–419.

Kotler, J. D. (2002). *Seizing the moment: Redefining state mental health agency role in time of budget uncertainty.* Alexandria, VA: National Technical Assistance Center for State Mental Health Planning. Retrieved June 30, 2007, from *www.nasmhpd.org/publications.cfm#techpap.*

Kouzis, A. C., & Eaton, W. W. (2000). Psychopathology and the initiation of disability payments. *Psychiatric Services, 51*, 908–913.

Kraepelin, E. (1896). *Psychiatrie* (5th ed.). Leipzig: Barth.

Kraeplin, E. (1919/1971). *Dementia praecox and paraphrenia.* (R. M. Barclay, Trans.). New York: Robert E. Krieger.

Kreisman, D., & Blumenthal, R. (1995). Emotional overinvolvement: A review and explanation of its role in expressed emotion. *Research in Community and Mental Health, 8*, 3–39.

Krepp, J. K. (2000). *Lodge magic: Real life adventures in mental health recovery.* Minneapolis, MN: Tasks Unlimited.

Krizay, J. (1989). *Partial hospitalization: Facilities, cost, and utilization.* Washington, DC: American Psychiatric Association Office of Economic Affairs.

Krueger, J. (1996). Personal beliefs and cultural stereotypes about racial characteristics. *Journal of Personality and Social Psychology, 71*, 536–548.

Krumholz, H. M., Douglas, P. S., Lauer, M. S., & Pasternak, R. C. (1992). Selection of patients for coronary angiography and coronary revascularization early after myocardial infarction: Is there evidence for gender bias? *Annals of Internal Medicine, 116*, 785–790.

Krupa, T. (1998). The consumer-run business: People with psychiatric disabilities as entrepreneurs. *Work, 11*, 3–10.

Krupa, T., Eastbrook, S., Hern, L., Lee, D., North, R., Percy, K., et al. (2005). How do people who receive assertive community treatment experience the service? *Psychiatric Rehabilitation Journal, 29*, 18–24.

Krupa, T., McLean, H., Eastabrook, S., Bonham, A., & Baksh, L. (2003). Daily time use as a measure of community adjustment for clients of assertive community treatment. *American Journal of Occupational Therapy, 57*, 558–565.

Kuhn, E., Blanchard, E. B., & Hickling, E. J. (2003). Posttraumatic stress disorder and psychosocial functioning within two samples of MVA survivors. *Behaviour Research and Therapy, 41*, 1105–1112.

Kuipers, E., Garety, P., Fowler, D., Dunn, G., Bebbington, P., Freeman, D., et al. (1997). London-East Anglia randomised controlled trial of cognitive-behavioural therapy for psychosis: I. Effects of the treatment phase. *British Journal of Psychiatry, 171*, 319–327.

Kuipers, L., Leff, J., & Lam, D. (2002). *Family work for schizophrenia: A practical guide* (2nd ed.). London: Gaskell.

Kuntz, C. (1995). *Persons with severe mental illness: How do they fit into long-term care?* Rockville, MD: Office of Disability, Aging and Long-Term Care Policy with the U.S. Department of Health and Human Services.

Kurtz, L. (1988). Mutual aid for affective disorders: The manic depressive and depressive association. *American Journal of Orthopsychiatry, 58*, 152–155.

Kurtz, L., & Chambon, A. (1987). Comparison of self help groups for mental health. *Health and Social Work, 12*, 275-283.

Kurtz, M. M., Moberg, P. J., Gur, R. C., & Gur, R. E. (2001). Approaches to cognitive remediation of neuropsychological deficit in schizophrenia: A review and meta-analysis. *Neuropsychological Review, 11*, 197–210.

Lab, D. D., & Moore, L. (2005). Prevalence and denial of sexual abuse in a male psychiatric inpatient population. *Journal of Traumatic Stress, 18*, 323–330.

Laberge, D., & Morin, D. (1995). The overuse of criminal justice dispositions: Failure of diversionary policies in the management of mental health problems. *International Journal of Law and Psychiatry, 4*, 389–414.

LaGrange, T. (2000, November). *Distinguishing between the criminal and the "crazy": Decisions to arrest in police encounters with mentally disordered*. Paper presented at The American Society of Criminology, San Francisco, CA.

Laine, C., & Davidoff, F. (1996). Patient-centered medicine. A professional evolution. *Journal of the American Medical Association, 275*, 152–156.

Lally, S. J. (1989). "Does being in here mean there is something wrong with me?" *Schizophrenia Bulletin, 15*(2), 253–265.

Lam, D. (1991). Psychosocial family intervention in schizophrenia: A review of empirical studies. *Psychological Medicine, 21*, 423–441.

Lam, D. H., Bright, J., Jones, S., Hayward, P., Schuck, N., Chisholm, D., et al. (2000). Cognitive therapy for bipolar illness: A pilot study of relapse prevention. *Cognitive Therapy and Research, 24*, 503–520.

Lam, D. H., Hayward, P., Watkins, E. R., Wright, K., & Sham, P. (2005). Relapse prevention in patients with bipolar disorder: Cogniitive therapy outcome after two years. *American Journal of Psychiatry, 162*, 324–329.

Lam, D. H., Jones, S. H., Hayward, P., & Bright, J. A. (1999). *Cognitive therapy for bipolar disorder: A therapist's guide to concepts, methods and practice*. Chichester: Wiley.

Lam, D. H., McCrone, P., Wright, K., & Kerr, N. (2005). Cost-effectiveness of relapse-prevention cognitive therapy for bipolar disorder: 30-month study. *British Journal of Psychiatry, 186*, 500–506.

Lam, D. H., Watkins, E. R., Hayward, P., Bright, J. A., Wright, K., Kerr, N., et al. (2003). A randomized controlled study of cognitive therapy for relapse prevention for bipolar affective disorder. *Archives of General Psychiatry, 60*, 145–152.

Lam, J. A., & Rosenheck, R. (1998). The effect of victimization on clinical outcomes of homeless persons with serious mental illness. *Psychiatric Services, 49*, 678–683.

Lamb, H., & Grant, R. (1982). The mentally ill in an urban county jail. *Archives of General Psychiatry, 39*, 17–22.

Lamb, H., & Grant, R. (1983). Mentally ill women in a county jail. IArchives of General Psychiatry, 40, 363–368.

Lamb, H. R. (1976). *Community survival for the long-term patient*. San Francisco: Jossey-Bass.

Lamb, H. R. (1980). Therapist-case managers: More than brokers of services. *Hospital and Community Psychiatry, 31*, 762–764.

Lamb, H. R., & Bachrach, L. L. (2001). Some perspectives on deinstitutionalization. *Psychiatric Services, 52*(8), 1039–1045.

Lamb, H. R., Shaner, R., Elliott, D., DeCuir, W. J., & Foltz, J. (1995). Outcome for psychiatric emergency patients seen by an outreach police mental health team. *Psychiatric Services, 46*, 1267–1271.

Lamb, H. R., & Weinberger, L. E. (1998). Persons with severe mental illness in jails and prisons: A review. *Psychiatric Services, 49*, 483–492.

Lamb, H. R., Weinberger, L. E., & DeCuir, W. J. (2002). The police and mental health. *Psychiatric Services, 53*, 1266–1271.

Lamb, H. R., Weinberger, L. E., & Gross, B. (1999). Community treatment of severely mentally ill offenders under the jurisdiction of the criminal justice system: A review. *Psychiatric Services, 50*, 907–913.

Lamb, H. R., Weinberger, L., & Reston-Parham, C. (1996). Court intervention to address the mental health needs of mentally ill offenders. *Psychiatric Services, 47*, 275–281.

Lamberg, L. (2004, August 4). Efforts grow to keep mentally ill out of jails. *Journal of the American Medical Association, 292*, 555–556.

Lambert, T. J., Velakoulis, D., & Pantelis, C. (2003). Medical comorbidity in schizophrenia. *Medical Journal of Australia, 178*(Suppl.), S67–S70.

Lamberti, J. S., Weisman, R. L., & Faden, D. (2004). Forensic assertive community treatment: Preventing incarceration of adults with severe mental illness. *Psychiatric Services, 55*, 1285–1293.

Lamberti, J. S., Weisman, R. L., Schwartzkopf, S. B., Price, N., Ashton, R., & Trompeter, J. (2001). The mentally ill in jails and prisons: Toward an integrated model of prevention. *Psychiatric Quarterly, 72*, 63–77.

Larsen, S. F., & Fromholt, P. (1976). Mnemonic organization and free recall in schizophrenia. *Journal of Abnormal Psychology, 85*, 61–65.

Latimer, E. (1999). Economic impacts of assertive community treatment: A review of the literature. *Canadian Journal of Psychiatry, 44*, 443–454.

Latimer, E., Lecomte, T., Becker, D., Drake, R., Duclos, I., Piat, M., et al. (2006). Generalizability of the Individual Placement and Support model of supported employment: Results of a Canadian randomized controlled trial. *British Journal of Psychiatry, 189*, 65–73.

Latimer, E. A. (2001). Economic impacts of supported employment for persons with severe mental illness. *Canadian Journal of Psychiatry, 46*, 496–505.

Latimer, E. A., Bush, P. W., Becker, D. R., Drake, R. E., & Bond, G. R. (2004). The cost of high-fidelity supported employment programs for people with severe mental illness. *Psychiatric Services, 55*, 401–406.

Laudet, A. B., Magura, S., Vogel, H. S., & Knight, E. L. (2003). Participation in 12-step-based fellowships among dually-diagnosed persons. *Alcoholism Treatment Quarterly, 21*, 19–39.

Leaf, P. J., Bruce, M. L., & Tischler, G. L. (1986). The differential effect of attitudes on the use of mental health services. *Social Psychiatry, 21*, 187–192.

Leaf, P. J., Bruce, M. L., Tischler, G. L., & Holzer, C. E. (1987). The relationship between demographic factors and attitudes toward mental health services. *Journal of Community Psychology, 15*, 275–284.

Leazenby, L. (1997). Confidentiality as a barrier to treatment. *Psychiatric Services, 48*, 1467–1468.

Lee, M. L. (1998). Clozapine and substance abuse in patients with schizophrenia. *Canadian Journal of Psychiatry, 45*, 855–856.

Lefley, H. (1987). Aging parents as caregivers of mentally ill adult children: An emerging social problem. *Hospital and Community Psychology, 38*, 1063–1070.

Lefley, H. (1996). *Family caregiving in mental illness*. Thousand Oaks, CA: Sage.

Lefley, H. (2003). Advocacy, self-help, and consumer operated services. In A. Tasman, J. Kay, & J. Lieberman (Eds.), *Psychiatry* (2nd ed., pp. 2274–2288). West Sussex, UK: Wiley.

Lehman, A. F. (1988). A Quality of Life Interview for the chronically mentally ill. *Evaluation and Program Planning, 11*(1), 51–62.

Lehman, A. F. (1995). Vocational rehabilitation in schizophrenia. *Schizophrenia Bulletin, 21*, 645–656.

Lehman, A. F., & Cordray, D. S. (1993). Prevalence of alcohol, drug, and mental disorders among the homeless: One more time. *Contemporary Drug Problems, 20*, 355–383.

Lehman, A. F., Goldberg, R. W., Dixon, L. B., McNary, S., Postrado, L., Hackman, A., et al. (2002). Improving employment outcomes for

persons with severe mental illness. *Archives of General Psychiatry, 59*, 165–172.

Lehman, A. F., Kernan, E., & Postrado, L. (1995). *Toolkit for evaluating quality of life for persons with severe mental illness*. Baltimore: The Evaluation Center at HSRI.

Lehman, A. F., Kreyenbuhl, J., Buchanan, R., Dickerson, F. B., Dixon, L., Goldberg, R. W., et al. (2004). The Schizophrenia Patient Outcomes Research Team (PORT): Updated treatment recommendations 2003. *Schizophrenia Bulletin, 30*, 193–217.

Lehman, A. F., Myers, C. P., Thompson, J. W., & Corty, E. (1993). Implications of mental and substance use disorders: A comparison of single and dual diagnosis patients. *Journal of Nervous and Mental Disease, 181*, 365–370.

Lehman, A. F., Steinwachs, D. M., & PORT Co-Investigators. (1998a). At issue: Translating research into practice: The Schizophrenia Patient Outcomes Research Team (PORT) treatment recommendations. *Schizophrenia Bulletin, 24*, 1–10.

Lehman, A. F., Steinwachs, D. M., & PORT Co-Investigators. (1998b). Patterns of usual care for schizophrenia: Initial results from the Schizophrenia Patient Outcomes Research Team (PORT) client survey. *Schizophrenia Bulletin, 24*, 11–20.

Lehman, S., Joy, V., Kreisman, D., & Simmens, S. (1976). Responses to viewing symptomatic behaviors and labeling of prior mental illness. *Journal of Counseling Psychology, 4*, 327–334.

Lennox, D. B., Miltenberger, R. G., Spengler, P., & Erfanian, N. (1988). Decelerative treatment practices with persons who have mental retardation: A review of five years of the literature. *American Journal on Mental Retardation, 92*, 492–501.

Leong, F. T., & Lau, A. S. (2001). Barriers to providing effective mental health services to Asian Americans. *Mental Health Services Research, 3*, 201–214.

Lerman, D. C., & Vorndran, C. M. (2002). On the status of knowledge for using punishment: Implications for treating behavior disorders. *Journal of Applied Behavior Analysis, 35*, 431–464.

Levenstein, J. H., McCracken, E. C., McWhinney, I. R., Stewart, M. A., & Brown, J. B. (1986). The patient-centered clinical method: 1. A model for the doctor–patient interaction in family medicine. *Family Practice, 3*, 24–30.

Levstek, D. A., & Bond, G. R. (1993). Housing cost, quality, and satisfaction among formerly homeless persons with serious mental illness in two cities. *Innovations and Research, 2*(3), 1–8.

Lewin Group. (2001). *Draft report: Implementing*

assertive community treatment programs: A policy guide for state officials (Prepared for SAMHSA and CMS). Falls Church, VA: Author.

Lewine, R. R. J. (2005). Social class of origin, lost potential, and hopelessness in schizophrenia. *Schizophrenia Research, 76*, 329–335.

Lezak, M. D. (2004). *Neuropsychological Assessment* (4th ed.). New York: Oxford University Press.

Liberman, R. P. (1988). Behavioral family management. In R. P. Liberman (Ed.), *Psychiatric rehabilitation of chronic mental patients* (pp. 199–244). Washington, DC: American Psychiatric Association.

Liberman, R. P. (2002). Future directions for research studies and clinical work on recovery from schizophrenia: Questions with some answers. *International Review of Psychiatry, 14*(4), 337–342.

Liberman, R. P., Corrigan, P. W., & Schade, M. L. (1989a). Drug and psychosocial treatment interactions in schizophrenia. *International Review of Psychiatry, 1*, 283–295.

Liberman, R. P., DeRisi, W. J., & Mueser, K. T. (1989b). *Social skills training for psychiatric patients.* Needham Heights, MA: Allyn & Bacon.

Liberman, R. P., Kopelowicz, A., Ventura, J., & Gutkind, D. (2002). Operational criteria and factors related to recovery from schizophrenia. *International Review of Psychiatry, 14*(4), 256–272.

Liberman, R. P., Mueser, K. T., Wallace, C. J., Jacobs, H. E., Eckman, T., & Massel, H. K. (1986). Training skills in the psychiatrically disabled: Learning coping and competence. *Schizophrenia Bulletin, 12*, 631–647.

Liberman, R. P., Wallace, C. J., Blackwell, G., Eckman, T. A., Vaccaro, J. V., & Kuehnel, T. G. (1993). Innovations in skills training for the seriously mentally ill: The UCLA Social and Independent Living Skills modules. *Innovations and Research, 2*, 43–59.

Liberman, R. P., Wallace, C. J., Blackwell, G., Kopelowicz, A., Vaccaro, J. V., & Mintz, J. (1998). Skills training versus psychosocial occupational therapy for persons with persistent schizophrenia. *American Journal of Psychiatry, 155*, 1087–1091.

Liberman, R. P., Wallace, C. J., Teigen, J., & Davis, J. (1974). *Interventions with psychotic behaviors.* New York: Wiley.

Liberman, R. P., & Wong, S. E. (1984). *Behavioral analysis and therapy procedures related to seclusion and restraint.* Washington, DC: American Psychiatric Association.

Liberman, R. R., Blair, K., Glynn, S. M., Marden, S., Wirshing, W., & Wirshing, D. A. (2001).

Generalization of skills training to the natural environment. In H. D. Brenner, B. Wolfgang, & R. Genner (Eds.), *The treatment of schizophrenia: Status and emerging trends* (pp. 104–128). Ashland, OH: Hogrefe & Huber.

Lieberman, A., Gowdy, E., & Knutson, L. (1991). The mental health outreach project: A case study in self-help. *Psychosocial Rehabilitation Journal, 14*, 100–113.

Lieberman, J. A., Stroup, T., & McEvoy, J. P. (2005). Effectiveness of antipsychotic drugs in patients with chronic schizophrenia. *New England Journal of Medicine, 353*, 1209–1223.

Lieberman, M. (1990). A group therapist perspective on self-help groups. *International Journal of Group Psychotherapy, 40*, 251–279.

Lieberman, M. A., & Snowden, L. R. (1993). Problems in assessing prevalence and membership characteristics of self-help group participants. *Journal of Applied Behavioral Science, 29*, 166–180.

Lieberman, M. A., & Snowden, L. (1994). Problems in assessing prevalence and membership characteristics of self-help group participation. In T. J. Powell (Ed.), *Understanding the self-help organization: Frameworks and findings* (pp. 32–49). Thousand Oaks, CA: Sage.

Lindamer, L. A., Bailey, A., Hawthorne, W., Folsom, D. P., Gilmer, T. P., Garcia, P., et al. (2003). Gender differences in characteristics and service use of public mental health patients with schizophrenia. *Psychiatric Services, 54*, 1407–1409.

Lindberg, N., Tani, P., Appelberg, B., Naukkarinen, H., Rimón, R., Porkka-Heiskanen, T., et al. (2003). Human impulsive aggression: A sleep research perspective. *Journal of Psychiatric Research, 37*, 313–324.

Linehan, M. M. (1993a). *Skills training manual for treating borderline personality disorder.* New York: Guilford Press.

Linehan, M. M. (1993b). *Cognitive-behavioral treatment of borderline personality disorder.* New York: Guilford Press.

Linehan, M. M., Armstrong, H. E., Suarez, A., Allmon, D., & Heard, H. L. (1991). Cognitive behavioral treatment of chronically parasuicidal borderline patients. *Archives of General Psychiatry, 48*, 1060–1064.

Linehan, M. M., Dimeff, L. A., Reynolds, S. K., Comtois, K. A., Welch, S. S., Heagerty, P., et al. (2002). Dialectical behavior therapy versus comprehensive validation therapy plus 12-step for the treatment of opioid dependent women meeting criteria for borderline personality disorder. *Drug and Alcohol Dependence, 67*, 13–26.

Linehan, M. M., Schmidt, H., III, Dimeff, L. A.,

Craft, J. C., Kanter, J., & Comtois, K. A. (1999). Dialectical behavior therapy for patients with borderline personality disorder and drug-dependence. *American Journal on Addictions, 8,* 279–292.

Link, B. (1982). Mental patient status, work, and income: An examination of the effects of a psychiatric label. *American Sociological Review, 47,* 202–215.

Link, B., Andrews, H., & Cullen, F. (1992). The violent and illegal behavior of mental patients reconsidered. *American Sociological Review, 57,* 275–292.

Link, B., & Cullen, F. (1983). Reconsidering the social rejection of ex-mental patients: Levels of attitudinal response. *American Journal of Community Psychology, 11,* 261–273.

Link, B. G. (1987). Understanding labeling effects in the area of mental disorders: An assessment of the effects of expectations of rejection. *American Sociological Review, 52,* 96–112.

Link, B. G., & Cullen, F. T. (1986) Contact with the mentally ill and perceptions of how dangerous they are. *Journal of Health and Social Behavior, 27,* 289–302.

Link, B. G., Cullen, F. T., Frank, J., & Wozniak, J. F. (1987). The social rejection of former mental patients: Understanding why labels matter. *American Journal of Sociology, 92,* 1461–1500.

Link, B. G., Cullen, F. T., Struening, E. L., Shrout, P. E., & Dohrenwend, B. P. (1989). A modified labeling theory approach to mental disorders: An empirical assessment. *American Sociological Review, 54,* 400–423.

Link B. G., Mirotznik J., & Cullen F. T. (1991). The effectiveness of stigma coping orientations: Can negative consequences of mental illness labeling be avoided? *Journal of Health and Social Behavior, 32*(3), 302–320.

Link, B. G., & Phelan, J. C. (2001). Conceptualizing stigma. *Annual Review of Sociology, 27,* 363–385.

Link, B. G., Phelan, J. C., Bresnahan, M., Stueve, A., & Pescosolido, B. A. (1999). Public conceptions of mental illness: Labels, causes, dangerousness, and social distance. *American Journal of Public Health, 89*(9), 1328–1333.

Link, B. G., & Stueve, A. (1994). Psychotic symptoms and the violent/illegal behavior of mental patients compared to community controls. In J. Monahan & H. J. Steadman (Eds.), *Violence and mental disorder: Developments in risk assessment* (pp. 137–159). The John D. and Catherine T. MacArthur Foundation Series on Mental Health and Development. Chicago: University of Chicago Press.

Linn, M. W. (1981). Can foster care survive? *New Directions for Mental Health Services, 11,* 35–47.

Linszen, D. H., Dingemans, P. M., & Lenior, M. E. (1994). Cannabis abuse and the course of recent-onset schizophrenic disorders. *Archives of General Psychiatry, 51*(4), 273–279.

Lipschitz, D. S., Kaplan, M. L., Sorkenn, J. B., Faedda, G. L., Chorney, P., & Asnis, G. M. (1996). Prevalence and characteristics of physical and sexual abuse among psychiatric outpatients. *Psychiatric Services, 47,* 189–191.

Lipton, F. R., Siegel, C., Hannigan, A., Samuels, J., & Baker, S. (2000). Tenure in supportive housing for homeless persons with severe mental illness. *Psychiatric Services, 51,* 479–486.

Liraud, F., & Verdoux, H. (2001). Association between temperamental characteristics and medication adherence in subjects presenting with psychotic or mood disorders. *Psychiatry Research, 102,* 91–95.

Litzelman, D. K., Dittus, R. S., & Miller, M. E. (1993). Requiring physicians to respond to computerized reminders improves their compliance with preventive care protocols. *Journal of General Internal Medicine, 3,* 311–317.

Llewelyn, S., & Haslett, A. (1986). Factors perceived as helpful by members of self-help groups: An exploratory study. *British Journal of Guidance and Counseling, 14,* 252–262.

Loder, A., & Glover, R. (1992). New frontiers: Pioneer diaglogue between consumers/survivors and commissioners. *Mental health statistics improvement program updates.* Fort Lauderdale, FL: Peer Center.

Loebel, A. D., Lieberman, J. A., Alvir, J. M., Mayerhoff, D. I., et al. (1992). Duration of psychosis and outcome in first-episode schizophrenia. *American Journal of Psychiatry, 149*(9), 1183–1188.

Lögdberg, B., Nilsson, L.-L., Levander, M. T., & Levander, S. (2004). Schizophrenia, neighborhood, and crime. *Acta Psychiatrica Scandinavica, 110,* 92–97.

Longman, P. (2005, January/February). The best care anywhere. *Washington Monthly,* 1–15.

Looper, K., Fielding, A., Latimer, E., & Amir, E. (1998). Improving access to family support organizations: A member survey of the AMI-Quebec alliance for the mentally ill. *Psychiatric Services, 49,* 1491–1492.

Loranger, A. W. (1999). *International Personality Disorder Examination (IPDE) manual.* Odessa, FL: Psychological Assesssment Resources.

Lovell, D., Allen, D., Johnson, C., & Jemelka, R. (2001). Evaluating the effectiveness of residential treatment for persons with mental illness. *Criminal Justice and Behavior, 28,* 83–104.

Lovell, D., Gagliardi, G., & Peterson, P. (2002). Recidivism and use of services among persons with mental illness after release from prison. *Psychiatric Services, 53,* 1290–1296.

Lovell, D., & Jemelka, R. (1998). Coping with mental illness in prisons. *Community Health, 21,* 54–66.

Low, A. A. (1950). *Mental health through will-training: A system of self-help psychotherapy as practiced by Recovery, Incorporated.* Winnetka, IL: Willett.

Low, A. A. (1967). *Mental health through will training* (15th ed.). Boston: Christopher.

Lucca, A. M., & Allen, G. J. (2001). A statewide assessment of psychosocial rehabilitation programs: General characteristics and services. *Psychosocial Rehabilitation Journal, 24,* 205–213.

Luke, D., Roberts, L., & Rappaport, J. (1993). Individual group context and individual group fit predictors of self-help group attendance. *Journal of Applied Behavioral Science, 29,* 216–238.

Lukens, E., Thorning, H., & Lohrer, S. (2004). Sibling perspectives on severe mental illness: Reflections on self and family. *American Journal of Orthopsychiatry, 74,* 489–501.

Lukoff, D., Nuechterlein, K. H., & Ventura, J. (1986). Manual for the Expanded Brief Psychiatric Rating Scale (BPRS). *Schizophrenia Bulletin, 12,* 594–602.

Lurigio, A. (2000). Persons with serious mental illness in the criminal justice system: Background, prevalence, and principles of care. *Criminal Justice Policy Review, 11,* 312–328.

Lurigio, A. (2001). Effective services for persons with mental illness. *Crime and Delinquency, 47,* 446–461.

Lurigio, A., Fallon, J., & Dincin, J. (2000). Helping the mentally ill in jails adjust to community life: A description of postrelease ACT Program and its clients. *International Journal of Offender Therapy and Comparative Criminology, 44,* 450–466.

Lynde, D. W. (2005). Supported employment. In R. E. Drake, M. R. Merrens, & D. W. Lynde (Eds.), *Evidence-based mental health practice: A textbook* (pp. xix–xxvii). New York: Norton.

Lyon, H. M., Kaney, S., & Bentall, R. P. (1994). The defensive function of persecutory delusions: Evidence from attribution tasks. *British Journal of Psychiatry, 164,* 637–646.

Lyons, J. S., Cook, J. A., Ruth, A. R., Karver, M., & Slagg, N. B. (1996). Service delivery using consumer staff in a mobile crisis assessment team. *Community Mental Health Journal, 32,* 33–40.

Lysaker, P. H., Bell, M., & Beam-Goulet, J. (1995).

Wisconsin Card Sorting Test and work performance in schizophrenia. *Psychiatry Research, 56,* 45–51.

Lysaker, P. H., Bell, M. D., Bioty, S. M., & Zito, W. S. (1995). The frequency of associations between positive and negative symptoms and dysphoria in schizophrenia. *Comprehensive Psychiatry, 36,* 113–117.

Lysaker, P. H., Bell, M. D., Bryson, G. J., & Zito, W. (1993). *Raters' guide for the Work Behavior Inventory.* West Haven, CT: Rehabilitation, Research, and Development Service, Department of Veterans Affairs.

Maccoby, E., & Jacklin, C. N. (1974). Myth, reality and shades of gray: What we know and don't know about sex differences. *Psychology Today, 8,* 109–112.

MacDonald-Wilson, K. L., Rogers, E. S., Ellison, M. L., & Lyass, A. (2003). A study of the Social Security work incentives and their relation to perceived barriers to work among persons with psychiatric disability. *Rehabilitation Psychology, 48,* 301–309.

MacDonald-Wilson, K. L., Rogers, E. S., Massaro, J. M., Lyass, A., & Crean, T. (2002). An investigation of reasonable workplace accommodations for people with psychiatric disabilities: Quantitative findings from a multi-site study. *Community Mental Health Journal, 38,* 35–50.

MacGregor, P. (1994). Grief: The unrecognized parental response to mental illness in a child. *Social Work, 39,* 160–166.

Machon, R. A., Huttunen, M. O., Mednick, S. A., Sinivuo, J., Tanskanen, A., Watson, J. B., et al. (2002). Adult schizotypal personality characteristics and prenatal influenza in a Finnish birth cohort. *Schizophrenia Research, 54*(1–2), 7–16.

Macias, C., Jackson, R., Schroeder, C., & Wang, Q. (1999). What is a clubhouse? Report on the ICCD 1996 survey of USA clubhouses. *Community Mental Health Journal, 35,* 181–190.

Mackinnon, A., Copolov, D. L., & Trauer, T. (2004). Factors associated with compliance and resistance to command hallucinations. *Journal of Nervous and Mental Disease, 192,* 357–362.

Macrae, C. N., Bodenhausen, G. V., Milne, A. B., & Jetten, J. (1994). Out of mind but back in sight: Stereotypes on the rebound. *Journal of Personality and Social Psychology, 67*(5), 808.

Madara, E. (1997). Mutual-aid self-help online revolution. *Social Policy, 27,* 20–26.

Madara, E. J. (1988, May 3–4). Seven principles in self help: Understanding how self-help groups help. *New Program Initiatives in Mental Health.*

Madianos, M. G., Madianou, D., Vlachonikolis, J., & Stefanis, C. N. (1987). Attitudes towards mental illness in the Athens area: Implications for community mental health intervention. *Acta Psychiatrica Scandinavica, 75,* 158–165.

Magliano, L., Fadden, G., Fiorillo, A., Malangone, C., Sorrentino, D., Robinson, A., et al. (1999). Family burden and coping strategies in schizophrenia: Are key relatives really different to other relatives? *Acta Psychiatrica Scandinavica, 99,* 10–15.

Magliano, L., Fiorillo, A., Malangone, C., Marasco, C., Guarneri, M., Maj, M., et al. (2003). The effect of social network on burden and pessimism in relatives of patients with schizophrenia. *Journal of Orthopsychiatry, 73,* 302–309.

Maguire, K., & Pastore, A. (Eds.). (1997). Sourcebook of criminal justice statistics 1996. Washington, DC: Bureau of Justice Statistics.

Magura, S., Laudet, A., Mahmood, D., Rosenblum, A., Vogel, H., & Knight, E. (2003). Role of self-help processes in achieving abstinence among dually diagnosed persons. *Addictive Behaviors, 28,* 399–413.

Maher, B. A., & Spitzer, M. (1993). Delusions. In P. Sutker & H. Adams (Eds.), *Comprehensive handbook of psychology.* New York: Plenum Press.

Maier, G., & Fulton, L. (1998). Inpatient treatment of offenders with mental disorders. In R. Wettstein (Ed.), *Treatment of offenders with mental disorders* (pp. 126–167). New York: Guilford Press.

Malgady, R., Lloyd, H., & Tryon, W. (1992). Issues of validity in the Diagnostic Interview Schedule. *Journal of Psychiatric Research, 26,* 59–67.

Malm, U., May, P. R., & Dencker, S. J. (1981). Evaluation of the quality of life of the schizophrenic outpatient: A checklist. *Schizophrenia Bulletin, 7*(3), 477–487.

Mancuso, L. L. (1995). Achieving reasonable accommodation for workers with psychiatric disabilities: Understanding the employer's perspective. *American Rehabilitation, 21,* 2–8.

Manderscheid, R., & Sonnenschein, M. (1997). *Mental health, United States, 1996.* Washington, DC: Substance Abuse and Mental Health Services Administration, U.S. Department of Health and Human Services.

Mandler, G. (1972). Organization and recognition. In E. Tulving & W. Donaldson (Eds.), *Organization of memory* (pp. 139–166). New York: Academic Press.

Mank, D. (1994). The underachievement of supported employment: A call for reinvestment. *Journal of Disability Policy Studies, 5*(2), 1–24.

Mann, C. (2002). *The new Medicaid and CHIP waiver initiatives.* Kaiser Commission on Medicaid and the Uninsured. Retrieved June 30, 2007, from *www.kff.org/medicaid/4028–index.cfm.*

Manning, S., & Suire, B. (1996). Consumers as employers in mental health: Bridges and roadblocks. *Psychiatric Services, 47,* 939–940, 943.

Mannion, E. (1996). Resilience and burden in spouses of people with mental illness. *Psychiatric Rehabilitation Journal, 20,* 13–23.

Mannion, E. (2000). *Training manual for the implementation of family education in the adult mental health system of Berks County, Pennsylvania.* Philadelphia: University of Pennsylvania, Center for Mental Health Policy and Services Research.

Mannion, E., Draine, J., Solomon, P., & Meisel, M. (1997). Applying research on family education about mental illness to development of a relatives' group consultation model. *Community Mental Health Journal, 33,* 555–574.

Mannion, E., Meisel, M., Solomon, P., & Draine, J. (1996). A comparative analysis of families with mentally ill adult relatives: Support group members versus non-members. *Psychiatric Rehabilitation Journal, 20,* 43–50.

Mannion, E., Mueser, K., & Solomon, P. (1994). Designing psychoeducational services for spouses of persons with serious mental illness. *Community Mental Health Journal, 30,* 117–190.

Manos, E. (1992). The patient's perspective: Prosumers. *Journal of Psychosocial Nursing, 30,* 3–4.

Manos, E. (1993). Prosumers. *Psychosocial Rehabilitation Journal, 16*(4), 117–120.

Maramba, G. G., & Hall, G. C. N. (2002). Meta-analysis of ethnic match as a predictor of dropout, utilization, and level of functioning. *Cultural Diversity and Ethnic Minority Psychology, 8,* 290–297.

Marder, S. R., Essock, S. M., & Miller, A. L. (2004). Physical health monitoring of patients with schizophrenia. *American Journal of Psychiatry, 161,* 1334–1349.

Marder, S. R., Mebane, A., & Chien, C. P. (1983). A comparison of patients who refuse and consent to neuroleptic treatment. *American Journal of Psychiatry, 140,* 470–472.

Marder, S. R., Wirshing, W. C., Mintz, J., McKenzie, J., Johnston, K., Eckman, T. A., et al. (1996). Two-year outcome for social skills training and group psychotherapy for outpatients with schizophrenia. *American Journal of Psychiatry, 153,* 1585–1592.

Mares, A. S., & Rosenheck, R. A. (2004). One-year housing arrangements among homeless adults with serious mental illness in the ACCESS Program. *Psychiatric Services, 55*, 566–574.

Mari, J., & Streiner, D. (1994). An overview of family intervention and relapse on schizophrenia: Meta-analysis of research findings. *Psychological Medicine, 24*, 565–578.

Mark, T., & Mueller, C. (1996). Access to care in HMOS and traditional insurance plans. *Health Affairs, 15*, 81–87.

Mark, T. L., Coffey, R. M., McKusick, D. R., Harwood, H., King, E., Bouchery, E., et al. (2005). *National estimates of expenditures for mental health services and substance abuse treatment, 1991–2001* (SAMHSA Publication No. SMA 05-3999). Rockville, MD: Substance Abuse and Mental Health Services Administration.

Marks, I., Lovell, K., Noshirvani, H., Livanou, M., & Thrasher, S. (1998). Treatment of posttraumatic stress disorder by exposure and/or cognitive restructuring. *Archives of General Psychiatry, 55*, 317–325.

Marlatt, G. A., & Gordon, J. R. (Eds.). (1985). *Relapse prevention: Maintenance strategies in the treatment of addictive behaviors.* New York: Guilford Press.

Marley, J. A., & Buila, S. (1999). When violence happens to people with mental illness: Disclosing victimization. *American Journal of Orthopsychiatry, 69*, 398–402.

Marrelli, A. F., Tondora, J., & Hoge, M. A. (2005). Strategies for developing competency models. *Administration and Policy in Mental Health, 32*, 533–561.

Marsh, D. (1992). *Families and mental illness: New directions in professional practice.* New York: Praeger.

Marsh, D. (1998). *Serious mental illness and the family: The practitioner's guide.* New York: Wiley.

Marsh, D. Lefley, H., Evans-Rhodes, D., Ansell, V., Doerzbacher, B., LaBarbera, L., et al. (1996). The family experience of mental illness: Evidence for resilence. *Psychiatric Rehabilitation Journal, 20*, 3–12.

Marshak, L. E., Bostick, D., & Turton, L. J. (1990). Closure outcomes for clients with psychiatric disabilities served by the vocational rehabilitation system. *Rehabilitation Counseling Bulletin, 33*, 247–250.

Marshall, M., & Creed, F. (2000). Assertive community treatment: Is it the future of community care in the UK? *International Review of Psychiatry, 12*, 191–196.

Marshall, M., Crowther, R., Almaraz-Serrano, A., Creed, F., Sledge, W., Kluiter, H., et al. (2001). Systematic reviews of the effectiveness of day care for people with severe mental disorders: (1) Acute day hospital versus admission; (2) vocational rehabilitation; (3) day hospital versus outpatient care. *Health Technology Assessment, 5*(21), 1–75.

Marshall, M., Gray, A., Lockwood, A., & Green, R. (2004). *Case management for people with severe mental disorders.* The Cochrane Library, 2000, Issue 2.

Marshall, M., Hogg, L. I., Gath, G. H., & Lockwood, A. (1995). The Cardinal Needs Schedule: A modified version of the MRC Needs for Care Assessment Schedule. *Psychological Medicine, 25*, 603–617.

Marshall, M., & Lockwood, A. (1999). Assertive community treatment for people with severe mental disorders. *Cochrane Review*, 1–51.

Marshall, T., & Solomon, P. (2000). Releasing information to families of persons with severe mental illness: A survey of NIMH members. *Psychiatric Services, 51*, 1006–1011.

Marshall, T., & Solomon, P. (2003). Professionals' responsibilities in releasing information to families of adults with severe mental illness. *Psychiatric Services, 54*, 1622–1628.

Marshall, T., & Solomon, P. (2004a). Confidentiality intervention: Effects on provider–consumer–family collaboration. *Research on Social Work Practice, 14*, 3–13.

Marshall, T., & Solomon, P. (2004b). Provider contact with families of adults with severe mental illness: Taking a closer look. *Family Process, 43*, 209–216.

Marshall, T., Solomon, P., Steber, S., & Mannion, E. (2003). Provider and family beliefs regarding the causes of severe mental illness. *Psychiatric Quarterly, 74*, 223–236.

Martell, D. A., Rosner, R., & Harmon, R. B. (1995). Base rate estimates of criminal behavior by homeless mentally ill persons in New York City. *Psychiatric Services, 46*, 596–600.

Martin, J. K., Pescosolido, B. A., & Tuch, S. A. (2000). Of fear and loathing: The role of "disturbing behavior," labels, and causal attributions in shaping public attitudes toward people with mental illness. *Journal of Health and Social Behavior, 41*, 208–223.

Marx, A., Test, M., & Stein, L. (1973). Extra-hospital management of severe mental illness. *Archives of General Psychiatry, 29*, 505–511.

Maslow, A. H. (1970). *Motivation and personality* (2nd ed.). New York: Harper & Row.

Mason, K., Olmos-Gallo, A., Bacon, D., McQuilken, M., Henley, A., & Fisher, S. (2004). Exploring the consumer's and provider's perspective on service quality in community mental health care. *Community Mental Health Journal, 40*, 33–46.

Mastrofski, S. D., Snipes, J. B., Parks, R. B., & Maxwell, C. D. (2000). The helping hand of the law: Police control of citizens on request. *Criminology, 38*, 307–342.

Masur, F. T. (1981). Adherence to health care regimens. In C. K. Prokop & L. A. Bradley (Eds.), *Medical psychology: Contributions to behavioral medicine.* New York: Academic Press.

Maurin, J., & Boyd, C. (1990). Burden of mental illness on the family: A critical review. *Archives of Psychiatric Nursing, IV*, 99–107.

Maxwell, S., & Shinderman, M. S. (1997). Use of naltrexone in the treatment of dually diagnosed patients. *Journal of Addictive Diseases, 16*, 125.

Maxwell, S., & Shinderman, M. S. (2000). Use of naltrexone in the treatment of alcohol use disorders in patients with concomitant major mental illness. *Journal of Addictive Diseases, 19*, 61–69.

May, P. R. (1968). *Treatment of schizophrenia: A comparative study of five treatments.* New York: Science House.

Mayfield, D., McCleod, G., & Hall, P. (1974). The CAGE questionnaire: Validation of a new alcoholism screening questionnaire. *American Journal of Psychiatry, 131*, 1121–1123.

McAlpine, D. D., & Warner, L. (2000). *Barriers to employment among persons with mental illness: A review of the literature.* New Brunswick, NJ: Center for Research on the Organization and Financing of Care for the Severely Mentally Ill, Institute for Health, Health Care Policy and Aging Research, Rutgers University.

McCabe, S. S., Edgar, E. R., Mancuso, L. L., King, D., Ross, E. C., & Emery, B. D. (1993). A national study of housing affordability for recipients of Supplemental Security Income. *Hospital and Community Psychiatry, 44*, 494–495.

McCarrick, A. K., Bertolucci, D. E., Goldman, H., & Tessler, R. C. (1986). Chronic medical problems in the chronic mentally ill. *Hospital and Community Psychiatry, 37*, 289–291.

McCoy, M. L., Devitt, T., Clay, R., Davis, K. E., Dincin, J., Pavick, D., et al. (2003). Gaining insight: Who benefits from residential, integrated treatment for people with dual diagnoses? *Psychiaric Rehabilitation Journal, 27*, 140–150.

McDonagh-Coyle, A., Friedman, M. J., McHugo, G. J., Ford, J. D., Sengupta, A., Mueser, K. T., et al. (2005). Randomized trial of cognitive behavioral therapy for chronic PTSD in adult female childhood sexual abuse survivors. *Journal of Consulting and Clinical Psychology, 73*, 515–524.

McDonald, C. J., Hui, S. L., & Smith, D. M. (1984). Reminders to physicians from an introspective computer medical record: A two-year

randomized trial. *Annals of Internal Medicine, 100*, 130–138.

McEvoy, J., Scheifler, P., & Frances, A. (Eds.). (1999). The expert consensus guideline series: Treatment of schizophrenia. *Journal of Clinical Psychiatry, 60*(Suppl. 11), 1–80.

McEvoy, J. P., & Freudenreich, O. (1999). Smoking and therapeutic response to clozapine in patients with schizophrenia. *Biological Psychiatry, 46*, 125–129.

McEvoy, J. P., Freudenreich, O., McGee, M., VanderZwaag, C., Levin, E., & Rose, J. (1995). Clozapine decreases smoking in patients with schizophrenia. *Psychopharmacology, 37*, 550–552.

McFall, R. M. (1982). A review and reformulation of the concept of social skills. *Behavioral Assessment, 4*, 1–33.

McFarland, B. H. (1994). Health maintenance organizations and persons with severe mental illness. *Community Mental Health Journal, 30*, 221–242.

McFarlane, A. C., Bookless, C., & Air, T. (2001). Posttraumatic stress disorder in a general psychiatric inpatient population. *Journal of Traumatic Stress, 14*, 633–645.

McFarlane, W. (2002). *Multifamily groups in the treatment of severe psychiatric disorders.* New York: Guilford Press.

McFarlane, W., Dixon, L., Lukens, E., & Lucksted, A. (2003). Family psychoeducation and schizophrenia: A review of the literature. *Journal of Marital and Family Therapy, 29*, 223–245.

McFarlane, W., Dushay, R., Statsny, P., Deakins, S., & Link, B. (1996). A comparison of two levels of family-aided assertive community treatment. *Psychiatric Services, 47*, 744–750.

McFarlane, W. R., Stastny, P., & Deakins, S. (1995, October 6–10). *Employment outcomes in family-aided assertive community treatment (FACT).* Paper presented at the Institute on Psychiatric Services, Boston.

McGill, C., & Patterson, C. (1990). Former patients as peer counselors on locked psychiatric inpatient units. *Hospital and Community Psychiatry, 4*, 1017–1019.

McGlashan, T. H. (1984). The Chestnut Lodge follow-up study: II. Long-term outcome of schizophrenia and the affective disorders. *Archives of General Psychiatry, 41*, 586–601.

McGorry, P., Kaplan, I., Dossetor, C., Copolov, D. L., & Singh, B. S. (1988). *The Royal Park Multidiagnostic Instrument for Psychosis (RPMIP): A comprehensive assessment procedure for the acute psychotic episode.* Melbourne, Australia: Department of Psychological Medicine, Monash University.

McGorry, P. D., Chanen, A., McCarthy, E., Van Riel, R., McKenzie, D., & Singh, B. S. (1991). Posttraumatic stress disorder following recent-onset psychosis: An unrecognized postpsychotic syndrome. *Journal of Nervous and Mental Disease, 179,* 253–258.

McGovern, M. P., Wrisley, B. R., & Drake, R. E. (2005). Substance use disorder relapse and its prevention: Implications for persons with comorbid psychiatric disorders. *Psychiatric Services, 56,* 1270–1273.

McGrew, J., Bond, G., Dietzen, & Saylers, M. (1994). Measuring the fidelity of implementation of a mental health program model. *Journal of Consulting and Clinical Psychology, 62,* 670–678.

McGrew, J., Wilson, R., & Bond, G. (1996). Client perspectives on helpful ingredients of assertive community treatment. *Psychiatric Rehabilitation Journal, 19,* 13–21.

McGrew, J. H., Wright, E. R., Pescosolido, B. A., & McDonel, E. C. (1999). The closing of Central State Hospital: Long-term outcomes for persons with severe mental illness. *Journal of Behavioral Health Services and Research, 26,* 246–261.

McGurk, S. R., & Mueser, K. T. (2004). Cognitive functioning, symptoms, and work in supported employment: A review and heuristic model. *Schizophrenia Research, 70,* 147–173.

McGurk, S. R., Mueser, K. T., Feldman, K., Wolfe, R., & Pascaris, A. (2007). Cognitive training for supported employment: 2–3 year outcomes of a randomized controlled trial. *American Journal of Psychiatry, 164,* 437–441.

McGurk, S. R., Mueser, K. T., Harvey, P. D., LaPuglia, R., & Marder, J. (2003). Cognitive and symptom predictors of work outcomes for clients with schizophrenia in supported employment. *Psychiatric Services, 54,* 1129–1135.

McGurk, S. R., Mueser, K. T., & Pascaris, A. (2005). Cognitive training and supported employment for persons with severe mental illness: One year results from a randomized controlled trial. *Schizophrenia Bulletin, 31,* 898–909.

McHugo, G., Drake, R., Teague, G., & Xie, H. (1999). Fidelity to assertive community treatment and client outcomes in the New Hampshire Dual Disorders Study. *Psychiatric Services, 50,* 818–824.

McHugo, G. J., Bebout, R. R., Harris, M., Cleghorn, S., Herring, G., Xie, H., et al. (2005). A randomized controlled trial of integrated versus parallel housing services for homeless adults with severe mental illness. *Schizophrenia Bulletin, 30,* 969–982.

McHugo, G. J., Drake, R. E., & Becker, D. R. (1998). The durability of supported employment effects. *Psychiatric Rehabilitation Journal, 22*(1), 55–61.

McHugo, G. J., Drake, R. E., Burton, H. L., & Ackerson, T. H. (1995). A scale for assessing the stage of substance abuse treatment in persons with severe mental illness. *Journal of Nervous and Mental Disease, 183,* 762–767.

McHugo, G. J., Drake, R. E., Whitley, R., Bond, G. R., Campbell, K., Rapp, C. A., et al. (in press). Fidelity outcomes in the National Evidence-Based Practices Project. *Psychiatric Services.*

McKellar, P. (1968). *Experience and Behaviour.* Harmondsworth, UK: Penguin Books.

McKenzie, K., van Os, J., & Fahy, T. (1995). Psychosis with good prognosis in Afro-Caribbean people now living in the United Kingdom. *British Medical Journal, 311,* 1325–1328.

McKibbin, C. L., Brekke, J. S., Sires, D., Jeste, D. V., & Patterson, T. L. (2004). Direct assessment of functional abilities: Relevance to persons with schizophrenia. *Schizophrenia Research, 72,* 53–67.

McKinney Act. (1987). Stuart B. McKinney Homess Assistance Act (1987). Public Law 100-77.

McLean, A. (1995). Empowerment and the psychiatric consumer/ex-patient movement in the United States: Contradictions, crisis and change. *Social Science and Medicine, 40,* 1053–1071.

McLellan, A. T., Kushner, H., Metzger, D., Peters, R., Smith, I., Grissom, G., et al. (1992). The fifth edition of the Addiction Severity Index: Historical critique and normative data. *Journal of Substance Abuse Treatment, 9,* 199–213.

McLellan, A. T., Lewis, D. C., O'Brien, C. P., & Kleber, H. D. (2000). Drug dependence, a chronic mental illness: Implications for treatment and outcome. *Journal of the American Medical Association, 284,* 1689–1695.

McNally, R. J. (1999). EMDR and Mesmerism: A comparative historical analysis. *Journal of Anxiety Disorders, 13,* 225–236.

McNeil, D., Binder, R., & Robinson, J. (2005). Incarceration associated with homelessness, mental disorder, and co-occurring substance abuse. *Psychiatric Services, 56,* 840–846.

McNeil, D. E. (1994). Hallucinations and violence. In J. Monahan & H. J. Steadman (Eds.), *Violence and mental disorder: Developments in risk assessment* (pp. 183–202). Chicago: Chicago University Press.

McNeil, D. E. (1997). Correlates of violence in psychotic patients. *Psychiatric Annals, 27,* 683–690.

McNeil, D. E., Eisner, J. P., & Binder, R. L. (2000). The relationship between command hallucinations and violence. *Psychiatric Services, 51,* 1288–1292.

McQuilken, M., Zahniser, J. H., Novak, J., Starks, R. D., Olmos, A., & Bond, G. R. (2003). The Work Project Survey: Consumer perspectives on work. *Journal of Vocational Rehabilitation, 18,* 59–68.

Mead, S., & Copeland, M. E. (2000). What recovery means to us: Consumers' perspectives. *Community Mental Health Journal, 36,* 315–328.

Meade, S., Hilton, D., & Curtis, L. (2001). Peer support: A theoretical perspective. *Psychiatric Rehabilitation Journal, 25,* 134–141.

Mechanic, D. (2003). Policy challenges in improving mental health services: Some lessons from the past. *Psychiatric Services, 54,* 1227–1232.

Mechanic, D., & Aiken, L. H. (1989). Capitation in mental health: Potentials and cautions. In D. Mechanic & L. H. Aiken (Eds.), *Paying for services: Promises and pitfalls of capitation* (pp. 5–18). San Francisco: Jossey-Bass.

Mechanic, D., & McAlpine, D. D. (2000). Use of nursing homes in the care of persons with severe mental illness: 1985 to 1995. *Psychiatric Services, 51,* 354–358.

Mechanic, D., McAlpine, D. D., Rosenfield, S., & Davis, D. (1994). Effects of illness attribution and depression on the quality of life among persons with serious mental illness. *Social Science and Medicine, 39,* 155–164.

Medalia, A., Aluma, M., Tryon, W., & Merriam, A. E. (1998). Effectiveness of attention training in Schizophrenia. *Schizophrenia Bulletin, 24,* 147–152.

Medalia, A., Gold, J., & Merriam, A. (1988). The effects of neuroleptics on neuropsychological test results in schizophrenia. *Archives of Clinical Neurology, 3,* 249–271.

Medalia, A., & Revheim, N. (1999). Computer assisted learning in psychiatric rehabilitation. *Psychiatric Rehabilitation Skills, 3,* 77–98.

Meeks, S., & Murrell, S. A. (1997). Mental illness in late life: Socioeconomic conditions, psychiatric symptoms, and adjustment of long-term sufferers. *Psychology and Aging, 12*(2), 298–308.

Mehta, S., & Farina, A. (1997). Is being "sick" really better? Effect of the disease view of mental disorder on stigma. *Journal of Social and Clinical Psychology, 16,* 405–419.

Meichenbaum, D., & Cameron, R. (1973). Training schizophrenics to talk to themselves: A means of developing attentional controls. *Behavior Therapy, 4,* 515–534.

Meiselman, K. C. (1973). Broadening dual modality cue utilization in chronic nonparanoid schizophrenics. *Journal of Consulting and Clinical Psychology, 41,* 447–453.

Meisler, N., Blankertz, L., Santos, A. B., & McKay, C. (1997). Impact of assertive community treatment on homeless persons with co-occurring severe psychiatric and substance use disorders. *Community Mental Health Journal, 33,* 113—122.

Melick, M. E., Steadman, H., & Cocozza, J. (1979). The medicalization of criminal behavior among mental patients. *Journal of Health and Social Behavior, 20,* 228–237.

Mellman, T. A., Miller, A. L., Weissman, E. M., Crismon, M. L., Essock, S. M., & Marder, S. R. (2001). Evidence-based pharmacologic treatment for people with severe mental illness: A focus on guidelines and algorithms. *Psychiatric Services, 52,* 619–625.

Meltzer, H. Y., Alphs, L., Green, A. I., Cltamura, C., Anand, R., Bertoldi, A., et al. (2003). Clozapine treatment for suicidality in schizophrenia. *Archives of General Psychiatry, 60,* 82–91.

Meltzer, H. Y., & McGurk, S. R. (1999). The effects of clozapine, risperidone, and olanzapine on cognitive function in schizophrenia. *Schizophrenia Bulletin, 25,* 233–255.

Menditto, A. A., Baldwin, L. J., O'Neal, L. G., & Beck, N. C. (1991). Social-learning procedures for increasing attention and improving basic skills in severely regressed institutionalized patients. *Journal of Behavior Therapy and Experimental Psychiatry, 22,* 265–269.

Menditto, A. A., Beck, N. C., & Stuve, P. (2000). A social-learning approach to reducing aggressive behavior among chronically hospitalized psychiatric patients. In M. L. Crowner (Ed.), *Understanding and treating violent psychiatric patients: Progress in psychiatry* (p. 192). Washington, DC: American Psychiatric Association.

Mercer-McFadden, C., Drake, R. E., Brown, N. B., & Fox, T. S. (1997). The community support program demonstrations of services for young adults with severe mental illness and substance use disorders 1987–1991. *Psychiatric Rehabilitation Journal, 20,* 13–24.

Merinder, L. B. (2000). Patient education in schizophrenia: A review. *Acta Psychiatrica Scandinavica, 102,* 98–106.

Meyer, H., Taimenen, T., Vuori, T., Aijala, A., & Helenius, H. (1999). Posttraumatic stress disorder symptoms related to psychosis and acute involuntary hospitalization in schizophrenic and delusional patients. *Journal of Nervous and Mental Disease, 187,* 343–352.

Meyer, I. H., Muenzenmaier, K., Cancienne, J., & Struening, E. L. (1996). Reliability and validity of a measure of sexual and physical abuse histories among women with serious mental illness. *Child Abuse and Neglect, 20,* 213–219.

Michaels, D., Zoloth, S. K., Alcabes, P., Braslow, C. A., & Sayer, S., et al. (1992). Homelessness and indicators of mental illness among inmates in New York City's correctional system. *Hospital and Community Psychiatry, 43,* 150–155.

Middelboe, T., Mackeprang, T., Hansson, L., Werdelin, G., Karlsson, H., Bjarnason, O., et al. (2001). The Nordic study on schizophrenic patients living in the community: Subjective needs and perceived help. *European Psychiatry, 16,* 207–214.

Miklowitz, D. J. (2002). *The bipolar disorder survival guide: What you and your family need to know.* New York: Guilford Press.

Miller, A. L., Chiles, J. A., Chiles, J. K., Crismon, M. L., Rush, A. J., & Shon, S. P. (1999). The Texas Medication Algorithm Project (TMAP) schizophrenia algorithms. *Journal of Clinical Psychiatry, 60,* 649–657.

Miller, A. L., Crismon, M. L., Rush, A. J., Chiles, J., Kashner, T. M., Toprac, M., et al. (2004). The Texas Medication Algorithm Project: Clinical results for schizophrenia. *Schizophrenia Bulletin, 30,* 627–647.

Miller, F., Dworkin, J., Ward, M., & Barone, D. (1990). A preliminary study of unresolved grief in families of seriously mentally ill patients. *Hospital and Community Psychiatry, 41,* 1321–1325.

Miller, G. A. (1956). The magical number seven, plus or minus two: Some limits on our capacity for processing information. *Psychological Review, 63,* 81–97.

Miller, I., & Miller, L. (1997). A.N.G.E.L.S., Inc.: Consumer-run supported employment agency. *Psychiatric Rehabilitation Journal, 21,* 160–163.

Miller, W. R., & Rollnick, S. (2002). *Motivational interviewing: Preparing people for change* (2nd ed.). New York: Guilford Press.

Millet, K. (1991). *The loony bin trip.* London: Virago Press.

Millon, T. (1982). *Millon Clinical Multiaxial Inventory—II.* Minneapolis: National Computer Systems.

Millon, T., Davis, R., Millon, C., Escovar, L., & Meagher, S. (2000). *Personality disorders in modern life.* Hoboken, NJ: Wiley.

Mills, C. W. (1967). *The sociological imagination.* New York: Oxford University Press.

Mingyuan, Z., Hegin, Y., Chengde, Y., Jianlin, Y., Qingfeng, Y., et al. (1993). Effectiveness of psychoeducation of relatives of schizophrenic patients: A prospective cohort study in five cities of China. *International Journal of Mental Health, 22,* 47–59.

Minkoff, K. (1989). An integrated treatment model for dual diagnosis of psychosis and addiction. *Hospital and Community Psychiatry, 40,* 1031–1036.

Minsky, S., Gubman, G., & Duffy, M. (1995). The eye of the beholder: Housing preferences of inpatients and their treatment teams. *Psychiatric Services, 46,* 173–176.

Minth, H. (2005). The St. Louis Empowerment Center, St. Louis Missouri. In S. Clay (Ed.), *On our own, together* (pp. 108–122). Nashville, Vanderbilt University Press.

Miotto, P., Preti, A., & Frezza, M. (2001). Heroin and schizophrenia: Subjective responses to abused drugs in dually diagnosed patients. *Journal of Clinical Psychopharmacology, 21,* 111–113.

Miranda, J., Nakamura, R., & Bernal, G. (2003). Including ethnic minorities in mental health intervention research: A practical approach to a long-standing problem. *Culture, Medicine and Psychiatry, 27,* 467–486.

Mishara, A. L., & Goldberg, T. E. (2004). A meta-analysis and critical review of the effects of conventional neuroleptic treatment on cognition in schizophrenia: Opening a closed book. *Biological Psychiatry, 55,* 1013–1022.

Modestin, J., Huber, A., Satirli, E., Malti, T., & Hell, D. (2003). Long-term course of schizophrenic illness: Bleuler's study reconsidered. *American Journal of Psychiatry, 160*(12), 2202–2208.

Moeller, H., & von Zerssen, D. (1995). Self-rating procedures in the evaluation of antidepressants: Review of the literature and results of our studies. *Psychopathology, 28*(6), 291–306.

Moggi, F., Hirsbrunner, H. P., Brodbeck, J., & Bachmann, K. M. (1999). One-year outcome of an integrative inpatient treatment for dual diagnosis patients. *Addictive Behaviors, 24,* 589–592.

Mojtabai, R. (2005). Perceived reasons for loss of housing and continued homelessness among homeless persons with mental illness. *Psychiatric Services, 56,* 172–178.

Monahan, J. (1973). The psychiatricization of criminal behavior: A reply. *Hospital and Community Psychiatry, 24,* 105–107.

Monahan, J. (1992). Mental disorder and violent behavior: Perceptions and evidence. *American Psychologist, 47,* 511–521.

Monahan, J. (1997). Clinical and acturial predictions of violence. In D. Faigman, D. Kaye, M. Saks, M. Saks, & M. Sanders (Eds.), *Modern scientific evidence: The law and science of expert testimony* (p. 315). St. Paul, MN: West Group.

Monahan, J. (2000). Violence and mental disorder: Recent research. In M. L. Crowner (Ed.), *Understanding and treating violent psychiatric patients. Progress in psychiatry* (pp. 167–178). Washington, DC: American Psychiatric Association.

Monahan, J., Steadman, H. J., Applebaum, P. S., Robbins, P. C., Mulvey, E. P., Silver, E., et al. (2000). Developing a clinically useful actuarial tool for assessing violence risk. *British Journal of Psychiatry, 176,* 312–319.

Monahan, J. C., Steadman, H., Silver, E., Appelbaum, P., Robbins, P. C., Mulvey, E., Roth, L. H., et al. (2001). *Rethinking risk assessment.* New York: Oxford University Press.

Monson, C. M. (2005). PTSD and intimate relationships. *PTSD Research Quarterly, 16*(4), 1–8.

Montini, T. (2000). Compulsory closets and the social context of disclosure. *Sociological Perspectives, 43*(4), S121.

Moore, A., Sellwood, W., & Stirling, J. (2000). Compliance and psychological reactance in schizophrenia. *British Journal of Clinical Psychology, 39,* 287–296.

Mor-Barak, M. E., Miller, L. S., & Syme, L. S. (1991). Social networks, life events, and health of the poor, frail elderly: A longitudinal study of the buffering versus the direct effect. *Family and Community Health, 14*(2), 1–13.

Morris, S., Steadman, H., & Veysey, B. (1997). Mental health services in United States jails. A survey of innovative practices. *Criminal Justice and Behavior, 24,* 3–19.

Morrison, A. P., Bowe, S., Larkin, W., & Nothard, S. (2001). The psychological impact of psychiatric admission: Some preliminary findings. *Journal of Nervous and Mental Disease, 189,* 250–253.

Morrison, A. P., Renton, J. C., Dunn, H., Williams, S., & Bentall, R. P. (2004). *Cognitive therapy for psychosis: A formulation-based approach.* New York: Brunner-Routledge.

Morrison, J. K. (1980). The public's current beliefs about mental illness: Serious obstacle to effective community psychology. *American Journal of Community Psychology, 8,* 697–707.

Morrison, J. K., Becker, R. E., & Bourgeois, C. A. (1979). Decreasing adolescents' fear of mental patients by means of demythologizing. *Psychological Reports, 44,* 855–859.

Morrison, J. K., & Teta, D. C. (1979). Impact of a humanistic approach on students' attitude, attributions and ethical conflicts. *Psychological Reports, 45,* 863–866.

Morrison, J. K., & Teta, D. C. (1980). Reducing students' fear of mental illness by means of seminar-induced belief change. *Journal of Clinical Psychology, 36,* 275–276.

Morrison, P., Meehan, T., Gaskill, D., Lunney, P., & Collings, P. (2000). Enhancing case managers skills on the assessment and management of antipsychotic medication side effects. *Australian and New Zealand Journal of Psychiatry, 34,* 814–821.

Morrissey, J. P., & Goldman, H. H. (1984). Cycles of reform in the care of the chronically mentally ill. *Hospital and Community Psychiatry, 35,* 785–793.

Morse, G. A., Calsyn, R. J., Klinkenberg, W. D., Helminiak, T. W., Wolff, N., Drake, R. E., et al. (2006). Treating homeless clients with severa mental illness and substance use disorders: Costs and outcomes. *Community Mental Health Journal, 42,* 377–404.

Mortensen, P. B., & Juel, K. (1990). Mortality and causes of death in schizophrenic patients in Denmark. *Acta Psychiatrica Scandinavica, 81,* 372–377.

Moser, L. L., DeLuca, N. L., Bond, G. R., & Rollins, A. L. (2004). Implementing evidence based psychosocial practices: Lessons learned from statewide implementation of two practices. *CNS Spectrums, 9,* 926–936.

Moss, K., Ullman, M., Starrett, B. E., Burris, S., & Johnsen, M. C. (1999). Outcomes of employment discrimination charges filed under the Americans with Disabilities Act. *Psychiatric Services, 50,* 1028–1035.

Mowbray, C. (1997). Benefits and issues created by consumer role innovation in psychiatric rehabilitation. In C. Mowbray, D. Moxley, C. Jasper, & L. Howell (Eds.), *Consumers as providers in psychiatric rehabilitation* (pp. 45–63). Columbia, MD. International Association of Psychosocial Rehabilitation Services.

Mowbray, C. T. (1985). Homelessness in America: Myths and realities. *American Journal of Orthopsychiatry, 55,* 4–8.

Mowbray, C. T. (Ed.). (2000). *Supported education and psychiatric rehabilitation: Models and methods.* Columbia, MD: International Association of Psychosocial Rehabilitation Services.

Mowbray, C. T., Brown, K. S., Furlong-Norman, K., & Sullivan Soydan, A. (Eds.). (2000). *Supported education and psychiatric rehabilitation.* Columbia, MD: International Association of Psychosocial Rehabilitation Services.

Mowbray, C. T., Bybee, D., & Collins, M. E. (2000). Integrating vocational services on case management teams: Outcomes from a research demonstration project. *Mental Health Services Research, 2,* 51–66.

Mowbray, C. T., Chamberlin, P., Jennings, M., &

Reed, C. (1988). Consumer-run mental health services: Results from five demonstration projects. *Community Mental Health Journal, 24,* 151–156.

Mowbray, C. T., Collins, M. E., Bellamy, C. D., Megivern, D. A., Bybee, D., & Szilvagyis, S. (2005a). Supported education for adults with psychiatric disabilities: An innovation for social work and psychosocial rehabilitation practice. *Social Work, 50*(1), 7–21.

Mowbray, C. T., Holter, M., Stark, L., Pfeffer, C., & Bybee, D. (2005b). A fidelity rating instrument for consumer-run drop-in centers (FRI-CRDI). *Research on Social Work Practice, 15,* 278–290.

Mowbray, C. T., & Moxley, D. (1997). A framework for organizing consumer roles as providers of psychiatric rehabilitation. In C. Mowbray, D. Moxley, C. Jasper, & L. Howell (Eds.), *Consumers as providers in psychiatric rehabilitation* (pp. 35–44). Columbia, MD: International Association of Psychosocial Rehabilitation Services.

Mowbray, C. T., Moxley, D. P., & Collins, M. E. (1998). Consumers as mental health providers: First-person accounts of benefits and limitations. *Journal of Behavioral Health Services and Research, 25*(4), 397–412.

Mowbray, C. T., Moxley, D., Thrasher, S., Bybee, D., McCrohan, N., Harris, S., et al. (1996). Consumers as community support providers: Issues created by innovation. *Community Mental Health Journal, 32,* 47–67.

Mowbray, C. T., Oyserman, D., Bybee, D., MacFarlane, P., & Rueda-Riedle, A. (2001). Life circumstances of mothers with serious mental illness. *Psychiatric Rehabilitation Journal, 25,* 114–123.

Mowbray, C. T., Oyserman, D., & Ross, S. (1995a). Parenting and the significance of children for women with a serious mental illness. *Journal of Mental Health Administration, 22,* 189–200.

Mowbray, C. T., Oyserman, D., Zemencuk, M., Ross, S., & Scott, R. (1995b). Motherhood for women with serious mental illness: Pregnancy, childbirth, and the postpartum period, *American Journal of Orthopsychiatry, 65,* 21–38.

Mowbray, C. T., Robinson, E., & Holter, M. (2002). Consumer drop-in centers: Operations, services, and consumer involvement. *Health and Social Work, 27,* 248–261.

Mowbray, C. T., Schwartz, S., Bybee, D., Spong, J., Rueda-Riedle, A., & Oyserman, D. (2000). Mothers with a mental illness: Stressors and resources for parenting and living. *Families in Society, 81,* 118–129.

Mowbray, C. T., & Tan, C. (1992). Evaluation of an innovative consumer-run service model: The drop-in center. *Innovation and Research, 1,* 19–24.

Mowbray, C. T., & Tan, C. (1993). Consumer operated drop-in centers: Evaluation of operations and impact. *Journal of Mental Health Administration, 20,* 8–19.

Moxley, D., & Mowbray, C. (1997). Consumers as providers: Forces and factors legitimizing role innovation in psychiatric rehabilitation. In C. Mowbray, D. Moxley, C. Jasper, & L. Howell (Eds.), *Consumers as providers in psychiatric rehabilitation* (pp. 2–34). Columbia, MD: International Association of Psychosocial Rehabilitation Services.

Muenzenmaier, K., Meyer, I., Struening, E., & Ferber, J. (1993). Childhood abuse and neglect among women outpatients with chronic mental illness. *Hospital and Community Psychiatry, 44,* 666–670.

Mueser, K. (2005). Family intervention for schizophrenia. In L. D. Vandecreek (Ed.), *Innovations in clinical practice* (pp. 219–233). Sarasota, FL: Professional Resources Press.

Mueser, K. T. (1998). Social skill and problem solving. In A. S. Bellack & M. Hersen (Eds.), *Comprehensive clinical psychology* (Vol. 6, pp. 183–201). New York: Pergamon.

Mueser, K. T., Aalto, S., Becker, D. R., Ogden, J., Wolfe, R., Schiavo, D., et al. (2005a). A randomized controlled trial of the effectiveness of skills training in improving outcomes in supported employment. *Psychiatric Services, 56,* 1254–1260.

Mueser, K. T., Becker, D. R., Torrey, W. C., Xie, H., Bond, G. R., Drake, R. E., et al. (1997a). Work and nonvocational domains of functioning in persons with severe mental illness: A longitudinal analysis. *Nervous and Mental Disease, 185,* 419–426.

Mueser, K. T., & Bellack, A. S. (1998). Social skills and social functioning. In K. T. Mueser & N. Tarrier (Eds.), *Handbook of social functioning in schizophrenia* (pp. 79–96). Needham Heights, MA: Allyn & Bacon.

Mueser, K. T., Bellack, A. S., Douglas, M. S., & Morrison, R. L. (1991a). Prevalence and stability of social skill deficits in schizophrenia. *Schizophrenia Research, 5,* 167–176.

Mueser, K. T., Bellack, A. S., Douglas, M. S., & Wade, J. H. (1991b). Prediction of social skill acquisition in schizophrenic and major affective disorder patients from memory and symptomatology. *Psychiatry Research, 37,* 281–296.

Mueser, K. T., Bellack, A. S., Morrison, R. L., & Wixted, J. T. (1990a). Social competence in schizophrenia: Premorbid adjustment, social skill, and domains of functioning. *Journal of Psychiatric Research, 24*, 51–63.

Mueser, K. T., Bellack, A., Wade, J., Sayers, S., & Rosenthal, C. (1992). An assessment of the educational needs of chronic psychiatric patients and their relatives. *British Journal of Psychiatry, 160*, 674–680.

Mueser, K. T., Bennett, M., & Kushner, M. (1995a). Substance abuse disorders among persons with chronic mental illness. In A. Lehman & L. Dixon (Eds.), *Double jeopardy: Chronic mental illness and substance abuse* (pp. 9–25). Chur, Switzerland: Harwood.

Mueser, K. T., Blanchard, J. J., & Bellack, A. S. (1995b). Memory and social skill in schizophrenia: The role of gender. *Psychiatry Research, 57*, 141–153.

Mueser, K. T., Bolton, E. E., Carty, P. C., Bradley, M. J., Ahlgren, K. F., DiStaso, D. R., et al. (2007). The trauma recovery group: A cognitive-behavioral program for PTSD in persons with severe mental illness. *Community Mental Health Journal, 43*, 281–304.

Mueser, K. T., Bond, G., Drake, R., & Resnick, S. (1998a). Models of community care for severe mental illness. A review of research on case management. *Schizophrenia Bulletin, 24*, 27–74.

Mueser, K. T., & Butler, R. W. (1987). Auditory hallucinations in combat-related chronic posttraumatic stress disorder. *American Journal of Psychiatry, 144*, 299–302.

Mueser, K. T., Clark, R. E., Haines, M., Drake, R. E., McHugo, G. J., Bond, G. R., et al. (2004a). The Hartford study of supported employment for persons with severe mental illness. *Journal of Consulting and Clinical Psychology, 72*, 479–490.

Mueser, K. T., Corrigan, P. W., Hilton, D. W., Tanzman, B., Schaub, A., Gingerich, S., Copeland, M. E., et al. (2002a). Illness management and recovery for severe mental illness: A review of the research. *Psychiatric Services, 53*, 1272–1284.

Mueser, K. T., Crocker, A. G., Frisman, L. B., Drake, R. E., Covell, N. H., & Essock, S. M. (2006a). Conduct disorder and antisocial personality disorder in persons with severe psychiatric and substance use disorders. *Schizophrenia Bulletin, 32*, 626–636.

Mueser, K. T., Douglas, M. S., Bellack, A. S., & Morrison, R. L. (1991c). Assessment of enduring deficit and negative symptom subtypes in schizophrenia. *Schizophrenia Bulletin, 17*, 565–582.

Mueser, K. T., Drake, R. E., Ackerson, T. H., Alterman, A. I., Miles, K. M., & Noordsy, D. L. (1997b). Antisocial personality disorder, conduct disorder, and substance abuse in schizophrenia. *Journal of Abnormal Psychology, 106*, 473–477.

Mueser, K. T., Drake, R. E., & Bond, G. R. (1997c). Recent advances in psychiatric rehabilitation for patients with severe mental illness. *Harvard Review of Psychiatry, 5*, 123–137.

Mueser, K. T., Drake, R. E., Sigmon, S. C., & Brunette, M. (2005b). Psychosocial interventions for adults with severe mental illnesses and co-occurring substance use disorders: A review of specific interventions. *Journal of Dual Diagnosis, 1*, 57–82.

Mueser, K. T., & Fox, L. (2002). A family intervention program for dual disorders. *Community Mental Health Journal, 38*, 253–270.

Mueser, K. T., Foy, D. W., & Carter, M. J. (1986). Social skills training for job maintenance in a psychiatric patient. *Journal of Counseling Psychology, 33*, 360–362.

Mueser, K. T., & Gingerich, S. (2006). *The complete family guide to schizophrenia: Helping your loved one get the most out of life.* New York: Guilford Press.

Mueser, K. T., & Glynn, S. M. (1999). *Behavioral family therapy for psychiatric disorders* (2nd ed.). Oakland, CA: New Harbinger.

Mueser, K. T., Goodman, L. A., Trumbetta, S. L., Rosenberg, S. D., Osher, F. C., Vidaver, R., et al. (1998b). Trauma and posttraumatic stress disorder in severe mental illness. *Journal of Consulting and Clinical Psychology, 66*, 493–499.

Mueser, K. T., Hiday, V. A., Goodman, L. A., & Valenti-Hein, D. (2003a). People with mental and physical disabilities. In B. L. Green, M. J. Friedman, J. T. V. M. de Joop, S. D. Solomon, T. M. Keane, J. A. Fairbank, et al. (Eds.), *Trauma interventions in war and peace: Prevention, practice, and policy* (pp. 129–154). New York: Kluwer Academic/Plenum Press.

Mueser, K. T., Levine, S., Bellack, A. S., Douglas, M. S., & Brady, E. U. (1990b). Social skills training for acute psychiatric patients. *Hospital and Community Psychiatry, 41*, 1249–1251.

Mueser, K. T., Meyer, P. S., Penn, D. L., Clancy, R., Clancy, D. M., & Salyers, M. P. (2006b). The Illness Management and Recovery program: Rationale, development, and preliminary findings. *Schizophrenia Bulletin, 32*(Suppl. 1), S32–S43.

Mueser, K. T., Noordsy, D. L., Drake, R. E., & Fox, L. (2003b). *Integrated treatment for dual disorders: A guide to effective practice.* New York: Guilford Press.

Mueser, K. T., Noordsy, D. L., Fox, L., & Wolfe, R. (2003c). Disulfiram treatment for alcoholism in severe mental illness. *American Journal of Addictions, 12,* 242–252.

Mueser, K. T., & Penn, D. L. (2004). A rush to judgment on social skills training: A comment on Pilling et al. (2002). *Psychological Medicine, 34,* 1365–1369.

Mueser, K. T., Penn, D. L., Blanchard, J. J., & Bellack, A. S. (1997d). Affect recognition in schizophrenia: A synthesis of findings across three studies. *Psychiatry: Interpersonal and Biological Processes, 60,* 301–308.

Mueser, K. T., & Rosenberg, S. R. (2003). Treating the trauma of first episode psychosis: A PTSD perspective. *Journal of Mental Health, 12,* 103–108.

Mueser, K. T., Rosenberg, S. D., Goodman, L. A., & Trumbetta, S. L. (2002b). Trauma, PTSD, and the course of severe mental illness: An interactive model. *Schizophrenia Research, 53*(1–2), 123–143.

Mueser, K. T., Rosenberg, S. D., Jankowski, M. K., Hamblen, J., & Descamps, M. (2004b). A cognitive-behavioral treatment program for posttraumatic stress disorder in persons with severe mental illness. *American Journal of Psychiatric Rehabilitation, 7,* 107–146.

Mueser, K. T., Rosenberg, S. R., Xie, H., Jankowski, M. K., Bolton, E. E., Lu, W., et al. (2007). *A randomized controlled trial of cognitive-behavioral treatment of posttraumatic stress disorder in severe mental illness.* Manuscript under review.

Mueser, K. T., Salyers, M. P., & Mueser, P. R. (2001a). A prospective analysis of work in schizophrenia. *Schizophrenia Bulletin, 27,* 281–296.

Mueser, K. T., Salyers, M. P., Rosenberg, S. D., Ford, J. D., Fox, L., & Cardy, P. (2001b). A psychometric evaluation of trauma and PTSD assessments in persons with severe mental illness. *Psychological Assessment, 13,* 110–117.

Mueser, K. T., Salyers, M. P., Rosenberg, S. D., Goodman, L. A., Essock, S. M., Osher, F. C., et al. (2004c). Interpersonal trauma and posttraumatic stress disorder in patients with severe mental illness: Demographic, clinical, and health correlates. *Schizophrenia Bulletin, 30,* 45–57.

Mueser, K. T., Sengupta, A., Schooler, N. R., Bellack, A. S., Xie, H., Glick, I. D., et al. (2001c). Family treatment and medication dosage reduction in schizophrenia: Effects on patient social functioning, family attitudes, and burden. *Journal of Consulting and Clinical Psychology, 69,* 3–12.

Mueser, K. T., & Tarrier, N. (Eds.). (1998). *Handbook of social functioning in schizophrenia.* Boston: Allyn & Bacon.

Mueser, K. T., & Taylor, K. L. (1997). A cognitive-behavioral approach. In M. Harris & C. L. Landis (Eds.), *Sexual abuse in the lives of women diagnosed with serious mental illness* (pp. 67–90). Amsterdam: Harwood.

Mueser, K. T., Torrey, W. C., Lynde, D., Singer, P., & Drake, R. E. (2003d). Implementing evidence-based practices for people with severe mental illness. *Behavior Modification, 27,* 387–411.

Mueser, K. T., Valentiner, D. P., & Agresta, J. (1997e). Coping with negative symptoms of schizophrenia: Patient and family perspectives. *Schizophrenia Bulletin, 23,* 329–339.

Mueser, K. T., Webb, C., Pfeiffer, M., Gladis, M., & Levinson, D. (1996). Family burden of schizophrenia and bipolar disorder: Perceptions of relatives and professionals. *Psychiatric Services, 47,* 507–511.

Mulick, J. A. (1990). The ideology and science of punishment in mental retardation. *American Journal on Mental Retardation, 95,* 142–156.

Mullen, B., Rozell, D., & Johnson, C. (1996). The phenomenology of being in a group: Complexity approaches to operationalizing cognitive representation. In J. L. Nye & A. M. Brower (Eds.), *What's social about social cognition? Research on socially shared cognition in small groups* (pp. 205–229). Thousand Oaks, CA: Sage.

Mulvey, E. (1994). Assessing the evidence of a link between mental illness and violence. *Hospital and Community Psychiatry, 45,* 663–668.

Munroe-Blum, H., Collins, E., McCleary, L., & Nuttall, S. (1996). The Social Dysfunction Index (SDI) for patients with schizophrenia and related disorders. *Schizophrenia Research, 20,* 211–219.

Murray-Swank, A. B., & Dixon, L. (2004). Family psychoeducation as an evidence-based practice. *CNS Spectrums, 9,* 905–912.

Myers, J., & Bean, L. (1968). *A decade later: A follow-up of social class and mental illness.* New York: Wiley.

Najavits, L. M. (2002). *Seeking safety: A treatment manual for PTSD and substance abuse.* New York: Guilford Press.

NAMI E-News. (2002). White House issues report on "New Freedom Initiative" and implementation of the U.S. Supreme Court's *Olmstead* decision. *NAMI E-News, 02-43.*

NAMI E-News. (2005, August 22). *Medicaid reform commission endorses higher co-payments for prescription drugs, medication access restrictions, rejects bid to narrow definition of rehabilitation and case management services.* Retrieved June 30, 2007, from *www.nami.org.*

NAMI StigmaBusters. (2002). NAMI Stigma

Busters alert. Retrieved May 18, 2002, from *www.nami.org/campagin/20000405.htm*.

National Association of State Mental Health Program Directors. (2000). *Position statement on the repeal of the Medicaid IMD exclusion*. Alexandria, VA: Author.

National Center for Cultural Competence. (2006). Conceptual frameworks/models, guiding values and principles. Retrieved January 16, 2006, from *gucchd.georgetown.edu/nccc/framework.html*.

National Institute on Aging. (1987). *Personnel for health needs of the elderly through the year 2020*. Bethesda, MD: U.S. Department of Health and Human Services.

National Mental Health Campaign. (2002). Retrieved May 18, 2002, from *www.nostigma.org*.

Neale, M., & Rosenheck, R. (2000). Therapeutic limit setting in an assertive community treatment program, *Psychiatric Services, 51*, 499–505.

Nelson, A. A., Gold, B. H., Huchinson, R. A., & Benezra, E. (1975). Drug default among schizophrenic patients. *American Journal of Hospital Pharmacy, 32*, 1237–1242.

Nelson, G., Hall, G. B., & Walsh-Bowers, R. (1998). The relationship between housing characteristics, emotional well-being, and the personal empowerment of psychiatric consumer/ survivors. *Community Mental Health Journal, 34*, 57–69.

Nelson, G., & Smith Fowler, H. (1987). Housing for the chronically mentally disabled: II. Process and outcome. *Canadian Journal of Community Mental Health, 6*, 79–91.

Neria, Y., Bromet, E. J., Sievers, S., Lavelle, J., & Fochtmann, L. J. (2002). Trauma exposure and posttraumatic stress disorder in psychosis: Findings from a first-admission cohort. *Journal of Consulting and Clinical Psychology, 70*, 246–251.

New Freedom Commission on Mental Health (2003). *Achieving the promise: Transforming mental health care in America: Final Report* (DHHS Publication No. SMA-033832). Rockville, MD: Author.

Newman, C. F., Leahy, R. L., Beck, A. T., Reilly-Harrington, N. A., & Gyulai, L. (2002). *Bipolar disorder: A cognitive therapy approach*. Washington, DC: American Psychological Association.

Newman, S. J. (2001a). *Housing and mental illness: A critical review of the literature*. Washington, DC: Urban Institute.

Newman, S. J. (2001b). Housing attributes and serious mental illness: Implications for research and practice. *Psychiatric Services, 52*, 1309–1317.

Newman, S. J., & Ridgely, M. S. (1994). Organization and delivery of independent housing for persons with chronic mental illness. *Administration and Policy in Mental Health, 21*, 199–216.

Newman, S. X., & Bland, R. C. (1991). Mortality in a cohort of patients with schizophrenia: A record linkage study. *Canadian Journal of Psychiatry, 36*, 239–245.

New York Office of Mental Health. (2005). *Final report on the status of assisted outpatient treatment*. Albany, NY: New York Office of Mental Health.

News & Notes. (1999). President Clinton announces an array of initiatives at First White House Conference on Mental Health. *Psychiatric Services, 50*, 980–981.

NIAAA, NIDA, NIMH, & Workshop. (2006, February 23–March 1). *Methodology of conducting pharmacologic clinical trials in patients with alcohol/drug dependence and psychiatric comorbidity*, Bethesda, MD.

Nicholson, J., Biebel, K., Katz-Leavy, J., & Williams, V. (2002). The prevalence of parenthood in adults with mental illness: Implications for state and federal policy makers, programs, and providers. In R. Manderscheid & M. Henderson (Eds.), *Mental health, United States, 2002*. Rockville, MD: U.S. Department of Health and Human Services, Substance Abuse and Mental Health Services Administration, Center for Mental Health Services.

Nicholson, J., & Blanch, A. (1994). Rehabilitation for parenting roles for people with serious mental illness. *Psychosocial Rehabilitation, 18*, 109–119.

Nicholson, J., & Henry, A. (2003). Achieving the goal of evidence based psychiatric rehabilitation practices for mothers with mental illness. *Psychiatric Rehabilitation Journal, 27*, 122–130.

Nicholson, J., Geller, J., Fisher, W., & Dion, G. (1993). State policies and programs that address the needs of mentally ill mothers in the public sector. *Hospital and Community Psychiatry, 44*, 484–489.

Nicholson, J., Sweeney, E., & Geller, J. (1998a). Mothers with mental illness: I. The competing demands of parenting and living with mental illness. *Psychiatric Services, 49*, 635–642.

Nicholson, J., Sweeney, E., & Geller, J. (1998b). Mothers with mental illness: II. Family relationships and the context of parenting. *Psychiatric Services, 49*, 643–649.

Nikkel, R., Smith, G., & Edwards, D. (1992). A consumer-operated case management project. *Hospital and Community Psychiatry, 43*, 577–579.

Nimgaonkar, V., Ward, S., Agarde, H., Weston, N.,

& Ganguli, R. (1997). Fertility in schizophrenia: Results for a contemporary U.S. cohort. *Acta Psychiatrica Scandinavica, 95*, 364–369.

Nishith, P., Hearst, D. E., Mueser, K. T., & Foa, E. B. (1995). PTSD and major depression: Methodological and treatment considerations in a single case design. *Behavior Therapy, 26*, 319–335.

Nishith, P., Mechanic, M. B., & Resick, P. A. (2000). Prior interpersonal trauma: The contribution to current PTSD symptoms in female rape victims. *Journal of Abnormal Psychology, 109*, 20–25.

Noble, J. H., Honberg, R. S., Hall, L. L., & Flynn, L. M. (1997). *A legacy of failure: The inability of the federal–state vocational rehabilitation system to serve people with severe mental illness.* Arlington, VA: National Alliance for the Mentally Ill.

Noordsy, D., Schwab, B., Fox, L., & Drake, R. (1996). The role of self-help programs in the rehabilitation of persons with severe mental illness and substance use disorders. *Community Mental Health Journal, 32*, 71–81.

Noordsy, D. L., O'Keefe, C., Mueser, K. T., & Xie, H. (2001). Six month outcomes for patients who switched to olanzapine treatment. *Psychiatric Services, 52*, 501–507.

Nordstroem, A., & Kullgren, G. (2003). Victim relations and victim gender in violent crimes committed by offenders with schizophrenia. *Social Psychiatry and Psychiatric Epidemiology, 38*, 326–330.

Norton, S., Wanderman, A., & Goldman, C. (1993). Perceived costs and benefits of membership in self-help groups: Comparison of members and non-members of the Alliance for the Mentally Ill. *Community Mental Health Journal, 29*, 143–160.

Nuechterlein, K. H., Dawson, M. E., Gitlin, M., Ventura, J., Goldstein, M. J., Snyder, K. S., et al. (1992). Developmental processes in schizophrenic disorders: Longitudinal studies of vulnerability and stress. *Schizophrenia Bulletin, 18*(3), 387–425.

Nuechterlein, K. H., Subotnik, K. L., Ventura, J., Gitlin, M. J., Green, M. F., Wallace, C. J., et al. (2005). Advances in improving and predicting work outcome in recent-onset schizophrenia. *Schizophrenia Bulletin, 31*, 530.

Nuttbrock, L. A., Rahav, M., Rivera, J. J., Ng-Mak, D. S., & Link, B. G. (1998). Outcomes of homeless mentally ill chemical abusers in community residences and a therapeutic community. *Psychiatric Services, 49*, 68–76.

O'Brien, W. F., & Anthony, W. A. (2002). Avoiding the "any models trap." *Psychiatric Rehabilitation Journal, 25*, 213–214.

O'Connor, A. M., Rostom, A., & Fiset, V. (1999). Decision aids for patients facing health treatment or screening decisions. *British Medical Journal, 319*, 731–734.

O'Day, B. L., Killeen, M. B., Sutton, J., & Iezzoni, L. I. (2005). Primary care experiences of people with psychiatric disabilities: Barriers to care and potential solutions. *Psychiatric Rehabilitation Journal, 28*, 339–345.

O'Donnell, C., Donohoe, G., Sharkey, L., Owens, N., Migone, M., Harries, R., et al. (2003). Compliance therapy: A randomised controlled trial in schizophrenia. *British Medical Journal, 327*, 834.

Ogawa, K., Miya, M., Watarai, A., Nakazawa, M., Yuasa, S., & Utena, H. (1987). A long-term follow-up study of schizophrenia in Japan with special reference to the course of social adjustment. *British Journal of Psychiatry, 151*, 758–765.

Ogilvie, R. J. (1997). The state of supported housing for mental health consumers: A literature review. *Psychiatric Rehabilitation Journal, 21*, 122–131.

Okazaki, S. (2000). Treatment delay among Asian-American patients with severe mental illness. *American Journal of Orthopsychiatry, 70*, 58–64.

O'Keefe, C., Potenza, D. P., & Mueser, K. T. (1997). Treatment outcomes for severely mentally ill patients on conditional discharge to community-based treatment. *Journal of Nervous and Mental Disease, 185*, 409–411.

Oldman, J., Thomson, L., Calsaferri, K., Luke, A., & Bond, G. R. (2005). A case report of the conversions of sheltered employment to evidence-based supported employment in Canada. *Psychiatric Services, 56*, 1436–1440.

Oldridge, M., & Hughes, I. (1992). Psychological well-being in families with a member suffering from schizophrenia. *British Journal of Psychiatry, 147*, 183–186.

Olfson, M. (1990). Assertive community treatment: An evaluation of experimental evidence. *Hospital and Community Psychiatry, 41*, 634–641.

Olfson, M., Mechanic, D., Hansell, S., Boyer, C. A., Walkup, J., & Weiden, P. J. (2000). Predicting medication noncompliance after hospital discharge among patients with schizophrenia. *Psychiatric Services, 51*, 216–222.

Oliver, C. (1992). The antecedents of deinstitutionalization. *Organization Studies, 13*, 563–588.

Oliver, J. P. J. (1991). The social care directive: Development of a quality of life profile for use in community services for the mentally ill. *Social Work and Social Sciences Review, 3*, 5–45.

Oliver, M., & Kuipers, E (1996). Stress and its relationship to expressed emotion in community mental health workers. *International Journal of Social Psychiatry, 42*, 150–159.

Ollendick, T. H., & Matson, J. L. (1978). Overcorrection: An overview. *Behavior Therapy, 9*, 830–842.

Olshansky, S., Grob, S., & Ekdahl, M. (1960). Survey of employment experience of patients discharged from three mental hospitals during the period 1951–1953. *Mental Hygiene, 44*, 510–521.

Olvera, R. L. (2002). Intermittent explosive disorder: Epidemiology, diagnosis and management. *CNS Drugs, 16*, 517–526.

Ortega, A. N., & Rosenheck, R. (2002). Hispanic client–case manager matching: Differences in outcomes and service use in a program for homeless persons with severe mental illness. *Journal of Nervous and Mental Disease, 190*, 315–323.

Osher, F., Steadman, H., & Barr, H. (2003). A best practice approach to community re-entry from jails for inmates with co-occurring disorders: The APIC model. *Crime and Delinquency, 49*, 79–96.

Osher, F. C., & Dixon, L. B. (1996). Housing for persons with co-occurring mental and addictive disorders. In R. E. Drake & K. T. Mueser (Eds.), *Dual diagnosis of major mental illness and substance abuse: II. Recent research and clinical implications: New directions for mental health services* (pp. 53–64). San Francisco: Jossey-Bass.

Osher, F. C., & Kofoed, L. L. (1989). Treatment of patients with psychiatric and psychopactive substance use disorders. *Hospital and Community Psychiatry, 40*, 1025–1030.

Oshima, I., Cho, N., & Takahashi, K. (2004). Effective components of a nationwide case management program in Japan for individuals with severe mental illness. *Community Mental Health Journal, 40*, 525–537.

Ouimette, P. C., & Brown, P. (2002). *Trauma and substance abuse: causes, consequences, and treatment of comribid disorders.* Washington, DC: American Psychological Association.

Owen, R. R., Fischer, E. P., Booth, B. M., & Cuffel, B. J. (1996). Medication noncompliance and substance abuse among patients with schizophrenia. *Psychiatric Services, 47*, 853–858.

Oyserman, D., Mowbray, C., & Zemencuk, J. (1994). Resources and supports for mothers with severe medical illness. *Health and Social Work, 19*, 132–142.

Pachet, A. K., & Wisniewski, A. M. (2003). The effects of lithium on cognition: An updated review. *Psychopharmacology, 170*(3), 225–234.

Page, S. (1977). Effects of the mental illness label in attempts to obtain accommodation. *Canadian Journal of Behavioural Science, 9*, 85–90.

Page, S. (1983). Psychiatric stigma: Two studies of behaviour when the chips are down. *Canadian Journal of Community Mental Health, 2*, 13–19.

Page, S. (1995). Effects of the mental illness label in 1993: Acceptance and rejection in the community. *Journal of Health and Social Policy, 7*, 61–68.

Palermo, G., Gumz, E., & Liska, F. J. (1992). Mental illness and criminal behavior revisited. *International Journal of Offender Therapy and Comparative Criminology, 36*, 53–61.

Palmer, B. W., Heaton, R. K., Paulsen, J. S., Kuck, J., Braff, D., Harris, M. J., et al. (1997). Is it possible to be schizophrenic yet neuropsychologically normal? *Neuropsychology, 11*, 437–446.

Park, J. M., Solomon, P., & Mandell, D. S. (2006). Involvement in the child welfare system among mothers with serous mental illness. *Psychiatric Services, 57*, 493–497.

Parker, S., & Knoll, J. L. (1990). Partial hospitalization: An update. *American Journal of Psychiatry, 147*, 156–160.

Parkinson, S., Nelson, G., & Horgan, S. (1999). From housing to homes: A review of the literature on housing approaches for psychiatric consumer/survivors. *Canadian Journal of Community Mental Health, 18*, 145–164.

Pate, G. S. (1988). Research on reducing prejudice. *Social Education, 52*, 287–289.

Patterson, T. L., Bucardo, J., McKibbin, C. L., Mausbach, B. T., Moore, D., Barrio, C., et al. (2005). Development and pilot testing of a new psychosocial intervention for older Latinos with chronic psychosis. *Schizophrenia Bulletin, 31*, 922–930.

Patterson, T. L., Moscona, S., McKibbin, C. L., Hughs, T., & Jeste, D. V. (2001). UCSD Performance-based Skills Assessment (UPSA): Development of a new measure of everyday functioning for severely mentally ill adults. *Schizophrenia Bulletin, 27*, 235–245.

Paul, G. L., & Lentz, R. J. (1977). *Psychosocial treatment of chronic mental patients: Milieu versus social learning programs.* Cambridge, MA: Harvard University Press.

Paul, G. L., & Menditto, A. A. (1992). Effectiveness of inpatient treatment programs for mentally ill adults in public psychiatric facilities. *Applied and Preventive Psychology, 1*, 41–63.

Paulson, R. (1991). Professional training for consumers and family members: One road to empowerment. *Psychosocial Rehabilitation Journal, 14*, 69–80.

Paulson, R., Herinckx, H., Demmler, J., Clarke, G., Cutler, D., & Birecree, E. (1999). Comparing practice patterns of consumer and non-consumer mental health service providers. *Community Mental Health Journal, 35,* 251–269.

Pearlin, L., & Schooler, C. (1978). The structure of coping. *Journal of Health and Social Behavior, 19,* 2–21.

Peniston, E. G. (1988). Evaluation of long-term therapeutic efficacy of behavior modification program with chronic male psychiatric inpatients. *Journal of Behavior Therapy and Experimental Psychiatry, 19,* 95–101.

Penn, D. L., Addington, J., & Pinkham, A. (2006). Social cognitive impairments. In J. A. Lieberman, T. S. Stroup, & D. O. Perkins (Eds.), *The American Psychiatric Publishing textbook of schizophrenia* (pp. 261–274). Arlington, VA: American Psychiatric Association.

Penn, D. L., Corrigan, P. W., Bentall, R. P., Racenstein, J. M., & Newman, L. (1997a). Social cognition in schizophrenia. *Psychological Bulletin, 121,* 114–132.

Penn, D. L., Guynan, K., Daily, T., Spaulding, W. D., Garbin, C. P., & Sullivan, M. (1994). Dispelling the stigma of schizophrenia: What sort of information is best? *Schizophrenia Bulletin, 20,* 567–578.

Penn, D. L., Kommana, S., Mansfield, M., Link, B. G. (1999). Dispelling the stigma of schizophrenia: II. The impact of information on dangerousness. *Schizophrenia Bulletin, 25,* 437–446.

Penn, D. L., & Martin, J. (1998). The stigma of severe mental illness: Some potential solutions for a recalcitrant problem. *Psychiatric Quarterly, 69,* 235–247.

Penn, D. L., & Mueser, K. T. (1996). Research update on the psychosocial treatment of schizophrenia. *American Journal of Psychiatry, 153,* 607–617.

Penn, D. L., Mueser, K. T., & Doonan, R. (1997b). Physical attractiveness in schizophrenia: The mediating role of social skill. *Behavior Modification, 21,* 78–85.

Penn, D. L., Mueser, K. T., & Spaulding, W. (1996). Information processing, social skill, and gender in schizophrenia. *Psychiatry Research, 59,* 213–220.

Penn, D. L., Mueser, K. T., Spaulding, W., Hope, D. A., & Reed, D. (1995). Information processing and social competence in chronic schizophrenia. *Schizophrenia Bulletin, 21*(2), 269–281.

Penn, D. L., Van Der Does, A. W., Spaulding, W. D., Garbin, C. P., Linszen, D., & Dingemans, P. (1993). Information processing and social cognitive problem solving in schizophrenia: Assessment of interrelationships and changes over time. *Journal of Mental and Nervous Disease, 181,* 13–20.

Penn, P. E., & Brooks, A. J. (1999). *Comparing substance abuse treatments for dual diagnosis: Final report.* Tucson, AZ: La Frontera Center.

Pennebaker, J. W., Barger, S. D., & Tiebout, J. (1989). Disclosure of traumas and health among Holocaust survivors. *Psychosomatic Medicine, 51,* 577–589.

Pennebaker, J. W., Kiecolt-Glaser, J. K., & Glaser, R. (1988). Disclosure of traumas and immune function: Health implications for psychotherapy. *Journal of Consulting and Clinical Psychology, 56,* 239–245.

Penrose, L. (1939). Mental disease and crime: Outline of a comparative study of European statistics. *British Journal of Medical Psychology, 18,* 1–15.

Pepper, B., Krishner, M. C., & Ryglewicz, H. (1981). The young adult chronic patient: Overview of a population. *Hospital and Community Psychiatry, 32,* 463–469.

Perez, A., Leifman, S., & Estrada, A. (2003). Reversing the criminalization of mental illness. *Crime and Delinquency, 49,* 62–78.

Perkins, R., & Buckfield, R. (1997). Access to employment: A supported employment project to enable mental health users to obtain jobs. *Journal of Mental Health, 6,* 307–319.

Perky, C. W. (1910). An experimental study of imagination. *American Journal of Psychology, 21,* 422–452.

Pernell-Arnold, A., & Finley, L. (1999). Integrating multicultural competence into psychosocial rehabilitation. In R. Hughes & D. Weinstein (Eds.), *Best practices in psychosocial rehabilitation* (pp. 213–244). Columbia, MD: International Association of Psychosocial Rehabilitation Services.

Perron, B. (2002). Online support for caregivers of people with mental illness. *Psychiatric Rehabilitation Journal, 26,* 70–77.

Perry, A., Tarrier, N., Morriss, R., McCarthy, E., & Limb, K. (1999). Randomised controlled trial of efficacy of teaching patients with bipolar disorder to identify early symptoms of relapse and obtain treatment. *British Medical Journal, 318,* 149–153.

Persaud, R. (2000). Psychiatrists suffer from stigma too. *Psychiatric Bulletin, 24,* 284–285.

Pescosolido, B. A., Monahan, J., Link, B. G., Stueve, A., & Kikuzawa, S. (1999). The public's view of the competence, dangerousness, and need for legal coercion of persons with mental health problems. *American Journal of Public Health, 89,* 1339–1345.

Pescosolido, B. A., Wright, E. R., & Lutfey, K.

(1999). The changing hopes, worries, and community supports of individuals moving from a closing long-term care facility. *Journal of Behavioral Health Services and Research, 26*, 276–288.

Petersillia, J., & Turner, S. (1993, May). Evaluating intensive supervision probation/parole: Results of a nationwide experiment. *National Institute of Justice: Research in Brief*. Washington, DC: U.S. Department of Justice, Office of Justice Programs.

Petrakis, I. L., Nich, C., & Ralevski, E. (2006). Psychotic spectrum disorders and alcohol abuse: A review of pharmacotherapeutic strategies and a report on the effectiveness of naltrexone and disulfiram. *Schizophrenia Bulletin, 32*, 644–654.

Petrila, J. (2003). An introduction to special jurisdiction court. *International Journal of Law and Psychiatry, 26*, 3–12.

Petrila, J., Poythress, N., McGaha, A., & Boothroyd, R. (2001, Winter). Preliminary observations from an evaluation of the Broward County Florida Mental Health Court. *Court Review*, 14–22.

Pettigrew, T. F., & Tropp, L. R. (2000). Does intergroup contact reduce prejudice: Recent meta-analytic findings. In S. Oskamp (Ed.), *Reducing prejudice and discrimination* (pp. 93–114). Mahwah, NJ: Erlbaum.

Pfohl, B., & Zimmerman, M. (1995). *The structured interview for DSM-IV personality: SIDP-IV*. Iowa City: University of Iowa.

Pharoah, F., Rathbone, J., Mari, J., & Streiner, D. (2004). *Family intervention for schizophrenia*. The Cochrane Library (Issue 2). Oxford, UK: Wiley.

Phelan, J. C., Bromet, E. J., & Link, B. G. (1998). Psychiatric illness and family stigma. *Schizophrenia Bulletin, 24*, 115–126.

Phelan, J. C., Link, B. G., Moore, R. E., & Stueve, A. (1997). The stigma of homelessness: The impact of the label "homeless" on attitudes toward poor persons. *Social Psychology Quarterly, 60*, 323–337.

Phelan, J. C., Link, B. G., Stueve, A., & Pescosolido, B. A. (2000). Public conceptions of mental illness in 1950 and 1996: What is mental illness and is it to be feared? *Journal of Health and Social Behavior, 41*, 188–207.

Phelan, M., Slade, M., Thornicroft, G., Dunn, G., Holloway, F., Wykes, T., et al. (1995). The Camberwell Assessment of Need: The validity and reliability of an instrument to assess the needs of people with severe mental illness. *British Journal of Psychiatry, 167*, 589–595.

Phillips, E. S., Barrio, C., & Brekke, J. S. (2001a). The impact of ethnicity on prospective functional outcomes from community based psychosocial rehabilitation for persons with schizophrenia. *Journal of Community Psychology, 29*, 657–673.

Phillips, S. D., & Burns, B. J. (2002). Information for public mental health authorities. In S. D. Phillips & B. J. Burns (Eds.), *Assertive community treatment implementation resource kit*. Rockville, MD: Center for Mental Health Services, Substance Abuse and Mental Health Services Administration.

Phillips, S. D., Burns, B. J., Edgar, E., Mueser, K., Jenkins, K., Rosenheck, R., et al. (2001b). Moving assertive community treatment into standard practice. *Psychiatric Services, 52*, 771–779.

Physicians' Desk Reference. (2005). (59th ed.), Montvale, NH: Thomson PDR.

Pi, E. H., & Simpson, G. M. (2005). Psychopharmacology: Cross-cultural psychopharmacology: A current clinical perspective. *Psychiatric Services, 56*, 31–33.

Pickett, S., Cook, J., Cohler, B., & Solomon, M. (1997). Positive parent/adult child relationships: Impact of severe mental illness and caregiving burden. *American Journal of Orthopsychiatry, 67*, 220–230.

Pickett, S., Greenley, J., & Greenberg, J. (1995). Off-timedness as a contributor to subjective burden for parents of offspring with severe mental illness. *Family Relations, 44*, 185–201.

Pickett, S., Vraniak, D., Cook, J., & Cohler, B. (1993). Strength in adversity: Blacks bear burden better than whites. *Professional Psychology: Research and Practice, 24*, 460–467.

Pickett-Schenk, S., Cook, J., & Laris, A. (2000). Journey of hope: Program outcomes. *Community Mental Health Journal, 36*, 413–424.

Pickett-Schenk, S., Steigman, P., Bennett, C., & Lippincott, R. (2005).*Journey of Hope education course outcomes project*. Chicago: University of Illinois, Center on Mental Health Services Research and Policy.

Pilling, S., Bebbington, P., Kuipers, E., Garety, P., Geddes, J. R., Martindale, B., et al. (2002a). Psychological treatments in schizophrenia: II. Meta-analyses of randomized controlled trials of social skills training and cognitive remediation. *Psychological Medicine, 32*, 783–791.

Pilling, S., Bebbington, P., Kuipers, E., Garety, P., Geddes, J., Orbach, G., et al. (2002b). Psychological treatments in schizophrenia: I. Meta-analysis of family intervention and cognitive behavior therapy. *Psychological Medicine, 32*, 763–782.

Pincus, F. L. (1996). Discrimination comes in many

forms: Individual, institutional, and structural. *American Behavioral Scientist, 40,* 186–194.

Pincus, F. L. (1999). From individual to structural discrimination. In F. L. Pincus & H. J. Ehrlich (Eds.), *Race and ethnic conflict: Contending views on prejudice, discrimination and ethnoviolence* (pp. 120–124). Boulder, CO: Westview Press.

Pinfold, V., Huxley, P., Thornicroft, G., Farmer, P., Toulmin, H., & Graham, T. (2002). *Reducing psychiatric stigma and discrimination: Evaluating an education intervention with the police force in England.* Unpublished manuscript.

Pitschel-Walz, G., Leucht, S., Bäuml, J., Kissling, W., & Engel, R. R. (2001). The effect of family interventions on relapse and rehospitalization in schizophrenia: A meta-analysis. *Schizophrenia Bulletin, 27,* 73–92.

Platman, S. R. (1983). Family caretaking and expressed emotion: An evaluation. *Hospital and Community Psychiatry, 34,* 921–925.

Pogue-Geile, M. F. (1989). The prognostic significance of negative symptoms in schizophrenia. *British Journal of Psychiatry* (Suppl. 7), *162,* 123–127.

Polak, P., & Warner, R. (1996). The economic life of seriously mentally ill people in the community. *Psychiatric Services, 47,* 270–274.

Polak, P. R., & Kirby, M. W. (1976). A model to replace psychiatric hospitals. *Journal of Nervous and Mental Disease, 162,* 13–22.

Pompili, M., Girardi, P., Ruberto, A., & Tatarelli, R. (2004). Toward a new prevention of suicide in schizophrenia. *World Journal of Biological Psychiatry, 5,* 201–210.

Porter, J. R., & Washington, R. E. (1979). Black identity and self-esteem: A review of studies of black self-concept, 1968–1978. *Annual Review of Sociology, 5.*

Porterfield, J. K., Herbert-Jackson, E., & Risley, T. R. (1976). Contingent observation: An effective and acceptable procedure for reducing disruptive behavior of young children in a group setting. *Journal of Applied Behavior Analysis, 9,* 55–64.

Posey, T. B., & Losch, M. E. (1983). Auditory hallucinations of hearing voices in 375 normal subjects. *Imagination, Cognition and Personality, 3,* 99–113.

Posner, C., Wilson, K., Kral, M., Lander, S., & McIlwraith, R. (1992). Family psychoeducation support groups in schizophrenia. *American Journal of Orthopsychiatry, 62,* 206–218.

Posner, M. I., Nissen, M. J., & Klein, R. M. (1976). Visual dominance: An information-processing account of its origins and significance. *Psychological Review, 83*(2) 157–171.

Powell, G., Caan, W., & Crowe, M. (1994). What events precede violent incidents in psychiatric hospitals? *British Journal of Psychiatry, 165,* 107–112.

Powell, T. (1985). Improving the effectiveness of self-help. *Social Policy, 16,* 22–29.

Powell, T., Silk, K., & Albeck, J. (2000). Psychiatrist's referrals to self-help groups for people with mood disorders. *Psychiatric Services, 51,* 809–811.

Powell, T., Yeaton, W., Hill, E., & Silk, K. (2001). Predictors of psychosocial outcomes for patients with mood disorders: The effects of self-help group participation. *Psychiatric Rehabilitation Journal, 25,* 3–11.

Pratt, C. W., & Gill, K. J. (2001). Psychiatric rehabilitation education: A government, service provider, and academic collaboration. *Rehabilitation Education, 15,* 191–199.

Pratt, C. W., Gill, K. J., Barrett, N. M., & Roberts, M. M. (1999). *Psychiatric rehabilitation.* New York: Academic Press.

Pratt, C. W., Gill, K. J., Barrett, N. M., & Roberts, M. M. (2006). *Psychiatric rehabilitation* (2nd ed.). Burlington, MA: Elsevier Science & Technology.

Pratt, S. I., Bartels, S. J., Mueser, K. T., & Forester, B. (in press). Helping Older People Experience Success (HOPES): An Integrated Model of Psychosocial Rehabilitation and Health Care Management for Older Adults with Serious Mental Illness. *American Journal of Psychiatric Rehabilitation.*

Pratt, S. I., & Mueser, K. T. (2005). *Helping older people experience success: An integrated social and health care skills program for older persons with severe mental illness.* Concord: New Hampshire–Dartmouth Psychiatric Research Center.

Pratt, S. I., Mueser, K. T., Driscoll, M., Wolfe, R., & Bartels, S. J. (2006). Medication nonadherence in older people with serious mental illness: Prevalence and correlates. *Psychiatric Rehabilitation Journal, 29,* 299–310.

Pratt, S. I., Rosenberg, S. D., Mueser, K. T., Brancato, J., Salyers, M. P., Jankowski, M. K., et al. (2005). Evaluation of a PTSD psychoeducational program for psychiatric inpatients. *Journal of Mental Health, 14,* 121–127.

President's Commission on Mental Health (1978). *Report to the president.* Washington, DC, U.S. Government Printing Office.

President's New Freedom Commission on Mental Health. (2003). *Achieving the promise: Transforming mental health care in America. Final Report* (DHHS Publication No. SMA-03–3832). Rockville, MD: Substance Abuse and Mental Health Services Administration.

Press, A. N., Marty, D., & Rapp, C. A. (2003). *Consumer outcome monitoring package* (Kansas version with modifications for Indiana). Lawrence: University of Kansas. Retrieved June 30, 2007, from *research. socwel.ku.edu/ebp/*.

Priebe, S., Broker, M., & Gunkel, S. (1998). Involuntary admission and posttraumatic stress disorder symptoms in schizophrenia patients. *Comprehensive Psychiatry, 39*, 220–224.

Pritchard, M. (Ed.). (1995). *Dare to vision: Shaping the national agenda for women, abuse and mental health services.* Holyoke, MA: Human Rescource Association of the Northeast.

Prochaska, J. O., & Diclemente, C. C. (1984). *The transtheoretical approach: Crossing the traditional boundaries of therapy.* Homewood, IL: Dow-Jones/Irwin.

Propst, R. N. (1992). Standards for clubhouse programs: Why and how they were developed. *Psychosocial Rehabilitation Journal, 16*(2), 25–30.

Pruegger, V. J., & Rogers, T. B. (1994). Cross-cultural sensitivity training: Methods and assessment. *International Journal of Intercultural Relations, 18*, 369–387.

Pryce, I. (1982). An expanding "stage army" of long-stay psychiatric day-patients. *British Journal of Psychiatry, 141*, 595–601.

Pudlinski, C. (2001). Contrary themes on three peer-run warm lines. *Psychiatric Rehabilitation Journal, 24*, 397–400.

Pudlinski, C. (2004). The pros and cons of different warm line settings. *Psychiatric Rehabiltiation Journal, 28*, 72–74.

Quanbeck, C., Frye, M., & Altshuler, L. (2003). Mania and the law in California: Understanding the criminalization of the mentally ill. *American Journal of Psychiatry, 160*, 1245–1250.

Quimby, E., Drake, R. E., & Becker, D. R. (2001). Ethnographic findings from the Washington, DC, Vocational Services Study. *Psychiatric Rehabilitation Journal, 24*, 368–374.

Rabinowitz, J. C., Mandler, G., & Patterson, K. E. (1977). Determinants of recognition and recall: Accessibility and generation. *Journal of Experimental Psychology: General, 106* 302–329.

Rabkin, J. (1974). Public attitudes toward mental illness: A review of the literature. *Schizophrenia Bulletin, 10*, 9–33.

Rabkin, J. (1979). Criminal behavior of discharged mental patients: A critical appraisal of the research. *Psychological Bulletin, 86*, 1–27.

Raiff, N. (1982). Self-help participation and quality of life: A study of the staff of Recovery. *Prevention in the Human Services, 1*, 79–89.

Raiff, N. (1984). Some health related outcomes of self-help participation: Recovery, Inc. as a case example of a self help organization in mental health In A. Gardner & F. Reissman (Eds.), *The self-help revolution* (pp. 183–193). New York: Human Sciences Press.

Rajkumar, S., & Thara, R. (1989). Factors affecting relapse in schizophrenia. *Schizophrenia Research, 2*, 403–409.

Rakis, J., & Monroe, R. (1989). Monitoring and managing the suicidal prisoner. *Psychiatric Quarterly, 60*, 151–160.

Ralph, R. O. (1998). Recovery. In *Contribution to the Surgeon General's Report on Mental Health.* Portland: Edmund S. Muskie School of Public Service, University of Southern Maine.

Ralph, R. O. (2000). *Review of recovery literature: A synthesis of a sample of recovery literature 2000.* Portland: Edmund S. Muskie Institute of Public Affairs, University of Southern Maine.

Ralph, R. O. (2000). Recovery. *Psychiatric Rehabilitation Skills, 4*, 480–517.

Randolph, E. T. (1998). Social networks and schizophrenia. In K. T. Mueser & N. Tarrier (Eds.), *Handbook of social functioning in schizophrenia* (pp. 238–246). Boston: Allyn & Bacon.

Randolph, F., Blasinsky, M., Morrissey, J. P., Rosenheck, R. A., Cocozza, J., & Goldman, H. H. (2002). Overview of the ACCESS program. *Psychiatric Services, 53*, 945–948.

Randolph, F. L., Ridgway, P., Sanford, C., Simoneau, D., & Carling, P. J. (1988). *A national survey of community residential programs for persons with prolonged mental illness.* Burlington: Center for Community Change through Housing and Support, University of Vermont.

Rapp, C. A. (1993a). Theory, principles, and methods of the strengths model of case management. In M. Harris & H. Bergman (Eds.), *Case management for mentally ill patients* (pp.143–164). Langhorne, PA: Harwood.

Rapp, C. A. (1993b). Client-centered performance management for rehabilitation and mental health services. In R. W. Flexer & P. L. Solomon (Eds.), *Psychiatric rehabilitation in practice* (pp. 173–192). Boston: Andover.

Rapp, C. A. (1998a). The active ingredients of effective case management: A research synthesis. *Community Mental Health Journal, 34*, 363–380.

Rapp, C. A. (1998b). *The strengths model: Case management with people suffering from severe and persistent mental illness.* New York: Oxford University Press.

Rapp, C. A., Bond, G. R., Becker, D. R., Carpinello, S. E., Nikkel, R. E., & Gintoli, G. (2005). The role of state mental health authorities in promoting improved client outcome through evidence-based practice. *Community Mental Health Journal, 41*, 347–363.

Rapp, C. A., & Goscha, R. J. (2004). The principles of effective case management of mental health services. *Psychiatric Rehabilitation Journal, 27*, 319–333.

Rapp, C. A., & Goscha, R. J. (2005). What are the common features of evidence-based practices? In R. E. Drake, M. R. Merrens, & D. W. Lynde (Eds.), *Evidence-based mental health practice: A textbook* (pp. 189–215). New York: Norton.

Rapp, C. A., & Goscha, R. J. (2006). *The strengths model: Case management with people with psychiatric disabilities* (2nd ed.). New York: Oxford University Press.

Rapp, C. A., Huff, S., & Hansen, K. (2003). The New Hampshire financing policy. *Psychiatric Rehabilitation Journal, 26*, 385–391.

Rapp, C. A., & Poertner, J. (1992). *Social administration: A client-centered approach*. White Plains, NY: Longman.

Rappaport, J. (1987). Terms of empowerment/exemplars of prevention: Toward a theory for community psychology. *American Journal of Community Psychology, 15*, 121–148.

Rappaport, J. (1993). Narrative studies, personal stories, and identity transformation in the mutual help context. *Journal of Applied Behavioral Science, 29*, 239–256.

Rappaport, J., Seidman, E., Toro, P., McFadden, L., Reischl, T., Roberts, L., et al. (1985). Collaborative research with a self-help organization. *Social Policy, 15*, 12–24.

Rasanen, P., Tiihonen, J., Isohanni, M., Rantakallio, P., Lehttonen, J., & Moring, J. (1998). Schizophrenia, alcohol abuse, and violent behavior. A 26-year follow-up study of an unselected birth cohort. *Schizophrenia Bulletin, 24*, 437–441.

Razali, M. S., & Yahya, H. (1995). Compliance with treatment in schizophrenia: A drug intervention program in a developing country. *Acta Psychiatrica Scandinavica, 91*, 331–335.

Read, J. (1997). Child abuse and psychosis. *Professional Psychology: Research and Practice, 28*, 448–456.

Read, J., & Fraser, A. (1998). Staff responses to abuse histories of psychiatric inpatients. *Australian and New Zealand Journal of Psychiatry, 32*, 206–213.

Read, J., & Law, A. (1999). The relationship of causal beliefs and contact with users of mental health services to attitudes to the mentally ill. *International Journal of Social Psychiatry, 45*, 216–229.

Read, J., Perry, B. D., Moskowitz, A., & Connolly, J. (2001). The contribution of early traumatic events to schizophrenia in some patients: A traumagenic neurodevelopmental model. *Psychiatry, 64*, 319–345.

Read, J., van Os, J., Morrison, A. P., & Ross, C. A. (2005). Childhood trauma, psychosis and schizophrenia: A literature review with theoretical and clinical implications. *Acta Psychiatrica Scandinavica, 112*, 330–350.

Rector, N. A., & Beck, A. T. (2001). Cognitive behavioral therapy for schizophrenia: An empirical review. *Journal of Nervous and Mental Disease, 189*, 278–287.

Redko, C., Durbin, J., Wasylenki, D., & Krupa, T. (2004). Participant perspectives of satisfaction with assertive community treatment. *Psychiatric Rehabilitation Journal, 27*, 283–286.

Reiger, D. A., Boyd, J. H., Burke, J. D., Jr., Rae, D. S., Myers, J. K., Kramer, M., et al. (1988). One-month prevalence of mental disorders in the United States based on five Epidemiologic Catchment Area sites. *Archives of General Psychiatry, 45*, 977–986.

Regier, D. A., Farmer, M. E., Rae, D. S., Locke, B. Z., Keith, S. J., Judd, L. L., et al. (1990). Comorbidity of mental disorders with alcohol and other drug abuse: Results from the Epidemiologic Catchment Area (ECA) study. *Journal of the American Medical Association, 264*, 2511–2518.

Regier, D. A., Narrow, W. E., Rae, D. S., Manderscheid, R. W., Locke, B. Z., & Goodwin, F. K. (1993). The de facto US mental and addictive disorders service system: Epidemiologic Catchment Area prospective 1-year prevalence rates of disorders and services. *Archives of General Psychiatry, 50*, 85–94.

Reid, D. H., & Parsons, M. B. (2000). Organizational behavior management in human service settings. In J. Austin & J. E. Carr (Eds.), *Handbook of applied behavior analysis* (pp. 275–294). Reno, NV: Context Press.

Reinhard, S. (1994). Burden assessment scale for families of the seriously mentally ill. *Evaluation and Program Planning, 17* 261–269.

Reinke, R., & Corrigan, P. W. (2002). *Examining media's use of contact on the stigma of mental illness*. Unpublished manuscript.

Reitan, R. M., & Wolfson, D. (1993). *The Halstead-Reitan Neuropsychological Test Battery: Theory and clinical interpretation*. Tucson, AZ: Neuropsychology Press.

Resick, P. A., & Schnicke, M. K. (1993). *Cognitive processing therapy for rape victims: A treatment manual*. Newbury Park, CA: Sage.

Resnick, H. S., Kilpatrick, D. G., Dansky, B. S., Saunders, B. E., & Best, C. E. (1993). Prevalence of civilian trauma and post-traumatic stress disorder in a representative national sample of women. *Journal of Consulting and Clinical Psychology, 61,* 984–991.

Resnick, S. G., Armstrong, M., Sperrazza, M., Harkness, L., & Rosenheck, R. A. (2004). A model of consumer–provider partnership: Vet-to-vet. *Psychiatric Rehabilitation Journal, 28,* 185–187.

Resnick, S. G., Bond, G. R., & Mueser, K. T. (2003). Trauma and posttraumatic stress disorder in people with schizophrenia. *Journal of Abnormal Psychology, 112,* 415–423.

Richardson, C. R., Faulkner, G., McDevitt, J., Skrinar, G. S., Hutchinson, D. S., & Piette, J. D. (2005). Integrating physical activity into mental health services for persons with serious mental illness. *Psychiatric Services, 56,* 324–331.

Ridgely, M. S., Osher, F. C., Goldman, H. H., & Talbott, J. A. (1987). *Chronic mentally ill young adults with substance abuse problems: A review of research, treatment, and training issues.* Baltimore: University of Maryland Press.

Ridgway, P., & Rapp, C. A. (1997). *The active ingredients of effective supported housing: A research synthesis.* Lawrence: University of Kansas School of Social Welfare.

Ridgway, P., & Zipple, A. M. (1990). The paradigm shift in residential services: From the linear continuum to supported housing approaches. *Psychosocial Rehabilitation Journal, 13*(4), 11–31.

Rielly, J., Rohrbough, M., & Lackner, J. (1988). A controlled evaluation of psychoeducation workshops for relatives of state hospital patients. *Journal of Marital and Family Therapy, 14,* 429–432.

Ries, R. K., & Comtois, K. A. (1997). Managing disability benefits as part of treatment for persons with severe mental illness and comorbid drug/alcohol disorders. *American Journal of Addictions, 6,* 330–337.

Ries, R. K., Dyck, D. G., Short, R., Srebnik, D., Fisher, A., & Comtois, K. A. (2004). Outcomes of managing disability benefits among patients with substance dependence and severe mental illness. *Psychiatric Services, 55,* 445–447.

Riessman, C. K. (2000). Stigma and everyday resistance practices: Childless women in South India. *Gender and Society, 14*(1), 111.

Riessman, F. (1965). The "helper therapy principle." *Social Work, 10,* 27–32.

Riggs, R. T. (1996). HMOs and the seriously mentally ill: A view from the trenches. *Community Mental Health Journal, 32,* 213–218.

Rimmerman, A., & Keren, N. (1995). Letting go: Patient attitudes toward out-of-home placement

of their children with psychiatric disability. *Psychiatric Rehabilitation Journal, 19,* 3–8.

Rinaldi, M., McNeil, K., Firn, M., Koletsi, M., Perkins, R., & Singh, S. P. (2004). What are the benefits of evidence-based supported employment for patients with first-episode psychosis? *Psychiatric Bulletin, 28,* 281–284.

Ring, N., Tantam, D., Montague, L., Newby, D., Black, D., & Morris, J. (1991). Gender differences in the incidence of definite schizophrenia and atypical psychosis: Focus on negative symptoms of schizophrenia. *Acta Psychiatrica Scandinavica, 84*(6), 489–496.

Roach, J. (1993). Clinical case management with severely mentally ill adults. In M. Harris & H. Bergman (Eds.), *Case management for mentally ill* (pp. 17–40). Langhorne, PA: Harwood.

Roberts, L. J., Salem, D., Rappaport, J., Toro, P. A., Luke, D. A., & Seidman, E. (1999). Giving and receiving help: Interpersonal transactions in mutual-help meetings and psychosocial adjustment of members. *American Journal of Community Psychology, 27,* 841–868.

Roberts, L. J., Shaner, A., & Eckman, T. A. (1999). *Overcoming addictions: Skills training for people with schizophrenia.* New York: Norton.

Robertson, G., Pearson, R., & Gibb, R. (1996). The entry of mentally disordered people to the criminal justice system. *British Journal of Psychiatry, 169,* 172–180.

Robertson, M. J. (1992). The prevalence of mental disorder among homeless people. In R. I. Jahiel (Ed.), *Homelessness: A preventative approach* (pp. 57–86). Baltimore: Johns Hopkins University Press.

Robins, C. S., Sauvageot, J. A., Cusack, K. J., Suffoletta-Maierle, S., & Frueh, B. C. (2005). Consumers' perceptions of negative experiences and "sanctuary harm" in psychiatric settings. *Psychiatric Services, 56,* 1134–1138.

Robins, L. N. (1966). *Deviant children grown up.* Huntington, NY: Robert E. Krieger.

Robins, L. N. (1978). Psychiatric epidemiology. *Archives of General Psychiatry, 35*(6), 697–702.

Robins, L. N. (1995). *Diagnostic Interview Schedule, Version IV.* St. Louis: Washington University School of Medicine.

Robins, L. N., Helzer, J. E., Croughan, J., & Ratcliff, K. S. (1981). National Institute of Mental Helath Diagnsotic Interview Schedule: Its history, characteristics, and validity. *Archives of General Psychiatry, 38,* 381–389.

Roder, V., Mueller, D. R., Mueser, K. T., & Brenner, H. D. (2006). Integrated psychological therapy (IPT) for schizophrenia: Is it effective? *Schizophrenia Bulletin, 32,* S81–S93.

Roe, D. (2001). Progressing from patienthood to

personhood across the multidimensional outcomes in schizophrenia and related disorders. *Journal of Nervous and Mental Disease, 189,* 691–699.

Rog, D. J. (2004). The evidence on supported housing. *Psychiatric Rehabilitation Journal, 27,* 334–344.

Rog, D. J., & Raush, H. L. (1975). The psychiatric halfway house: How is it measuring up? *Community Mental Health Journal, 11,* 155–162.

Rogers, E., Anthony, W. A., Toole, J., & Brown, M. A. (1991a). Vocational outcomes following psychosocial rehabilitation: A longitudinal study of three programs. *Journal of Vocational Rehabilitation, 1*(3), 21–29.

Rogers, E. S., Chamberlin, J., Ellison, M., & Crean, T. (1997a). A consumer-constructed scale to measure empowerment. *Psychiatric Services, 48,* 1042–1047.

Rogers, E. S., Walsh, D., Masotta, L., & Danley, K. (1991b). *Massachusetts survey of client preferences for community support services: Final report.* Boston: Center for Psychiatric Rehabilitation.

Rogers, J. A. (1995). Work is key to recovery. *Psychosocial Rehabilitation Journal, 18,* 5–10.

Rogers, R. (2001). *Handbook of diagnostic and structured interviewing.* New York: Guilford Press.

Rogers, S. E., Anthony, W. A., Cohen, M., & Davies, R. R. (1997b). Prediction of vocational outcome based on clinical and demographic indicators among vocationally ready clients. *Community Mental Health Journal, 33*(2), 99–113.

Rogler, L. H. (1999). Methodological sources of cultural insensitivity in mental health research. *American Psychologist, 54,* 424–433.

Roman, P., & Floyd, H. (1981). Social acceptance of psychiatric illness and psychiatric treatment. *Social Psychiatry, 16,* 16–21.

Romans, S., Belaise, C., Martin, J., Morris, E., & Raffi, A. (2002). Childhood abuse and later medical disorders in women: An epidemiological study. *Psychotherapy and Psychosomatics, 71,* 141–150.

Rose, L. (1996). Families of psychiatric patients: A critical review and future research directions. *Archives of Psychiatric Nursing, 10,* 67–76.

Rose, S. M., Peabody, C. G., & Stratigeas, B. (1991). Undetected abuse among intensive case management clients. *Hospital and Community Psychiatry, 42,* 499–503.

Rosen, A., Hadzi-Pavlovic, D., & Parker, G. (1989). The Life Skills Profile: A measure assessing function and disability in schizophrenia. *Schizophrenia Bulletin, 15,* 325–337.

Rosenberg, M. (1965). *Society and the adolescent self image.* Princeton, NJ: Princeton University Press.

Rosenberg, S. D., Brunette, M. F., Oxman, T. E., Marsh, B. J., Dietrich, A., Mueser, K. T., et al. (2004b). The STIRR model of best practices for blood-borne diseases among clients with serious mental illness. *Psychiatric Services, 55,* 660–664.

Rosenberg, S. D., Drake, R. E., Wolford, G. L., Mueser, K. T., Oxman, T. E., Vidaver, R. M., et al. (1998). Dartmouth Assessment of Lifestyle Instrument (DALI): A substance use disorder screen for people with severe mental illness. *American Journal of Psychiatry, 155,* 232–238.

Rosenberg, S. D., Goodman, L. A., Osher, F. C., Swartz, M. S., Essock, S. M., Butterfield, M. I., et al. (2001a). Prevalence of HIV, hepatitis B, and hepatitis C in people with severe mental illness. *American Journal of Public Health, 91*(1), 31–37.

Rosenberg, S. D., Mueser, K. T., Friedman, M. J., Gorman, P. G., Drake, R. E., Vidaver, R. M., et al. (2001b). Developing effective treatments for post-traumatic disorders: A review and proposal. *Psychiatric Services, 52,* 1453–1461.

Rosenberg, S. D., Mueser, K. T., Jankowski, M. K., Salyers, M. P., & Acker, K. (2004a). Cognitive-behavioral treatment of posttraumatic stress disorder in severe mental illness: Results of a pilot study. *American Journal of Psychiatric Rehabilitation, 7,* 171–186.

Rosenfield, S. (1992). Factors contributing to the subjective quality of life of the chronic mentally ill. *Journal of Health and Social Behavior, 33,* 299–315.

Rosenheck, R. (2005). *Mental health and substance abuse services for veterans: Experience with performance evaluation in the Department of Veterans Affairs.* West Haven, CT: VA Northeast Program Evaluation Center.

Rosenheck, R., & Neale, M. (2004). Therapeutic limit setting and six month outcomes in a Veterans Affairs assertive community treatment program. *Psychiatric Services, 55,* 139–144.

Rosenheck, R., Neale, M., Leaf, P., Milstein, R., & Frisman, L. (1995). Multisite experimental cost study of intensive psychiatric community care. *Schizophrenia Bulletin, 21,* 129–140.

Rosenheck, R. A., Lam, J., Morrissey, J. P., Calloway, M. O., Stolar, M., & Randolph, F. (2002). Service systems integration and outcomes for mentally ill homeless persons in the ACCESS program. *Psychiatric Services, 53,* 958–966.

Rosenstock, I. M. (1975). Patients' compliance with health regimens. *Journal of the American Medical Association, 234,* 402–403.

Rosie, J. S. (1987). Partial hospitalization: A review of recent literature. *Hospital and Community Psychiatry, 38,* 1291–1299.

Ross, C. A., Anderson, G., & Clark, P. (1994). Childhood abuse and the positive symptoms of schizophrenia. *Hospital and Community Psychiatry, 45,* 489–491.

Rounsaville, B. J., Carroll, K. M., & Onken, L. S. (2001). A stage model of behavioral therapies research: Getting started and moving on from stage I. *Clinical Psychology: Science and Practice, 8,* 133–142.

Rubin, A. (1992). Is case management effective for people with severe mental illness? A research review. *Health and Social Work, 17,* 138–150.

Rubin, A., Cardenas, J., Warren, K., Pike, C., & Wambach, K. (1998). Outdated practitioner views about family culpability and severe mental disorders. *Social Work, 43,* 412–422.

Rubin, S. E., & Roessler, R. T. (2001). *Foundations of the vocational rehabilitation process* (5th ed.). Austin, TX: PRO-ED.

Rubinstein, D. (1994). The social construction of opportunity. *Journal of Socio-Economics, 23,* 61–79.

Rund, B. R., & Borg, N. E. (1999). Cognitive deficits and cognitive training in schizophrenic patients: A review. *Acta Psychiatrica Scandinavica, 100,* 85–95.

Rupp, K., & Bell, S. H. (2003). *Paying for results in vocational rehabilitation: Will provider incentives work for Ticket to Work?* Washington, DC: Urban Institute.

Rupp, K., & Scott, C. G. (1996). Trends in the characteristics of DI and SSI disability awardees and duration of program participation. *Social Security Bulletin, 59,* 3–21.

Rupp, K., & Scott, C. (1998). Determinants of duration on the disability rolls and program trends. In K. Rupp & D. Stapleton (Eds.), *Growth in income entitlement benefits for disability: Explanations and policy implications.* Kalamazoo, MI: Upjohn Institute.

Ruscher, S. M., de Wit, R., & Mazmanian, D. (1997). Psychiatric patients' attitudes about medication and factors affecting noncompliance. *Psychiatric Services, 48,* 82–85.

Rush, A. J., Rago, W. V., Crismon, M. L., Toprac, M. G., Shon, S. P., Suppes, T., et al. (1999). Medication treatment for the severely and persistently mentally ill: The Texas Medication Algorithm Project. *Journal of Clinical Psychiatry, 60,* 284–291.

Rutman, I. D. (1987). The psychosocial rehabilitation movement in the United States. In A. T. Meyerson & T. Fine (Eds.), *Psychiatric disability: Clinical, legal, and administrative dimensions* (pp. 197–220). Washington, DC: American Psychiatric Association.

Rutman, I. D. (1993). And now, the envelope please . . . *Psychosocial Rehabilitation Journal, 16*(3), 1–3.

Rutman, I. D. (1997). What is psychiatric rehabilitation? In R. Hughes & D. Weinstein (Eds.), *Best practices in psychosocial rehabilitation* (pp. 4–8). Columbia, MD: International Association of Psychosocial Rehabilitation.

Ryan, M. C., & Thakore, J. H. (2002). Physical consequences of schizophrenia: The metabolic syndrome. *Life Sciences, 71,* 239–257.

Sabin, J. E., & Daniels, N. (2003). Strengthening the consumer voice in managed care: VII. The Georgia peer specialist program. *Psychiatric Services, 54,* 497–498.

Sackett, D. L., Richardson, W. S., Rosenberg, W., & Haynes, R. B. (1997). *Evidence-based medicine.* New York: Churchill Livingstone.

Sacks, F. M. (2004). Metabolic syndrome: Epidemiology and consequences. *Journal of Clinical Psychiatry, 65*(Suppl. 18), 3–12.

Sacks, S. (1997). *Final report: Therapeutic community-oriented supported housing for MICAs.* New York: Center for Therapeutic Community Research.

Sacks, S., Sacks, J. Y., McKendrick, K., Banks, S. M., & Stommel, J. (2004). Modified therapeutic community for MICA offenders: Crime outcomes. *Behavioral Sciences and the Law, 22,* 477–501.

Sajatovic, M., Davies, M., & Hrouda, D. R. (2004). Enhancement of treatment adherence among patients with bipolar disorder. *Psychiatric Services, 55,* 264–269.

Saks, E. R. (2002). *Refusing care: Forced treatment and the rights of the mentally ill.* Chicago: University of Chicago Press.

Salter, A. (1949). *Conditioned reflex therapy.* New York: Farrar, Strauss.

Salyers, H., Masterton, T., Fekete, D., Picone, J., & Bond, G. (1998). Transferring clients from intensive case management: Impact on client functioning. *American Journal of Orthopsychiatry, 68,* 233–245.

Salzer, M., & Mental Health Association of Southeastern Pennsylvania Best Practices Team. (2002). Consumer delivered services as a best practice in mental health care delivery and the development of practice guidelines. *Psychiatric Rehabilitation Skills, 6,* 355–382.

Salyers, M., & Mueser, K. T. (2001). Social functioning, psychopathology, and medication side effects in relation to substance use and abuse in schizophrenia. *Schizophrenia Research, 48,* 109–123.

Salzer, M., Rappaport, J., & Segre, L. (2001). Mental health professionals support of self help groups. *Journal of Community and Applied Social Psychology, 11*, 1–10.

Salzer, M., & Shear, L. (2002). Identifying consumer-provider benefits in evaluations of consumer-delivered services. *Psychiatric Rehabilitation Journal, 25*, 281–288.

Salyers, M. P., Becker, D. R., Drake, R. E., Torrey, W. C., & Wyzik, P. F. (2004a). Ten-year follow-up of a supported employment program. *Psychiatric Services, 55*, 302–308.

Salyers, M. P., Evans, L. J., Bond, G. R., & Meyer, P. S. (2004b). Barriers to assessment and treatment of posttraumatic stress disorder and other trauma-related problems in people with severe mental illness: Clinician perspectives. *Community Mental Health Journal, 40*, 17–31.

Salyers, M. P., Godfrey, J. L., Mueser, K. T., & Labriola, S. (in press). Measuring illness management outcomes: A psychometric study of clinician and consumer rating scales for illness self-management and recovery. *Community Mental Health Journal.*

Sands, R. (1995). The parenting experience of low-income single women with serious mental disorders. *Families in Society, 76*, 86–96.

Sands, R. (2001). *Clinical social work practice in behavioral mental health*. Boston: Allyn & Bacon.

Sands, R., Koppelmon, N., & Solomon, P. (2004). Maternal custody status and living arrangements of children of women with severe mental illness. *Health and Social Work, 29*, 317–325.

Sanguineti, V., Samuel, S., Schwartz, S., & Robeson, M. (1999). Retrospective study of 2,200 involuntary psychiatric admissions and readmissions. *American Journal of Psychiatry, 153*, 392–396.

Sarason, I., Levine, H., Basham, R., & Sarason, B. (1983). Assessing social support: The social support questionnaire. *Journal of Personality and Social Psychology, 44*, 127–139.

Sautter, F. J., Brailey, K., Uddo, M. M., Hamilton, M. F., Beard, M. G., & Borges, A. H. (1999). PTSD and comorbid psychotic disorder: Comparison of veterans diagnosed with PTSD or psychotic disorder. *Journal of Traumatic Stress, 12*, 73–88.

Sautter, F. J., Cornwell, J., Johnson, J. J., Wiley, J., & Faraone, S. V. (2002). Family history study of posttraumatic stress disorder with secondary psychotic symptoms. *American Journal of Psychiatry, 159*, 1775–1777.

Sayers, S. L., Curran, P. J., & Mueser, K. T. (1996). Factor structure and construct validity of the Scale for the Assessment of Negative Symptoms. *Psychological Assessment, 8*, 269–280.

Schaedle, R., & Epstein, I. (2000). Specifying intensive case management: A multiple stakeholder approach. *Mental Health Services Research, 2*, 95–105.

Schaefer, N., & Stefancic, A. (2003). "Alternative to prison" programs for the mentally ill offender. *Journal of Offender Rehabilitation, 38*, 41–55.

Schatzberg, A. F., Cole, J. O., & DeBattista, C. (2007). *Manual of clinical psychopharmacology* (6th ed.). Washington, DC: American Psychiatric Press.

Schatzberg, A. F., & Nemeroff, C. B. (Eds.). (1998). *American Psychiatric Press Textbook of Psychopharmacology* (2nd ed.). Washington, DC: American Psychiatric Press.

Schatzberg, A. F., & Nemeroff, C. B. (Eds.). (2001). *Essentials of clinical psychopharmacology*. Washington, DC: American Psychiatric Press.

Scheel, K. R. (2000). The empirical basis of dialectical behavior therapy: Summary, critique, and implications. *Clinical Psychology Science and Practice, 7*, 68–86.

Scheff, T. (1974). The labelling theory of mental illness. *American Sociological Review, 39*, 444–452.

Scheff, T. J. (1966). Users and non-users of a student psychiatric clinic. *Journal of Health and Human Behavior, 7*, 114–121.

Scheff, T. J. (1972). Decision rules, types of error and their consequences in medical diagnosis. In E. Freidson & J. Lorber (Eds.), *Medical men and their work* (pp. 296–305). Chicago: Aldine-Atherton.

Scheff, T. J. (Ed.). (1975). *Labeling madness*. Oxford, UK: Prentice-Hall.

Scheffler, R., & Miller, A. (1989). Demand analysis of mental health service use among ethnic subpopulations. *Inquiry, 26*, 202–215.

Scheffler, R. M., & Adams, N. (2005, May 3). Millionaires and mental health: Proposition 63 in California. *Health Affairs Web Exclusive* (10.1377/hlthaff.w5.212).

Scheifler, P. L. (2000). *Team Solutions: A comprehensive psychoeducational program designed to help you educate your clients with schizophrenia* (Instructors' Guide and Patient Workbooks). Indianapolis: Eli Lilly and Company.

Schenkel, L. S., Spaulding, W. D., DiLillo, D., & Silverstein, S. M. (2005). Histories of childhood maltreatment in schizophrenia: Relationships with premorbid functioning, symptomatology, and cognitive deficits. *Schizophrenia Research, 76*, 273–286.

Schiraldi, G. R. (2000). *The post-traumatic stress disorder sourcebook: A guide to healing, recovery, and growth.* Los Angeles: Lowell House.

Schmidt, L. (2005). *Comparison of services outcomes of case management teams with and without a consumer provider.* Unpublished doctoral dissertation, Univeristy of Medicine and Dentistry of New Jersey.

Schmook, A. (2000). *Prosumers as PSR staff: Recruitment, hiring, supervision and supports: Hiring qualified people with mental health consumer experience.* Illinois Department of Human Services, Office of Mental Health. Retrieved November 3, 2003, from *www. State.il.u.s./agency/dhs/mental health_pdf.chapter.PDF.*

Schnapp, W., & Cannedy, R. (1998). Offenders with mental illness: Mental health and criminal justice best practices. *Administration and Policy in Mental Health, 25,* 463–466.

Schneider, B., Scissons, H., Arney, L., Benson, G., Derry, J., Lucas, K., et al. (2004). Communication between people with schizophrenia and their medical professionals: A participatory research project. *Qualitative Health Research, 14,* 562–577.

Schneider, K. (1959). *Clinical psychopathology* (5th ed.). (M. W. Hamilton, Trans.). New York: Grune and Stratton.

Schneider, L. C., & Struening, E. L. (1983). SLOF: A behavioral rating scale for assessing the mentally ill. *Social Work Research and Abstracts, 19*(3), 9–21.

Schneider, W., & Shiffrin, R. M. (1977). Controlled and automatic human information processing: I. Detection, search, and attention. *Psychological Review, 84,* 1–66.

Schnurr, P. P., Vielhauer, M. J., Weathers, F., & Findler, M. (1999). *Brief Trauma Questionnaire.* White River Junction, VT: National Center for PTSD.

Schooler, N., Hogarty, G., & Weissman, M. (1979). Social Adjustment Scale II (SAS-II). In W. A. Hargreaves, C. C. Atkisson, & J. E. Sorenson (Eds.), *Resource materials for community mental health program evaluations* (pp. 290–303). Rockville, MD: National Institute of Mental Health.

Schreiber, J. L., Breier, A., & Pickar, D. (1995). Expressed emotion: Trait or state? *British Journal of Psychiatry, 166*(5), 647–649.

Schubert, M., & Borkman, T. (1991). An organizational typology for self-help groups. *American Journal of Community Psychology, 19,* 769–787.

Schubert, M., & Borkman, T. (1994). Identifying the experiential knowledge developed within a self-help group. In T. Powell (Ed.), *Understanding the self-help organization* (pp. 227–247). Thousand Oaks, CA: Sage.

Schuckit, M., Herman, G., & Schuckit, J. (1977). The importance of psychiatric illness in newly arrested prisoners. *Journal of Nervous and Mental Disease, 165,* 118–125.

Schutt, R. K., Weinstein, B., & Penk, W. E. (2005). Housing preferences of homeless veterans with dual diagnoses. *Psychiatric Services, 56,* 350–352.

Schwab, B., Drake, R. E., & Burghardt, E. M. (1988). Health care of the chronically mentally ill: The culture broker model. *Community Mental Health Journal, 24,* 174–184.

Scott, J., & Dixon, L. (1995). Assertive community treatment and case management of schizophrenia. *Schizophrenia Bulletin, 21,* 657–668.

Scott, J., Garland, A., & Moorhead, S. (2001). A pilot study of cognitive therapy in bipolar disorders. *Psychological Medicine, 31,* 459–467.

Scott, J., Paykel, E. S., Morriss, R., Bentall, R. P., Kinderman, P., Johnson, T., et al. (2006). Cognitive-behavioural therapy for severe and recurrent bipolar disorders. *British Journal of Psychiatry, 188,* 313–320.

Scott, R. (2000). Evaluation of a mobile crisis program: Effectiveness, efficiency, and consumer satisfaction. *Psychiatric Services, 51,* 1153–1156.

Scott, R. W. (1995). *Institutions and organizations.* Thousand Oaks, CA: Sage.

Sechrest, L., & Pion, G. (1990). Developing cross-discipline measures of clinical competencies in diagnosis, treatment, and case management. In D. L. Johnson (Ed.), *Service needs of the seriously mentally ill: Training implications for psychology* (pp. 29–31). Washington, DC: American Psychological Association.

Segal, S. (1995). Characteristics and service base of long-term members of self-help agencies for mental health clients. *Psychiatric Services, 46,* 269–274.

Segal, S. P., & Aviram, U. (1978). *The mentally ill in community-based sheltered care: A study of community care and social integration.* New York: Wiley.

Segal, S. P., Baumohl, J., & Moyles, E. W. (1980). Neighborhood types and community reaction to the mentally ill: A paradox of intensity. *Journal of Health and Social Behavior, 21,* 345–359.

Segal, S. P., & Kotler, P. L. (1993). Sheltered care residence: Ten-year personal outcomes. *American Journal of Orthopsychiatry, 63,* 80–91.

Segal, S. P., Silverman, C., & Temkin, T. (1995). Characteristics and service use of long-term members of self-help agencies for mental health clients. *Psychiatric Services, 46,* 269–274.

Sells, D. J., Rowe, M., Fisk, D., & Davidson, L. (2003). Violent victimization of persons with co-occurring psychiatric and substance use disorders. *Psychiatric Services, 54*, 1253–1257.

Sellwood, W., Tarrier, N., Quinn, J., & Barrowclough, C. (2003). The family and compliance in schizophrenia: The influence of clinical variables, relatives' knowledge and expressed emotion. *Psychological Medicine, 33*, 91–96.

Seltzer, M., Greenberg, J., Floyd, F., & Hong, J. (2004). Accommodating coping and wellbeing of midlife parents of children with mental health problems or developmental disabilities. *American Journal of Orthopsychiatry, 74*, 187–195.

Selzer, M. L. (1971). The Michigan Alcoholism Screening Test: The quest for a new diagnostic instrument. *American Journal of Psychiatry, 127*, 1653–1658.

Semke, J., Fisher, W. H., Goldman, H. H., & Hirad, A. (1996). The evolving role of the state hospital in the care and treatment of older adults: State trends, 1984 to 1993. *Psychiatric Services, 47*(10), 1082–1087.

Sengupta, A., Drake, R. E., & McHugo, G. J. (1998). The relationship between substance use disorder and vocational functioning among persons with severe mental illness. *Psychiatric Rehabilitation Journal, 22*, 41–45.

Shadish, W. R., & Bootzin, R. R. (1981). Nursing homes and chronic mental patients. *Schizophrenia Bulletin, 7*, 488–498.

Shafer, M., Arthur, B., & Franczak, M. (2004). An analysis of post-booking jail diversion programming for persons with co-occurring disorders. *Behavioral Sciences and the Law, 22*, 771–785.

Shain, R., & Phillips, J. (1991). The stigma of mental illness: Labeling and stereotyping in the news. In L. Wilkins & P. Patterson (Eds.), *Risky business: Communicating issues of science, risk, and public policy* (pp. 61–74). New York: Greenwood Press.

Shaner, A., Eckman, T. A., Roberts, L. J., Wilkins, J. N., Tucker, D. E., Tsuang, J. W., et al. (1995). Disability income, cocaine use, and repeated hospitalization among schizophrenic cocaine abusers—A government-sponsored revolving door? *New England Journal of Medicine, 333*, 777–783.

Shaner, A., & Eth, S. (1989). Can schizophrenia cause posttraumatic stress disorder? *American Journal of Psychotherapy, 43*, 588–597.

Shaner, A., Roberts, L. J., Eckman, T. A., Tucker, D. E., Tsuang, J. W., Wilkins, J. N., et al. (1997). Monetary reinforcement of abstinence from cocaine among mentally ill patients with cocaine dependence. *Psychiatric Services, 48*, 807–810.

Shapiro, F. (1995). *Eye movement desensitization and reprocessing: Basic principles, protocols, and procedures.* New York: Guilford Press.

Sharfstein, S. S. (2000). Whatever happened to community mental health? *Psychiatric Services, 51*, 616–620.

Shea, S. C. (1988). *Psychiatric interviewing: The art of understanding.* Philadelphia: W. B. Saunders.

Sheehan, D. V., Lecrubier, Y., Sheehan, K. H., Amorim, P., Janavis, J., Weiller, E., et al. (1998). The Mini-International NeuropsychiatricInterview (M.I.N.I): The development and validation of a structured diagnostic psychiatric interview for DSM-IV and ICD 10. *Journal of Clinical Psychiatry, 59*(Suppl. 20), 22–33.

Sheline, Y. I., & Nelson, T. (1993). Patient choice: Deciding between psychotropic medication and physical restraints in an emergency. *Bulletin of the American Academy of Psychiatry and the Law, 21*, 321–329.

Shelton, R., & Ressmeyer, D. (1991). Involving consumers in the discharge process. *Psychosocial Rehabilitation Journal, 12*, 19–28.

Shepherd, M., & Lavender, T. (1999). Putting aggression into context: An investigation into contextual factors influencing the rate of aggressive incidents in a psychiatric hospital. *Journal of Mental Health, 8*, 159–170.

Sherer, M., & Adams, C. H. (1983). Construct validation of the Self-efficacy Scale. *Psychological Reports, 53*, 899–902.

Sherman, P., & Porter, R. (1991). Mental health consumers as case management aides. *Hospital and Community Psyhiatry, 42*, 494–498.

Shern, D., Surles, R., & Wiazer, J. (1989). Designing community treatment systems for the most seriously mentally ill: A state administrative perspective. *Journal of Social Issues, 45*, 105–117.

Shern, D. L., Felton, C. J., Hough, R. L., Lehman, A. F., Goldfinger, S., Valencia, E., et al. (1997). Housing outcomes for homeless adults with mental illness: Results from the second-round McKinney program. *Psychiatric Services, 48*, 239–241.

Shern, D. L., Tsemberis, S., Anthony, W. A., Lovell, A. M., Richmond, L., Felton, C. J., et al. (2000). Serving street-dwelling individuals with psychiatric disabilities: Outcomes of a psychiatric rehabilitation clinical trial. *American Journal of Public Health, 90*, 1873–1878.

Shore, J. H. (1996). Psychiatry at a crossroad: Our role in primary care. *American Journal of Psychiatry, 153*, 1398–1403.

Shurka, E. (1983). The evaluation of ex-mental patients by other ex-mental patients. *Interna-*

tional Journal of Social Psychology, 29, 286–291.

Siegel, C. (2002). Statement on cultural competence. In R. E. Drake (Ed.), *Evidence-based practices implementation resource kits.* Retrieved January 15, 2006, from *www.mentalhealth.samhsa.gov/cmhs/communitysupport/toolkits/.*

Siegel, C., Haugland, G., & Schore, R. (2005). The interface of cultural competency and evidence-based practices. In R. E. Drake, M. R. Merrens, & D. W. Lynde (Eds.), *Evidence-based mental health practice: A textbook* (pp. 273–299). New York: Norton.

Sigmon, S., Steingard, S., Badger, G. J., Anthony, S. L., & Higgins, S. T. (2000). Contingent reinforcement of marijuana abstinence among individuals with serious mental illness: A feasibility study. *Experimental and Clinical Psychopharmacology, 8*, 509–517.

Signorelli, N. (1989). Television and conceptions about sex roles: Maintaining conventionality and the status quo. *Sex Roles, 21*, 341–360.

Sigurdson, C. (2000). The mad, the bad, and the abandoned: The mentally ill in prisons and jails. *Corrections Today, 62*(7), 70–78.

Silberberg, J., Vital, T., & Brakel, J. (2001). Breaking down barriers to mandated outpatient treatment for mentally ill offenders. *Psychiatric Annals, 31*, 433–440.

Silver, J. M., & Yudofsky, S. C. (1987). Documentation of aggression in the assessment of the violent patient. *Psychiatric Annals, 17*, 375–384.

Silver, T. (2004). Staff in mental health agencies: Coping with the dual challenges as providers with psychiatric disabilities. *Psychiatric Rehabilitation Journal, 28*, 165–171.

Silverman, E. K., Lu, F., & O'Neill, P. (1994). Developing a primary care role for psychiatrists. *Bulletin of the Association for Academic Psychiatry, 22*, 4A.

Silverstein, S. M., Hitzel, H., & Schenkel, L. (1998). Identifying and addressing cognitive barriers to rehabilitation readiness. *Psychiatric Services, 49*, 34–36.

Silverstein, S. M., Menditto, A. A., & Stuve, P. (1999). Shaping procedures as cognitive retraining techniques in individuals with severe and persistent mental illness. *Psychiatric Rehabilitation Skills, 3*, 59–76.

Silverstein, S. M., Menditto, A. A., & Stuve, P. (2001). Shaping attention span: An operant conditioning procedure to improve neurocognition and functioning in schizophrenia. *Schizophrenia Bulletin, 27*, 247–257.

Silverstein, S. M., Schenkel, L. S., Valone, C., & Nuernberger, S. W. (1998). Cognitive deficits and psychiatric rehabilitation outcomes in schizophrenia. *Psychiatric Quarterly, 69*, 169–191.

Simmonds, S., Coid, J., Philip, J., Marriott, S., & Tyrer, P. (2001). Community mental health team management in severe mental illness: A systematic review. *British Journal of Psychiatry, 178*, 497–502.

Simpson, G. M., & Angus, J. W. S. (1970). A rating scale for extrapyramidal side effects. *Acta Psychiatrica Scandinavica, 212*(Suppl.), 11–19.

Simpson, J. C., & Tsuang, M. T. (1996). Mortality among patients with schizophrenia. *Schizophrenia Bulletin, 22*, 485–499.

Singh, N. N., Singh, S. D., Davis, C. M., Latham, L. L., & Ayers, J. G. (1999). Reconsidering the use of seclusion and restraints in inpatient child and adult psychiatry. *Journal of Child and Family Studies, 8*, 243–253.

Sirey, J., Bruce, M. L., Alexopoulos, G. S., Perlick, D., Friedman, S. J., & Meyers, B. S. (2001). Perceived stigma and patient-rated severity of illness as predictors of antidepressant drug adherence. *Psychiatric Services, 52*, 1615–1620.

Sisley, A., Jacobs, L. M., Poole, G., Campbell, S., & Esposito, T. (1999). Violence in America: A public health crisis—domestic violence. *Journal of Trauma, 46*, 1105–1112.

Skantze, K., Malm, U., Dencker, S. J., May, P. R., & Corrigan, P. (1992). Comparison of quality of life with standard of living in schizophrenic outpatients. *British Journal of Psychiatry, 161*, 797–801.

Skeem, J., & Emke-Francis, P. (2004, September). Probation and mental health: Defining and responding to the challenge. *Perspectives*, 123–126.

Skeem, J., Encandela, J., & Louden, J. (2003). Perspectives on probation and mandated mental health treatment in specialized and traditional probation departments. *Behavioral Sciences and the Law, 21*, 429–458.

Skeem, J., & Petrila, J. (2004). Problem-solving supervision: Speciality probation for individuals with mental illness. *Court Review, 40*, 8–15.

Skinner, B. F. (1938). *The behavior of organisms.* New York: Appleton-Century-Crofts.

Skinner, H. A. (1982). The Drug Abuse Screening Test. *Addictive Behaviors, 7*, 363–371.

Skitka, L. J., & Tetlock, P. E. (1992). Allocating scarce resources: A contingency model of distributive justice. *Journal of Experimental Social Psychology, 28*, 491–522.

Skitka, L. J., & Tetlock, P. E. (1993). Of ants and grasshoppers: The political psychology of allocating public assistance. In B. Mellers & J. Baron (Eds.), *Psychological Perspectives on jus-*

tice: Theory and applications. New York: Cambridge University Press.

Skovholt, T. (1974) The client as helper: A means to promote psychological growth. *Counseling Psychologist, 13,* 58–64.

Slawson, D. C., & Shaughnessy, A. F. (2005). Teaching evidence-based medicine: Should we be teaching information management instead? *Academic Medicine, 80,* 685–689.

Sledge, W., Astrachan, B., Thompson, K., Rakfeldt, J., & Leaf, P. (1995). Case management in psychiatry: An analysis of tasks. *American Journal of Psychiatry, 152,* 1259–1265.

Smith, A. (1990). Social influence and antiprejudice training programs. In J. Edwards, R. S. Tindale, L. Health, & E. J. Posavac (Eds.), *Social influence processes and prevention* (pp. 183–196). New York: Plenum Press.

Smith, G. (2004). Predictors of the stage of residential planning among aging families of adults with severe mental illness. *Psychiatric Services, 55,* 804–810.

Smith, G., Kennedy, C., Knipper, S., O'Brien, J., & O'Keeffe, J. (2005). *Using Medicaid to support working age adults with serious mental illness in the community: A handbook.* Washington, DC: Office of Disability, Aging, and Long-Term Care Policy, Office of the Assistant Secretary for Planning and Evaluation, U.S. Department of Health and Human Services. Retrieved June 30, 2007, from *aspe.hhs.gov/daltcp/reports/handbook.pdf.*

Smith, G. J. (1999). Teaching a long sequence of a behavior using whole task training, forward chaining, and backward chaining. *Perceptual and Motor Skills, 89,* 951–965.

Smith, J., & Birchwood, M. (1987). Specific and non-specific educational intervention with effects of families living with a schizophrenic relative. *British Journal of Psychiatry, 150,* 645–652.

Smith, J. A., Hughes, I. C., & Budd, R. J. (1999a). Non-compliance with anti-psychotic depot medication: Users' views on advantages and disadvantages. *Journal of Mental Health, 8*(3), 287–296.

Smith, T. B., Constantine, M. G., Dunn, T. W., Dinehart, J. M., & Montoya, J. A. (2006). Multicultural education in the mental health professions: A meta-analytic review. *Journal of Counseling Psychology, 53,* 132–145.

Smith, T. E., Bellack, A. S., & Liberman, R. P. (1996). Social skills training for schizophrenia: Review and future directions. *Clinical Psychology Review, 16,* 599–617.

Smith, T. E., Hull, J. W., Romanelli, S., Fertuck, E., & Weiss, K. A. (1999b). Symptoms and neurocognition as rate limiters in skills training for psychotic patients. *American Journal of Psychiatry, 156,* 1817–1818.

Snow, D. A., Barker, S. G., & Anderson, L. (1989). Criminality and homeless men: An empirical assessment. *Social Problems, 36,* 532–549.

Snowden, L. R. (2001). Barriers to effective mental health services for African Americans. *Mental Health Services Research, 3,* 181–187.

Snowden, L. R., & Hu, T. W. (1997). Ethnic differences in mental health services use among the severely mentally ill. *Journal of Community Psychology, 25,* 235–247.

Sobell, L. C., & Sobell, M. B. (1992). Timeline Follow-Back: A technique for assessing self-reported alcohol consumption. In R. Z. Litten & J. Allen (Eds.), *Measuring alcohol consumption: Psychosocial and biological methods* (pp. 41–72). Totowa, NJ: Humana Press.

Sobsey, D. (1994). *Violence and abuse in the lives of people with disabilities.* Baltimore: Paul H. Brookes.

Socall, D. W., & Holtgraves, T. (1992). Attitudes toward the mentally ill: The effects of label and beliefs. *Sociological Quarterly, 33,* 435–445.

Sohler, N. L., Bromet, E. J., Lavelle, J., Craig, T. J., & Mojtabai, R. (2004). Are there racial differences in the way patients with psychotic disorders are treated at their first hospitalization? *Psychological Medicine, 34,* 705–718.

Sokal, J., Messias, E., Dickerson, F. B., Kreyenbuhl, J., Brown, C. H., Goldberg, R. W., et al. (2004). Comorbidity of medical illnesses among adults with serious mental illness who are receiving community psychiatric services. *Journal of Nervous and Mental Disease, 192,* 421–427.

Solomon, M., Jonikas, J., Cook, J., & Kerouac, J. (1998). *Positive partnerships: How consumers and nonconsumers can work together as service providers* (2nd ed.). Chicago: UICC National Research and Training Center on Psychiatric Disability.

Solomon, P. (1988a). Racial factors in mental health service utilization. *Psychosocial Rehabilitation Journal, 11*(3), 3–12.

Solomon, P. (1988b). Services to severely mentally disabled homeless persons and to emergency food and shelter providers. *Psychosocial Rehabilitation Journal, 12,* 3–13.

Solomon, P. (1992). The efficacy of case management services for severely mentally disabled clients. *Community Mental Health Journal, 28,* 163–180.

Solomon, P. (1994). Family views of service delivery: An empirical assessment. In H. Lefley & M. Wasow (Eds.), *Helping families cope with men-*

tal illness (pp. 259–274). Chur, Switzerland: Harwood.

Solomon, P. (1996). Moving from psychoeducation to family education for families of adults with severe mental illness. *Psychiatric Services, 47,* 1364–1370.

Solomon, P. (1998a). The conceptual and empirical base of case management for adults with severe mental illness. In J. Williams & K. Ell (Eds.), *Mental health research: Implications for practice.* (pp. 482–497). Washington, DC: NASW Press.

Solomon, P. (1998b). The cultural context of interventions for family members with a seriously mentally ill relative. In H. Lefley (Ed.), *Families coping with mental illness: The cultural context. Vol. 70. New directions for mental health services* (pp. 516). San Francisco: Jossey-Bass.

Solomon, P. (1999). Evolution of service innovation for adults with severe mental illness. In D. Biegel & A. Blum (Eds.), *Innovation in practices and service delivery across the life span* (pp. 147–168). New York: Oxford University Press.

Solomon, P. (2000). Interventions for families of individuals with schizophrenia: Maximizing outcomes for their relatives. *Disease Management and Health Outcomes, 8,* 211–221.

Solomon, P. (2003). Case management and the forensic client. In W. Fischer (Ed.), *Community-based interventions for criminal offenders with severe mental illness* (pp. 53–71). Amsterdam: Elsevier.

Solomon, P. (2004). Peer support/peer provided services underlying processes, benefits, and critical ingredients. *Psychiatric Rehabilitation Journal, 27,* 392–401.

Solomon, P., Beck, S., & Gordon, B. (1988a). A comparison of perspectives on discharge of extended care facility clients: Views of families, hospital staff, community mental health workers, and clients. *Administration in Mental Health, 15,* 166–174.

Solomon, P., Beck, S., & Gordon, B. (1988b). Family members' perspectives on psychiatric hospitalization and discharge. *Community Mental Health Journal, 24,* 108–117.

Solomon, P., Cavanaugh, M., & Gelles, R. (2005). Family violence among adults with severe mental illness: A neglected area of research. *Trauma, Violence and Abuse, 6,* 40–54.

Solomon, P., & Draine, J. (1994a). Satisfaction with mental health treatment in a randomized trial of consumer case management. *Journal of Nervous and Mental Disease, 182,* 179–184.

Solomon, P., & Draine, J. (1994b). Family perspectives on consumers as case managers. *Community Mental Health Journal, 30,* 165–176.

Solomon, P., & Draine, J. (1995a). The efficacy of a consumer case management team: 2 year outcomes of a randomized trial. *Journal of Mental Health Administration, 22,* 135–146.

Solomon, P., & Draine, J. (1995b). One year outcomes of a randomized trial of consumer case management. *Evaluation and Program Planning, 18,* 117–127.

Solomon, P., & Draine, J. (1995c). Issues in serving the forensic client. *Social Work, 40,* 25–33.

Solomon, P., & Draine, J. (1995d). Jail recidivism in a forensic case management program. *Health and Social Work, 20,* 167–173.

Solomon, P., & Draine, J. (1995e). One year outcome of a randomized trial of case management with seriously mentally ill clients leaving jail. *Evaluation Review, 19,* 256–273.

Solomon, P., & Draine, J. (1995f). Subjective burden among family members of mentally ill adults: Relation to stress, coping, and adaptation. *American Journal of Orthopsychiatry, 65,* 419–427.

Solomon, P., & Draine, J. (1996). Examination of grief among family members of individuals with serious and persistent mental illness. *Psychiatric Quarterly, 67,* 221–234.

Solomon, P., & Draine, J. (1998). Consumers as providers in psychiatric rehabilitation. *New Directions for Mental Health Services, 79,* 65–77.

Solomon, P., & Draine, J. (1999). Using clinical and criminal involvement factors to explain homelessness among clients of a psychiatric probation and parole service. *Psychiatric Quarterly, 70,* 75–87.

Solomon, P., & Draine, J. (2001). The state of knowledge of the effectiveness of consumer provided services. *Psychiatric Rehabilitation Journal, 25*(1), 20–28.

Solomon, P., Draine, J., & Delaney, M. (1995a). The use of restraining orders by families of severely mentally ill adults. *Administration and Policy in Mental Health, 23,* 157–161.

Solomon, P., Draine, J., & Delaney, M. A. (1995b). The working alliance and consumer case management. *Journal of Mental Health Administration, 22,* 126–134.

Solomon, P., Draine, J., Mannion, E., & Meisel, M. (1996a). The impact of individualized consultation and group workshop family education and interventions on ill relative outcomes. *Journal of Nervous and Mental Disease, 184,* 252–254.

Solomon, P., Draine, J., Mannion, E., & Meisel, M. (1996b). Impact of brief family psychoeducation on self efficacy. *Schizophrenia Bulletin, 22,* 41–50.

Solomon, P., Draine, J., Mannion, E., & Meisel, M. (1997). Effectiveness of two models of brief family education: Retaining gains of family members of adults with serious mental illness. *American Journal of Orthopsychiatry, 67,* 177–186.

Solomon, P., Draine, J., & Marcus, S. (2002). Predicting incarceration rates of clients of a psychiatric probation and parole service. *Psychiatric Services, 33,* 50–56.

Solomon, P., & Marcenko, M. (1992). Families of adults with severe mental illness: Their satisfaction with impatient and outpatient treatment. *Psychosocial Rehabilitation Journal, 16,* 121–134.

Solomon, P., Marshall, T., Mannion, E., & Farmer, J. (2002). Social workers as consumers and family consultants. In K. Bentley (Ed.), *Social work practice in mental health: Contemporary roles, tasks, and techniques* (pp. 230–253). Pacific Grove, CA: Brooks/Cole.

Solomon, P., & Meyerson, A. (2003). Social stabilization: Achieving satisfactory community adaptation for persons with severe mental illness. In A. Tasman, J. Kay, & J. Lieberman (Eds.), *Psychiatry* (2nd ed., pp. 2253–2275). West Sussex, UK: Wiley.

Sommers, I., & Baskin, D. (1995). Social selection and mental health service utilization among mentally ill parolees: A research agenda. *Psychiatric Quarterly, 66,* 185–200.

Spaniol, L., & Zipple, A. (1998). Family and professional perceptions of family needs and coping strengths. *Rehabilitation Psychology, 33,* 37–45.

Spaulding, W., Harig, R., & Schwab, L. O. (1987). Preferred clinical skills for transitional living specialists. *Psychosocial Rehabilitation Journal, 11*(1), 5–21.

Spaulding, W., Polland, J., Elbogen, E., & Ritchie, A. J. (2000). Applications of therapeutic jurisprudence in rehabilitation for people with severe and disabling mental illness. *Thomas M. Cooley Law Review, 17,* 135–170.

Spaulding, W. D., Fleming, S. K., Reed, D., Sullivan, M., Storzbach, D., & Lam, M. (1999). Cognitive functioning in schizophrenia: Implications for psychiatric rehabilitation. *Schizophrenia Bulletin, 25,* 275–289.

Spaulding, W. D., Storms, L., Goodrich, V., & Sullivan, M. (1986). Applications of experimental psychopathology in psychiatric rehabilitation. *Schizophrenia Bulletin, 12*(4), 560–577.

Spaulding, W. D., Sullivan, M. E., & Poland, J. S. (2003). *Treatment and rehabilitation of severe mental illness.* New York: Guilford Press.

Sperling, A. (2005). Housing update: Consumers need a borad range of options to meet their needs. *NAMI Advocate, 3*(2), 16.

Sperling, G. (1960). The information available in brief visual presentations. *Psychological Monographs, 74,* 1–29.

Spohn, H. E., & Strauss, M. E. (1989). Relation of neuroleptic and anticholinergic medication to cognitive functions in schizophrenia. *Journal of Abnormal Psychology, 98,* 367–380.

Stangor, C., & McMillan, D. (1992). Memory for expectancy-congruent and expectancy-incongruent information: A review of the social and social developmental literatures. *Psychological Bulletin, 111,* 42–61.

Stanton, M. D., & Shadish, W. R. (1997). Outcome, attrition, and family-couples treatment for drug abuse: A meta-analysis and review of the controlled, comparative studies. *Psychological Bulletin, 122,* 170–191.

Star, S. (1955, November 5). *The public's ideas about mental illness.* Paper presented at the Annual Meeting of the National Association for Mental Health, Indianapolis, IN.

Steadman, H., Cocozza, J., & Veysey, B. (1999a). Comparing outcomes for diverted and non-diverted jail detainees with mental illness. *Law and Human Behavior, 23,* 615–627.

Steadman, H., Davidson, S., & Brown, C. (2001a). Mental health courts: Their promise and unanswered questions. *Psychiatric Services, 52,* 457–458.

Steadman, H., Deane, M. W., Borum, R., & Morrissey, J. (2000). Comparing outcomes of major models of police responses to mental health emergencies. *Psychiatric Services, 51,* 645–649.

Steadman, H., Deane, M. W., Morrissey, J., Westcott, M., Salasin, S., & Shapiro, S. (1999b). A SAMHSA Research Initiative assessing the effectiveness of jail diversion programs for mentally ill persons. *Psychiatric Services, 50,* 1620–1623.

Steadman, H., Holohean, E., & Dvoskin, J. (1991). Estimating mental health needs and service utilization among prison inmates. *Bulletin of the American Academy of Psychiatry and the Law, 19,* 297–307.

Steadman, H., Morris, S., & Dennis, D. (1995). The diversion of mentally ill persons from jails to community based services: A profile of programs. *American Journal of Public Health, 85,* 1630–1635.

Steadman, H., Stainbrook, K., Griffin, P., Draine, J., Dupont, R., & Horey, C. (2001b). A specialized crisis response site as a core element of police-based diversion programs. *Psychiatric Services, 52,* 219–222.

Steadman, H., & Veysey, B. (1997, January). Providing services for jail inmates with mental disorders. *National Institute of Justice: Research in*

Brief. Washington, DC: U.S. Department of Justice, Office of Justice Programs, National Institute of Justice.

Steadman, H. J., McCarthy, D. W., & Morrissey, J. P. (1989). *The mentally ill in jail: Planning for essential services.* New York: Guilford Press.

Steadman, H. J., Mulvey, E. P., Monahan, J., Robbins, P. C., Appelbaum, P. S., Grisso, T., et al. (1998). Violence by people discharged from acute psychiatric inpatient facilities and by others in the same neighborhoods. *Archives of General Psychiatry, 55,* 393–401.

Steele, K., & Berman, C. (2001). *The day the voices stopped: Memoir of madness and hope.* New York: Basic Books.

Stefan, S. (2001). *Unequal rights: Discrimination against people with mental disabilities and the Americans with Disabilities Act.* Washington DC: American Psychological Association.

Stein, L. (1992). Perspective: On the abolishment of the case manager. *Health Affairs, 11,* 172–177.

Stein, L., & Test, M. (1980b). Alternative to the hospital: A controlled study. *American Journal of Psychiatry, 132,* 517–522.

Stein, L. I., & Santos, A. B. (1998). *Assertive community treatment of persons with severe mental illness.* New York: Norton.

Stein, L. I., & Test, M. A. (1980a). Alternatives to mental hospital treatment: I. Conceptual, model, treatment program and clinical evaluation. *Archives of General Psychiatry, 37,* 392–397.

Steinmeyer, E. M., Marneros, A., Deister, A., Rohde, A., & Junemann, H. (1989). Long-term outcome of schizoaffective and schizophrenic disorders, a comparative study, II: Casual-analytical investigations. *European Archives of Psychiatry and Neurological Sciences, 238,* 126–134.

Sternberg, D. (1986). Testing for physical illness in psychiatric patients. *Journal of Clinical Psychiatry, 47*(Suppl.), 3–9.

Sternberg, S. (1966). High-speed scanning in human memory. *Science, 153,* 652–654.

Sternberg, S. (1967). Two operations in character recognition: Some evidence from reaction-time measurements. *Perception and Psychophysics, 2,* 45–53.

Sternhell, P. S., & Corr, M. J. (2002). Psychiatric morbidity and adherence to antiretroviral medication in patients with HIV/AIDS. *Australian and New Zealand Journal of Psychiatry, 36,* 528–533.

Storzbach, D. M., & Corrigan, P. W. (1996). Cognitive rehabilitation for schizophrenia. In P. W. Corrigan (Ed.), *Cognitive rehabilitation for neuropsychiatric disorders* (pp. 299–328). Washington, DC: American Psychiatric Press.

Strachan, A. (1986). Family interventions for the rehabilitation of schizophrenia: Toward protection and coping. *Schizophrenia Bulletin, 12,* 678–698.

Strachan, A., Leff, J., Goldstein, M., & Doane, J. (1986). Emotional attributes and direct communication in the families of schizophrenics: A cross national replication. *British Journal of Psychiatry, 149,* 279–287.

Strassnig, M., Brar, J. S., & Ganguli, R. (2005). Dietary fatty acid and antioxidant intake in community-dwelling patients suffering from schizophrenia. *Schizophrenia Research, 76,* 343–351.

Straube, E. R., & Öhman, A. (1990). Functional role of the different autonomic nervous system activity patterns found in schizophrenia: A new model. In E. R. Straube & K. Hahlweg (Eds.), *Schizophrenia: Concepts, vulnerability, and intervention* (pp. 135–157). Berlin: Springer-Verlag.

Straus, M. A., Hamby, S. L., Boney-McCoy, S., & Sugarman, D. B. (1996). The Revised Conflict Tactics Scales (CTS2): Development and preliminary psychometric data. *Journal of Family Issues, 17,* 283–316.

Strauss, J. S. (1969) Hallucinations and delusions as points on continua of function. *Archives of General Psychiatry, 21,* 581–586.

Strauss, J. S. (1989). Subjective experiences of schizophrenia: Toward a new dynamic psychiatry: II. *Schizophrenia Bulletin, 15,* 179–187.

Strauss, J. S., & Carpenter, W. T. (1972). The prediction of outcome in schizophrenia: I. Characteristics of outcome. *Archives of General Psychiatry, 27,* 739–746.

Strauss, J. S., & Carpenter, W. T. (1974). The prediction of outcome in schizophrenia: II. Relationships between predictor and outcome variables: A report from the WHO International Pilot Study of Schizophrenia. *Archives of General Psychiatry, 31*(1), 37–42.

Strauss, J. S., & Carpenter, W. T. (1977). Prediction of outcome in schizophrenia: III. Five-year outcome and its predictors. *Archives of General Psychiatry, 34,* 159–163.

Strauss, J. S., Carpenter, W. T. J., & Bartko, J. J. (1974). The diagnosis and understanding of schizophrenia: III. Speculations on the processes that underlie schizophrenic symptoms and signs. *Schizophrenia Bulletin, 11,* 61–69.

Strauss, J. S., Hafez, H., Lieberman, P., & Harding, C. M. (1985). The course of psychiatric disorder: III. Longitudinal principles. *American Journal of Psychiatry, 142,* 289–296.

Stringfellow, J., & Muscari, K. (2003). A program

of support for consumer participation in systems change. *Journal of Disability Policy Studies, 14,* 142–147.

Stroul, B. (1993). Rehabilitation in community support systems. In R. Flexer & P. Solomon (Eds.), *Psychiatric rehabilitation in practice* (pp. 45–61). Boston: Andover Medical.

Stroul, B. A. (1986). *Models of community support services: Approaches to helping persons with long-term mental illness.* Boston: Center for Psychiatric Rehabilitation.

Stroul, B. A. (1988). Residential crisis services: A review. *Hospital and Community Psychiatry, 39,* 1095–1099.

Stroup, S., Appelbaum, P., Swartz, M. S., Patel, M., Davis, S., Jeste, D. V., et al. (2005). Decision-making capacity for research participation among individuals in the CATIE schizophrenia trial. *Schizophrenia Research, 80,* 1–8.

Strous, S. E., Richardson, W. S., Glasziou, P., & Haynes, R. B. (2005). Evidence-based medicine: How to practice and teach EBM. New York: Elsevier, Churchill, and Livingston.

Stueve, A., Vine, P., & Struening, E. (1997). Perceived burden among caregivers of adults with serious mental illness. Comparison of black, Hispanic, and white families. *American Journal of Orthopsychiatry, 67,* 199–209.

Substance Abuse and Mental Health Services Administration (SAMHSA). (1998). *Cooperative agreements to evaluate consumer operated human service programs for persons with serious mental illness.* Catalog of Federal Domestic Assistance No. 93.230. Rockville, MD: Author.

Substance Abuse and Mental Health Services Administration. (2005). *Building a foundation for recovery: How states can establish Medicaid-funded peer support services.* DHHS Publication No. (SMA) 05-8088. Rockville, MD: Center for Mental Health Services, Substance Abuse and Mental Health Services Administration.

Substance Abuse and Mental Health Services Administration. (2006). *Cultural competence standards in managed care mental health services: Four underserved/underrepresented racial/ethnic groups.* Retrieved January 7, 2006, from *www.mentalhealth.samhsa.gov/publications/allpubs/SMA00–3457/ch3.asp.*)

Sue, D. W. (2004). Whiteness and ethnocentric monoculturalism: Making the "invisible" visible. *American Psychologist, 59,* 761–769.

Sue, D. W., Arredondo, P., & McDavis, R. J. (1992). Multicultural counseling competencies and standards: A call to the profession. *Journal of Multicultural Counseling and Development, 20,* 64–88.

Sue, D. W., Bingham, R. P., Porché-Burke, L., &

Vasquez, M. (1999). The diversification of psychology: A multicultural revolution. *American Psychologist, 54,* 1061–1069.

Sue, S. (2003). In defense of cultural competency in psychotherapy and treatment. *American Psychologist, 58,* 964–970.

Sue, S., & Zane, N. (1987). The role of culture and cultural technique in psychotherapy. *American Psychologist, 42,* 37–45.

Sullivan, W. P., & Rapp, C. A. (2002). Social workers as case managers. In K. J. Bentley (Ed.), *Social work practice in mental health* (pp. 182–210). Pacific Shore, CA: Brooks/Cole.

Surles, R., & McGinn, M. (1987). Increased use of psychiatric emergency services by young chronic mentally ill patients. *Hospital and Community Psychiatry, 38,* 401–405.

Susser, E., Valencia, E., Berkman, A., Sohler, N., Conover, S., Torres, J., et al. (1998). Human immunodeficiency virus sexual risk reduction in homeless men with mental illness. *Archives of General Psychiatry, 55,* 266–272.

Susser, E. S., & Wanderling, J. (1994). Epidemiology of nonaffective acute remitting psychosis vs. schizophrenia: Sex and sociocultural setting. *Archives of General Psychiatry, 51*(4), 294–301.

Suzuki, L. A., Meller, P. J., & Ponterotto, J. G. (Eds.). (1996). *Handbook of multicultural assessment: Clinical, psychological, and educational applications.* San Francisco: Jossey-Bass.

Swanson, A. J., Pantalon, M. V., & Cohen, K. R. (1999). Motivtional interviewing and treatment adherence among psychiatric and dually diagnosed patients. *Journal of Nervous and Mental Disease, 187,* 630–635.

Swanson, J. (1994). Mental disorder, substance abuse, and community violence: An epidemiological approach. In J. Monahan & H. Steadman (Eds.), *Violence and mental disorder: Developments in risk assessment* (pp. 101–136). Chicago: University of Chicago Press.

Swanson, J. W., Borum, R., Swartz, M., & Monahan, J. (1996). Psychotic symptoms and disorders and the risk of violent behaviour in the community. *Criminal Behaviour and Mental Health, 6,* 309–329.

Swanson, J. W., Borum, R., Swartz, M., & Hiday, V. A. (1999). Violent behavior preceding hospitalization among persons with severe mental illness. *Law and Human Behavior, 23,* 185–204.

Swanson, J. W., Holzer, C. E., Ganju, V. K., & Jono, R. T. (1990). Violence and psychiatric disorder in the community: Evidence from the Epidemiologic Catchment Area Surveys. *Hospital and Community Psychiatry, 41*(7), 761–770.

Swanson, J. W., Swartz, M. S., Borum, R., Hiday, V. A., Wagner, H. R., & Burns, B. J. (2000). Involuntary out-patient commitment and reduction of violent behavior in persons with severe mental illness. *British Journal of Psychiatry, 176*, 324–331.

Swanson, J., Swartz, M., Estroff, S., Borum, R., Wagner, R., & Hiday, V. (1998). Psychiatric impairment, social contact, and violent behavior: Evidence from a study of outpatient-committed persons with severe mental disorder. *Social Psychiatry and Psychiatric Epidemiology, 33*, S86–S94.

Swartz, M., Swanson, J., Hiday, V., Borum, R., Wagner, H. R., & Burns, B. (1998). Violence and severe mental illness: The effects of substance abuse and nonadherence to medication. *American Journal of Psychiatry, 155*, 226–231.

Swartz, M. S., Swanson, J. W., Wagner, H. R., Burns, B. J., & Hiday, V. A. (2001). Effects of involuntary outpatient commitment and depot antipsychotics on treatment adherence in persons with severe mental illness. *Journal of Nervous and Mental Disease, 189*, 583–592.

Swezey, R. L., & Swezey, A. M. (1976). Educational theory as a basis for patient education. *Journal of Chronic Diseases, 29*, 417–422.

Switzer, G. E., Dew, M. A., Thompson, K., Goycoolea, J. M., Derricott, T., & Mullins, S. D. (1999). Posttraumatic stress disorder and service utilization among urban mental health center clients. *Journal of Traumatic Stress, 12*, 25–39.

Swofford, C. D., Kasckow, J. W., Scheller-Gilkey, G., & Inderbitzin, L. B. (1996). Substance use: A powerful predictor of relapse in schizophrenia. *Schizophrenia Research, 20*(1–2), 145–151.

Szmukler, G. (1996). From family "burden" to caregiving. *Psychiatric Bulletin, 20*, 449–451.

Szmukler, G., Burgess, P., Herrman, H., Benson, A., Colusa, S., & Bloch, S. (1996). Caring for relatives with serious mental illness: The development of the Experience of Caregiving Inventory. *Social psychiatry and Psychiatric Epidemiolgy, 31*, 137–148.

Talbott, J. A. (Ed.). (1978). *The chronic mental patient*. Washington, DC: American Psychiatric Press.

Talbot, N. L., Houghtalen, R. P., Cyrulik, S., Betz, A., Barkun, M., Duberstein, P. R., et al. (1998). Women's safety in recovery: Group therapy for patients with a history of childhood sexual abuse. *Psychiatric Services, 49*, 213–217.

Talley, N. J., Fett, S. L., Zinsmeister, A. R., & Melton, L. J. R. (1994). Gastrointestinal tract symptoms and self-reported abuse: A population-based study. *Gastroenterology, 107*, 1040–1049.

Tanzman, B. (1993). An overview of surveys of mental health consumers' preferences for housing and support services. *Hospital and Community Psychiatry, 44*, 450–455.

Tarrier, N., Beckett, R., Harwood, S., Baker, A., Yusupoff, L., & Ugarteburu, I. (1993). A trial of two cognitive-behavioural methods of treating drug-resistant residual psychotic symptoms in schizophrenic patients: I. Outcome. *British Journal of Psychiatry, 162*, 524–532.

Tarrier, N., & Wykes, T. (2004). Is there evidence that cognitive behaviour therapy is an effective treatment for schizophrenia?: A cautious or cautionary tale? *Behaviour Research and Therapy, 42*, 1377–1401.

Tarutis, G., & Boyd, M. (2001, Summer). The Supplemental Special Needs Trust. *NAMI Advocate, 22*–25.

Tattan, T., & Tarrier, N. (2000). The expressed emotion of case mangers of the seriously mentally ill: The influence of expressed emotion on clinical outcomes. *Psychological Medicine, 30*, 195–204.

Tauber, R., Wallace, C. J., & Lecomte, T. (2000). Enlisting indigenous community supporters in skills training programs for persons with severe mental illness. *Psychiatric Services, 51*, 1428–1432.

Taylor, M. A., & Abrams, R. (1975). Acute mania: Clinical and genetic study of responders and nonresponders to treatments. *Archives of General Psychiatry, 32*, 863–865.

Teague, G., Drake, R., & Ackerson, T. (1995). Evaluating use of continuous treatment teams for persons with mental illness and substance abuse. *Psychiatric Services, 46*, 689–695.

Teague, G. B., Bond, G. R., & Drake, R. E. (1998). Program fidelity in assertive community treatment: Development and use of a measure. *American Journal of Orthopsychiatry, 68*, 216–232.

Telles, C., Karno, M., Mintz, J., Paz, G., Arias, M., Tucker, D., et al. (1995). Immigrant families coping with schizophrenia: Behavioral family intervention with a low-income Spanish speaking population. *British Journal of Psychiatry, 167*, 473–479.

Tengstrom, A., Hodgins, S., Grann, M., Langstrom, N., & Kullgren, G. (2004). Schizophrenia and criminal offending: The role of psychopathy and substance use disorders. *Criminal Justice and Behavior, 31*, 367–391.

Teplin, L. (1983). The criminalization of the mentally ill: Specialization in search of data. *Psychological Bulletin, 94*, 54–67.

Teplin, L. (1985). The criminality of the mentally ill: A dangerous misconception. *American Journal of Psychiatry, 142*, 593–599.

Teplin, L. (1990). The prevalence of severe mental disorder among male urban jail detainees: Comparison with Epidemiological Catchment Area Program. *American Journal of Public Health, 80,* 663–669.

Teplin, L. (1991). The criminalization hypothesis: Myth, misnomer, or management strategy. In S. Shah & B. Sales (Eds.), *Law and mental health: Major developments and research needs* (pp. 149–183). Rockville, MD: U.S. Department of Health and Human Services.

Teplin, L. (1994). Psychiatric and substance abuse disorders among male urban jail detainees. *American Journal of Public Health, 84,* 290–293.

Teplin, L., & Pruett, N. (1992). Police as streetcorner psychiatrist: Managing the mentally ill. *International Journal of Law and Psychiatry, 15,* 139–156.

Teplin, L. A. (1984). Criminalizing mental disorder: The comparative arrest rate of the mentally ill. *American Psychologist, 39,* 794–803.

Teplin, L. A., Abram, K. M., & McClelland, G. M. (1996). Prevalence of psychiatric disorders among incarcerated women: Pretrial jail detainees. *Archives of General Psychiatry, 53,* 505–512.

Terkelson, K. (1990). A historical perspective on family–provider relationships. In H. P Lefley & D. Johnson (Eds.), *Families as allies in the treatment of the mentally ill.* Washington, DC: American Psychological Association.

Tessler, R. E., & Gamache, G. (1996). *Toolkit for evaluating family experiences with severe mental illness.* Amherst, MA: The Evaluation Center at HSRI.

Tessler, R. E., & Gamache, G. (2000). *Family experiences with mental illness.* Wesptport, CT: Auburn House.

Test, M. A. (1979). Continuity of care in community treatment. *New Directions for Mental Health Services, 2,* 15–23.

Test, M. A. (1998). Community-based treatment models for adults with severe and persistent mental illness. In J. Williams & K. Ell (Eds.), *Mental health research: Implications for practice* (pp. 420–436). Washington, DC: NASW Press.

Test, M. A., & Stein, L. (2001). In reply. *Psychiatric services, 52,* 1396–1397.

Thakore, J. H. (2004). Metabolic disturbance in first-episode schizophrenia. *British Journal of Psychiatry, 184*(Suppl. 47), S76–S79.

Thampanichawat, W. (1999). *Thai mothers living with HIV infection in urban areas.* Unpublished doctoral dissertation, University of Washington.

Thompson, K., Kulkarni, J., & Sergejew, A. A. (2000a). Reliability and validity of a new Medication Adherence Rating Scale (MARS) for the psychoses. *Schizophrenia Research, 42,* 241–247.

Thompson, M., Reuland, M., & Souweine, D. (2003). Criminal justice/mental health consensus: Improving responses to people with mental illness. *Crime and Delinquency, 49,* 30–51.

Tidey, J. W., O'Neill, S. C., & Higgins, S. T. (2002). Contingent monetary reinforcement of smoking reductions, with and without transdermal nicotine, in outpatients with schizophrenia. *Experimental and Clinical Psychopharmacology, 10,* 241–247.

Timko, C., & Sempel, J. (2004). Intensity of acute services, self-help attendance and one-year outcomes among dually diagnosed patients. *Journal of Studies on Alcohol, 65,* 274–282.

Tokar, D. M., & Swanson, J. L. (1991). An investigation of the validity of Helms's (1984) model of white racial identity development. *Journal of Counseling Psychology, 38,* 296–301.

Ton, H., Koike, A., Hales, R. E., Johnson, J. A., & Hilty, D. (2005). A qualitative needs assessment for development of a cultural consultation service. *Transcultural Psychiatry, 42,* 491–504.

Torrey, E. E. (1995). Editorial: Jails and prisons—America's new mental hospitals. *American Journal of Public Health, 85,* 1611–1612.

Torrey, E. E., Steiber, J., Ezekiel, J., Wolfe, S., Sharfstein, J., Noble, J., et al. (1992). *Criminalizing the serious mentally ill: The abuse of jails as mental hospitals.* Washington, DC: Public Citizens Research Group.

Torrey, E. F. (1983). *Surviving schizophrenia: A family manual* (rev. ed.). New York: Harper & Row.

Torrey, E. F. (1988). *Nowhere to go.* New York: Harper & Row.

Torrey, E. F. (2001). *Surviving schizophrenia: A manual for families, consumers, and providers* (4th ed.). New York: HarperCollins.

Torrey, E. F., Bowler, A. E., & Clark, K. (1997). Urban birth and residence as risk factors for psychoses: An analysis of 1880 data. *Schizophrenia Research, 25,* 169–176.

Torrey, E. F., Erdman, K., Wolfe, S. M., & Flynn, L. M. (1990). *Care of the seriously mentally ill: A rating of state programs* (3rd ed.). Arlington, VA: National Alliance for the Mentally Ill.

Torrey, W. C., Clark, R. E., Becker, D. R., Wyzik, P. F., & Drake, R. E. (1997). Switching from rehabilitative day treatment to supported employment. In L. L. Kennedy (Ed.), *Continuum, developments in ambulatory mental health care* (Vol. 4, pp. 27–38). San Francisco: Jossey-Bass.

Torrey, W. C., Drake, R. E., Cohen, M., Fox, L. B., Lynde, D., Gorman, P., et al. (2002). The challenge of implementing and sustaining integrated dual disorders treatment programs. *Community Mental Health Journal, 38,* 507–521.

Torrey, W. C., Drake, R. E., Dixon, L., Burns, B. J., Rush, A. J., Clark, R. E., et al. (2001). Implementing evidence-based practices for persons with severe mental illness. *Psychiatric Services, 52,* 45–50.

Torrey, W. C., Finnerty, M., Evans, A., & Wyzik, P. F. (2003). Strategies for leading the implementation of evidence-based practices. *Psychiatric Clinics of North America, 26,* 883–897.

Torrey, W. C., & Wyzik, P. (2000). The recovery vision as a service improvement guide for community mental health center providers. *Community Mental Health Journal, 36,* 209–216.

Toussaint, D. W., VanDeMark, N. R., Bornemann, A., & Graeber, C. J. (2006). *Modifications to the Trauma Recovery and Empowerment Model (TREM) for substance-abusing women with histories of violence: Outcomes and lessons learned at a Colorado substance abuse treatment center.* Unpublished manuscript.

Tracy, B. (2003). Evidence-based practices or value-based services. *Psychiatric Services, 54,* 1437.

Trainor, J., Shepherd, M., Boydell, K. M., Leff, A., & Crawford, E. (1997). Beyond the service paradigm: The impact and implications of consumer/survivor initiatives. *Psychiatric Rehabilitation Journal, 21*(2), 132–140.

Travis, J. (1997, September). *The mentally ill offender: Viewing crime and justice through a different lens.* U.S. Dept. of Justice speech to the National Association of State Forensic Mental Health Directors. (Available at *www.ojp.usdoj.gov/nij/speeches.htm*)

Tremblay, T., Smith, J., Xie, H., & Drake, R. E. (2004). The impact of specialized benefits counseling services on Social Security Administration disability beneficiaries in Vermont. *Journal of Rehabilitation, 70*(2), 5–11.

Trivedi, M. H., Kern, J. K., Grannemann, B. D., Altshuler, K. L., & Sunderajan, P. (2004). A computerized clinical decision support system as a means of implementing depression guidelines. *Psychiatric Services, 55,* 879–885.

Trochim, W. M., & Cook, J. (1993). *Workforce competencies for psychosocial rehabilitation workers: A concept mapping project (Final report).* Columbia, MD: International Association of Psychosocial Rehabilitation Services.

Trower, P., Birchwood, M., Meaden, A., Byrne, S., Nelson, A., & Ross, K. (2004). Cognitive therapy for command hallucinations: Randomised controlled trial. *British Journal of Psychiatry, 184,* 312–320.

Trower, P., Bryant, B., & Argyle, M. (1978). *Social skills and mental health.* London: Methuen.

Trupin, E., & Richards, H. (2003). Seattle's mental health courts: Early indicators of effectiveness. *International Journal of Law and Psychiatry, 26,* 33–53.

Tsang, H. W., & Pearson, V. (2001). Work-related social skills training for people with schizophrenia in Hong Kong. *Schizophrenia Bulletin, 27,* 139–148.

Tse, W. S., & Bond, A. J. (2004). The impact of depression on social skills: A review. *Journal of Nervous and Mental Disease, 192,* 260–268.

Tsemberis, S., & Asmussen, S. (1999). From streets to homes: The pathways to housing consumer preference supported housing model. *Alcoholism Treatment Quarterly, 17,* 113–131.

Tsemberis, S., & Eisenberg, R. F. (2000). Pathways to housing: Supported housing for street-dwelling homeless individuals with psychiatric disabilities. *Psychiatric Services, 51,* 487–493.

Tsemberis, S., Gulcur, L., & Nakae, M. (2004). Housing First, consumer choice, and harm reduction for homeless individuals with a dual diagnosis. *American Journal of Public Health, 94,* 651–656.

Tsuang, M. T., Perkins, K., & Simpson, J. C. (1983). Physical disease in schizophrenia and affective disorder. *Journal of Clinical Psychiatry, 44,* 42–46.

Tsuang, M. T., Tohen, M., & Zahner, G. E. P. (Eds.). (1995). *Textbook in psychiatric epidemiology.* Hoboken, NJ: Wiley.

Tsuang, M. T., & Winokur, G. (1975). The Iowa 500: Field work in a 35-year follow-up of depression, mania, and schizophrenia. *Canadian Psychiatric Association Journal, 20,* 359–365.

Tsuang, M. T., & Woolson, R. F. (1978). Excess mortality in schizophrenia and affective disorders: Do suicides and accidental deaths solely account for this excess? *Archives of General Psychiatry, 35,* 1181–1185.

Tsuang, M. T., Woolson, R. F., & Fleming, J. A. (1980a). Premature deaths in schizophrenia and affective disorders: An analysis of survival curves and variables affecting the shortened survival. *Archives of General Psychiatry, 37,* 979–983.

Tsuang, M. T., Woolson, R. F., & Fleming, J. A. (1980b). Causes of death in schizophrenia and manic-depression. *British Journal of Psychiatry, 136,* 239–242.

Turner, C. F. (1998). Adolescent sexual behavior, drug use, and violence: Increased reporting with computer technology. *Science, 280,* 867–873.

Turner, J. C., & TenHoor, W. J. (1978). The NIMH community support program: Pilot approach to a needed social reform. *Schizophrenia Bulletin, 4,* 319–348.

Twamley, E. W., Bartels, S. J., & Becker, D. R. (2004, May 18–21). *Individual placement and support for middle-aged and older clients with schizophrenia.* Paper presented at the International Association of Psychosocial Services, San Diego.

Twamley, E. W., Jeste, D. V., & Bellack, A. S. (2003). A review of cognitive training in schizophrenia. *Schizophrenia Bulletin, 29,* 359–382.

Tyrer, P. (1998). Whither community care? *British Journal of Psychiatry, 173,* 359–360.

Tyson, P. D. (1998). Physiological arousal, reactive aggression, and the induction of an incompatible relaxation response. *Aggression and Violent Behavior, 3,* 143–158.

Ullman, M. D., Johnsen, M. C., Moss, K., & Burris, S. (2001). The EEOC charge priority policy and claimants with psychiatric disabilities. *Psychiatric Services, 52,* 644–649.

Unger, K. V. (1990, Summer). Supported postsecondary education for people with mental illness. *American Rehabilitation,* 2–6.

Unzicker, R. (1989). On my own: A personal journey through madness and re-emergence. *Psychosocial Rehabilitation Journal, 13,* 71–77.

U.S. Congress. (1963, October 31). Public Law 88-164—*Mental Retardation Facilities and Community Mental Health Centers Construction Act of 1963.*

U.S. Department of Health and Human Services, Substance Abuse and Mental Health Services Administration, Center for Mental Health Services, National Institutes of Health, National Institute of Mental Health (1999). *Mental Health: A Report of the Surgeon General.* Rockville, MD. Author.

U.S. Department of Health and Human Services. (2002). *Report to Congress on the Prevention and Treatment of Co-occurring Substance Abuse Disorders and Mental disorders.* Washington, DC: Author.

U.S. Department of Health and Human Services. (2003a). *Assertive Community Treatment Implementation Resource Kit.* Rockville, MD: Substance Abuse and Mental Health Services Administration, Center for Mental Health Services.

U.S. Department of Health and Human Services. (2003b). *Family Psychoeducation Implementation Resource Kit.* Rockville, MD: Substance Abuse and Mental Health Services Administration, Center for Mental Health Services.

U.S. Department of Health and Human Service. (2003c). *New Freedom Commission on Mental Health: Achieving the promise: Transforming mental health care in America. Final Report.* (DHHS Publication No. SMA-03-3832). Rockville, MD: Author.

U.S. General Accounting Office. (1993). *Vocational rehabilitation: Evidence for federal program's effectiveness is mixed* (Vol. PEMD-93-19). Washington, DC: Author.

U.S. General Accounting Office. (1996). *SSA disability: Program redesign necessary to encourage return to work: Report to the chairman, Special Committee on Aging and the U.S. Senate (GAO/HEHS 96–62).* Washington, DC: Author.

U.S. Psychiatric Rehabilitation Association. (2005). *CPRP program fact sheet.* Linthicum, MD: Author.

U.S. Surgeon General. (1999). *Mental health: A report of the surgeon general.* Washington, DC: Department of Health and Human Services.

U.S. Surgeon General. (2001). *Mental health: Culture, race, and ethnicity: A supplement to Mental Health: A Report of the Surgeon General.* Rockville, MD: U.S. Department of Health and Human Services.

Van der Does, A. W., & Van den Bosch, R. J. (1992). What determines Wisconsin Card Sorting performance in schizophrenia? *Clinical Psychology Review, 12*(6), 567–583.

Van der Gaag, M., Kern, R. S., Van den Bosch, R. J., & Liberman, R. P. (2002). A controlled trial of cognitive remediation in schizophrenia. *Schizophrenia Bulletin, 28,* 167–176.

van der Kolk, B. A. (1987). The psychological consequences of overwhelming life experiences. In v. d. Kolk (Ed.), *Psychological trauma* (pp. 1–30). Washington, DC: American Psychiatric Press.

Vandiver, B. J., Cross, W. E., Worrell, F. C., & Fhagen-Smith, P. E. (2002). Validating the Cross Racial Identity Scale. *Journal of Counseling Psychology, 49,* 71–85.

Van Dongen, C. J. (1996). Quality of life and self-esteem in working and nonworking persons with mental illness. *Community Mental Health Journal, 32,* 535–548.

Van Dongen, C. J. (1998). Self-esteem among persons with severe mental illness. *Issues in Mental Health Nursing, 19,* 29–40.

Van Os, J. (2004). Does the urban environment cause psychosis? *British Journal of Psychiatry, 184,* 287–288.

Van Os, J., McKenzie, K., & Jones, P. (1997). Cultural differences in pathways to care, service use and treated outcomes. *Current Opinion in Psychiatry, 10,* 178–182.

Van Putten, T. (1974). Why do schizophrenic patients refuse to take their drugs? *Archives of General Psychiatry, 31,* 67–72.

Van Tosh, L., & DelVecchio, P. (1998). *Consumer-operated self-help programs: A technical report.* Rockville, MD., Center for Mental Health Services.

Van Tosh, L., Ralph, R., & Campbell, J. (2000). The rise of consumerism. *Psychiatric Rehabilitation Skills, 4*, 383–409.

Van Wijngaarden, B., Schene, A., Koeter, M., Becker, T., Knapp, M., Knudson, H., et al. (2003). People with schizophrenia in five countries: Conceptual similarities and intercultural differences in family caregiving. *Schizophrenia Bulletin, 29*, 573–586.

Vega, W. A., & Lopez, S. R. (2001). Priority issues in Latino mental health services research. *Mental Health Services Research, 3*, 189–200.

Velligan, D., & Bow-Thomas, C. (2000). Two case studies of cognitive adaptation training for outpatients with schizophrenia. *Psychiatric Services, 51*, 25–29.

Velligan, D. I., Bow-Thomas, C. C., Huntzinger, C., Ritch, J. L., Ledbetter, N., Prihoda, T. J., et al. (2000). Randomized controlled trial of the use of compensatory strategies to enhance adaptive functioning in outpatients with schizophrenia. *American Journal of Psychiatry, 157*, 1317–1323.

Velligan, D. I., DiCocco, M., Bow-Thomas, C. C., Cadle, C., Glahn, D. C., Miller, A. L., et al. (2004). A brief cognitive assessment for use with schizophrenia patients in community clinics. *Schizophrenia Research, 71*, 273–283.

Velligan, D. I., Lam, F., Ereshefsky, L., & Miller, A. L. (2003). Psychopharmacology: Perspectives on medication adherence and atypical antipsychotic medications. *Psychiatric Services, 54*, 665–667.

Velligan, D. I., Mahurin, R. K., Hazleton, D. C., Eckert, S. L., & Miller, A. L. (1997). The functional significance of symptomatology and cognitive function in schizophrenia. *Schizophrenia Research, 25*, 21–31.

Velligan, D. I., Prihoda, T. J., Ritch, J. L., Maples, N., Bow-Thomas, C. C., & Dassori, A. (2002). A randomized single-blind pilot study of compensatory strategies in schizophrenia outpatients. *Schizophrenia Bulletin, 28*, 283–292.

Ventura, L., Cassel, J. C., Jacoby, J., & Huang, B. (1998). Case management and recidivism of mentally ill persons released from jail. *Psychiatric Services, 49*, 1330–1337.

Ventura, J., Nuechterlein, K. H., Lukoff, D., & Hardesty, J. P. (1989). A prospective study of stressful life events and schizophrenic relapse. *Journal of Abnormal Psychology, 98*(4), 407–411.

Ventura, J., Nuechterlein, K. H., Subotnik, K. L., Hardesty, J. P., & Mintz, J. (2000). Life events can trigger depressive exacerbation in the early course of schizophrenia. *Journal of Abnormal Psychology, 109*(1), 139–144.

Verdoux, H., Maurice-Tison, S., Gay, B., van Os, J., Salamon, R., & Bourgeois, M. (1998). A survey of delusional ideation in primary care patients. *Psychological Medicine, 28*, 127–134.

Verheul, R., Van Den Bosch, L. M. C., Koetter, M. W. J., De Ridder, M. A. J., Stijnen, T., & Van Den Brink, W. (2003). Dialectical behaviour therapy for women with borderline personality disorder: 12-month, randomised clinical trial in the Netherlands. *British Journal of Psychiatry, 182*, 135–140.

Verkuyten, M. (1994). Self-esteem among ethnic minority youth in western countries. *Social Indicators Research, 32*, 21–47.

Verkuyten, M. (1995). Self-esteem, self-concept stability, and aspects of ethnic identity among minority and majority youth in the Netherlands. *Journal of Youth and Adolescence, 24*, 155–175.

Veysey, B. (1994). Challenges for the future. In National Institute of Corrections, *Topics in community corrections: Annual issue: Mentally ill offenders in the community* (pp. 3–10). Washington, DC: U. S. Department of Justice, National Institute of Corrections.

Veysey, B., Steadman, H., Morrissey, J., & Johnson, M. (1997). In search of the missing linkages: Continuity of care in U.S. jails. *Behavioral Sciences and the Law, 15*, 383–397.

Visher, C., & Travis, J. (2003). Transitions from the prison to the community: Understanding individual pathways. *Annual Review of Sociology, 29*, 89–113.

Vitale, J. H., & Steinbach, M. (1965). The prevention of relapse of chronic mental patients. *International Journal of Social Psychiatry, 11*, 85–95.

Vogel, H. W., Knight, E., Laudet, A. B., & Magura, S. (1998). Double trouble in recovery: Self-help for people with dual diagnoses. *Psychiaric Rehabilitation Journal, 21*, 356–364.

Vorspan, R. (1988). Activities of daily living in the clubhouse: You can't vacuum in a vacuum. *Psychosocial Rehabilitation Journal, 12*(2), 15–21.

Vreeland, B., Minsky, S., Yanos, P. T., Gara, M., Menza, M., Kim, E., et al. (2006). Efficacy of a modular psychoeducational program for increasing patient knowledge of illness management and treatment: The Team Solutions Program. *Psychiatric Services, 57*, 822–828.

Wagner, B. R. (1968). The training of attending and abstracting responses in chronic schizophrenia. *Journal of Experimental Research in Personality, 3*, 77–88.

Wagner, J., & Gartner, C. (1999). *Highlights of the 1998 Institute on Psychiatric Services, 50*, 15–20.

Wahl, O. (1995). *Media madness: Public images of mental illness*. New Brunswick, NJ: Rutgers University Press.

Wahl, O. (1997). *Consumer experience of stigma*. Fairfax, VA: George Mason University, Department of Psychology.

Wahl, O. F. (1999a). Mental health consumers' experience of stigma. *Schizophrenia Bulletin, 25*, 467–478.

Wahl, O. F. (1999b). *Telling is risky business: Mental health consumers confront stigma*. New Brunswick, NJ: Rutgers University Press.

Wahl, O. F., & Harman, C. R. (1989). Family views of stigma. *Schizophrenia Bulletin, 15*, 131–139.

Wahl, O. F., Wood, A., & Richards, R. (2002). Newspaper coverage of mental illness: Is it changing? *Psychiatric Rehabilitation Skills, 6*, 9–31.

Wallace, C. J. (1998). Social skills training in psychiatric rehabilitation: Recent findings. *International Review of Psychiatry, 10*, 9–19.

Wallace, C. J., Lecomte, T., Wilde, J., & Liberman, R. P. (2001). CASIG: A consumer-centered assessment for planning individualized treatment and evaluating program outcomes. *Schizophrenia Research, 50*, 105–109.

Wallace, C. J., Liberman, R. P., MacKain, S. J., Blackwell, G., & Eckman, T. (1992). Effectiveness and replicability of modules for teaching social and instrumental skills to the severely mentally ill. *American Journal of Psychiatry, 149*, 654–658.

Wallace, C. J., Liberman, R. P., Tauber, R., & Wallace, J. (2000). The Independent Living Skills Survey: A comprehensive measure of the community functioning of severely and persistently mentally ill individuals. *Schizophrenia Bulletin, 26*, 631–658.

Wallace, C. J., Nelson, C. J., Liberman, R. P., Aitchison, R. A., Lukoff, D., Elder, J. P., et al. (1980). A review and critique of social skills training with schizophrenic patients. *Schizophrenia Bulletin, 6*, 42–63.

Wallace, C. J., & Tauber, R. (2004). Supplementing supported employment with workplace skills training. *Psychiatric Services, 55*, 513–515.

Wallace, C. J., Tauber, R., & Wilde, J. (1999). Teaching fundamental workplace skills to persons with serious mental illness. *Psychiatric Services, 50*, 1147–1153.

Walls, R. T., Dowler, D. L., & Fullmer, S. L. (1990). Incentives and disincentives to supported employment. In F. R. Rusch (Ed.), *Supported employment: Models, methods, and issues* (pp. 251–269). Sycamore, IL: Sycamore.

Walsh, E., Moran, P., Scott, C., McKenzie, K., Burns, T., Creed, F., et al. (2003). Prevalence of violent victimisation in severe mental illness. *British Journal of Psychiatry, 183*, 233–238.

Walsh, E. R. (2000a). *Women's decision-making experiences regarding disclosure of HIV seropositivity: A qualitative study*. Unpublished doctoral dissertation, University of Michigan.

Walsh, J. (2000b). *Clinical case management with persons having mental illness*. Scarborough, CA: Brooks/Cole.

Walsh, J., & Connelly, P. (1996). Supportive behaviors in natural support networks of people with serious mental illness. *Health and Social Work, 21*, 296–303.

Wang, P., Berglund, P., & Kessler, R. (2000). Recent care of common mental disorders in the United States: Prevalence and conformance with evidence-based recommendations. *Journal of General Internal Medicine, 15*, 284–292.

Ware, N. C., Dickey, B., Tugenberg, T., & McHorney, C. A. (2003). CONNECT: A measure of continuity of care in mental health services. *Mental Health Services Research, 5*, 209–221.

Warner, R., Taylor, D., Wright, J., Sloat, A., Springett, G., Arnold, S., et al. (1994). Substance use among the mentally ill: Prevalence, reasons for use, and effects on illness. *American Journal of Orthopsychiatry, 64*, 30–39.

Warr, P. (1987). *Work, unemployment, and mental health*. Oxford, UK: Oxford University Press.

Warren, R., & McLellarn, R. W. (1982). Systematic desensitization as a treatment for maladaptive anger and aggression: A review. *Psychological Reports, 50*, 1095–1102.

Wasow, M. (1986). The need for asylum for the chronically mentally ill. *Schizophrenia Bulletin, 12*(2), 162–167.

Wastell, C. A. (2002). Exposure to trauma: The long-term effects of suppressing emotional reactions. *Journal of Nervous and Mental Disease, 190*, 839–845.

Watson, A., Hanrahan, P., Luchins, D., & Lurigio, A. (2001). Mental health courts and complex issue of mentally ill offenders. *Psychiatric Services, 52*, 477–481.

Watson, A., Ottati, V., Corrigan, P., & Heyrman, M. (in press). Mental illness stigma and police decision making. *Community Mental Health Journal*.

Watts, D., Bindman, J., Slade, M., Halloway, F., Rosen, A., & Thornicroft, G. (2004). Clinical assessment of risk decision support (CARDS): The development and evaluation of a feasible violence risk assessment for routine psychiatry practice. *Journal of Mental Health, 13*, 569–581.

Watts, D., Leese, M., Thomas, S., Atakan, Z., & Wykes, T. (2003). The prediction of violence in acute psychiatric units. *International Journal of Forensic Mental Health, 2*, 173–180.

Wearden, A., Tarrier, N., Barrowclough, C., Zastowny, T., & Rahill, A. (2000). A review of express emotion research in health care. *Clinical Psychology Review, 20*, 633•666.

Webb, C., Pfeiffer, M., Mueser, K., Gladis, M., Mensch, E., DeGirolamo, J., et al. (1998). Burden and well-being of caregivers for the severely mentally ill: The role of coping style and social support. *Schizophrenia Research, 34*, 169–180.

Webber, A., & Orcutt, J. D. (1984). Employers' reactions to racial and psychiatric stigmata: A field experiment. *Deviant Behavior, 5*, 327–336.

Weber, R., & Crocker, J. (1983). Cognitive processes in the revision of stereotypic beliefs. *Journal of Personality and Social Psychology, 45*, 961–977.

Wehman, P. (1988). Supported employment: Toward zero exclusion of persons with severe disabilities. In P. Wehman & M. S. Moon (Eds.), *Vocational rehabilitation and supported employment* (pp. 3–14). Baltimore: Paul Brookes.

Wehman, P., & Kregel, J. (1995). At the crossroads: Supported employment a decade later. *Journal of the Association of Persons with Severe Handicaps, 20*, 286–299.

Wehman, P., & Moon, M. S. (Eds.). (1988). *Vocational rehabilitation and supported employment*. Baltimore: Paul Brookes.

Wehman, P., Revell, W. G., & Brooke, V. (2003). Competitive employment: Has it become the "first choice" yet? *Journal of Disability Policy Studies, 14*(3), 163–173.

Weiden, P. J. (Ed.). (1999). *TeamCare Solutions*. Trenton, NJ: Eli Lilly and Company.

Weiden, P. J., Mott, T., & Curcio, N. (1995). Recognition and management of neuroleptic noncompliance. In C. L. Shriqui & H. A. Nasrallah (Eds.), *Contemporary issues in the treatment of schizophrenia* (pp. 411–433). Washington, DC: American Psychiatric Press.

Weiden, P. J., & Olfson, M. (1995). Cost of relapse in schizophrenia. *Schizophrenia Bulletin, 21*, 419–429.

Weiden, P. J., Rapkin, B., Mott, T., Zygmunt, A., Goldman, D., Horvitz-Lennon, M., et al. (1994). Rating of Medication Influences (ROMI) Scale in schizophrenia. *Schizophrenia Bulletin, 20*, 297–310.

Weiner, B. (1995). *Judgments of responsibility: A foundation for a theory of social conduct*. New York: Guilford Press.

Weiner, E., & Ball, M. P. (2001). Effects of sustained-release bupropion and supportive group therapy on cigarette consumption in patients with schizophrenia. *American Journal of Psychiatry, 158*, 635–637.

Weingarten, R., Chinman, M., Tworkowski, S., Stayner, D., & Davidson, L. (2000). The Welcome Basket project: Consumers reaching out to consumers. *Psychiatric Rehabilitation Journal, 24*(1), 65–69.

Weinstein, D., & Hughes, R. (1997). What is psychosocial rehabilitation? In R. Hughes & D. Weinstein (Eds.), *Best practices in psychosocial rehabilitation* (pp. 35–62). Columbia, MD: International Association of Psychosocial Rehabilitation.

Weisbrot, D. M., & Ettinger, A. B. (2002). Aggression and violence in mood disorders. *Child and Adolescent Psychiatric Clinics of North America, 11*, 649–672.

Weisman, A., Lopez, S., Karno, M., & Jenkins, J. (1993). An attributional analysis of expressed emotion in Mexican-American families with schizophrenia. *Journal of Abnormal Psychology, 102*, 601–606.

Weisman, A., Nuechterlein, K., Goldstein, M., & Snyder, K. (1998). Expressed emotion, attributions and schizophrenia symptom dimensions. *Journal of Abnormal Psychology, 107*, 355–359.

Weisman, R., Lamberti, J., & Price, N. (2004). Integrating criminal justice, community healthcare, and support services for adults with severe mental disorders. *Psychiatric Quarterly, 75*, 71–85.

Weiss, K. A., Smith, T. E., Hull, J. W., Piper, A. C., & Huppert, J. D. (2002). Predictors of risk of nonadherence in outpatients with schizphrenia and other psychotic disorders. *Schizophrenia Bulletin, 28*, 341–349.

Weiss, R. D., Greenfield, S. F., Najavits, L. M., Soto, J. A., Wyner, D., Tohen, M., et al. (1998). Medication compliance among patients with bipolar disorder and substance use disorder. *Journal of Clinical Psychiatry, 59*, 172–174.

Weiss, R. D., Griffin, M. L., Greenfield, S. F., Najavits, L. M., Wyner, D., Soto, J. A., et al. (2000). Group therapy for patients with bipolar and substance dependence: Results of a pilot study. *Journal of Clinical Psychiatry, 61*, 361–367.

Weiss, R. D., Griffin, M. L., Kolodziej, M. E., Ray, H., & Hennen, J. A. (2004). *Randomized controlled trial of integrated group therapy for patients with bipolar disorder and substance dependence*. Paper presented at the 66th Annual Scientific Meeting of the College on Problems of Drug Dependence, San Juan, Puerto Rico.

Weisssman, M., & Bothwell, S. (1976). Assessment

of social adjustment by patient self -report. *Archives of General Psychiatry, 33,* 1111–1115.

Wells, K., Miranda, J., Bruce, M. L., Alegria, M., & Wallerstein, N. (2004). Bridging community intervention and mental health services research. *American Journal Psychiatry, 161,* 955–963.

Wells, K. B. (1999). Treatment research at the crossroads: The scientific interface of clinical trials and effectiveness research. *American Journal of Psychiatry, 156,* 5–10.

Welsh, A., & Ogloff, J. (2003). The development of a Canadian prison based program for offenders with mental illness. *International Journal of Forensic Mental Health, 2,* 59–71.

Wennberg, J. E. (1988). Improving the medical decision-making process. *Health Affairs, 7,* 99–105.

Wennberg, J. E. (1991). Outcomes research, patient preference, and the primary care physician. *Journal of the American Board of Family Practice, 4,* 365–367.

Wenneker, M. B., & Epstein, A. M. (1989). Racial inequalities in the use of procedures for patients with ischemic heart disease in Massachusetts. *Journal of the American Medical Association, 261*(2), 253–257.

Werneke, U., Taylor, D., Sanders, T., & Wessely, S. (2003). Behavioral management of antipsychotic-induced weight gain: A review. *Acta Psychiatrica Scandinavica, 108,* 252–259.

Wessely, S., Castle, D., Douglas, A., & Taylor, P. (1994). The criminal careers of incident cases of schizophrenia. *Psychological Medicine, 24,* 483–502.

West, D. J. (1948). A mass observation questionnaire on hallucinations. *Journal of the Society for Psychical Research, 34,* 187–196.

West, J. C., Wilk, J. E., Olfson, M., Rae, D. S., Marcus, S., Narrow, W. E., et al. (2005). Patterns and quality of treatment for patients with schizophrenia in routine psychiatric practice. *Psychiatric Services, 56,* 283–291.

Wewiorski, N. J., & Fabian, E. S. (2004). Association between demographic and diagnostic factors and employment outcomes for people with psychiatric disabilities: A synthesis of recent research. *Mental Health Services Research, 6,* 9–21.

Wexler, D., & Winick, B. (1991a). Therapeutic jurisprudence as a new research tool. In D. Wexler & B. Winick (Eds.), *Essays in therapeutic jurisprudence* (pp. 303–320). Durham, NC: Carolina Academic Press.

Wexler, D., & Winick, B. (1991b). *Essays in therapeutic jurisprudence.* Durham, NC: Carolina Academic Press.

Whaley, A. L. (2001a). Cultural mistrust of white mental health clinicians among African Americans with severe mental illness. *American Journal of Orthopsychiatry, 72,* 252–256.

Whaley, A. L. (2001b). Cultural mistrust: An important psychological construct for diagnosis and treatment of African Americans. *Professional Psychology: Research and Practice, 32,* 555–562.

Whaley, A. L. (2004). A two-stage method for the study of cultural bias in the diagnosis of schizophrenia in African Americans. *Journal of Black Psychology, 30,* 167–186.

White, C., Nicholson, J., Fisher, W., & Geller, J. (1995). Mothers with severe mental illness caring for young children. *Journal of Nervous and Mental Disease, 183*(6), 398–403.

Whitecraft, J., Scott, J., Rogers, J., Burns-Lynch, B., Means, T., & Salzer, M. (2005). The Friends Connection, Philadelphia, Pennsylvania. In S. Clay (Ed.), *On our own, together* (pp. 159–176). Nashville: Vanderbilt University Press.

Whitmer, G. E. (1980). From hospitals to jails: The fate of California's deinstitutionalized mentally ill. *American Journal of Orthopsychiatry, 50,* 65–75.

Widiger, T. A., Mangine, S., Corbitt, E. M., Ellis, C. G., & Thomas, G. V. (1995). *Personality Disorder Interview-IV.* Odessa, FL: Psychological Assessment Resources.

Wiersma, D., Nienhuis, F. J., Giel, R., & Sloof, C. J. (1998). Stability and change in needs of patients with schizophrenic disorders: A 15- and 17-year follow-up from first onset of psychosis, and a comparison between "objective" and "subjective" assessments of needs for care. *Social Psychiatry and Psychiatric Epidemiology, 33,* 49–56.

Wildgoose, J., Briscoe, M., & Lloyd, K. (2003). Psychological and emotional problems in staff following assaults by patients. *Psychiatric Bulletin, 27,* 295–297.

Wilkinson, G., Hedson, B., Wild, D., Cookson, R., Farina, C., Sharma, V., et al. (2000). Self-report quality of life measure for people with schizophrenia: The SQLS. *British Journal of Psychiatry, 177,* 42–46.

William, J. M., Ziedonis, D. M., & Foulds, J. (2004). A case series of nicotine nasal spray in the treatment of tobacco dependence among patients with schizophrenia. *Psychiatric Services, 55,* 1064–1066.

Williams-Keeler, L., Milliken, H., & Jones, B. (1994). Psychosis as precipitating trauma for PTSD: A treatment strategy. *American Journal of Orthopsychiatry, 64*(3), 493–498.

Willy, N. R., & McCandless, B. R. (1973). Social stereotypes for normal educable mentally retarded, and orthopedically handicapped children. *Journal of Special Education, 7*, 283–288.

Wilson, A. E., Calhoun, K. S., & Bernat, J. A. (1999). Risk recognition and trauma-related symptoms among sexually revictimized women. *Journal of Consulting and Clinical Psychology, 67*, 705–710.

Wilson, B. (1939). *Alcoholics Anonymous*. New York, Alcoholics Anonymous World Services.

Wilson, D., Tien, G., & Eaves, D. (1995). Increasing the community tenure of mentally disordered offenders: An assertive case management program. *International Journal of Law and Psychiatry, 18*, 61–69.

Wilson, W. J. (1987). *The truly disadvantaged: The inner city, the underclass and public policy*. Chicago: University of Chicago Press.

Winerip, M. (1994). *9 Highland Road*. New York: Pantheon Books.

Wing, J. K., & Brown, G. W. (1970). *Institutionalism and schizophrenia*. Cambridge, UK: Cambridge University Press.

Winick, B. (1997). The jurisprudence of therapeutic jurisprudence. *Psychology, Public Policy, and Law, 3*, 184–186.

Winokur, G., Coryell, W., Keller, M., Endicott, J., & Akiskal, H. (1993). A prospective follow-up of patients with bipolar and primary unipolar affective disorder. *Archives of General Psychiatry, 50*(6), 457–465.

Winokur, G., Pfohl, B., & Tsuang, M. (1987). A 40-year follow-up of hebephrenic-catatonic schizophrenia. In N. E. Miller & G. D. Cohen (Eds.), *Schizophrenia and aging: Schizophrenia, paranoia, and schizophreniform disorders in later life* (pp. 52–60). New York: Guilford Press.

Winstanley, S., & Whittington, R. (2002). Anxiety, burnout and coping styles in general hospital staff exposed to workplace aggression: A cyclical model of burnout and vulnerability to aggression. *Work and Stress, 16*, 302–315.

Wirshing, W. C., Marder, S. R., Eckman, T., Liberman, R. P., & Mintz, J. (1992). Acquisition and retention of skills training methods in chronic schizophrenic outpatients. *Psychopharmacology Bulletin, 28*, 241–245.

Witheridge, T. F. (1990). Assertive community treatment as a supported housing approach. *Psychosocial Rehabilitation Journal, 13*(4), 69–75.

Witheridge, T. F., Dincin, J., & Appleby, L. (1982). *The Bridge: An asertive home-visitng program for the most frequent psychiatric recidivists (Final Report to the NIMH Hospital Improvement Program)*. Chicago: Thresholds.

Witkiewitz, K., & Marlatt, G. (2004). Relapse prevention for alcohol and drug problems: That was Zen, this is Tao. *American Psychologist, 59*, 224–235.

Wolff, N. (2002). Courts on therapeutic agents: Thinking past the novelty of mental health courts. *Journal of the American Academy of Psychiatry and Law, 30*, 431–437.

Wolff, N. (2003). Courting the court: Courts as agents for treatment and justice. *Community-based interventions for criminal offenders with severe mental illness, 12*, 143–197.

Wolff, N., Helminiak, T., Morse, G., Caslyn, R., Klinkenberg, W. D., & Trusty, M. (1997). Cost-effectiveness evaluation of three approaches to case management for homeless mentally ill clients. *American Journal of Psychiatry, 154*, 341–348.

Wolpe, J. (1958). *Psychotherapy by reciprocal inhibition*. Stanford, CA: Stanford University Press.

Wong, K. K., Chiu, L., Tang, S., Kan, H., Kong, C., Chu, H., et al. (2004). A supported employment program for people with mental illness in Hong Kong. *American Journal of Psychiatric Rehabilitation, 7*, 83–96.

Wong, K. K., Chiu, R., Tang, B., Chiu, S. N., & Tang, J. L. (2005). *A randomized controlled trial of a supported employment program on vocational outcomes of individuals with chronic mental illness*. Hong Kong: Health Services Research Committee.

Wong, S. E., Woolsey, J. E., Innocent, A., & Liberman, R. P. (1988). Behavioral treatment of violent psychiatric patients. *Psychiatric Clinics of North America, 11*, 569–580.

Wong, Y. I. (2005). *Supported independent living programs for persons withserious mental illness in Philadelphia: A description*. Philadelphia: University of Pennsylvania Press.

Wong, Y. I., & Solomon, P. L. (2002). Community integration of persons with psychiatric disabilities in supportive independent housing: A conceptual model and methodological considerations. *Mental Health Services Research, 4*, 13–28.

World Health Organization. (1992). *The ICD-10 classification of mental and behavioural disorders: Clinical descriptions and diagnostic guidelines*. Geneva: Author.

World Health Organization. (1997). *The Composite International Diagnostic Interview (Version 2, 12 month)*. Geneva: Author.

World Schizophrenia Fellowship. (1997, September 4–5). *Strategy development family interventions work: Putting the research into practice*. Christchurch, New Zealand.

Worrell, F. C., Cross, W. E., & Vandiver, B. J. (2001). Nigrescence theory: Current status and challenges for the future. *Journal of Multicul-*

tural Counseling and Development, 29, 201–213.

Wright, E. R. (1997). The impact of organizational factors on mental health professionals involvement with families. Psychiatric Services, 48, 921–927.

Wright, E. R., Gronfein, W. P., & Owens, T. J. (2000). Deinstitutionalization, social rejection, and the self-esteem of former mental patients. Journal of Health and Social Behavior, 41, 68–90.

Wulsin, L. R. (1996). An agenda for primary care psychiatry. Psychosomatics, 37, 93–99.

Wykes, T., & Sturt, E. (1986). The measurement of social behaviour in psychiatric patients: An assessment of the reliability and validity of the SBS Schedule. British Journal of Psychiatry, 148, 1–11.

Wykes, T., Sturt, E., & Katz, R. (1990). The prediction of rehabilitative success after three years: The use of social, symptom and cognitive variables. British Journal of Psychiatry, 157, 865–870.

Wylie, R. (1979). The self-concept (Vol. 2). Lincoln: University of Nebraska Press.

Xiang, M. G., Ran, M., & Li, S. (1994). A controlled evaluation of psychoeducational family intervention in a rural Chinese community. British Journal of Psychiatry, 165, 544–548.

Xie, H., Drake, R., & McHugo, J. (2006). Are there distinctive trajectory groups in substance abuse remission over 10 years?: An application of the group-based modeling approach. Administration and Policy in Mental Health and Mental Health Services Research, 33, 423–432.

Xie, H., McHugo, G. J., Fox, L., & Drake, R. E. (2005). Substance abuse relapse in a ten-year prospective follow-up of clients with mental and substance use disorders. Psychiatric Services, 56, 1282–1287.

Yalom, I. (1985). The theory and practices of group psychotherapy (3rd ed.). New York: Basic Books.

Yang, J., Law, S., Chow, W., Andermann, L., Steinberg, R., & Sadavoy, J. (2005). Best practices: Assertive community treatment for persons with severe and persistent mental illness in ethnic minority groups. Psychiatric Services, 56, 1053–1055.

Youmans, R. (1992). The shortage of low-income housing: The role of the federal government. In R. I. Jahiel (Ed.), Homelessness: A preventative approach (pp. 255–268). Baltimore: Johns Hopkins University Press.

Young, A., Chinman, M., Forquer, S., Knight, E.,

Vogel, H., Miller, A., et al. (2005). Use of consumer-led intervention to improve provider competencies. Psychiatric Services, 56, 967–975.

Young, A., Sullivan, G., Burman, A., & Brook, R. (1998). Measuring the quality of outpatient treatment for schizophrenia. Archives of General Psychiatry, 55, 611–617.

Young, A. S., Forquer, S. L., Tran, A., Starzynski, M., & Shatkin, J. (2000). Identifying clinical competencies that support rehabilitation and empowerment in individuals with severe mental illness. Journal of Behavioral Health Services and Research, 27, 321–333.

Young, A. S., Mintz, J., Cohen, A. N., & Chinman, M. J. (2004). A network-based system to improve care for schizophrenia: The medical informatics network tool (MINT). Journal of the American Medical Informatics Association, 11, 3588–3367.

Young, J., & Williams, C. (1988). Whom do mutual-help groups help? Typology of members. Hospital and Community Psychiatry, 39, 1178–1182.

Young, M. A., Scheftner, W. A., Klerman, G. K., & Andreasen, N. C. (1986). The endogenous subtype of depression: A study of its internal construct validity. British Journal of Psychiatry, 148, 257–267.

Yuen, M., & Fossey, E. (2003). Working in a community recreation program: A study of consumer staff perspectives. Australian Occupational Therapy Journal, 50, 54–63.

Zahn, T. P. (1986). Psychophysiological approaches to psychopathology. In M. G. H. Coles, E. Donchin, & S. W. Porges (Eds.), Psychophysiology: Systems, processes and applications (pp. 508–610). New York: Guilford Press.

Zhang, M., He, Y., Gittelman, M., Wong, Z., & Yan, H. (1998). Group psychoeducation of relatives of schizophrenic patients: Two-year experiences. Psychiatry and Clinical Neurosciences, 52(Suppl.), S344–S347.

Zhang, M., Wang, M., & Li, J. (1994). Randomized-control trial of family intervention for 78 first episode male schizophrenia patients: An 18-month study. British Journal of Psychiatry, 165(Suppl. 24), 96–102.

Ziedonis, D., Kosten, T., Glazer, W., & Frances, R. (1994). Nicotine dependence and schizophrenia. Hospital and Community Psychiatry, 45, 204–206.

Ziedonis, D., & Trudeau, K. (1997). Motivation to quit using substances among individuals with schizophrenia: Implications for a motivation-based treatment model. *Schizophrenia Bulletin, 23,* 229–238.

Ziedonis, D. M., & George, T. P. (1997). Schizophrenia and nicotine use: Report of a pilot smoking cessation program and review of neurobiological and clinical issues. *Schizophrenia Bulletin, 23,* 247–254.

Zigler, E., & Glick, M. (1986). *A developmental approach to adult psychopathology.* New York: Wiley.

Ziguras, S., & Stuart, G. (2000). A meta-analysis of the effectiveness of mental health case management over 20 years. *Psychiatric Services, 51,* 1410–1421.

Zimmermann, G., Favrod, J., Trieu, V. H., & Pomini, V. (2005). The effect of cognitive behavioral treatment on the positive symptoms of schizophrenia spectrum disorders: A metaanalysis. *Schizophrenia Research, 77,* 1–9.

Zimmerman, M., & Mattia, J. I. (2001a). The Psychiatric Diagnostic Screening Questionnaire: Development, reliability and validity. *Comprehensive Psychiatry, 42,* 175–189.

Zimmerman, M., & Mattia, J. I. (2001b). A self-report scale to help make psychiatric diagnoses: The Psychiatric Diagnostic Screening Questionnaire. *Archives of General Psychiatry, 58,* 787–794.

Zimmerman, M., Sheeran, T., Chelminski, I., & Young, D. (2004). Screening for psychiatric disorders in outpatients with DSM-IV substance use disorders. *Journal of Substance Abuse Treatment, 26,* 181–188.

Zimmet, S. V., Strous, R. D., Burgess, E. S., Kohnstamm, S., & Green, A. I. (2000). Effects of clozapine on substance use in patients with schizophrenia and schizoaffective disorders: A retrospective survey. *Journal of Clinical Psychopharmacology, 20,* 94–98.

Zinnbauer, B. J., Pargament, K. I., & Scott, A. B. (1999). The emerging meanings of religiousness and spirituality: Problems and prospects. *Journal of Personality, 67*(6), 889–919.

Zubin, J., & Spring, B. (1977). Vulnerability: A new view of schizophrenia. *Journal of Abnormal Psychology, 86,* 103–126.

Zucker, G. S., & Weiner, B. (1993). Conservatism and perceptions of poverty: An attributional analysis. *Journal of Applied Social Psychology, 23,* 925–943.

Zwerling, C., Whitten, P. S., Sprince, N. L., Davis, C. S., Wallace, R. B., Blanck, P., et al. (2003). Workplace accommodations for people with disabilities: National Health Interview Survey Disability Supplement, 1994–1995. *Journal of Occupational and Environmental Medicine, 45,* 517–525.

Zygmunt, A., Olfson, M., Boyer, C. A., & Mechanic, D. (2002). Interventions to improve medication adherence in schizophrenia. *American Journal of Psychiatry, 159,* 1653–1664.

Index